BIOMEDICAL ENGINEERING – FRONTIERS AND CHALLENGES

Edited by **Reza Fazel-Rezai**

INTECHOPEN.COM

Biomedical Engineering – Frontiers and Challenges
Edited by Reza Fazel-Rezai

CBS, Edition 2016

Published by InTech

Janeza Trdine 9, 51000 Rijeka, Croatia

Publishing Process Manager Davor Vidicl

Technical Editor Teodora Smiljanic

Cover Designer InTech Design Team

Image Copyright Alfred Bondarenko, 2010. Used under license from Shutterstock.com

Additional hard copies can be obtained from orders@intechopen.com

Biomedical Engineering – Frontiers and Challenges, Edited by Reza Fazel-Rezai
p. cm.
ISBN 978-953-307-309-5

INTECH

open science | open minds

Contents

Preface

There have been different definitions for Biomedical Engineering. One of them is the application of engineering disciplines, technology, principles, and design concepts to medicine and biology. As this definition implies, biomedical engineering helps closing the gap between"engineering" and "medicine".

There are many different disciplines in engineering field such as aerospace, chemical, civil, computer, electrical, genetic, geological, industrial, mechanical. On the other hand, in the medical field, there are several fields of study such as anesthesiology, cardiology, dermatology, emergency medicine, gastroenterology, orthopedics, neuroscience, pathology, pediatrics, psychiatry, radiology, and surgery. Biomedical engineering can be considered as a bridge connecting field(s) in engineering to field(s) in medicine. Creating such a bridge requires understanding and major cross - disciplinary efforts by engineers, researchers, and physicians at health institutions, research institutes, and industry sectors. Depending on where this connection has happened, different areas of research in biomedical engineering have been shaped.

In all different areas in biomedical engineering, the ultimate objectives in research and education are to improve the quality life, reduce the impact of disease on the everyday life of individuals, and provide an appropriate infrastructure to promote and enhance the interaction of biomedical engineering researchers. In general, biomedical engineering has several disciplines including, but not limited to, bioinstrumentation, biostatistics, and biomaterial, biomechanics, biosignal, biosystem, biotransportation, clinical, tissue, rehabilitation and cellular engineering. Experts in biomedical engineering, a young area for research and education, are working in various industry and government sectors, hospitals, research institutions, and academia. The U.S. Department of Labor estimates that the job market for biomedical engineering will increase by 72%, faster than the average of all occupations in engineering. Therefore, there is a need to extend the research in this area and train biomedical engineers of tomorrow.

This book is prepared in two volumes to introduce a recent advances in different areas of biomedical engineering such as biomaterials, cellular engineering, biomedical devices, nanotechnology, and biomechanics. Different chapters in both volumes are stand-alone and readers can start from any chapter that they are interested in. It is hoped that this book brings more awareness about the biomedical engineering field and helps in completing or establishing new research areas in biomedical engineering.

As the editor, I would like to thank all the authors of different chapters. Without your contributions, it would not be possible to have a quality book and help in the growth of biomedical engineering.

Dr. Reza Fazel-Rezai
University of North Dakota
Grand Forks, ND,
USA

1

Modern Synthesis and Thermoresponsivity of Polyphosphoesters

Yasuhiko Iwasaki
Kansai University
Japan

1. Introduction

There has been a great deal of interest in polyphosphoesters, which are biodegradable through hydrolysis and possibly through enzymatic digestion of phosphate linkages under physiological conditions (Renier et al., 1997). Biodegradable polyphosphoesters appear interesting for biological and pharmaceutical applications because of their biocompatibility and structural similarities to naturally occurring nucleic and teichoic acids. Recently, there have been interesting studies of polyphosphoesters used in biomedical applications (Wang et al., 2009). In particular, the advantages of polyphosphoesters for use in the field of tissue engineering as scaffolds and gene carriers was elucidated (Wan et al., 2001; Wang et al., 2002; Huang et al., 2004; Ren et al., 2010).

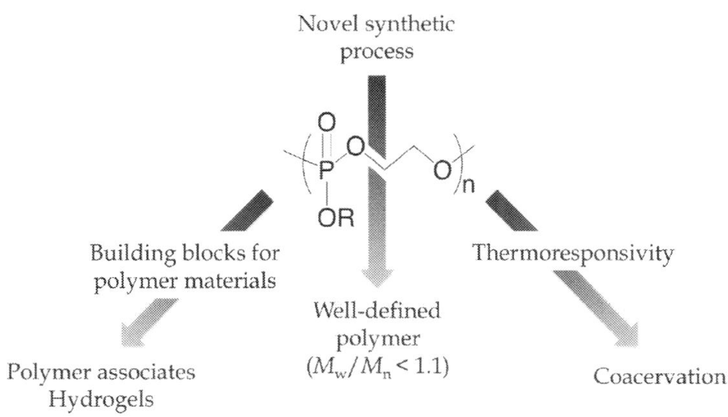

Fig. 1. Schematic contents of this chapter.

Figure 1 is a schematic representation of the contents of this chapter describing current research on polyphosphoesters. Although polyphosphoesters have a relatively long history, well-defined synthesis of the polymers has not been well explained. For use in medical applications such as drug delivery systems, understanding the synthetic process of polymers with narrow molecular weight distribution may be quite important to obtain reproducibility. The first part of this chapter discusses the controlled synthesis of polyphosphoesters.

In comparison with conventional biodegradable polymers, the molecular functionalization of polyphosphoesters is easier because varied cyclic phosphoesters, which work as monomers, can be obtained by a simple condensation reaction between alcohol and chloro cyclic phosphoesters. That is, theoretically, any alcohol can be introduced into polyphosphoesters. Here, a biodegradable macroinitiator and macrocrosslinker based on polyphosphoesters are described. They can be used as building blocks for preparing polymer blends and hydrogels.

We have also recently found that polyphosphoesters show thermoresponsivity in aqueous media. This polymer solution makes a lower critical solution temperature (LCST) type coacervate. The phenomenon is strongly influenced by the structure and molecular weight of the polymers and the solvent condition. The basic thermoresponsive properties of polyphosphoesters are summarized in this chapter. Enzyme-responsive polyphosphoesters are also introduced.

2. Synthesis of well-defied polyphosphoesters and incorporation of functional groups into polymers

A variety of synthetic routes for polyphosphoesters have been reported including ring-opening polymerization (ROP) (Libiszowski et al., 1978; Pretula et al., 1986), polycondensation (Richard et al, 1991), transesterfication (Pretula et al., 1999; Myrex et al., 2003), and enzymatic polymerization (Wen et al., 1998). Since the pioneering experiments by the Penczek group (Penczek & Klosinski, 1990), the ROP of cyclic phosphate has been studied for more than three decades and various polymers having a phosphoester backbone have been designed. The ROP of cyclic phosphoesters is the most common process used to obtain polyphosphoesters. This is because a variety of polyphosphoesters can be designed in comparison with conventional biodegradable polymers because cyclic phosphoesters are obtained as monomers from the condensation of alcohol and 2-chloro-2-oxo-1,3,2-dioxaphospholane (Katuiyhski et al., 1976).

2.1 Synthesis of polyphosphoesters using organocatalysts

For the ROP of cyclic phosphoesters, metallic compounds are commonly used as initiators or polymerization catalysts (Penczek et al., 1990; Libiszowski et al., 1978; Pretula et al., 1986; Xiao et al., 2006). Although the polymerization processes are very successful in producing polyphosphoesters, the metal compounds are environmentally sensitive and a lack of residual metal contaminants is required in biomedical applications. Recently, organocatalysts have been the focus of the modern synthetic processes of polyesters, polycarbonates, and silicones (Kamber et al., 2007). One of the most successful procedures for making biodegradable polymers is polymerization using guanidine and amidine bases, both in bulk and in solution. Nederberg and Hedrick prepared poly(trimethylene carbonate (TMC)) (PTMC) with the base catalysts in the presence of benzyl alcohol (Nederberg et al., 2007). Excellent controlled polymerization conditions were present with several catalysts, and PTMCs with relatively high molecular weight, narrow distribution, and high yield were obtained. We have recently recognized that organocatalysts have high potency for the ROP of cyclic phosphoesters (Iwasaki et al., 2010).

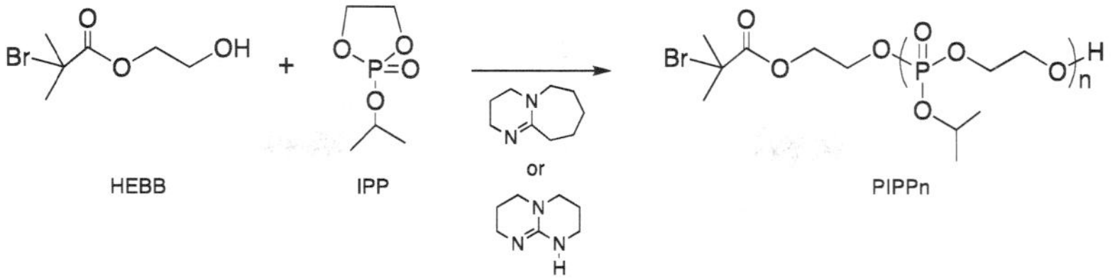

Scheme 1. Synthetic route of PIPP. (Reproduced from Iwasaki et al., (2010) *Macromolecules*, Vol. 40, No. 23, pp. 8136-8138, Copyright (2010), with permission from the American Chemical Society)

Poly(2-isopropoxy-2-oxo-1,3,2-dioxaphospholane) (PIPPn; n is degree of polymerization) was synthesized by ROP using an organocatalyst as an initiator in the presence of 2-hydroxyethyl-2′-bromoisobutyrate (HEBB) (Scheme 1). In the case of 1,8-diazabicyclo[5,4,0]undec-7-ene (DBU), polymerization was homogeneously performed in a solvent-free condition. In contrast, a small amount of toluene was used for dissolving 1,5,7-triazabicyclo[4,4,0]dec-5-ene (TBD) to make a homogeneous solution. The results of PIPP synthesis are summarized in Table 1. Twenty mmoles of IPP was first introduced into a polymerization tube under an argon gas atmosphere at 0°C, and then a given amount of HEBB was added to the tube. Finally, a given amount of organocatalyst was introduced. Polymerization was carried out at 0°C. The range of molecular weights was approximately 2.0 x 10^3 to 3.0 x 10^4 g/mol by gel-permeation chromatography (GPC) using a calibration curve based on linear polystyrene standards with chloroform as the mobile phase. In every case, the molecular weight distribution was lower than 1.10. Under each condition, the molecular weights of the synthetic polymers agreed with the theoretical values.

Code	Catalyst	$[M]_0/[I]$	HEBB (mmol)	Catalyst (mmol)	Time (min)	Conv. (%)	M_n x 10^{-3}	M_w/M_n	$M_{n(Theo)}$ x 10^{-3}
PIPP13	DBU	25	0.80	1.20	60	52.8	2.4	1.03	2.2
PIPP32	DBU	50	0.40	0.60	90	52.7	4.7	1.07	4.4
PIPP50	DBU	100	0.20	0.30	300	50.8	7.7	1.09	8.4
PIPP48	TBD	50	0.40	0.20	20	81.2	8.2	1.06	6.7
PIPP77	TBD	100	0.20	0.20	20	80.7	13.0	1.09	13.4
PIPP117	TBD	150	0.13	0.20	20	75.5	16.9	1.07	18.8
PIPP174	TBD	200	0.10	0.20	20	90.3	28.9	1.05	30.0

Table 1. Synthetic results of $PIPP_n$. (Reproduced from Iwasaki et al., (2010) *Macromolecules*, Vol. 40, No. 23, pp. 8136-8138, Copyright (2010), with permission from the American Chemical Society)

Figure 2 shows the number-averaged molecular weight (M_n) versus monomer conversion for the polymerization of IPP by using DBU as a catalyst. The plot of M_n vs. conversion was linear up to 60% conversion. The linearity of the plot suggests that the number of macromolecules in the reaction system was constant during polymerization. The molecular weight distribution of PIPP was narrow and stable during polymerization. The mechanism of ROP with organocatalysts was characterized using ^1H NMR by Hedrick and co-workers (Nederberg et al., 2007; Pratt et al., 2006). They indicated that DBU and TBD form hydrogen bonds to the alcohol of an initiator. ROP of IPP with DBU then occurs through a quasi-anionic polymerization mechanism by activation of the alcohol of the initiator. In contrast, the increase in monomer conversion for the polymerization of IPP between DBU and TBD was significantly different. When TBD was used as a catalyst, the conversion of PIPP reached a level of more than 75% within 20 min. The heightened activity of TBD for the polymerization of lactone and TMC was also observed (Nederberg et al., 2007).

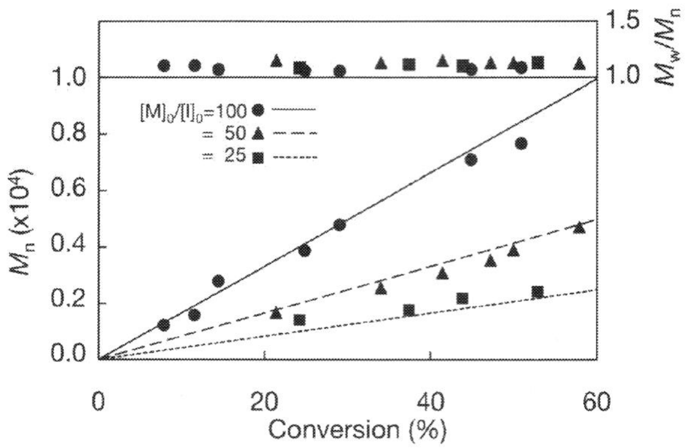

Fig. 2. Plot of M_w/M_n and M_n versus monomer conversion for the polymerization of 2-isopropoxy-2-oxo-1,3,2-dioxaphospholane by using 1,8-diazabicyclo[5,4,0]undec-7-ene as a catalyst. Lines suggest the theoretical amount of each polymerization condition. (Reproduced from Iwasaki et al., (2010) *Macromolecules*, Vol. 40, No. 23, pp. 8136-8138, Copyright (2010), with permission from the American Chemical Society)

2.2 Polyphosphoester macroinitiators

Atom transfer radical polymerization (ATRP) has great ability to control the molecular architecture of synthetic polymers and is an exceptionally robust method of producing block or graft copolymers (Matyjaszewski & Xia, 2001). However, the still limited design of biodegradable amphiphilic polymers has been performed via ATRP. Polyphosphoesters bearing 2-bromo-isobutyryl groups as novel biodegradable macroinitiators for ATRP were then synthesized and amphiphilic polymers with well-defined hydrophilic graft chains were prepared (Iwasaki & Akiyoshi, 2004).

A cyclic phosphoester bearing bromoisobutyrate, 2-(2-oxo,1,3,2-dioxaphospholoyloxy) ethyl-2′-bromoisobutyrate (OPBB), was obtained from the reaction of HEBB and 2-chloro-2-oxo-1,3,2-dioxaphosphorane (COP). Poly(IPP-co-OPBB) (PI_xBr_y (Scheme 2); x:IPP (mol%), y: OPBB (mol%)) was synthesized by ring-opening polymerization using triisobutyl aluminum (TIBA) as an initiator. The chemical structure and synthetic results of the polyphosphoesters are shown in Scheme 2 and Table 2, respectively. Polymerization was homogeneously performed by a solvent-free reaction. As indicated in Table 2, the composition of each monomer unit could be controlled by the feed. The M_w of the polyphosphoester was 3.1 x 10^4 to 3.9 x 10^4 g/mol. The absolute molecular weights of $PIBr_2$ and $PIBr_5$ determined by MALLS were 3.4 x 10^4 and 3.7 x 10^4, respectively.

ATRP of 2-methacryloyloxyethyl phosphorylcholine (MPC) from macroinitiator polyphosphoesters was carried out in an ethanol solution. Figure 3 shows the number of

MPC units in a graft chain of $PIBr_2$-g-PMPC and $PIBr_5$-g-PMPC as determined by ^1H NMR. The numbers were linearly increased with an increase in the duration of polymerization. The slope of the $PIBr_2$-g-PMPC was much greater than that of $PIBr_5$-g-PMPC. The rates of polymerization decreased with graft density.

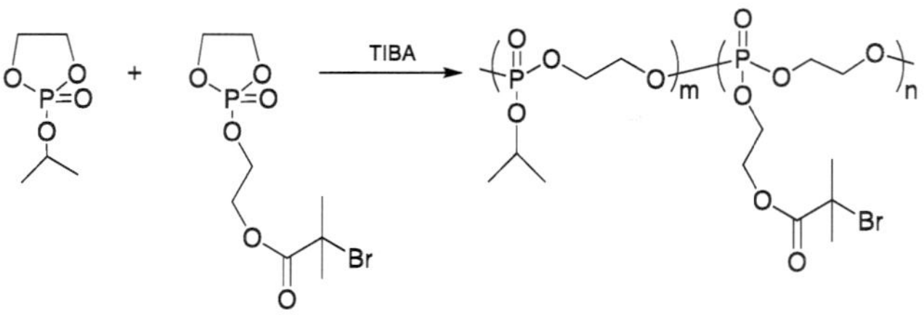

Scheme 2. Synthetic route of polyphosphoester bearing bromoisobutyrate (PIBr). (Reproduced from Iwasaki et al., (2004) *Macromolecules*, Vol. 37, No. 20, pp. 7637-7642, Copyright (2004), with permission from the American Chemical Society)

Polyphosphoesters	OPBB/IPP (mol%) In feed	OPBB/IPP (mol%) In copolymer	Yield (%)	Mw x 10^{-4}	M_w/M_n	No. of OPBB per PIBr molecule
$PI_{97}Br_3$	2.0/98.0	1.5/98.5	76.1	3.9 3.4	1.4	3.0
$PI_{95}Br_5$	6.0/94.0	5.0/95.0	49.2	3.1 3.7	1.4	10.5

Table 2. Synthetic results of PIBr. (Reproduced from Iwasaki et al., (2004) *Macromolecules*, Vol. 37, No. 20, pp. 7637-7642, Copyright (2004), with permission from the American Chemical Society)

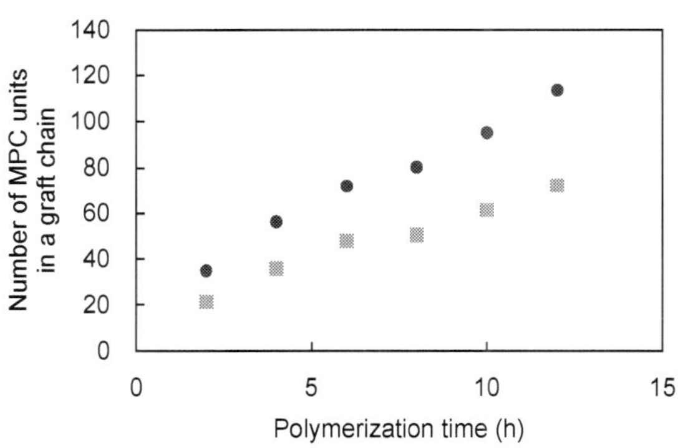

Fig. 3. Change in number of units of MPC in a graft chain during ATRP. (Circle): $PIBr_3$-g-PMPC; (Square): $PIBr_5$-g-PMPC. (Reproduced from Iwasaki et al., (2004) *Macromolecules*, Vol. 37, No. 20, pp. 7637-7642, Copyright (2004), with permission from the American Chemical Society)

The transition point of the surface tension increased with an increase in the molecular weight and density of PMPC. Typical examples for the concentrations of $PIBr_3$-g-PMPC71[1] and $PIBr_5$-g-PMPC115 were 8.6 x 10^{-3} g/dL and 2.3 x 10^{-3} g/dL, respectively. A decrease in surface tensions was observed on every graft copolymer. The surface tensions were influenced by the density and molecular weight of PMPC.
Based on MALLS analysis for associative $PIBr_3$-g-PMPC71, the molecular weight of the polymeric associate was 91.1 x 10^4. From the data in Figure 3, the molecular weight of $PIBr_3$-g-PMPC71 can be estimated at 13.6 x 10^4. Thus, the association number of the $PIBr_3$-g-PMPC71 was 6.7. For $PIBr_5$-g-PMPC, the association number was 1.5, that is, it is almost a "unimer-micelle." Figure 4 shows schematic representations of the polymeric associates of $PIBr_2$-g-$PMPC_{12}$ and $PIBr_5$-g-PMPC115.
In an acidic medium, the loss of molecular weight of the graft copolymer was observed as being less; degradation remarkably occurred after 50 days of soaking. Under physiological pH conditions, the molecular weight of the PIBr-g-PMPC decreased from 15.6 x 10^4 (GPC data) to 12.7 x 10^4 after 50 days. Under a basic condition, the polyphosphoester degraded almost completely within 3 days. After soaking in pH11.0, the $PIBr_2$-g-PMPC71 and $PIBr_5$-g-PMPC115 polymers had molecular weights of 2.4 x 10^{-4} and 3.1 x 10^{-4} (M_w/M_n=1.2), respectively, as determined by GPC. These polymers were identified as PMPC by ^{1}H NMR (data not shown). Although a basic condition (pH11.0) is not a physiological condition, we chose the optimal pH to characterize the degradation behavior of polyphosphoesters in a relatively short period. Under an acidic condition (pH 4.0), the hydrolysis of PIBr was slow. In contrast, under a basic condition (pH 11.0), the PIBr was completely degraded in only 3 days.

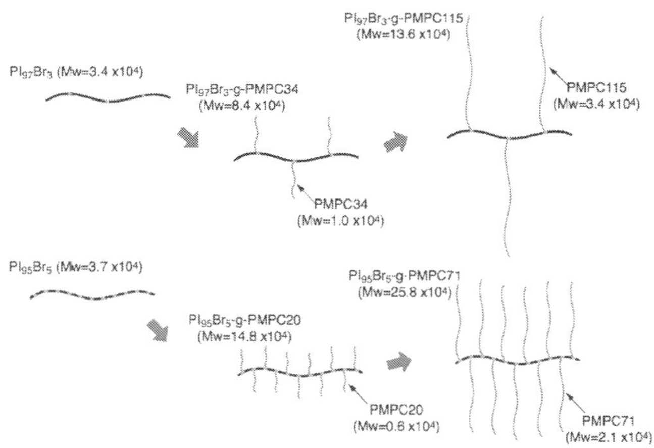

Fig. 4. Schematic representation of PIBr and PIBr-g-PMPC. (Reproduced from Iwasaki et al., (2004) *Macromolecules*, Vol. 37, No. 20, pp. 7637-7642, Copyright (2004), with permission from the American Chemical Society)

[1] The number after PMPC is degree of MPC polymerization in each graft chain.

The PIPPn shown in Scheme 1 also works as a macroinitiator because it has bromoisobutyrate at the end. Using PIPPn, well-defined block copolymers can be obtained by ATRP (Iwasaki et al., 2010).

2.3 Polyphosphoester macrocrosslinkers

Biomaterials have an enormous impact on human health care. They are widely used in biomedical applications, including drug delivery devices and tissue engineering matrices (Lin et al., 2003). Specifically, hydrogels are included in the more recent development of biomaterials because they can absorb significant amounts of water and are as flexible as soft tissue, which minimizes their potential for irritating surrounding tissue. In order to obtain synthetic cellular matrices offering both biocompatibility and biodegradability, a novel porous biodegradable MPC polymer hydrogel crosslinked with polyphosphoesters was prepared with a gas-forming technique (Iwasaki et al., 2003; Iwasaki et al., 2004; Wachiralarpphaithoon et al., 2007).

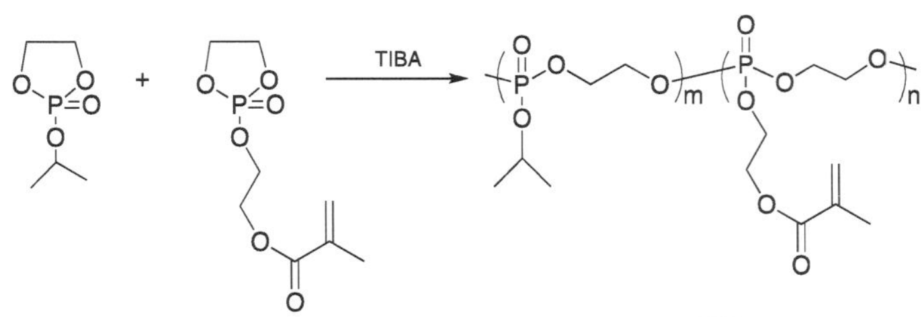

Scheme 4. Synthetic route of PIOP. (Reproduced from Wachiralarpphaithoon et al., (2007) *Biomaterials*, Vol. 28, No. 6, pp. 984-993, Copyright (2007), with permission from Elsevier)

Code	PIOP:MPC (%)	Potassium hydrogen carbonate size range (μm)	Swelling ratio (%)	Elastic modulus (x 10^4 Pa)	Porosity (%)
G1	0.5:99.5	-	1519±208	2.47±0.47	95.0±0.3
G1A	0.5:99.5	500-300	1576±191	0.06±0.01	98.4±0.4
G1B	0.5:99.5	300-250	1549±502	0.05±0.01	98.2±0.1
G1C	0.5:99.5	250-150	1547±665	0.04±0.00	97.8±0.2
G2	1:99	-	804±128	3.08±0.77	92.7±0.6
G2A	1:99	500-300	963±129	0.18±0.01	96.4±0.3
G2B	1:99	300-250	957±153	0.21±0.02	96.5±0.1
G2C	1:99	250-150	977±26	0.26±0.01	96.7±0.2
G3	2.5:97.5	-	357±103	10.10±3.26	86.0±1.3
G3A	2.5:97.5	500-300	518±40	2.61±0.23	96.2±0.1
G3B	2.5:97.5	300-250	523±183	2.61±0.25	95.8±0.1
G3C	2.5:97.5	250-150	512±133	2.65±0.01	94.8±0.2

Table 3. Synthetic condition and properties of hydrogels. (Reproduced from Wachiralarpphaithoon et al., (2007) *Biomaterials*, Vol. 28, No. 6, pp. 984-993, Copyright (2007), with permission from Elsevier)

The synthetic route of the macrocrosslinker, PIOP, was also synthesized using TIBA as an initiator (Scheme 4). The molecular weight of PIOP was 1.1 x 104 (M_w/M_n=1.1). The calculated number of 2-(2-oxo-1,3,2-dioxaphosphoroyloxy) ethyl methacrylate (OPEMA) units in a PIOP chain was 2.02.

The synthetic conditions and characterizations of the hydrogels are summarized in Table 3. Figure 5 shows macroscopic pictures of the swollen hydrogels prepared in this study. The hydrogels (G1, G2, and G3) shown in picture a) were prepared without porogen salts. When the crosslinking density is low, the hydrogels have a highly stretched network, which was experimentally observed as a large transparent appearance. With an increase in the composition of PIOP, the size of the hydrogels decreased and the transparency became poor because of the close distance of the PIOP molecules. Picture b) shows porous hydrogels (G1A, G2A, and G3A) prepared with the largest porogen salts (ϕ = 300-500 μm). The effect of PIOP composition on the macroscopic form was similarly observed as in picture a). This result indicates that PIOP works as a macromolecular crosslinking reagent in the preparation of hydrogels. Many small bubbles are observed in the hydrogels prepared with porogen salts. Macroscopic observation clarifies the difference in the inner structure between G1 and G1A.

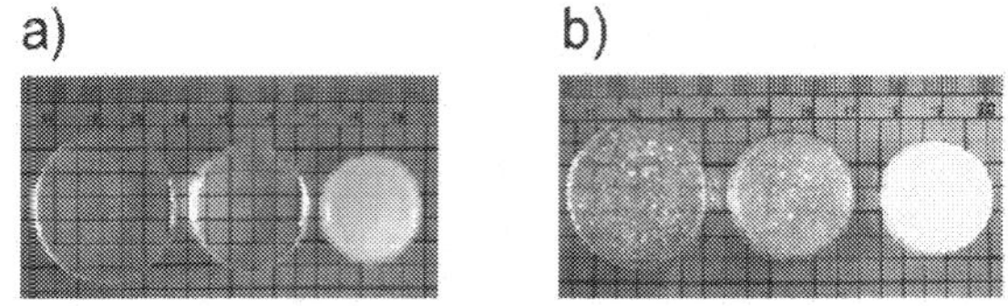

Fig. 5. Macroscopic pictures of swollen hydrogels. a) Hydrogels without porogen salts (G1, G2, and G3) b) Hydrogels with porogen salts (G1A, G2A, and G3A) after 24 h equilibration in water. (Reproduced from Wachiralarpphaithoon et al., (2007) *Biomaterials*, Vol. 28, No. 6, pp. 984-993, Copyright (2007), with permission from Elsevier)

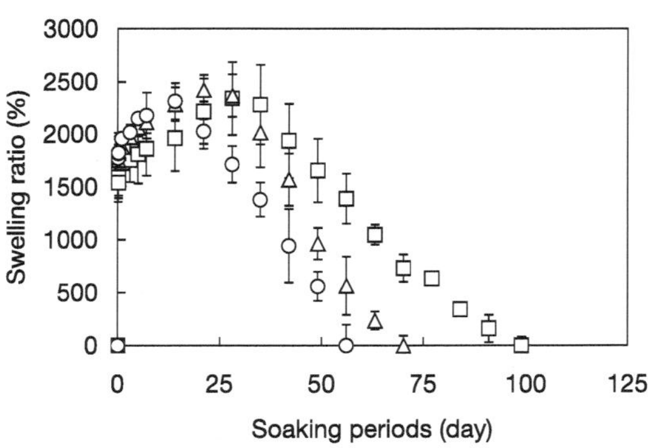

Fig. 6. Enzymatic degradation as a function of time for hydrogel G1A in ALP aqueous solution at 37°C; [ALP]= 0 U/L (□), 72.5 U/L (△), 220 U/L (○). Each point represents the average of three samples. (Reproduced from Wachiralarpphaithoon et al., (2007) *Biomaterials*, Vol. 28, No. 6, pp. 984-993, Copyright (2007), with permission from Elsevier)

Alkaline phosphatase (ALP) is an important enzyme produced in bone and liver cells. It catalyzes the hydrolysis of phosphate groups from monophosphate ester substrates mostly found in an alkaline state with a pH of 9 (Coburn et al., 1998). Although Zhao and co-workers reported that synthetic polyphosphoesters and polyphosphoesters are enzymatically degradable (Zhao et al., 2003), the process was not described in detail. The concentration of ALP for the degradation study was adjusted to 72.5 and 220 U/L, which is the concentration in healthy adults and children, respectively (Takeshita et al., 2004; Rafan et al., 2000). Figure 6 is an enzymatic degradation profile of G1A hydrogels by changing the concentration of ALP. G1A took about 100 days to reach complete dissolution at pH 9.0. The degradation was accelerated with a higher concentration of ALP; G1A completely degraded after 60 days in 220 U/L of ALP. The degradation period was shortened with an increase in the concentration of the enzyme. The digestion of a hydrogel might be regulated by varying the density of cells secreting an enzyme in the hydrogel.

MC3T3-E1 is a clonal osteogenic cell line derived from neonatal mouse calvaria. The cells are well characterized and provide a homogeneous source of osteoblastic cells for study. They were encapsulated in various biomaterial networks and remained viable (Burdick et al., 2005). MC3T3-E1 cells express high levels of alkaline phosphatase and differentiate into osteoblasts that can form calcified bone tissue *in vitro* (Choi et al., 1996). The response of MC3T3-E1 cells to many growth factors and hormones mimics that of primary cultures of rodent osteoblastic cells.

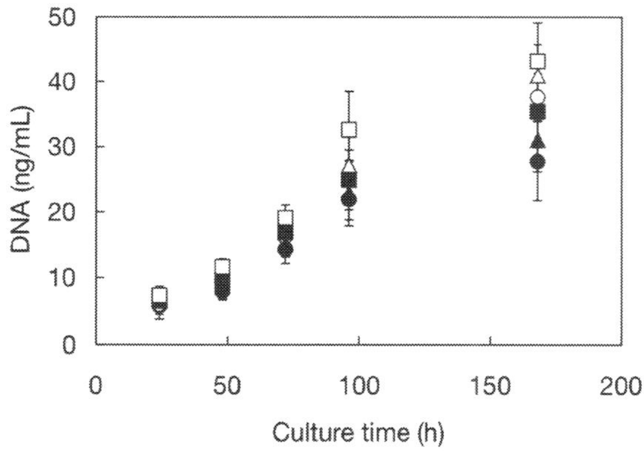

Fig. 7. Kinetics of MC3T3-E1 cell proliferation in hydrogels. (○) G1A, (△) G2A, (□) G3A with bFGF; (●) G1A, (▲) G2A, (■) G3A without bFGF. (Reproduced from Wachiralarpphaithoon et al., (2007) *Biomaterials*, Vol. 28, No. 6, pp. 984-993, Copyright (2007), with permission from Elsevier)

Figure 7 shows the time-dependent concentration of the DNA produced from the MC3T3-E1 cells in porous hydrogels. The concentration increment of DNA corresponds to the proliferation of cells in a hydrogel. Under every sample condition, the amount of DNA significantly increased ($p < 0.05$) with increased cultivation time. After culture for 168 h, the amount of DNA collected was significantly higher from G3A ($p = 0.036$) in comparison to G1A. Therefore, the density of PIOP influenced cell proliferation. When the bFGF was incorporated into a hydrogel, the rate of cell proliferation relatively increased with an increase in the concentration of PIOP (p = 0.017 and p = 0.107 G1A vs. G3A after culture for 96 h and 168 h, respectively). While MPC polymer provides a suitable condition for maintaining cell viability, this polymer is not effective for inducing cell adhesion on the surface (Wachiralarpphaithoon et al., 2007). Polyphosphoester might induce cell adhesion and proliferation in a hydrogel. Wang and co-workers have recently reported that poly(ethylene glycol) (PEG) hydrogel having a phosphoester linkage promotes gene expression of bone-specific markers and secretion of alkaline phosphatase, osteocalcin, and osteonectin protein from marrow-derived mesenchymal stem cells (Wang et al., 2005).

3. Thermoresponsive polyphosphoesters

Thermoresponsive polymers are widely studied in both research and technology because of their versatility in many fields. Recent trends in the application of polymer materials are drug delivery (Kikuchi & Okano, 2002), separation of bioactive molecules (Kobayashi et al., 2003), and tissue engineering (Kikuchi & Okano, 2005). *N*-Substituted acrylamide polymers have been found to have a phase separation characteristic with changes occurring in their properties upon heating above a certain lower critical solution temperature (LCST) (Monji et al., 1994; Yamazaki et al., 1999; Idziak et al., 1999). In particular, *N*-isopropyl acrylamide (NIPAAm) is one of the best monomers for accomplishing this; the homopolymer has LCST at 32°C in aqueous solution (Heskins et al., 1968). Although NIPAAm is a robust monomer for obtaining thermoresponsive polymer materials such as stimuli-responsive surfaces, particles, and hydrogels, the polymers are not biodegradable.
Besides the stimuli-responsive nature, biodegradability and biocompatibility are important characteristics for polymeric materials used in biomedical fields. While the thermoresponsivity of some biodegradable polymers such as aliphatic polyester block copolymers or polypeptides was recently advanced (Fujiwara et al., 2001; Kim et al., 2004; Tachibana et al., 2003; Shimokuri et al., 2006), the molecular design and synthetic processes of thermoresponsive biodegradable polymers are still limited.

3.1 Thermoresponsivity of polyphosphoesters

In current research, thermoresponsive polyphosphoesters are now being synthesized with simple copolymerization of cyclic phosphoester compounds and their properties are being investigated (Iwasaki et al., 2007). Poly(IPP-co-EP) (PI_xE_y (Scheme 4); x:IPP (mol%), y: EP (mol%)) was synthesized by ring-opening polymerization using TIBA as an initiator. The range of weight-averaged molecular weights was 1.2×10^4 to 1.5×10^4 g/mol (GPC analysis).

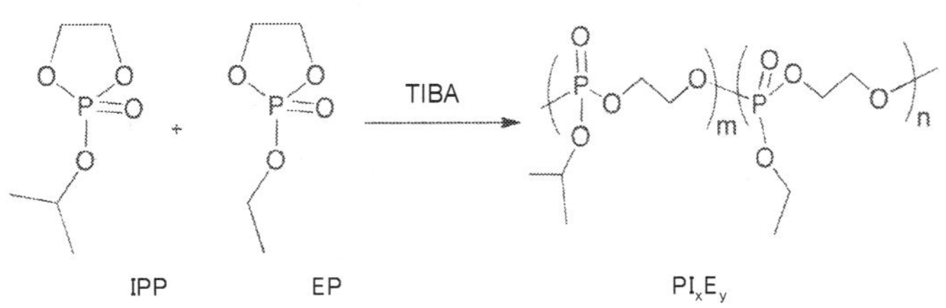

Scheme 4. Synthetic route of PI_xE_y (Reproduced from Iwasaki et al., (2007) *Macromolecules*, Vol. 40, No. 23, pp. 8136-8138, Copyright (2007), with permission from the American Chemical Society)

Figure 8 shows the LCST-type phase separation of $PI_{24}E_{76}$ aqueous solution. From the optical microscopic image, it is clear that the polymer solution was separated at the liquid-liquid phase above the cloud point. This appears to be coacervation. After several hours, the turbid solution spontaneously separated into two phases. The cloud point could be controlled by the ratio of IPP and EP, that is, it decreased with an increase in the molar fraction of hydrophobic IPP.

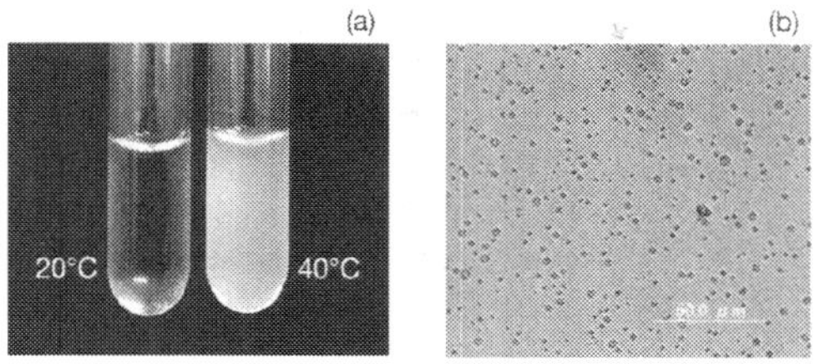

Fig. 8. LCST-type phase separation of polyphosphoester aqueous solution. (a) 1%- $PI_{24}E_{76}$ aqueous solution at 20 and 40°C. (b) Optical micrograph of 1%-$PI_{24}E_{76}$ aqueous solution at 40°C. (Reproduced from Iwasaki et al., (2007) *Macromolecules*, Vol. 40, No. 23, pp. 8136-8138,Copyright (2007), with permission from the American Chemical Society)]

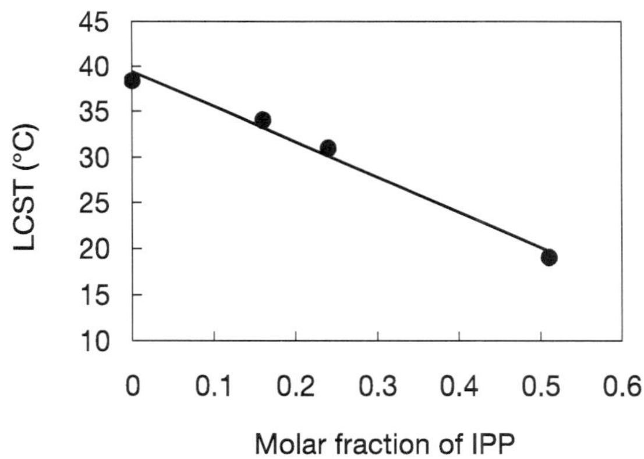

Fig. 9. Effect of molecular fraction of IPP on LCST of PIxEy (Reproduced from Iwasaki et al., (2007) *Macromolecules*, Vol. 40, No. 23, pp. 8136-8138. Copyright (2007), with permission from the American Chemical Society)

Figure 9 shows the effect of the composition of the monomer unit on the LCST of the copolymers. The LCST of poly(EP) (PEP) was 38°C and it linearly decreased with an increase in the ratio of IPP. IPP is relatively hydrophobic; the homopolymer of IPP is not soluble in water above 5°C. Dehydration of the polymer then preferably occurred with the addition of the hydrophobic IPP unit. It is reported that the LCST of thermoresponsive polymers can be controlled by the ratio of the hydrophobic and hydrophilic units (Takei et al., 1993; Tachibana et al., 2003). Thermoresponsivity under physiological conditions is

effective for drug delivery or tissue engineering applications (Okuyama et al., 1993; Nishida et al., 2004). The thermoresponsivity of polyphosphoesters can also be observed under physiological temperatures. Thus, the polymers are applicable in the biomedical field.
The effect of NaCl concentration on the cloud point on PEP and $PI_{24}E_{76}$ is shown in Figure 10. The cloud point of the polymer solution decreased with an increase in the concentration of NaCl in aqueous media. Under physiological conditions ([NaCl] = 100 mM), the cloud point of PEP and $PI_{24}E_{76}$ was 28 and 26°C, respectively. The solution property of nonionic polymer in water is sensitively influenced by the addition of salt because salt can alter polymer-water interaction (Foss et al., 1992).
Figure 11 shows the dependence of the cloud point of $PI_{24}E_{76}$ on polymer concentration in distilled water. The cloud point decreased with an increase in polymer concentration. Furthermore, the change in the transmittance of the polymer solution was more abrupt at a higher concentration. The effect of polymer concentration on phase separation temperature was also observed on poly(acryl amide) derivatives (Miyazaki & Kataoka, 1996). In their report, coacervate droplets could be condensed with centrifugation; the polymer concentration of the coacervate phase was much greater than that of the homogeneous solution.

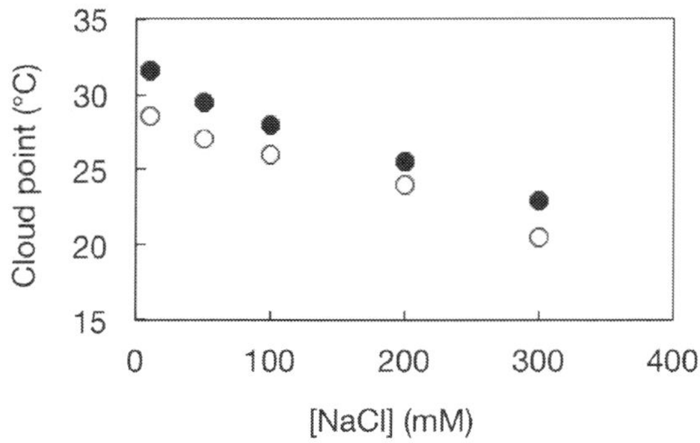

Fig. 10. Effect of NaCl concentration ([NaCl]) on cloud point of polyphosphoester aqueous solution. (●) PE, (○) $PI_{24}E_{76}$, [Polymer] = 1.0 wt%.

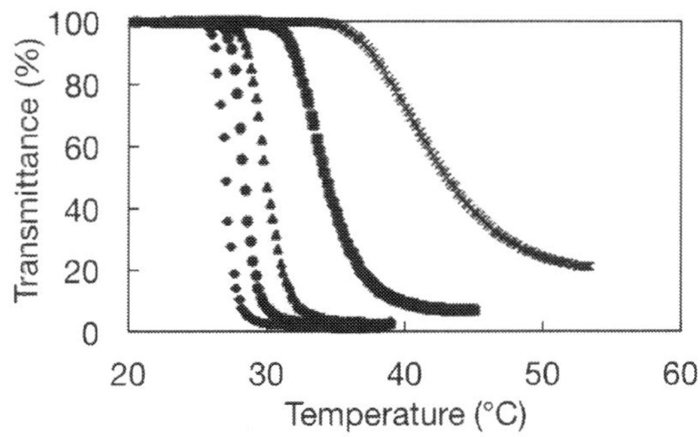

Fig. 11. Effect of polymer concentration on cloud point of $PI_{24}E_{76}$ aqueous solution. [Polymer] = 1.0 (◆), 0.75 (●), 0. 5 (▲), 0.25 (■), and 0.1 wt% (×).

Temperature (°C)	Relaxation time (ms) 4.1 ppm (main chain CH_2)	Relaxation time (s) 4.0 ppm (side chain CH_2)	Relaxation time (s) 1.2 ppm (side chain CH_3)
T_1			
19.0	577.314	1.721	1.493
39.0	671.000	2.022	1.889
T_2			
19.0	314.293	1.084	1.187
39.0	438.944	1.233	1.380

Table 4. Spin-lattice relaxation time (T_1) and spin-spin relaxation time (T_2) of proton in $PI_{24}E_{76}$.

To understand the molecular phenomenon for creating coacervates, we measured T_1 and T_2 of the protons in the main and side chains of $PI_{24}E_{76}$. Table 4 summarizes the typical data for relaxation times. It can be considered that a polymer in solution behaves as a liquid molecule with high mobility (Mao et al., 2000). As shown in Table 4, T_1 and T_2 of every proton contained in the main and side chains of $PI_{24}E_{76}$ increase as the temperature increases. Furthermore, a significant change of these relaxation times at the cloud point of $PI_{24}E_{76}$ was not observed. T_2 of the protons is mostly influenced by the dipole-dipole interaction of nuclear spin. The shorter the distance between protons, the slower the motion of the polymer chains and the stronger the interaction of the proton-proton dipolar coupling; thus the smaller T_2. The experimental results indicated that the mobility of the polymer thermodynamically increased with an increase in temperature regardless of the phase separation.

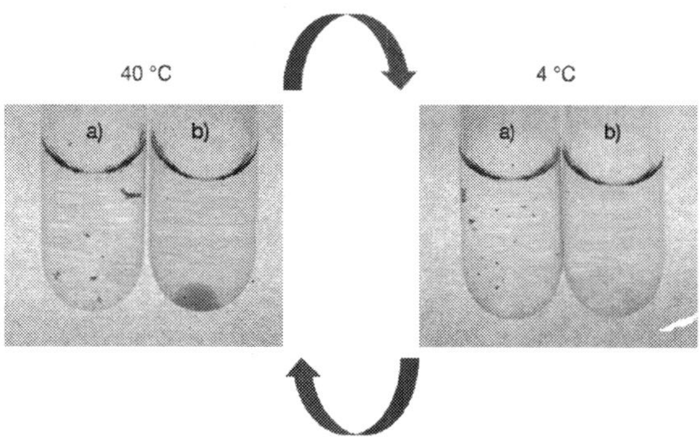

Fig. 12. Condensation of hydrophobic compound (Nile Red) from aqueous media. a) 150 mM NaCl aqueous solution, b) 150 mM NaCl aqueous solution containing 1-wt% $PI_{24}E_{76}$. [Nile Red] = 5 μg/mL.

The relaxation times of the protons of associated trigger groups normally decrease because of a decrease in mobility (Hsu et al., 2005). However, the results did not show this. In the coacervate phase with enriched polymers, solvent remained above the cloud point. Then, the polymers might loosely associate and their mobility was not reduced with an increase in temperature. While the mobility of the polymers in the coacervate phase was clarified, further study will be needed to show the molecular mechanism of coacervation.

We demonstrated the separation of hydrophobic molecules with thermoresponsive polyphosphoesters from aqueous media. Nile Red was used as a model compound; its solubility in water is very low. Nile Red dissolved in acetone was added to Dulbecco's phosphate buffered saline (PBS, calcium chloride- and magnesium chloride-free, Sigma). Polyphosphoester was then immediately introduced into the solution. Both PBS and that containing the polymer appear homogeneous before heating. When the solutions were incubated at 40°C, significant differences in solution behavior were observed, as shown in Figure 12. At 40°C, the polymer solution became turbid and then separated into two phases. Nile Red selectively condensed at the bottom layer, which contains the concentrated polymers. In contrast, the aggregation of Nile Red was observed in PBS at 40°C because the acetone evaporated and the Nile Red could not then disperse in the aqueous solution. After a decrease in temperature back to 4°C, the polymer solution appeared clear and homogeneous, but the aggregation of Nile Red remained in the PBS. The polyphosphoesters interact with hydrophobic Nile Red and help its dispersion. Furthermore, the precipitation of Nile Red was not observed even after the polymer solution was diluted 100 times with PBS. By using polyphosphoesters, we were able to improve the solubility of hydrophobic molecules in aqueous media and separate them with temperature increments.

Wang and co-workers also observed the thermoresponsivity of polyphosphoesters. They have synthesized well-defined block copolymers of poly(ethylene glycol) and polyphosphoester (Wang et al., 2009). Block copolymers can form core-shell type polymeric micelles in an aqueous medium with the effect of temperature caused by self-association of the polyphosphoester block. Although it is clear that polyphosphoester is the new candidate thermoresponsive polymer, its properties have only been partially evaluated. The effect of molecular weight on the cloud point of PIPPn (Scheme 1) has not been discussed. Figure 13 shows the dependence of the phase separation temperature of PIPP in phosphate buffered saline (PBS) on molecular weight.

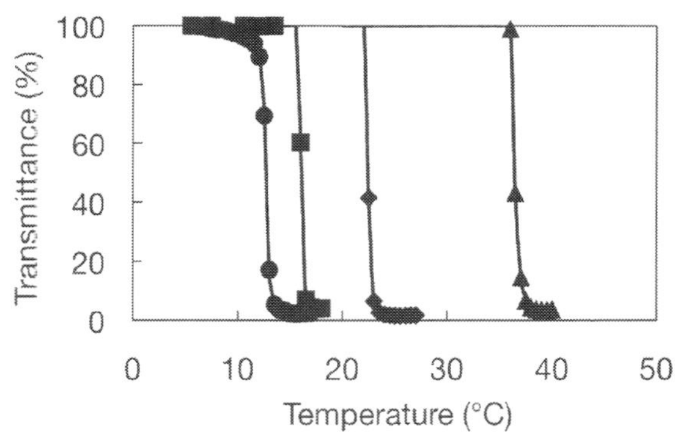

Fig. 13. Effect of molecular weight on cloud point of poly(2-isopropoxy-2-oxo-1,3,2-dioxaphospholane) (PIPP) (1 wt %) in PBS. (●) PIPP50(DBU), (■) PIPP48(TBD), (◆) PIPP32(DBU), (▲) PIPP13(DBU). (Reproduced from Iwasaki et al., (2010) *Macromolecules*, Vol. 40, No. 23, pp. 8136-8138, Copyright (2010), with permission from the American Chemical Society)

The cloud point of the polymer solution decreases with an increase in the molecular weight of PIPP. The result indicates that the type of organocatalyst does not influence the phase separation temperature. The phase separation temperature of polyphosphoesters is influenced by the chemical structure of the side chains, the concentration, and the ion strength of the aqueous media. In our previous report, PIPP that was synthesized using TIBA as an initiator was not soluble in water even when the molecular weight was less than 1.0 x 10^4 (Iwasaki & Akiyoshi, 2004). An uncontrolled reaction might occur when a metallic catalyst was used. Wang reported that long-term polymerization of cyclic phosphoesters with $Sn(Oct)_2$ makes some branch structures with high conversion rates (Xiao et al., 2006). In addition, some side reactions might occur in ring-opening polymerization of five-membered cyclic phosphoesters at high temperature (Liu et al., 2009). Furthermore, the molecular weight distribution of polyphosphoesters synthesized with an organocatalyst was significantly narrow compared with polymers that used metallic catalysts. The advantages of using organocatalysts can be observed on the synthesis of well-defined polymers with high conversion rates.

3.2 Polyphosphoester macroinitiators

Thermoresponsive polymers have great potential in bioscientific applications (Alarcon et al., 2005; Klouda et al., 2008). In particular, the selective delivery of drugs to target sites through hyperthermia could be performed (Chikoti et al., 2002). However, heat treatment might induce adverse effects on normal tissue and limitations remain in terms of selectivity. A polymer that can change its thermoresponsivity after contact with esterase has been synthesized. As shown in Scheme 5, polyphosphoesters bearing benzyl groups were synthesized. The synthetic results are listed in Table 5. The polymerization ability of BP and EP was similar. The ^{1}H NMR spectra of the polymers at each reaction step are summarized in Figure 14. After treatment with Pd/C in formic acid, a signal caused by the aromatic group at around 7.2 ppm disappeared. Deprotection of benzyl groups from PEB was completely accomplished and PEH was obtained. Then, PEH reacted with acetoxymethyl bromide in the presence of ethyldiisopropylamine. The ^{1}H NMR spectrum of PEHA clarified that the acetoxymethyl group was introduced at the deprotected position. No decrease in molecular weight was observed. No polymer degradation occurred during the introduction of the AM groups.

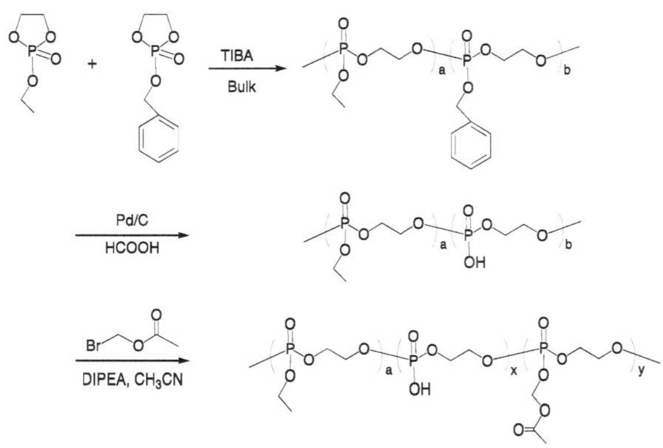

Scheme 5. Synthetic route of polyphosphoester bearing acetoxymethyl groups

The enzymatic digestion of acetoxymethyl esters from PEHA was evaluated in contact with porcine liver esterase for a specific time. Figure 15 shows the time dependence of the relative fraction of the acetoxymethyl groups on the EP units. The data are represented as the mean from 4 samples. When the enzyme was treated with PEHA, the decrease in the fraction of AM groups was dramatic compared to that soaked in PBS for 24 h. The fraction then gradually decreased over time. Esterase activity might influence this data. Geurtsen and co-worker reported that the activity of porcine liver esterase decreased during the first 24 h to approximately 40% and then remained constant for up to 6 days (Geurtsen et al., 1999). Even in synthetic polymer systems, the effect of esterase has been observed. The AM groups spontaneously degraded in PBS. The degradation rate at the early stage was much slower than that of the esterase treatment.

Polymer	Molar fraction		M_n x 10^{-3}	M_w/M_n
	In feed	In copolymer		
	0.90/0.10	0.92/0.08	6.31	1.43
		0.92/0.02/0.06	6.93	1.77

Table 5. Synthetic results of polyphosphoester bearing acetoxymethyl groups

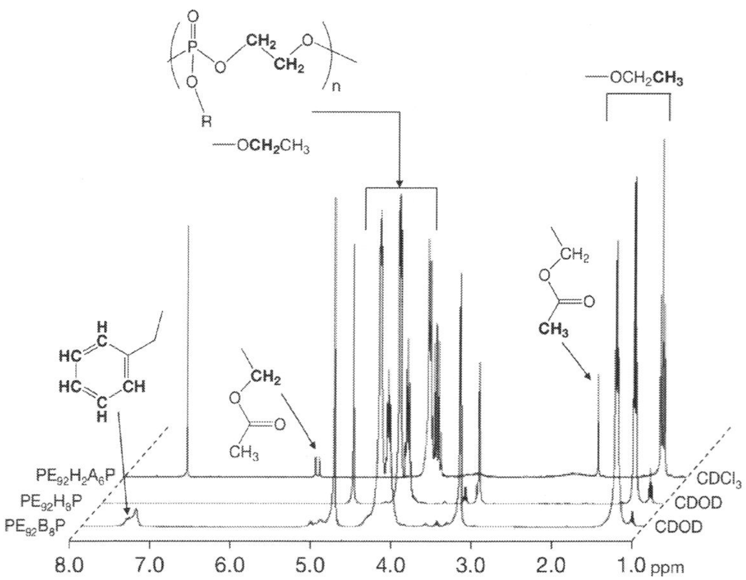

Fig. 14. ^{1}H NMR spectra of polyphosphoester bearing acetoxymethyl ester groups and the prepolymers.

Figure 16 shows the change in the number-averaged molecular weight (M_n) of PEHA incubated in PBS and that containing esterase. The decrease in molecular weight of PEHA was remarkable when the polymer was in contact with esterase. Digestion of the main chain was also accelerated with the esterase treatment.

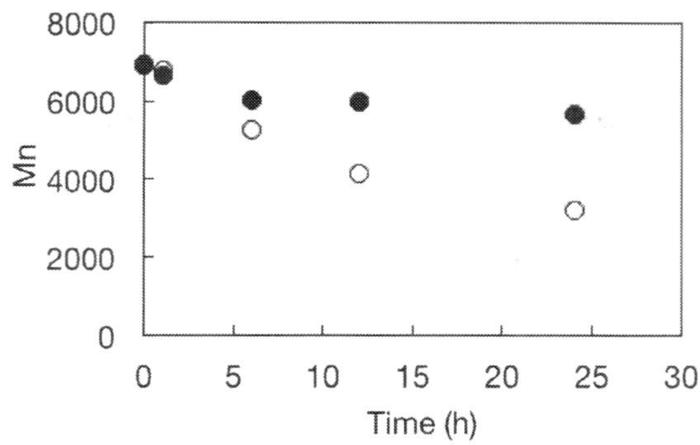

Fig. 15. Change in unit mole fraction of acetoxymethyl ester group of PEHA in contact with porcine liver esterase. (●) in PBS, (○) in esterase solution [Esterase] = 40 U/mL.

The thermoresponsivity of PEHA before and after contact with protease is shown in Figure 17. The PEHA/PBS showed LCST-type liquid-liquid phase separation and the cloud point was 40°C. In both PBS and that with esterase, the temperature of the phase separation increased with an increase in incubation time. In particular, the PEHA treated with esterase for 24 h did not have a cloud point between 20 and 65°C. The degree of AM groups on the polymer influenced its thermoresponsivity. That is, the phase separation phenomena could be controlled by acetoxymethylation of the polyphosphoesters. In addition, PEH, the polymer before acetoxymethylation, did not show any LCST-type liquid-liquid phase separation (data not shown). The influence of the change in molecular weight of PEHA with esterase treatment should also be of concern. While the cloud point of PEHA synthesized in this study was not in physiological conditions (>40°C), it could be adjusted by introducing more hydrophobic units into the polymer as described in previous literature (Iwasaki et al., 2004). Because the block copolymers composed of polyphosphoesters and poly(ethylene glycol) form a micelle structure above phase separation temperature (Wang et al., 2009), PEHA will work as building blocks for making enzyme-responsive micelles.

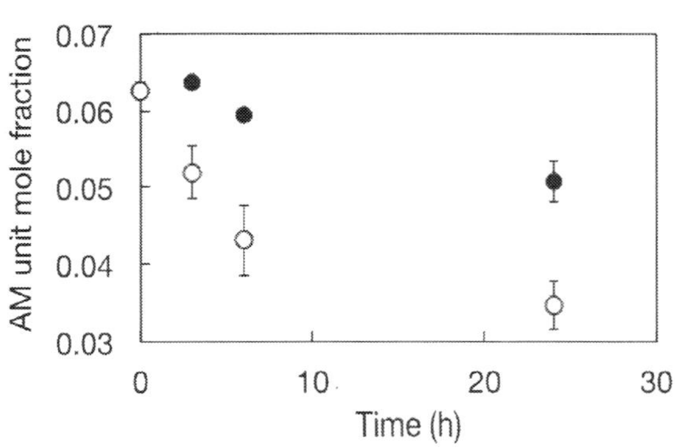

Fig. 16. Change in number-averaged molecular weight (Mn) of PEHA in contact with porcine liver esterase. (●) in PBS, (○) in esterase solution [Esterase] = 40 U/mL.

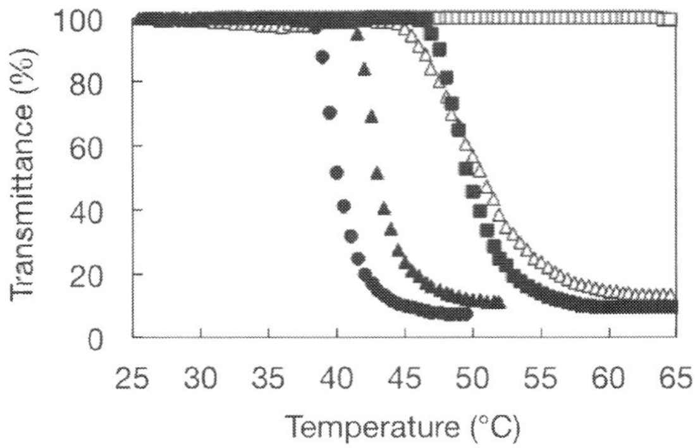

Fig. 17. Thermoresponsivity of PEHA in PBS before and after incubation with porcine liver esterase for 6 and 24 h. (●) 0, (▲) 6, and (■) 24 h in PBS; (△) 6 h and (□) 24 h in esterase solution.

The AM group is widely used for prodrugs and for fluorescence probes for cell imaging (Hecher et al., 2008; Takakusa et al., 2003). This group effectively induces cell membrane penetration and is rapidly cleaved intracellularly (Shultz et al., 1993; Yogo et al., 2004). Figure 18 is a fluorescence micrograph of HeLa cells in contact with Nile Red for 60 min with or without PEHA. The localization of Nile Red into the cells was improved by the presence of PEHA. At this concentration of PHEA, the polymer does not have a cloud point around 37°C. The solubilization capacity for hydrophobic molecules and the amphiphilic nature of the polymer might be improved by the cytoplasmic penetration of Nile Red. Although the mechanism of delivery of Nile Red into cells has not been fully clarified, the polyphosphoester bearing AM groups has the potential to induce penetration of hydrophobic drugs through the cell membrane.

To understand the interaction of PEHA and the cell membrane, we investigated the cytotoxicity of PEHA using Chinese hamster fibroblasts (V79), as described in a previous report (Iwasaki et al., 2004). There was no adverse effect of PEHA on cell viability when the PEHA concentration was below 0.01 g/dL (see supporting data). On the other hand, the cytotoxicity of PEHA was observed when the concentration was more than 0.1 g/dL. From the nature of this cytotoxicity test, it can be assumed that a high concentration of PEHA might damage the cell membrane. That is, that PHEA has an affinity for cell membrane.

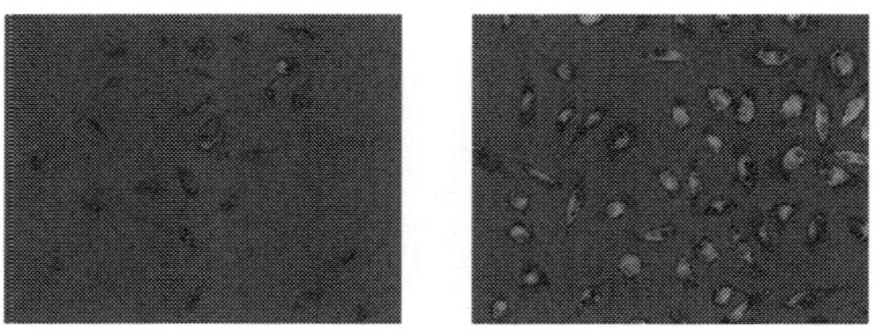

Fig. 18. Fluorescence micrographs of HeLa cells in contact with Nile Red in culture medium. a) Nile Red, b) Nile Red with PEHA. [PEHA] = 0.0025 mg/mL, [Nile Red] = 0.0125 μg/mL.

4. Conclusion

This chapter described current studies of new methods of syntheses and the characteristics of polyphosphoesters. Polymerization with a narrow molecular weight distribution is important to obtain the reproducible properties of polymers. In addition, the functionalization of the end or side groups of the polymers results in producing various types of polymer materials. The robustness of polyphosphoesters as biomedical materials has been clarified during the past decade (Zhao et al., 1003; Wang et al., 2009). However, the molecular and material designs of polyphosphoesters for biomedical applications are still limited. Polyphosphoesters have been explored as biomimetic to nucleic and teichoic acids. The study of the biological activity of polyphosphoesters will prove to be interesting.
As one of the unique properties of polyphosphoesters, LCST-type liquid-liquid phase separation of polyphosphoesters in aqueous media was introduced with a difference in the structure of their side chains. The aqueous solution of the polymers bearing alkyl groups became turbid with increments in temperature. From microscopic observation, liquid-liquid phase separation was observed in the turbid solution. The cloud points of the polymer solutions were influenced by polymer concentration, copolymerization ratio, and NaCl concentration. In addition, the copolymer effectively improved the solubility of the hydrophobic molecules in an aqueous medium and enabled separation of the molecules from the solution with increments in temperature.
Furthermore, thermoresponsive polyphosphoesters bearing AM groups as side chains were demonstrated as enzyme-responsive polymers. The thermoresponsivity of polymers in aqueous solution depended on the concentration of AM units and their molecular weight. Cleavage of the AM units and degradation of the polymer chain were accelerated with esterase treatment. The solubility of hydrophobic molecules and localization of the molecules into living cells were also improved by the synthetic polymers. To use polyphosphoesters bearing AM groups as drug carriers, further molecular design to achieve self-assembly, stealth, and targeting characteristics will be needed. However, the newly designed structure is interesting as a basic motif for applications.

5. Acknowledgments

Some activities described in this chapter were supported by a Grant-in-Aid for Scientific Research on Innovative Areas "Molecular Soft-Interface Science" (#21106520) and Young Scientists (A) (#21680043) from the Ministry of Education, Culture, Sports, Science and Technology of Japan. The author is grateful to Dr. Shin-ichi Yusa (University of Hyogo), Ms. Etsuko Yamaguchi (Kansai University), and Mr. Takashi Kawakita (Kansai University) for their assistance in the synthesis and characterization of the polyphosphoesters.

6. References

Alarcon, C.D.H.; Pennadam, S.; Alexander, C. (2005). Stimuli Responsive Polymers for Biomedical Applications. *Chemical Society Reviews*, Vol. 34, No. 4, (February 2005), pp. 276-285, ISSN 1460-4744

Burdick, J.A.; Chung, C.; Jia, X.; Randolph, M.A.; Langer, R. (2005). Controlled Degradation and Mechanical Behavior of Photopolymerized Hyaluronic Acid Networks. *Biomacromolecules*, Vol. 6, No. 1, (November 2004), pp. 386-391, ISSN 1526-4602

Coburn, S.P.; Mahuren, J.D.; Jain, M.; Zubovic. Y.; Wortsman, J. (1998). Alkaline Phosphatase (EC 3.1.3.1) in Serum is Inhibited by Physiological Concentrations of Inorganic Phosphate. *The Journal of Clinical Endocrinology and Metabolism*, Vol. 83, No. 11, (November 1998), pp. 3951-3957, ISSN 1945-7197

Chilkoti, A.; Dreher, M.R.; Meyer, D.E.; Raucher, D. (2002). Targeted Drug Delivery by Thermally Responsive Polymers. *Advanced Drug Delivery Reviews*, Vol. 54, No. 5, (September 2002), pp. 613-630, ISSN 0169-409X.

Choi, J.Y.; Lee, B.H.; Song, K.B.; Park, R.W.; Kim, I.S.; Sohn, K.Y.; Jo, J.S.; Ryoo, H.M. (1996). Expression Patterns of Bone-Related Proteins During Osteoblastic Differentiation in MC3T3-E1 Cells. *Journal of Cellular Biochemistry*, Vol. 61. No. 4, (June 1996), pp. 609-618, ISSN 1097-4644

Foss, C.A., Jr.; Hornyak, G.L.; Stockert, J.A.; Martin, C.R. (1992). Optical Properties of Composite Membranes Containing Arrays of Nanoscopic Gold Cylinders. *The Journal of Physical Chemistry*, Vol. 96, No. 19, (September 1992), pp. 7497-7499, ISSN 0022-3654

Fujiwara, T.; Mukose, T.; Yamaoka, T.; Yamane, H.; Sakurai, S.; Kimura, Y. (2001) Novel Thermo-Responsive Formation of a Hydrogel By Stereo-Complexation Between PLLA-PEG-PLLA and PDLA-PEG-PDLA Block Copolymers. *Macromolecular Bioscience*, Vol. 1, No. 5, (July 2001), pp. 204-208, ISSN 1616-5195

Geurtsen, W.; Leyhausen, G.; Garcia-Godoy, F. (1999) Effect of Storage Media on the Fluoride Release and Surface Microhardness of Four Polyacid-Modified Composite Resins ("Compomers"). Dental Materials, Vol. 15, No. 3, (May 1999), pp. 196-201, ISSN 0109-5641

Hecker, S.J.; Erion, M.D. (2008). Prodrugs of Phosphates and Phosphonates. *Journal of Medical Chemistry*, Vol. 51, No. 8, (Areil 2008), pp. 2328-2345, ISSN 1520-4804

Heskins, M.; Guillent, J.E.; James, E. (1968). Solution Properties of Poly(*N*-isopropylacrylamide). *Journal of Macromolecular Science, Part A*, Vol. 2, No. 8, (December 1968), pp. 1441–1455, ISSN 1520-5738

Hsu, Y.-H. ; Chiang, W.-H.; Chen, C.-H.; Chern, C.-S.; Chiu, H.-C. Thermally Responsive Interactions Between the PEG and Pnipaam Grafts Attached to the Paac Backbone and the Corresponding Structural Changes of Polymeric Micelles in Water. *Macromolecules*, Vol. 38, No. 23, (October 2005), pp. 9757-9765, ISSN 1520-5835

Huang, S.W.; Wang, J.; Zhang, P.C.; Mao, H.Q.; Zhuo, R.X.; Leong, K. W. (2004). Water-Soluble and Nonionic Polyphosphoester: Synthesis, Degradation, Biocompatibility and Enhancement of Gene Expression in Mouse Muscle. *Biomacromolecules*, Vol. 5, No. 2, (March-April 2004), pp. 306-311, ISSN 1526-4602

Idziak, I.; Avoce, D.; Lessard, D.; Gravel, D.; Zhu, X. X. (1999). Thermosensitivity of Aqueous Solutions of Poly(*N,N*-Diethylacrylamide). *Macromolecules*, Vol. 32, No. 4, (January 1999), pp. 1260-1263, ISSN 1520-5835

Iwasaki, Y. & Akiyoshi, K. (2004). Design of Biodegradable Amphiphilic Polymers: Well-Defined Amphiphilic Polyphosphates with Hydrophilic Graft Chains via ATRP. *Macromolecules*, Vol. 37, No. 20, (August 2004), pp. 7637-7642, ISSN 1520-5835

Iwasaki, Y. & Akiyoshi, K. (2006). Synthesis and Characterization of Amphiphilic Polyphosphates with Hydrophobic Graft Chains and Cholesteryl Groups as Nanocarriers. *Biomacromolecules*, Vol. 7, No. 5, (April 2006), pp. 1433-1438, ISSN 1526-4602

Iwasaki, Y.; Kawakita, T.; Yusa, S. (2009) Thermoresponsive Polyphosphoesters Bearing Enzyme-Cleavable Side Chains. *Chemistry Letters*, Vol. 38, No. 11, (November 200), pp. 1054-1055, ISSN 1348-0715

Iwasaki, Y.; Komatsu, S.; Narita T.; Ishihara, K.; Akiyoshi, K. (2003). Biodegradable Phosphorylcholine-Hydrogel Consist of Polyphosphate Cross-Linking Reagents. *Macromolecular Bioscience*, Vol. 3, No. 5, (May 2003), pp. 238-242, ISSN 1616-5195

Iwasaki, Y.; Nakagawa, C.; Ohtomi, M.; Ishihara, K.; Akiyoshi K. (2004). A Novel Biodegradable Polyphosphate Cross-Linker for Making Biocompatible Hydrogel. *Biomacromolecules*, Vol. 5, No. 3, (April 2004), pp. 1110-1115, ISSN 1526-4602

Iwasaki, Y.; Wachiralarpphaithoon, C.; Akiyoshi, K. (2007). Novel Thermoresponsive Polymers Having Biodegradable Phosphoester Backbone. *Macromolecules*, Vol. 40, No. 23, (October 2007), pp. 8136-8138, ISSN 1520-5835

Iwasaki, Y. & Yamaguchi, E. (2010). Synthesis of Well-Defined Thermoresponsive Polyphosphoester Macroinitiators Using Organocatalysts. *Macromolecules*, Vol. 43, No. 6, (February 2010), pp. 2664-2666, ISSN 1520-5835

Kamber, N. E.; Jeong, W.; Waymouth, R. M.; Pratt, R. C.; Lohmeijer, B. G. G.; Hedrick, J. L. (2007). Organocatalytic Ring-Opening Polymerization. *Chemical Reviews*, Vol. 107, No. 12, (December 2006), pp. 5813–5840, ISSN 1520-6890

Katuiyhski, K.; Libiszowski, J.; Penczek, S. (1976). A New Class of Synthetic Polyelectrolytes. Acidic Polyesters of Phosphoric Acid (Poly(hydroxyalkylene phosphates)). *Macromolecules*, Vol. 9, No. 2, (March 1976), pp. 365-367, ISSN 1520-5835

Kikuchi, A.; Okano, T. (2002). Pulsatile Drug Release Control Using Hydrogels. *Advanced Drug Delivery Reviews*, Vol. 54, No. 1, (January 2002), pp. 53-77, ISSN 0169-409X

Kikuchi, A.; Okano T. (2005) Nanostructured Designs of Biomedical Materials: Applications of Cell Sheet Engineering to Functional Regenerative Tissues and Organs. *Journal of Controlled Release*, Vol. 101, No. 1-3, (January 2005), pp. 69-84, ISSN 0168-3659

Kim, M.S.; Seo, K.S.; Khang, G.; Cho, S.H.; Lee, H.B. (2004). Preparation of Methoxy Poly(ethylene glycol)/Polyester Diblock Copolymers and Examination of The Gel-to-Sol Transition. *Journal of Polymer Science Part A: Polymer Chemistry*, Vol. 42, No. 22, (November 2004) pp. 5784-5793, ISSN 1099-0518

Klouda, L.A.; Mikos, G. (2008). Thermoresponsive Hydrogels in Biomedical Applications. *European Journal of Pharmaceutics and Biopharmaceutics*, Vol. 68, No. 1, (January 2008), pp. 34-45. ISSN 0928-0987

Kobayashi, J.; Kikuchi, A.; Sakai, K.; Okano T. (2003). Cross-Linked Thermoresponsive Anionic Polymer-Grafted Surfaces To Separate Bioactive Basic Peptides. *Analytical Chemistry*, Vol. 75, No. 13, (May 2003), pp. 3244-3249, ISSN 1520-6882

Libiszowski, J.; Kaluzynski, K.; Penczek, S. (1978). Polymerization of Cyclic Esters of Phosphoric Acid. VI. Poly(Alkyl Ethylene Phosphates). Polymerization of 2-Alkoxy-2-Oxo-1,3,2-Dioxaphospholans and Structure of Polymers. *Journal of Polymer Science Part A: Polymer Chemistry*, Vol. 16, No. 6, (June 1978), pp. 1275-1283, ISSN 1099-0518

Lin, A.S.P.; Barrows, T.H. ; Cartmell, S.H.; Guldberg, R.E. (2003). Microarchitectural and Mechanical Characterization of Oriented Porous Polymer Scaffolds. *Biomaterials*, Vol. 24, No. 3, (February 2003), pp. 481-489, ISSN 0142-9612

Liu, J.; Huang, W.; Zhou, Y.; Yan, D. (2009). Synthesis of Hyperbranched Polyphosphates by Self-Condensing Ring-Opening Polymerization of HEEP without Catalyst. *Macromolecules*, Vol. 42, No. 13, (June 2009), pp. 4394-4399, ISSN 1520-5835

Matyjaszewski, K.; Xia, J. (2001). Atom Transfer Radical Polymerization. *Chemical Reviews*, Vol. 101, No. 9, (September 2001), pp. 2921-2990, ISSN 1520-6890

Mao, S.-Z.; Zhang, X.-D.; Dereppe, J.-M.; Du, Y.-R. (2000). Nuclear magnetic resonance relaxation studies of polyacrylamide solution. *Colloid and Polymer Science*, Vol. 278, No. 3, (March 2000), pp. 264-269, ISSN 1435-1536

Miyazaki, H.; Kataoka, K. (1996). Preparation of Polyacrylamide Derivatives Showing Thermo-Reversible Coacervate Formation and Their Potential Application to Two-Phase Separation Processes. *Polymer*, Vol. 37, No. 4, (February 1996), pp. 681-685, ISSN 0032-3861

Monji, N.; Cole, C.A.; Hoffman, A.S. (1994). Activated, *N*-Substituted Acrylamide Polymers for Antibody Coupling: Application to a Novel Membrane-Based Immunoassay. *Journal of Biomaterials Science, Polymer Edition*, Vol. 5, No. 5, (October 1994), pp. 407-420, ISSN 1568-5624

Myrex, R.D.; Farmer, B.; Gray, G.M.; Wright, Y.-J.; Dees J.; Bharara, P.C.; Byrd, H.; Branham, K.E. (2003). 31P and 1H NMR Studies of the Transesterification Polymerization of Polyphosphonate Oligomers. *European Polymer Journal*, Vol. 39, No. 6, (June 2003) pp. 1105-1115, ISSN 0014-3057

Nederberg, F.; Lohmeijer, B.G.G.; Leibfarth, F.; Pratt, R.C.; Choi, J.; Dove, A.P.; Waymouth, R.M.; Hedrick, J.L. (2007). Organocatalytic Ring Opening Polymerization of Trimethylene Carbonate. *Biomacromolecules*, Vol. 8, No. 1, (December 2007), pp. 153-160, ISSN 1526-4602

Nishida, K.; Yamato, M.; Hayashida, Y.; Watanabe, K.; Yamamoto, K.; Adachi, E.; Nagai, S.; Kikuchi, A.; Maeda, N.; Watanabe, H.; Okano, T.; Tano, Y. N. (2004). Corneal Reconstruction with Tissue-Engineered Cell Sheets Composed of Autologous Oral Mucosal Epithelium. *The New England Journal of Medicine*, Vol. 351, pp. 1187-1196, (September 2004), ISSN 1533-4406

Okuyama, Y.; Yoshida, R.; Sakai, K,; Okano, T.; Sakurai, Y. (1993). Swelling Controlled Zero Order and Sigmoidal Drug Release from Thermo-Responsive Poly(*N*-Isopropylacrylamide-co-Butyl methacrylate) Hydrogel. *Journal of Biomaterials Science, Polymer Edition*, Vol. 4, No. 5, (October 1993), pp. 545-556, ISSN 1568-5624

Penczek, S. & Klosinski, P. (1990). Synthetic Polyphosphates Related to Nucleic Acid and Teichoic Acids, In: *Model of Biopolymer by Ring-opening Polymerization*; Penczek, S. Ed.; 291-378, CRC Press, Inc., ISBN0-8493-5077-8, Boca Raton

Pratt, R.C.; Lohmeijer, B.G.G.; Long, D.A.; Waymouth, R.M.; Hedrick J.L. (2006). Triazabicyclodecene: A Simple Bifunctional Organocatalyst for Acyl Transfer and Ring-Opening Polymerization of Cyclic Esters. *Journal of the American Chemical Society*, Vol. 128, No. 14, (April 2006), pp. 4556-4557, ISSN 0002-7863

Pretula, J.; Kaluzynski, K.; Penczek, S. (1986). Synthesis of poly(alkylene phosphates) with nitrogen-containing bases in the side chains. 1. Nitrogen- and carbon-substituted imidazoles. *Macromolecules*, Vol. 19, No. 7, (July 1986), pp. 1797-1799, ISSN 1520-5835

Pretula, J.; Kaluzynski, K.; Szymanski, R.; Penczek S. (1999). Transesterification of Oligomeric Dialkyl Phosphonates, Leading to the High-Molecular-Weight poly-H-

Phosphonates. *Journal of Polymer Science Part A: Polymer Chemistry*, Vol. 37, No. 9, (May 1999), pp. 1365-1381, ISSN 1099-0518

Rafanan, A.L.; Maurer, J.; Mehta, A.C.; Schilz, R. (2000). Progressive Portopulmonary Hypertension after Liver Transplantation Treated with Epoprostenol. *Chest*, Vol. 118, No. 5, (November 2000), pp. 1497-1500, ISSN 1931-3543

Ren, Y.; Jiang, X.; Pan, D.; Mao, H.-Q. (2010). Charge Density and Molecular Weight of Polyphosphoramidate Gene Carrier Are Key Parameters Influencing Its DNA Compaction Ability and Transfection Efficiency. *Biomacromolecules*, Vol. 11, No. 12, (November 2010), pp. 3432-3439, ISSN 1526-4602

Renier, M.L. & Kohn, D.H. (1997). Development and characterization of a biodegradable polyphosphate. *Journal of Biomedical Materials Research*, Vol. 34, No. 1, (January 1997), pp. 95-104, ISSN 1552-4965

Richards, M.; Dahiyat, B.I.; Arm, D.M.; Lin, S.; Leong, K.W. (1991). Interfacial polycondensation and characterization of polyphosphates and polyphosphonates. *Journal of Polymer Science Part A: Polymer Chemistry*, Vol. 29, No. 8, (July 1991), pp. 1157-1165, ISSN 1099-0518

Schultz, C.; Vajanaphanich, M.; Harootunian, A. T.; Sammak, P. J.; Barrett, K. E.; Tsien, R. Y. (1993). Acetoxymethyl Esters of Phosphates, Enhancement of the Permeability and Potency of cAMP. *The Journal of Biological Chemistry*, Vol. 268, No. 9, (March 1993), pp. 6316-6322, ISSN 1083-351X.

Shimokuri, T.; Kaneko, T.; Akashi, M. (2006). Effects of Thermoresponsive Coacervation on the Hydrolytic Degradation of Amphipathic Poly(γ-glutamate)s. *Macromolecular Bioscience*, Vol. 6,No. 11, (November 2006) pp. 942-951, ISSN 1616-5195

Tachibana, Y.; Kurisawa, M.; Uyama, H.; Kakuchi, T.; Kobayashi, S. (2003). Biodegradable Thermoresponsive Poly(Amino Acid)s. *Chemical Communications*, (January 2003), pp. 106-107, ISSN 1364-548X.

Takakusa, H.; Kikuchi, K.; Urano, Y.; Kojima, H.; Nagano, T. (2003). A Novel Design Method of Ratiometric Fluorescent Probes Based on Fluorescence Resonance energy Transfer Switching by Spectral Overlap Integral. *Chemistry - A European Journal*, Vol. 9, No. 7, (April 2003), pp. 1479-1485, ISSN 1521-376.

Takeshita, T.; Tanaka, H.; Harasawa, A.; Kaminaga, T.; Imamura, T.; Furui, S. (2003). Brown Tumor of the Sphenoid Sinus in a Patient with Secondary Hyperparathyroidism: CT and MR Imaging Findings. *Radiation Medicine*, Vol. 22, No. 4, (July-August 2004), pp. 265–268, ISSN 1862-5274

Takei, Y.G.; Aoki, T.; Sanui, K.; Ogata, N.; Okano, T.; Sakurai, Y. (1993). Temperature-Responsive Bioconjugates. 1. Synthesis of Temperature-Responsive Oligomers with Reactive End Groups and Their Coupling to Biomolecules. *Bioconjugate Chemistry*, Vol. 4, No. 1, (January 1993), pp. 341-346, ISSN 1520-4812

Wachiralarpphaithoon, C.; Iwasaki, Y.; Akiyoshi, K. (2007). Enzyme-Degradable Phosphorylcholine Porous Hydrogels Cross-Linked with Polyphosphoesters for Biocompatible Cell Matrices. *Biomaterials*, Vol. 28, No. 6, (February 2007), pp. 984-993, ISSN 1878-5905

Wan, A.C.; Mao, H.Q.; Wang, S.; Leong, K.W.; Ong, L.K.; Yu, H. (2001). Fabrication of Poly(Phosphoester) Nerve Guides by Immersion Precipitation and the Control of Porosity. *Biomaterials*, Vol. 22, No. 10, (May 2001), pp. 1147-1156, ISSN 1878-5905

Wang, D.A.; Williams, C.G.; Yang, F.; Cher, N.; Lee, H.; Elisseeff, J.H. (2005). Bioresponsive phosphoester hydrogels for bone tissue engineering. *Tissue Engineering*, Vol. 11, No. 1-2, (January-February 2005), pp. 201-213, ISSN 1557-8690

Wang, J.; Zhang, P.C.; Lu, H.F.; Ma, N.; Wang, S.; Mao, H.Q.; Leong, K.W. (2002). New polyphosphoramidate with a spermidine side chain as a gene carrier. *Journal of Controlled Release*, Vol. 83, No. 1, (September 2002), pp. 157-168, ISSN 0168-3659

Wang, Y.C.; Tang, L.Y.; Li, Y.; Wang, J. (2009). Thermoresponsive Block Copolymers of Poly(ethylene glycol) and Polyphosphoester: Thermo-Induced Self-Assembly, Biocompatibility, and Hydrolytic Degradation. *Biomacromolecules*, Vol. 10, No. 1, (January 2009), pp. 66-73, ISSN 1526-4602

Wang, Y.-C.; Yuan, Y.-Y.; Du, J.-Z.; Yang, X.-Z. ; Wang, J. (2009). Recent Progress in Polyphosphoesters: From Controlled Synthesis to Biomedical Applications. *Macromolecular Bioscience*, Vol. 9, No. 12, (December 2009), pp. 1154–1164, ISSN 1616-5195

Wen, J. & Zhuo, R.X. (1998). Enzyme-Catalyzed Ring-Opening Polymerization of Ethylene Isopropyl Phosphate. *Macromolecular Rapid Communications*, Vol. 19, No. 12, (December 1998), pp. 641-642, ISSN 1521-3927

Xiao, C.-S.; Wang, Y.-C.; Du, J.-Z.; Chen, X.-S.; Wang, J. (2006). Kinetics and Mechanism of 2-Ethoxy-2-oxo-1,3,2-dioxaphospholane Polymerization Initiated by Stannous Octoate. *Macromolecules*, Vol. 39, No. 20, (September 2006), pp. 6825-6831, ISSN 1520-5835

Yamazaki, A.; Winnik, F.M.; Cornelius, R.M.; Brash, J.L. (1999). Modification of Liposomes with N-Substituted Polyacrylamides: Identification of Proteins Adsorbed from Plasma. *Biochimica et Biophysica Acta (BBA) - Biomembranes*, Vol. 1421, No. 1, (September 1999), pp. 103-115, ISSN 0005-2736

Yogo, T.; Kikuchi, K.; Inoue, T.; Hirose, K.; Iino, M.; Nagano, T. (2004). Modification of Intracellular Ca2+ Dynamics by Laser Inactivation of Inositol 1,4,5-Trisphosphate Receptor Using Membrane-Permeant Probes. *Chemistry and Biology*, Vol. 11, No. 8, (August 2004), pp. 1053-1058, ISSN 1879-1301

Zhao, Z.; Wang, J.; Mao, H.Q.; Leong, K.W. (2003). Polyphosphoesters in Drug and Gene Delivery. *Advanced Drug Delivery Reviews*, Vol. 55, No. 4, (April 2003), pp. 483-499.

2

Inactivation of Bacteria by Non-Thermal Plasmas

R. Morent and N. De Geyter
Research Unit Plasma Technology - Department of Applied Physics
Faculty of Engineering and Architecture - Ghent University
Belgium

1. Introduction

In physical sciences, "plasma" refers to the forth state of matter, while in medicine and biology, plasma is known as the non-cellular component of blood (Fridman et al., 2008). Interestingly, the term "plasma" has been coined by Irving Langmuir to emphasize that the characteristics of ionic liquids ubiquitous in biology and medicine are analogous to plasma in the physical sciences (Fridman et al., 2008, Langmuir, 1928). Despite this historical connection, plasmas are mainly associated with the solid-state processing technology (Stoffels et al., 2003), while being rarely used in biomedical applications directly. This situation is however rapidly changing and multiple plasma applications in life sciences are recently emerging (Daeschlein et al., 2010, Vandamme et al., 2010, Kalghatgi et al., 2010, Kong et al., 2009, Nie et al., 2009, Kalghatgi et al., 2007).
The plasma state can be considered to be a gaseous mixture of oppositely-charged particles with a roughly zero net electrical charge (Denes&Manolache, 2004). Besides charged particles, plasmas also contain neutral atoms and molecules, excited atoms and molecules, radicals and UV photons. Generally, plasmas can be subdivided into 2 categories: thermal plasmas and non-thermal (or cold) plasmas (Denes&Manolache, 2004, Fridman et al., 2008, Bogaerts et al., 2002). Thermal plasmas are characterized by very high temperatures of electrons and heavy particles, both charged and neutral. In contrast, non-thermal plasmas are composed of low temperature particles (charged and neutral molecular and atomic species) and relatively high temperature electrons (Bogaerts et al., 2002, Denes&Manolache, 2004). Because the ions and the neutrals remain relatively cold, a non-thermal plasma does not cause any thermal damage to articles it comes in contact with. This characteristic opened up the possibility to use these non-thermal plasmas for the treatment of heat-sensitive materials including biological matter such as cells and tissues (Laroussi, 2009). Non-thermal plasmas are already routinely used in material processing applications, such as etching, activation and deposition (Borcia et al., 2006, Bruce et al., 2010, De Geyter et al., 2008, De Geyter et al., 2009, Morent et al., 2009a, Morent et al., 2009b, Maruyama et al., 2010). More recently, the biological and medical applications of these plasmas have witnessed a great interest from both plasma as well as medical research communities.
This review paper focuses on one specific fascinating application of non-thermal plasmas in biomedical science, namely the inactivation of bacteria, also called plasma sterilization

(Stoffels et al., 2008). We need to stress that the term sterilization is somewhat ambiguous since this term is only used when all initial micro-organisms are killed, which is however not always the case when applying non-thermal plasmas to contaminated surfaces (Boudam et al., 2006). Conventional sterilization methods include the use of dry heat (oven), moist heat (autoclave) or chemicals like gaseous ethylene oxide, liquid formaldehyde and glutaraldehyde (Kelly-Wintenberg et al., 1998, Moisan et al., 2001, Moisan et al., 2002, Park et al., 2003). Some major drawbacks of these conventional techniques are the high processing temperatures (ovens and autoclaves) which makes it impossible to sterilize heat-sensitive materials like polymers, the use of toxic chemicals and the long sterilization times needed (approximately 12 hours in the case of ethylene oxide exposure) (Park et al., 2003, Moisan et al., 2001, Montie et al., 2000). Another interesting sterilization method is the use of gamma irradiation, but this is an expensive technique and may cause the material to undergo undesirable changes during sterilization (Moisan et al., 2001, Henn et al., 1996, Ishigaki&Yoshii, 1992). The limitations of these conventional methods have encouraged the search for new approaches and an alternative method of sterilization is treatment with a non-thermal plasma (plasma sterilization). These plasmas operate under moderate temperatures and use non-toxic gases, therefore, thermal and chemical damage to the substrate is limited (Philip et al., 2002, Sladek&Stoffels, 2005). Moreover, plasmas are not only capable of killing bacteria and viruses, they can also remove these dead micro-organisms from the surfaces of the objects being sterilized (Chau et al., 1996). This chapter on plasma sterilization is organized as follows: a first part will focus on the inactivation of bacteria on non-living surfaces, which has reached a state of maturity. In this first section, the kinetics of bacterial inactivation processes will be described, followed by the effects of various plasma-generated agents on bacterial cells. Afterwards, a brief review on the inactivation of bacteria on non-living surfaces by vacuum and atmospheric pressure plasmas will be presented. A second part of the chapter will deal with state-of-the-art applications of non-thermal plasmas in bacterial inactivation, namely the sterilization of teeth and human/animal tissue, which are both relatively new research topics.

2. Plasma sterilization on non-living surfaces

2.1 Survival curves to determine the inactivation efficiency

Plasma effects on micro-organisms can be evaluated using various methods, however, a commonly used approach is the determination of survival curves (Stoffels et al., 2008, Boudam et al., 2006, Moisan et al., 2002). These curves are plots of the logarithm of the number of surviving micro-organisms as a function of exposure time to the sterilizing agent. Although the precise procedures to obtain these curves may vary, usually a suspension containing a well-defined concentration of micro-organisms is placed on a substrate and let to dry. After plasma exposure, the remaining micro-organisms are let to inoculate for several hours before counting. Considering that counting large numbers of cells is troublesome, the number of colony forming units (CFU) is determined instead of counting individual cells after inoculation (Stoffels et al., 2008). For conventional sterilization methods, the survival curve is usually a unique straight line: the inactivation process is an exponential function of time (Moisan et al., 2002, Cariou-Travers&Darbord, 2001). In contrast, plasma sterilization can provide survival curves with different shapes depending on the type of micro-organism, the type of medium supporting the micro-organisms and the method of plasma exposure (direct or remote) (Laroussi et al., 2000, Laroussi, 2002). In some cases, the survival curves after plasma exposure are straight lines (similar to conventional sterilization methods) (Laroussi et al., 2000, Herrmann et al., 1999, Yamamoto et al., 2001), however, in most cases, two or even three different linear segments occur, each segment being a different inactivation phase (Kelly-Wintenberg et al., 1998, Moisan et al., 2002, Laroussi et al., 2000). This implies that the number of surviving micro-organisms is also an exponential function of time, but with different time constants. To characterize the slope of each segment, an interesting parameter has been extensively used by several researchers studying plasma sterilization: the so-called "D-value" (decimal value) (Moisan et al., 2002, Laroussi, 2002, Fridman, 2008). This parameter is the time required to reduce an original concentration of micro-organisms by 90 % (one $\log_{10}$ reduction) and is expressed in the unit of time.

Single-slope survival curves have been observed in atmospheric pressure plasma sterilization by Herrmann et al. (Herrmann et al., 1999), Laroussi et al. (Laroussi et al., 2000) and Yamamoto et al. (Yamamoto et al., 2001) and an example of such a single-slope curve is presented in Figure 1.

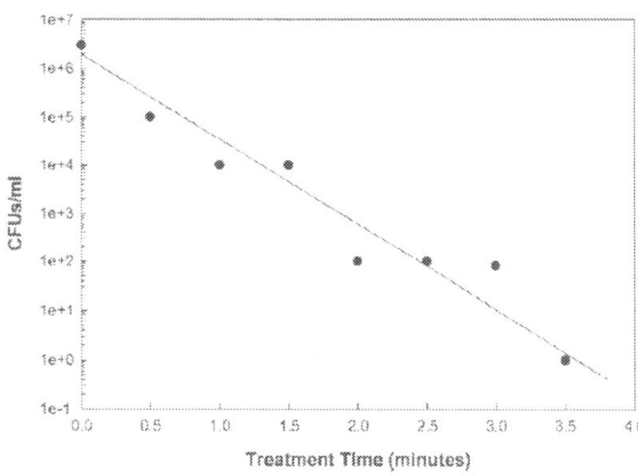

Fig. 1. Example of a single-slope survival curve: *E.coli* exposed to an atmospheric pressure glow discharge in a helium/air mixture [Reprinted with permission from (Laroussi, 2005)].

Herrmann et al. (Herrmann et al., 1999) employed a remote atmospheric pressure plasma jet in a helium/oxygen mixture to treat *Bacillus globigii* spores on glass coupons and found a D-value of 4.5 seconds. Laroussi et al. (Laroussi et al., 2000) and Yamamoto et al. (Yamamoto et al., 2001) utilized an atmospheric pressure glow discharge (DBD) in a helium/air mixture and an argon/H_2O_2 corona discharge respectively to treat *Escherichia coliphage* (*E. coli*). In these studies, single-slope survival curves were reported with D-values ranging from 15 seconds for the corona discharge to 5 minutes for the DBD-discharge (Laroussi et al., 2000, Laroussi, 2002, Yamamoto et al., 2001). More recently, Stoffels et al. (Sladek&Stoffels, 2005, Stoffels et al., 2008) and Choi et al. (Choi et al., 2006) presented results on plasma-induced deactivation of *E. coli* using a plasma needle operating in helium/air mixtures and a dielectric barrier discharge (DBD) in air respectively and also found a straight line as survival curve.

Two-slope survival curves can occur in both vacuum and atmospheric pressure plasma sterilization and were observed for the first time in 1998 by Hury et al. (Hury et al., 1998). These authors reported on the inactivation of different *Bacillus* spores in an oxygen plasma operating at low pressure (0.5 Pa) and did not observe a linear survival curve, but two successive lines with different slopes. According to their findings, the first slope has the smallest D-value (D_1), while the D-value of the second slope (D_2) is larger. As a result, the authors concluded that the inactivation of spores in their low pressure oxygen plasma is a two-step process: a fast process followed by a much slower one. Similar two-slope curves, as illustrated in Figure 2, were found in 2000 and 2002 by Moreau et al. (Moreau et al., 2000) and Philip et al. (Philip et al., 2002), who employed low pressure (133-933 Pa) microwave discharges in pure argon and N_2/O_2 mixtures (7 % oxygen) respectively for the inactivation of *Bacillus subtilis* spores. According to both Hury (Hury et al., 1998) and Moreau (Moreau et al., 2000), the first phase of their survival curve corresponds to the action of UV irradiation on isolated spores or on the first layers of stacked spores. The second phase, which is characterized by slower kinetics, represents spores that are shielded by others and thus require longer irradiation times to accumulate a lethal UV dose.

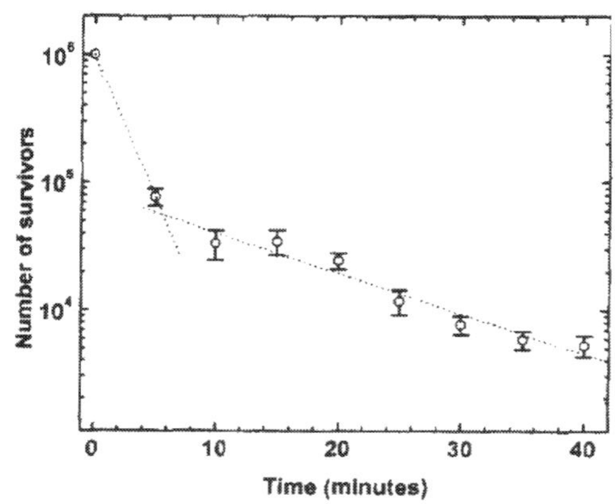

Fig. 2. Evolution as a function of time of the population of spores submitted to a pure argon afterglow at low pressure [Reprinted with permission from (Moreau et al., 2000)].

As previously mentioned, two-slope survival curves have also been observed in atmospheric pressure plasmas. Kelly-Wintenberg et al. (Kelly-Wintenberg et al., 1998) and Laroussi et al. (Laroussi et al., 2000) employed an atmospheric pressure glow discharge (DBD) for the inactivation of *E. coli*, *Staphylococcus aureus* and *Pseudomonas aeruginosa*. In contrast to the vacuum plasmas, the D-value of the observed second slope (D_2) was smaller than the D-value of the first slope (D_1) in these plasma systems. A general example of the observed survival curves is shown in Figure 3.

Montie et al. (Montie et al., 2000) found similar survival curves for the inactivation of *E. coli* and *B. subtilis* on glass, polypropylene and agar and claimed that the D_1-value depends on the species being treated, while the D_2-value depends on the type of surface supporting the micro-organisms (Laroussi, 2002, Fridman, 2008). A hypothesis for the two-slope survival curve was given by Kelly-Wintenberg et al. (Kelly-Wintenberg et al., 1998): during the first killing stage, active plasma species react with the outer membrane of the cells leading to damaging alterations. After this process has sufficiently advanced, the reactive species can quickly cause cell death, resulting in a very rapid second phase.

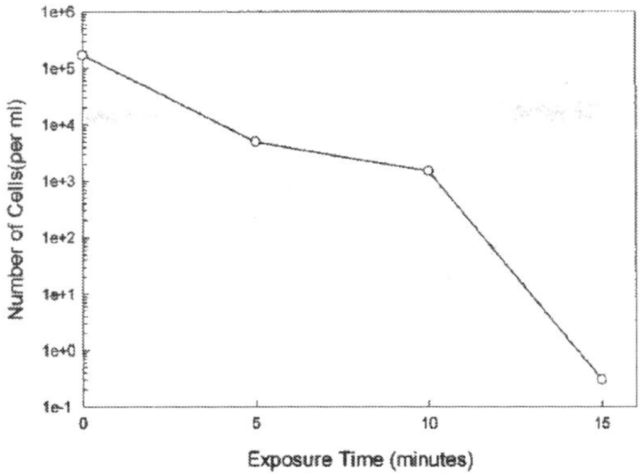

Fig. 3. Survival curve of *Pseudomonas aeruginosa* exposed to an atmospheric pressure glow discharge in a helium/air mixture [Reprinted with permission from (Laroussi et al., 2000)].

Multi-slope survival curves with three (or more) linear segments have also been observed in both vacuum as well as atmospheric pressure plasma sterilization. Moreau et al. (Moreau et al., 2000), Moisan et al. (Moisan et al., 2002) and Philip et al. (Philip et al., 2002) found three inactivation phases when employing a low pressure (133-933 Pa) microwave discharge in argon/oxygen and N_2/O_2 mixtures (0.7-2 % oxygen) respectively for the inactivation of *B. subtilis*. These authors claim that the first phase, which has the shortest D-value, is mainly due to the action of UV photons on isolated spores or on the first layers of stacked spores. The second phase (with the slowest kinetics) can be attributed to the erosion of the spores by active species, such as atomic oxygen. The third phase starts when the spores that were not inactivated during phases 1 and 2 have been sufficiently eroded, hence allowing UV photons to hit the genetic material of the still-living spores and finally kill them. A schematic illustration of the three-phase survival curve can be found in Figure 4.

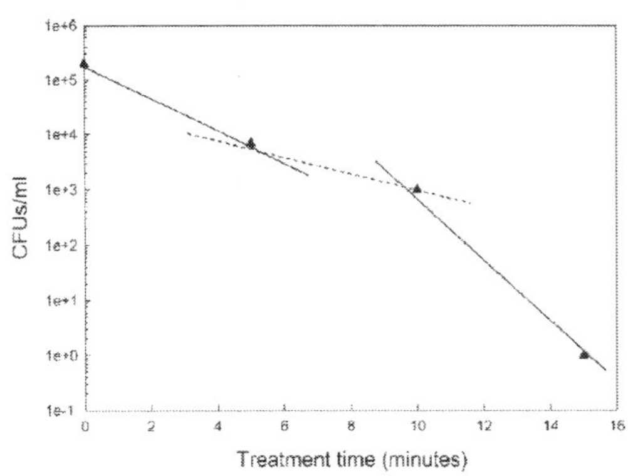

Fig. 4. Example of a three-phase survival curve: inactivation of *Pseudomonas aeruginosa* with an atmospheric pressure glow discharge in a helium/air mixture [Reprinted with permission from (Laroussi, 2005)].

These multi-slope survival curves were also recorded by Laroussi et al. (Laroussi et al., 2000) and Roth et al. (Roth et al., 2000) who employed atmospheric pressure plasma sources for sterilization, however, a clear elucidation for this type of survival curve is lacking for the moment. The explanation given earlier for low pressure plasma sterilization is most likely not applicable to atmospheric pressure plasmas, for which it has been shown that UV photons only play a secondary role in the killing process (Herrmann et al., 1999, Yamamoto et al., 2001, Kostov et al., 2010, Laroussi, 1996). Based on the above-mentioned bacterial inactivation kinetics, one can conclude that the mechanisms of sterilization by both vacuum and atmospheric pressure plasmas are very complex and far from understood at this moment.

2.2 Plasma species responsible for sterilization

As mentioned at the end of the previous section, plasma sterilization is a complex process since multiple plasma species, such as UV photons, excited species, reactive neutrals,... can interact with the bacterial cells being treated. This section tries to give an overview of the contributions of various plasma agents (heat, UV radiation, charged particles and reactive species) to the sterilization process.

2.2.1 Effect of heat

The first factor that usually comes to mind when discussing sterilization is the effect of heat. As previously mentioned, conventional sterilization methods are based on the use of either dry or moist heat. Moist heat (or autoclaving) is widely used for sterilization by subjecting objects to steam under pressure at temperatures of at least 120 °C for 15 minutes or longer (Gopal, 1978, Ratner et al., 1990). Dry heat sterilization requires even higher temperatures (close to 170 °C) with treatment times of about one hour (Laroussi, 2005). Most non-thermal plasmas operate at low temperatures (room temperature to approximately 70°C), therefore, no substantial thermal effects on bacterial cells are expected in plasma sterilization processes (Laroussi&Leipold, 2004). However, it should be noted that some non-thermal plasmas (like gliding arc discharges and dielectric barrier discharges) can be characterized by elevated temperatures in localized intervals in space or in time and for these discharges thermal effects should be sometimes also taken into account (Fridman, 2008). However, in general, heat is not a major contributor to the sterilization effect in non-thermal plasmas.

2.2.2 Effect of UV radiation

Non-thermal plasmas are a source of UV with different wavelengths, however, only UV radiation in the 200-300 nm wavelength range with doses of several mJ/cm^2 are known to cause lethal damage to cells (Fridman, 2008, Laroussi, 2005). This damage is mainly the dimerization of thymine bases in bacterial DNA strands, which inhibits the ability of bacteria to replicate properly (Fridman, 2008, Laroussi, 2005).

The presence of UV radiation in the plasma strongly depends on the operating pressure. It is well-known that vacuum plasma discharges are able to provide significant UV radiation in the range of wavelengths effective in sterilization. This can explain the important contribution of UV radiation in plasma sterilization at low pressures, as discussed in the previous section. In contrast, the great majority of papers published on the inactivation of micro-organisms by atmospheric pressure plasmas conclude that the contribution of UV radiation to the inactivation process is not important, when not at all relevant. By comparing the killing kinetics of UV radiation from a low pressure mercury-vapour lamp with that of a glow discharge plasma at atmospheric pressure, Laroussi et al. (Laroussi, 1996) concluded in 1996 that UV was not the main killing agent. In 1998, this claim was supported by Kelly-Wintenberg et al. (Kelly-Wintenberg et al., 1998) who exposed different types of micro-organisms to an atmospheric pressure glow DBD in air. These authors observed that there is no significant difference in the time needed to inactivate micro-organisms on polypropylene samples, whether exposed directly or sealed in bags. They concluded from this observation that UV is not a significant contributor to lethality since the opaque bags would have blocked much of the UV light (Kelly-Wintenberg et al., 1998). In the following years, several researchers (Laroussi, 2002, Laroussi, 2005, Choi et al., 2006, Laroussi&Leipold, 2004, Birmingham, 2004) have carried out various experiments that also supported the claim that UV plays a minor role in plasma sterilization. In 1999, Herrmann et al. (Herrmann et al., 1999) exposed *Bacillus globigii* to a remote atmospheric pressure plasma jet operating in helium/oxygen mixtures. When the reactive plasma effluent was blocked by a quartz window, allowing only UV radiation and heat to reach the spores, no substantial reduction in the initial concentration of bacteria was observed. In 2004, Laroussi and Leipold (Laroussi&Leipold, 2004) used the flowing afterglow of a DBD in air at atmospheric pressure to inactivate spores of the *Bacillus* genus. They quantified the UV emission from the discharge and observed no significant UV emission in the wavelength range effective in sterilization. Also in 2004, Birmingham (Birmingham, 2004) tested what he calls a "plasma blanket", which is an aluminium foil layer covered by a micro-machined dielectric polyimide layer. This structure provides small corona discharge spots in air and can be wrapped around a contaminated object. The author states that the "plasma blanket" does not generate sufficient photons of the appropriate wavelength and thus concludes that the inactivation process only results from the interaction of the ionized gas with the biological material. Choi et al. (Choi et al., 2006) subjected different samples to a DBD operated in air at atmospheric pressure and found no UV radiation below 290 nm. As a result, they concluded that UV plays no significant role in plasma sterilization. In an interesting review paper, Laroussi et al. (Laroussi, 2005) specifically concluded that there is no UV radiation in the 200-285 nm wavelength for dry air non-thermal plasmas at atmospheric pressure. Therefore, UV photons are not likely to take part in the inactivation of micro-organisms when air plasmas are used.

In contrast to the previous literature overview, some authors (Park et al., 2003, Heise et al., 2004, Lee et al., 2005, Trompeter et al., 2002) do mention the possible role of UV photons in plasma sterilization at atmospheric pressure, however, the arguments brought forward are quite often not fully convincing or incomplete (Boudam et al., 2006). For example, Trompeter et al. (Trompeter et al., 2002) employed an atmospheric pressure filamentary DBD in different gases and found that argon was the most efficient gas in terms of spore inactivation. As a result, they concluded that the inactivation process is purely due to UV radiation since argon is chemically inactive. Heise et al. (Heise et al., 2004) employed a similar discharge in argon and claimed that the inactivation of spores is partly due to UV-induced effects. Both Trompeter et al. (Trompeter et al., 2002) and Heise et al. (Heise et al., 2004) present their results as being performed in pure argon, nonetheless this is not the case since impurities are always present in the discharge gas (Boudam et al., 2006). This contamination can strongly reduce the UV emission (Boudam et al., 2006), therefore, the role of UV in the inactivation process might not be as large as mentioned by these authors. Recently, Boudam et al. (Boudam et al., 2006) subjected micro-organisms to an atmospheric pressure DBD operated in an N_2/N_2O_2 mixture. These authors claim that they have proven that UV photons, under specific operating conditions, can be the dominant inactivation species. The role of UV in atmospheric pressure plasma sterilization is thus still open for debate and further research should be definitely conducted before the controversy can be resolved.

2.2.3 Effect of reactive species

According to several authors (Laroussi, 2002, Laroussi, 2005, Fridman, 2008), reactive neutral species (such as O, O_2^*, O_3, $OH^•$, NO and NO_2) can make a significant contribution to the plasma sterilization process, especially at high pressures. To show the effect of these reactive species on the destruction of bacteria, Laroussi and Leipold (Laroussi&Leipold, 2004) employed an atmospheric pressure DBD in three different gases: pure helium, 97% helium-3% oxygen mixture and air to inactivate *Bacillus* spores. When helium is used as discharge gas, only very small concentrations of radicals originating from impurities are expected. When helium is mixed with oxygen, oxygen-based species such as O and O_3 will be present in the discharge. When air is used as discharge gas, both oxygen- and nitrogen-based species will be generated. Figure 5 shows a comparison between the inactivation kinetics in the case of pure helium and the helium/oxygen mixture.

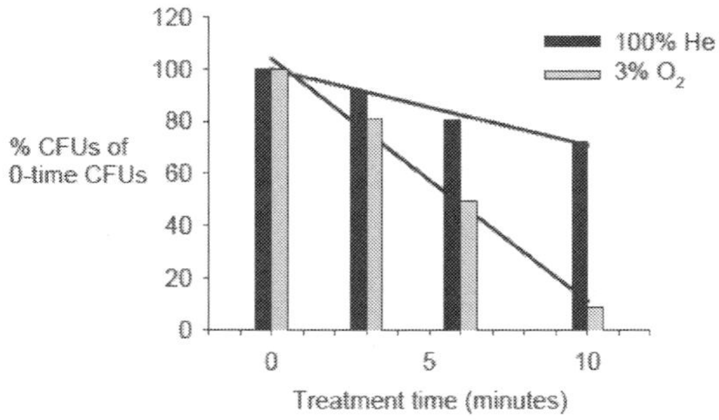

Fig. 5. Percent of surviving *Bacillus* spores as a function of plasma treatment time for pure helium (black) and a helium/oxygen mixture (97% He-3% O_2) (gray) [Reprinted with permission from (Laroussi&Leipold, 2004)].

When pure helium was used as discharge gas, the surviving spore population percentage was still much greater than 10% after 10 minutes of plasma treatment. In fact, in this case, the D-value was greater than 20 minutes. When a helium/oxygen mixture was employed, as shown in Figure 5, a D-value of 10 minutes was achieved. Laroussi and Leipold (Laroussi&Leipold, 2004) also showed that in the case of an air plasmas, the D-value could be even further decreased to approximately 20 seconds. According to these authors, this dramatic decrease in inactivation efficacy can thus be attributed to the presence of chemically reactive species such as NO, NO_2, O, O_3,... Besides Laroussi and Leipold, other authors (Herrmann et al., 1999, Moreau et al., 2000, Richardson et al., 2000) have also experimentally shown that discharges containing oxygen provide a strong germicidal effect. In particular, Herrmann et al. (Herrmann et al., 1999) compared results obtained by an atmospheric pressure plasma jet with and without oxygen. These authors found that the D-value in the case of absence of oxygen is higher than in the case when oxygen is added. Richardson et al. (Richardson et al., 2000) also showed that their resistive barrier discharge became more effective in killing *B. subtilis* when oxygen was added to the discharge gas helium. It is believed that the oxygen species attribute to the sterilization process due to their strong oxidative effects on the outer structures of cells (Fridman, 2008). Moreover, discharges containing oxygen also generate ozone (O_3) which interferes with the cellular respiration system and is known to have a strong bactericidal effect (Laroussi, 2002). After experimenting with different gas mixtures, Kuzmichev et al. (Kuzmichev et al., 2000) concluded that the best bactericidal effects were achieved in moistened oxygen and air. In the presence of moisture, hydroxyl (OH) radicals are generated in the plasma, which play a significant role by chemically attacking the outer structures of bacterial cells. In the case of air, the production of NO and NO_2 adds to the lethality of the process.

2.2.4 Effect of charged particles

In the discussion of the mechanisms of inactivation, a lot of attention is given to the effect of UV radiation and reactive species and most researchers have neglected to investigate the influence (if any) of charged particles. As a result, the exact role of electrons and ions is not yet fully resolved, but there are several indications of their importance. Fridman et al. (Fridman et al., 2007, Fridman, 2008) have stated that charged particles play an essential role in sterilization, especially in the case of direct plasma treatment, i.e. when the plasma is in direct contact with the micro-organisms. These authors employed an atmospheric pressure air DBD in direct mode and afterglow mode (so-called "plasma jet") at similar discharge powers and with the same amount of UV radiation and the results comparing the direct and indirect effects of plasma sterilization are illustrated in Figure 6. From this figure, it can be clearly seen that direct application of plasma yields a better sterilization efficiency than the treatment by plasma afterglow. Although this high efficiency in the direct mode cannot be solely described to the role of charged particles (the concentration of reactive species is also lower in case of indirect exposure), it could be possible that charged-induced mechanisms contribute to the sterilization process in direct plasma exposure.

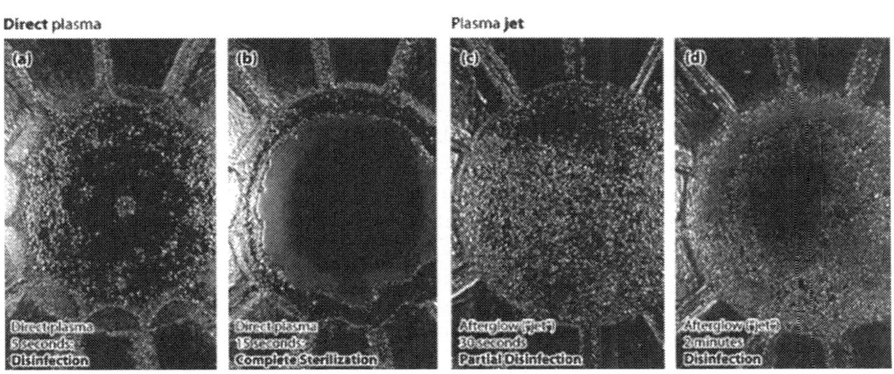

Fig. 6. Effect of direct application of plasma (a: 5 seconds, b: 15 seconds) and effect of plasma afterglow (c: 30 seconds, d: 2 minutes) [Reprinted with permission from (Fridman et al., 2007)].

Mendis et al. (Mendis et al., 2000) also suggested that charged particles might play a significant role in the rupture of outer cell membranes. According to these authors, charge accumulation on the outer surface of the membrane induces an electrostatic force, which can overcome the tensile strength of the membrane causing its rupture. They also state that this mechanism is only effective for Gram-negative bacteria, which posses thin outer membranes and a thin murein layer. The scenario will probably not occur for Gram-positive bacteria, which lack an outer membrane but have a much thicker murein layer thereby providing these bacteria higher strength and rigidity. Their conclusions can be supported by several experimental observations. Kelly-Wintenberg et al. (Kelly-Wintenberg et al., 1999) employed an atmospheric pressure glow discharge for the inactivation of the Gram-negative *E. coli* and used transmission electron microscopy (TEM) to visualize the plasma-induced physical damage to the micro-organisms. Figures 7 (a) and (b) show the cells before plasma exposure and after 30 seconds of plasma treatment respectively. As observed in these figures, plasma exposure rapidly disrupts the cell wall and leads to a release of cellular contents in the surrounding medium. Laroussi et al. (Laroussi, 2002) employed a similar discharge for the inactivation of the Gram-positive *B. Subtilis* and found intact cell walls after plasma sterilization, which clearly supports the claim of Mendis et al.. Based on the above-mentioned discussion, one can conclude that there may be a contribution of charged particles in bacterial inactivation, but most likely only in direct plasma treatment, however, this interesting possibility remains to be investigated in detail.

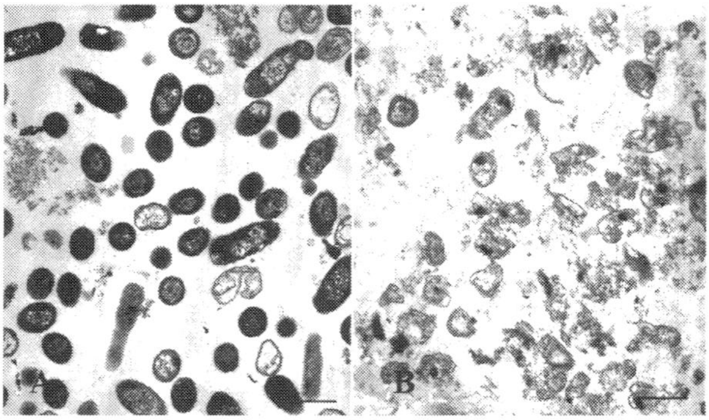

Fig. 7. TEM images of *E. coli* (A) before and (B) after 30 seconds of plasma exposure [Reprinted with permission from (Kelly-Wintenberg et al., 1999)].

2.3 Vacuum plasmas

Glow discharge plasmas operated in vacuum have been successfully employed to sterilize surfaces for quite some time. Patents written by Ashman and Menashi (Ashman&Menashi, 1972) as well as by Gut Boucher (Gut Boucher, 1980) showed that an electrical discharge in an appropriate gas can lead to sterilization. In these patents, samples are inserted within a chamber which is subsequently evacuated with a pump to 1-5 Pa. Afterwards, this chamber is filled with gas set at the required pressure, typically 5-300 Pa. The gas discharge is then achieved by applying an RF field to the gas by means of a coil located on the outside of the chamber. Ashman and Menashi (Ashman&Menashi, 1972) used different discharge gases, such as chlorine, bromine, iodine, water vapour, oxygen and nitrogen, but only observed an effective sterilizing effect when halogens were used as discharge gas. Gut Boucher (Gut Boucher, 1980) added aldehyde vapours to different carrier gases (oxygen, argon or nitrogen) and observed the best results with oxygen as carrier gas. In 1987, Jacobs and Lin (Jacobs&Lin, 1987) employed a similar RF discharge in a two-step process: (1) injection and contact of hydrogen peroxide (H_2O_2) with the item being sterilized; (2) application of an RF discharge to ensure that no toxic residues remain on the sterilized item. It is however important to note that the previously mentioned systems are not really plasma-based sterilization systems due to the use of gas mixtures that contain components with germicidal properties (such as H_2O_2 and aldehydes) before the plasma is ignited (Laroussi, 2005). Nevertheless, some of these sterilization systems have been commercially available since the 1990s (Montie et al., 2000, Rutala et al., 1998, Vassal et al., 1998).

One of the first reports on plasma sterilization where gases were used with no germicidal properties on their own was published in 1976 by Fraser et al. (Fraser et al., 1976). These authors employed a low pressure RF discharge in different gases (argon, nitrogen, oxygen, helium,...) and obtained reductions in spore populations of 99% after 2 minutes of plasma exposure. However, it was not specified for which discharge gas this result was obtained. A few years later, in 1982, Bithell (Bithell, 1982) observed that articles placed in a porous envelope could be sterilized in a low pressure (40 Pa) oxygen RF plasma after a plasma exposure time of 60 minutes. In 1989, Nelson and Berger (Nelson&Berger, 1989) also claimed that an oxygen RF plasma is very effective as biocidal medium.

Different authors have examined which discharge gas would be the most efficient to inactivate bacterial spores. Hury et al. (Hury et al., 1998) compared the mortality of *Bacillus subtilis* spores after exposure to low pressure argon, oxygen and CO_2 plasmas and concluded that oxygen and CO_2 plasmas are much more efficient in destroying *B. subtilis* spores than a pure argon plasma, most likely due to the presence of reactive oxygen species. A similar study was performed by Purevdorj et al. (Purevdorj et al., 2003) who used inert gas plasmas, oxygen-based plasmas and various moisturized air plasmas at low pressure for the inactivation of *B. pumilus* spores. These authors found that spore survival widely varied depending on the composition of the feed gas. In contrast to the results of Hury et al. (Hury et al., 1998), a pure oxygen plasma caused a lower spore mortality that an argon plasma, however, no clear explanation for this observation was given. Experiments also showed that a 50:50% oxygen-argon mixture leads to a much higher spore mortality, while the highest mortality could be achieved by employing moisturized air. Based on this latter result, the authors claim that the presence of water vapour enhances the inactivation process, most likely because of the generation of OH radicals.

Taking into account the high efficiency of oxygen-based plasmas, literature on low pressure sterilization has mainly focused on these kind of plasmas, nevertheless, inert gas plasmas are in some cases still employed for bacterial inactivation (Liu&Chen, 2008, Yang et al., 2009). Recently, many studies (Bol'shakov et al., 2004, Boscariol et al., 2008, Cvelbar et al., 2006, Liu et al., 2008, Nagatsu et al., 2003, Rossi et al., 2008, Singh et al., 2009, Vicoveanu et al., 2008) on the effects of pure oxygen vacuum plasmas on bacteria have been conducted. Bol'shakov et al. (Bol'shakov et al., 2004) published an interesting paper on the use of an oxygen RF plasma for sterilization purposes. The study was carried out for two operational modes: the inductively coupled mode and the capacitively coupled mode and it was found that the inductive mode offers a better efficiency in destroying bacterial cells. Rossi et al. (Rossi et al., 2008) also employed a low pressure oxygen RF discharge for the inactivation of

B. stearothermophilus. Figure 8 presents scanning electron microscopy (SEM) images of the untreated spores and spores exposed to the oxygen discharge.
As can be seen, the size of the spores is significantly reduced after 2 minutes of plasma treatment. According to the analysis of a statistically relevant number of spores done on the SEM pictures, it was found that in these conditions the mean length of the spores was reduced from 1.73 to 1.35 μm. Similar results were obtained by Nagatsu et al. (Nagatsu et al., 2003) and Singh et al. (Singh et al., 2009), who employed a low pressure oxygen microwave discharge. They experimentally confirmed that the *B. stearothermophilus* spores were sterilized after a plasma exposure time of 3 minutes. Moreover, based on SEM images of the spores, these authors found that the sterilized spores had different sizes and shapes compared to the untreated ones, which could be attributed to the interactions with reactive oxygen species.

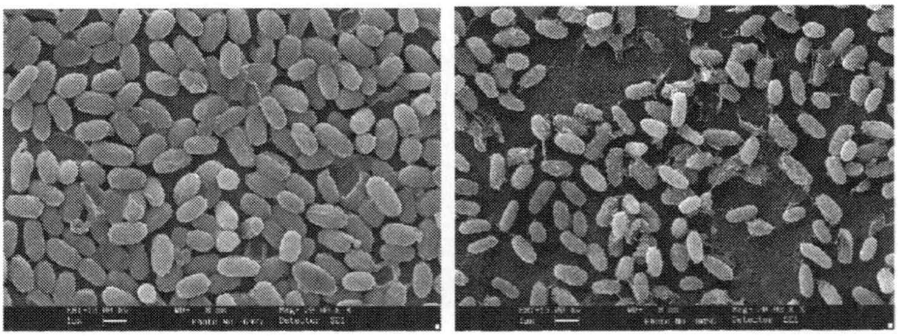

A) B)

Fig. 8. SEM images of (A) untreated and (B) oxygen plasma-treated spores [Reprinted with permission from (Rossi et al., 2008)].

Pure oxygen plasmas have also been employed by Cvelbar et al. (Cvelbar et al., 2006) and Vicoveanu et al. (Vicoveanu et al., 2008) for the inactivation of *B. subtilis* spores, who claimed that substrate heating might play a role in the inactivation process, especially at elevated discharge powers. In another study on pure oxygen plasmas, Boscariol et al. (Boscariol et al., 2008) shows the influence of discharge power on the bacterial inactivation of *B. subtilis* spores. Linear survival curves were experimentally obtained with D-values depending on discharge power. At 300 W, a D-value of approximately 8 minutes was found, while at higher discharge powers (350 and 400 W), the D-value decreased to approximately 3 minutes. Besides studying the influence of discharge power, Liu et al. (Liu et al., 2008) also examined the influence of other operating parameters on the inactivation of *E. coli* on poly(tetrafluoroethylene) (PTFE) films. These authors found, in accordance with Boscariol et al. (Boscariol et al., 2008), that the germicidal effect is higher at elevated discharge powers. They also experimentally confirmed that the inactivation effect increases with increasing plasma treatment time up to 50 seconds, after which it remains more or less stable. The authors also studied the difference between direct and remote plasma exposure by positioning the PTFE films at different distances varying from 0 to 80 cm from the centre of the induction coil. Samples placed in the region 0-30 cm from the centre of the coil are directly exposed to the plasma, while at larger distances, plasma treatment occurs in the afterglow mode. Figure 9 shows the germicidal effect as a function of distance from the induction coil and clearly shows that the oxygen plasma can effectively inactivate *E. coli* within a distance of 0-40 cm. In the afterglow zone at 40 cm from the coil centre, the concentration of ions and electrons is nearly zero, while the concentration of oxygen radicals is still approximately 70 % of the initial value. This afterglow treatment could be interesting to treat substrates prone to plasma-induced degradation.

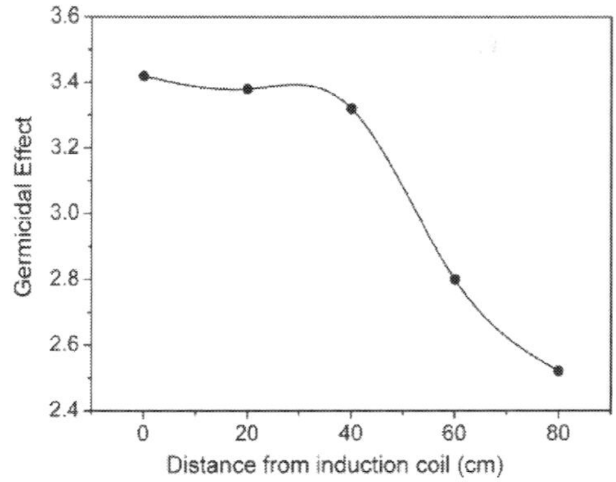

Fig. 9. Germicidal effect of an inductively coupled RF plasma sustained in oxygen at different distances from the induction coil [Reprinted with permission from (Liu et al., 2008)].

Besides pure oxygen plasmas, also low pressure N_2/O_2 plasmas have been widely investigated for the inactivation of bacteria (Moisan et al., 2002, Philip et al., 2002, Moreau et al., 2000, Rossi et al., 2006, Villeger et al., 2003, Villeger et al., 2005). Moreau et al. (Moreau et al., 2000) and Moisan et al. (Moisan et al., 2002) carried out detailed studies on the effects of a low pressure N_2/O_2 microwave plasma with biological samples placed in the afterglow of the discharge. Total inactivation of *B. subtilis* spores was achieved after 40 minutes of plasma exposure at 100 W. In a following set of experiments, Philip et al. (Philip et al., 2002) studied the influence of oxygen percentage added to the nitrogen carrier gas on *B. subtilis* inactivation. Sterilization was achieved in less than 40 minutes with 0.7, 1.5 and 2% of added oxygen. In contrast, sterility was only reached after 80 minutes with 4% of added oxygen, while it was not even attained after 120 minutes with 7% of oxygen. The authors claim that the short sterilization times (which occur at oxygen percentages below 2%) are due to the high UV intensity of the discharge, since the spores are only slightly eroded. Increasing the oxygen percentage in the mixture beyond this level increases the erosion rate of the spores, hence reducing more and more the dimensions of the spores. However, although the spores are heavily damaged, longer sterilization times are needed. The authors therefore state that the spores are mainly being inactivated by UV photons and not by erosion caused by reactive species. More recently, Rossi et al. (Rossi et al., 2006) claimed that the process determining the time to reach complete spore inactivation is etching rather than UV action, which is in contradiction with the paper written by Philip et al. (Philip et al., 2002). Rossi et al. (Rossi et al., 2006) employed an RF plasma for the inactivation of *G. stearothermophilus* spores and sterilization tests were performed in different N_2/O_2 mixtures ranging from a discharge in pure nitrogen to a pure oxygen one, which is a larger oxygen range than the one examined by Philip et al. (Philip et al., 2002). It was found that the best sterilization results were achieved in mixtures with high amounts of oxygen: complete sterilization was obtained in the 95% O_2 - 5% N_2 mixture within 5 minutes of plasma exposure and significant changes in the dimensions of the spores were observed for these discharges. In contrast, mixtures with low oxygen amounts, which produce high UV emission, resulted in low sterilization efficiencies and no variation in dimensions of the spores was found. The authors therefore claim that erosion caused by reactive species might after all be significant in the bacterial inactivation process. Recently, Kylian et al. (Kylian&Rossi, 2009) demonstrated that the application of $Ar/N_2/O_2$ plasmas offers the possibility to combine the advantageous properties of the binary mixtures, namely, the capability of an N_2/O_2 plasma to emit intense UV radiation needed for inactivation of bacterial spores together with high removal rates of biological substances from Ar/O_2 discharges.

2.4 Atmospheric pressure plasmas

Although the use of vacuum plasmas can be considered as a significant improvement over existing sterilization methods, there are still several drawbacks, including the need for batch processing, long processing times and high costs. As a result, in the past decades, interest has grown in applying atmospheric pressure plasmas for sterilization purposes and several methods have been developed that allowed researchers to easily generate non-thermal plasmas at high pressures, up to one atmosphere (Laroussi, 2005). In the following sections, the most commonly used atmospheric pressure plasmas sources for sterilization purposes will be briefly discussed together with some important results obtained for each of these discharge types.

2.4.1 Dielectric barrier discharge (DBD)

A widely used atmospheric pressure discharge for bacterial inactivation is the dielectric barrier discharge (DBD). In most cases, the plasma is created between closely spaced parallel plates, where one or two plates are covered by a dielectric layer (Kogelschatz et al., 1997, Kogelschatz, 2003). DBDs are generally driven by AC high voltages with frequencies in the kHz range and power consumptions between 10 and 100 W (Stoffels, 2007). Usually, a DBD operates in the filamentary mode: the breakdown starts at many points, followed by the development of independent current filaments, named microdischarges (Kogelschatz et al., 1997, Kogelschatz, 2003). However, it has been demonstrated that a homogeneous discharge can be obtained under special, quite restrictive conditions [83,84]. DBDs can be used for bacterial inactivation, but the narrow spacing between the electrodes makes it difficult to introduce thick samples. For these samples, remote DBD treatment can however be employed.

Laroussi et al. (Laroussi et al., 1999) demonstrated that a homogeneous helium/air DBD is effective for the inactivation of *E. coli* and observed that exposure times of 2 to 20 minutes can lead to complete inactivation. The authors also state that the treatment time necessary to obtain a complete kill depends on several parameters, such as plasma power, working gas, type of bacteria and type of medium. Using a similar pure air discharge, Kelly-Wintenberg et al. (Kelly-Wintenberg et al., 1999) reported on the inactivation of a broad spectrum of bacteria placed on a variety of surfaces. Experimental results have showed that at least a 5 log_{10} CFU reduction in bacteria can be achieved between 15 and 90 seconds of plasma

exposure. An exception to these very short exposure times were experiments with solid culture media in which 5 minutes of plasma exposure was necessary to achieve the same reduction in CFU. To enable the exposure of large or complex three-dimensional samples, Roth et al. (Roth et al., 2000) developed a so-called remote exposure reactor, in which samples can be sterilized in the afterglow of an atmospheric pressure glow DBD. These authors found that besides direct exposure, also remote plasma treatment can achieve effective bacterial inactivation (Roth et al., 2000, Ben Gadri et al., 2000, Montie et al., 2000).
Besides DBDs in the homogeneous mode, also filamentary discharges have been employed for the sterilization of various bacteria (Kostov et al., 2010, Heise et al., 2004, Trompeter et al., 2002, Hahnel et al., 2010, Yasuda et al., 2008). Kostov et al. (Kostov et al., 2010) and Yasuda et al. (Yasuda et al., 2008) were able to achieve sterilization of *E. coli* with their filamentary air DBD, while Trompeter et al. (Trompeter et al., 2002) focussed on the inactivation of *B. subtilis* and *Aspergillus Niger* with DBDs sustained in different working gases. Heise et al. (Heise et al., 2004) observed that the spore reduction of *B. subtilis* depends on which working gas is used to sustain the DBD: the efficiency of the discharge is the lowest when air is employed and the highest with argon as discharge gas. More recently, Hähnel et al. (Hahnel et al., 2010) observed that air humidity in a dielectric barrier surface discharge has a significant influence on the bacterial inactivation rate: higher concentration of water vapour in the process gas leads to higher killing rates of micro-organisms.
To enable the internal sterilization of complicated medical instruments, such as breathing circuits, catheders and endoscopes, different authors have developed special DBD configurations (Eto et al., 2008, Pointu et al., 2008, Sato et al., 2008). Eto et al. (Eto et al., 2008) developed a so-called "linear DBD" with a diameter of 0.2-3 mm and a length of 40 cm and found that 10^6 *B. stearothermophilus* spores could be killed inside a medical plastic tube at room temperature after 12 minutes of air plasma exposure. Sato et al. (Sato et al., 2008) also report on a special type of DBD and demonstrated the efficacy of their DBD for tube sterilization. A photograph of their discharge in a long flexible narrow tube can be found in Figure 10.

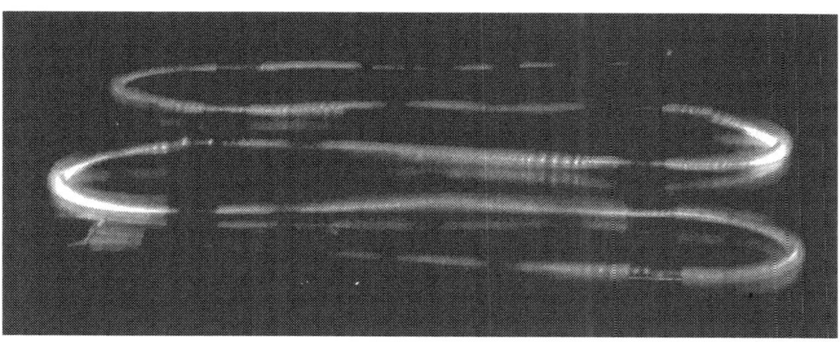

Fig. 10. Photograph of a DBD inside a tube for catheter sterilization [Reprinted with permission from (Sato et al., 2008)][91].

2.4.2 Atmospheric pressure plasma jets

Since the 1990s, an increasing interest in plasma jets for bacterial inactivation has been registered. Numerous plasma jets with different features have been developed and described in literature (Herrmann et al., 1999, Laroussi et al., 2006, Shimizu et al., 2008, Stoffels et al., 2006). These jets all differ in design, size, working gas, frequency of applied voltage,... but the principle is the same. The plasma is ignited inside a nozzle equipped with one or two electrodes and expands outside the nozzle via a gas flow. Atmospheric pressure plasmas jets are very practical due to their small size and light-weight plasma generation unit. They can be employed to treat small-sized objects, but can also be used for large-scale treatments by moving the jet over the selected area or by applying multiple nozzles next to each other. The following section will focus on the most important atmospheric pressure plasma jets employed for bacterial inactivation, however, it is important to mention that also other types of plasma jets have been developed for disinfection purposes (Shimizu et al., 2010, Chiang et al., 2010, Ikawa et al., 2010, Lee et al., 2005, Liu et al., 2010, Kim et al., 2009, Huang et al., 2007).

One type of plasma jet, which is actively employed for bacterial sterilization is the so-called "atmospheric pressure plasma jet (APPJ)". The design and operation of the APPJ have been already discussed in detail elsewhere (Jeong et al., 1998, Park et al., 2000, Schutze et al., 1998) and are only briefly summarized here for completeness. The APPJ consists of two coaxial electrodes between which a feed gas (mixtures of helium, oxygen and other gases) flows at high rate (50-100 litres per minute gas flow) and is schematically presented in Figure 11. By applying RF power (50-100 W) at 13.56 MHz to the inner electrode, a spatially uniform discharge is ignited. The chemically active species, such as excited atoms, excited molecules and free radicals exit the nozzle at high velocity (jet length of 10 mm) and impinge on the substrate being sterilized. Due to cooling by the high gas flow, the effluent temperature can be kept at moderate levels (100 °C). The ions and electrons quickly recombine outside the jet and are most likely not active in the bacterial inactivation process. Herrmann et al. (Herrmann et al., 1999) used the APPJ in a helium-oxygen mixture to inactivate spores of *B. globigii* and reported a reduction of seven orders of magnitude of the original concentration of *B. globigii* in approximately 30 seconds.

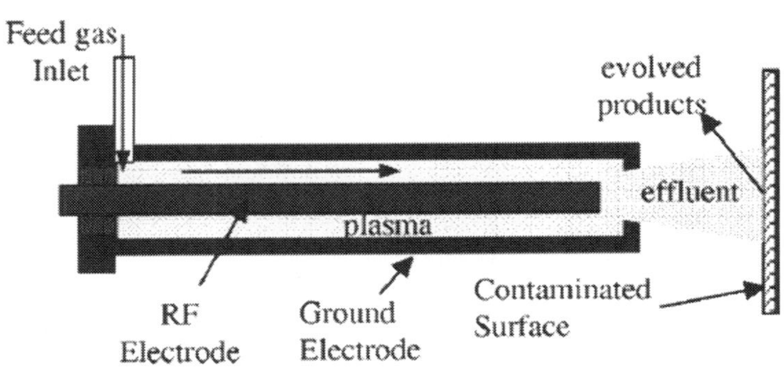

Fig. 11. Schematic representation of the atmospheric pressure plasma jet (APPJ) [Reprinted with permission from (Herrmann et al., 1999)].

A miniature jet was recently developed by Laroussi et al. (Laroussi et al., 2006, Lu&Laroussi, 2006), who named their new plasma source "plasma pencil". The plasma pencil is basically a 2.5 cm diameter dielectric tube where two disk electrodes of about the same diameter as the tube are inserted. The electrodes are separated by a gap that can be varied from 0.5 to 1.0 cm

and consist of a thin copper ring attached to the surface of a centrally perforated dielectric disk. To ignite the plasma, sub-microsecond square high voltage pulses at repetition rates in the 1-10 kHz range are applied between the two electrodes and a gas mixture (such as helium/oxygen) is flown through the holes of the electrodes (flow rates between 1 and 10 litres per minute). When the discharge is ignited, a plasma plume with lengths up to 5 cm is launched through the hole of the outer electrode in the surrounding air. Figure 12 shows a photograph of the plume emitted by the plasma pencil. This plasma plume remains stable and maintains at room temperature for extended operating times. As a result, the plume can be touched by bare hands without any harm.
Preliminary experiments (Laroussi et al., 2006) have been recently carried out to test the effectiveness of the plasma pencil to inactive bacteria. In this study, *E. coli* has been treated with the plasma pencil in two different operating gases (helium and helium with 0.75% admixture of oxygen) for different treatment times (30 seconds and 120 seconds). Figure 13 shows the results of these tests: from these photographs, it can be concluded that the area of the inactivated region increases with increasing plasma exposure time and that the area of the inactivated region is much greater when oxygen was added to helium, especially for long treatment times.
Recently, the biomedical team at the Eindhoven University of Technology has introduced another concept of a miniature atmospheric plasma jet: the "plasma needle" (Stoffels et al., 2002, Stoffels et al., 2006). The portable plasma needle consists of a metal wire (0.3 mm diameter) with a sharpened tip, confined in a Perspex tube (4 mm inner diameter). RF power at 13.05 MHz ranging between 10 mW and several watts can be applied to the needle resulting in the generation of a micro-plasma (0.1-2 mm glow size). In the 10-300 mW regime, the gas temperature is close to body temperature, while above 1 W, it can increase to 100°C and more (Stoffels, 2007). Because the voltage necessary to ignite the discharge is the lowest in helium, the plasma needle operates in helium-air mixtures. The Perspex tube is filled with helium at flow rates between 0.5 and 2.0 litres per minute, while the air content can be adjusted by pushing the needle in or out the Perspex tube: the more the needle protrudes from the tube, the more air can enter the plasma region (Sladek&Stoffels, 2005). A photograph of the portable plasma needle and a close-up of the metal wire inside the Perspex tube can be seen in Figure 14.

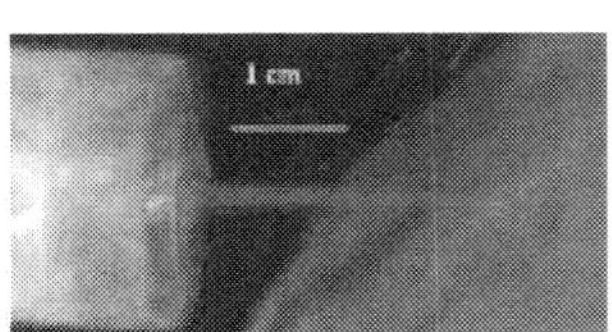

Fig. 12. Photograph of the plasma plume in contact with human skin [Reprinted with permission from (Lu&Laroussi, 2006)].

Sladek et al. (Sladek&Stoffels, 2005, Sladek et al., 2006) employed the plasma needle for the inactivation of *E. coli* films and observed that plasma treatment results in the formation of a bacteria-free void with a size up to 12 mm. 10^4-10^5 colony forming units could be destroyed after 10 seconds of plasma treatment at low power. The authors also state that prolongation of treatment time or usage of higher power does not significantly improve the destruction efficiency: short exposure at low plasma power is sufficient.

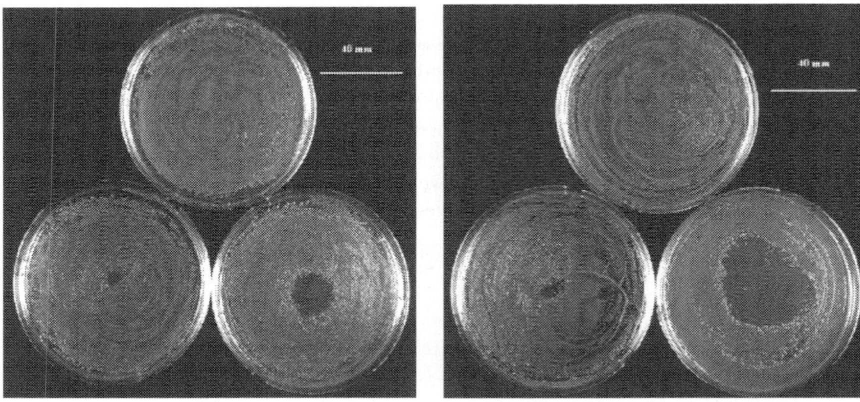

(a) (b)

Fig. 13. Photographs of Petri dishes showing the effects of the plasma pencil on *E. coli* cells for the case of (a) pure helium; (b) helium + 0.75% oxygen. Top Petri dishes are untreated samples, bottom Petri dishes were treated for 30 seconds (left) and 120 seconds (right) [Reprinted with permission from (Laroussi et al., 2006)].

An atmospheric pressure plasma jet with a special design has been developed by Shimizu et al. (Shimizu et al., 2008) and applied for the inactivation of *E. coli*. This so-called "microwave plasma torch" consists of 6 stainless steel electrodes placed inside an aluminium cylinder. The centres of the electrodes are equally distributed at a distance of 6 mm from the inner surface of the cylinder. Microwave power of approximately 85 W at 2.45 GHz is applied to the electrodes in flowing argon leading to the production of six plasma zones between each of the electrode tips and the inner surface of the cylinder, as shown in Figure 15. The authors observed that when an *E. coli* culture is placed for 2 minutes at 20 mm below the torch (where the gas temperature is sufficiently cool), the *E. coli* bacteria were almost completely killed within a 40 mm diameter.

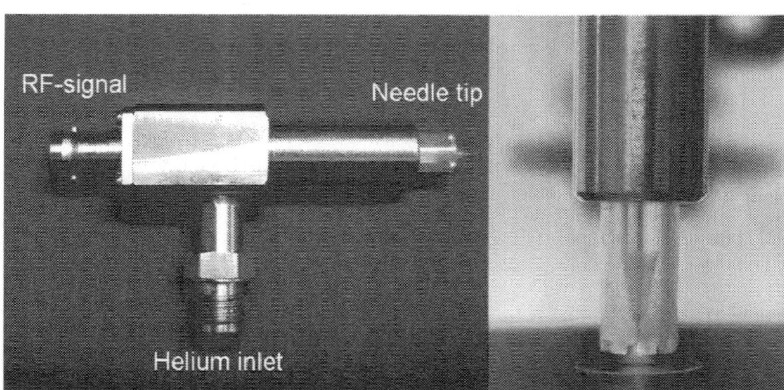

Fig. 14. Photograph of the portable plasma needle (left) and normal glow operation of the needle (right) [Reprinted with permission from (Sladek et al., 2006)].

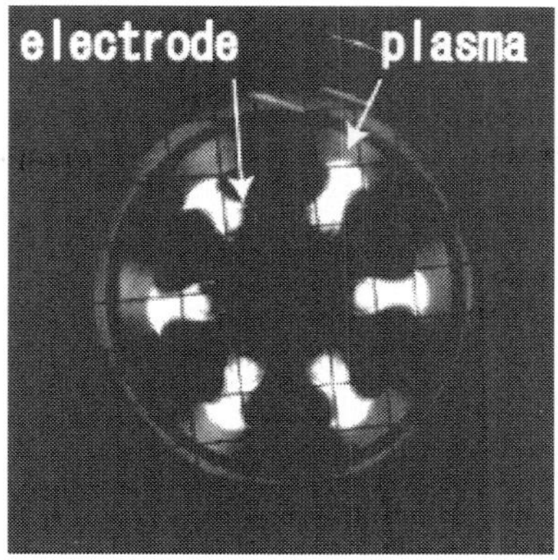

Fig. 15. Photograph of the microwave plasma torch with six plasma zones [Reprinted with permission from (Shimizu et al., 2008)].

3. Plasma sterilization of animal and human living tissue

3.1 Plasma sterilization in dentistry

Dental cavities, as the result of caries, are a common ailment and the improvement of current treatment methods is a major issue in dentistry (Sladek et al., 2004). Preparation of cavities prior to filling is done by removing necrotic, infected and non-remineralizable tissue by means of mechanical drilling or laser techniques (Banerjee et al., 2000). In both methods, heating takes place. Moreover, vibrations occur during mechanical drilling, which is usually quite painful for the patient since both heating as vibrations can stimulate the nerve (Banerjee et al., 2000). Moreover, these methods are often destructive: fractures can occur and an excess of healthy tissue must be removed to ensure that the cavity is free of bacteria (Sladek et al., 2004). A non-thermal atmospheric pressure plasma might offer a less destructive and less painful method to prepare dental cavities. These plasmas operate at room temperature and do not cause pain or bulk destruction of the tissue. Moreover, although the plasma is superficial, the active plasma species it produces can easily reach the inside of the cavity. Goree et al. (Goree et al., 2006b, Goree et al., 2006a) have employed the plasma needle to kill *S. mutans*, which is the main micro-organism causing dental caries. These authors found that the plasma needle can effectively kill these bacteria after 10 seconds of plasma treatment within a solid circle of 5 mm diameter, thereby demonstrating its site specific capabilities. As a result, the plasma needle can provide an attractive alternative for dental clinical treatment.

More recently, Jiang et al. (Jiang et al., 2009) have developed a hollow-electrode-based, 100ns-pulsed plasma dental probe that generates a tapered cylindrical plasma plume at room temperature in ambient atmosphere. This plasma plume causes minimal heating of biological materials and can be touched with bare hands without causing burning sensation or pain. After the developing phase, Jiang et al. (Jiang et al., 2009) used the plasma dental probe to disinfect root canals from extracted human teeth. For this purpose, two teeth were placed 5 mm below the plasma dental probe nozzle. One tooth was exposed to the helium/oxygen plasma for 5 minutes, while the other tooth, serving as control, was exposed to a similar helium/oxygen flow for the same amount of time, but with the plasma switched off. After treatment, the treated and control tooth were longitudinally and transversely split with a dental burr and subsequently examined with SEM, as shown in Figure 16. It can be clearly seen that in the case of the control tooth, biofilms cover the entire root canal surface. However, in the plasma-treated root canal, a distinct zone without biofilms (1 mm in depth) can be observed. However, the plasma failed to reach the lower zone. Nevertheless, the authors state that greater sterilization depth can be achieved by optimizing the width and the length of the plasma plume. Another solution to a better killing efficacy in root canals was provided by Lu et al. (Lu et al., 2009), who constructed a cold plasma jet device which is able to generate plasma inside the root canal. It was found that this device efficiently kills *Enterococcus faecalis* (one of the main types of bacteria causing failure of the root canal) within several minutes of plasma treatment. Although these preliminary results are very encouraging, a lot of basic issues still need more in-depth investigation before atmospheric pressure plasmas can be widely employed in dentistry.

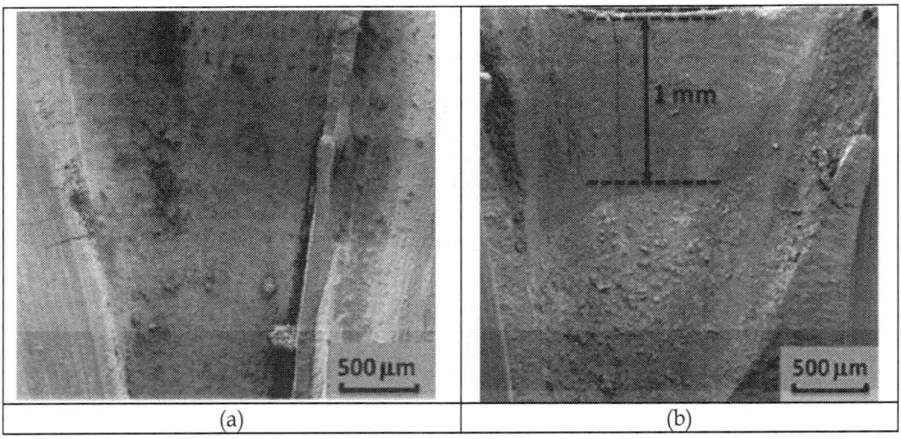

Fig. 16. (a) SEM image of the control split root canal and (b) SEM image of the split root canal after 5 minutes of plasma treatment [Reprinted with permission from (Jiang et al., 2009)].

3.2 Plasma sterilization of human/animal skin

Another interesting state-of-the-art application of non-thermal plasmas is the sterilization of human or animal skin, however, this is a recently developed research topic and has up to now only been examined by the research group of Alexander Fridman. In a hospital setting, sterilization of living animal or human tissue with minimal damage to this tissue is of great importance. Nowadays, chemical sterilization is commonly employed, however, this technique does not always offer a solution. For example, it cannot be used for the sterilization of open wounds, ulcers or burns due to the extent of damage they cause to punctured tissues. Transporting chemicals for sterilization can also become a major logistics problem for example in a military field hospital (Fridman, 2008). Non-thermal atmospheric pressure plasma sources can offer an interesting alternative since it is quite a potent disinfecting and sterilizing agent, as extensively discussed in the previous sections. As previously mentioned, it is crucial that the living tissue does not get damaged during plasma treatment, therefore, the discharge current should be limited below values acceptable for treatment of living tissue. Moreover, the discharge itself should be homogeneous enough to avoid local damage and discomfort (Fridman, 2008). The creation of special atmospheric pressure discharges effectively solving these problems is an important challenge and until now, only a few researchers succeeded in developing a non-thermal plasma suitable for living tissue sterilization. Fridman et al. (Fridman et al., 2006) especially developed a discharge for this purpose: the so-called floating-electrode DBD (FE-DBD). Similar to the classical DBDs, the set-up consist of two electrodes: a dielectric-protected powered electrode and a second active electrode, which can be human or animal skin or an organ. This latter electrode is not grounded and remains at a floating potential. The discharge ignites when the powered electrode approaches the surface to be treated at a distance of less than 3 mm, depending on the form, duration and polarity of the driving voltage. Figure 17 shows a photograph of the FE-DBD with human tissue as floating electrode.

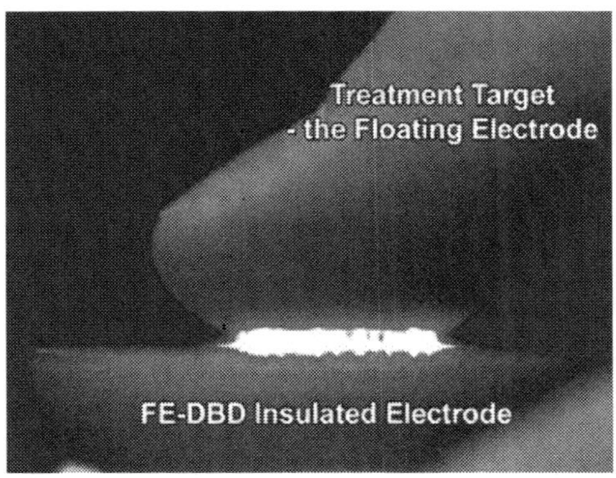

Fig. 17. FE-DBD for the sterilization of living tissue [Reprinted with permission from (Fridman et al., 2006)].

Recently, the FE-DBD has been further optimized to minimize the DBD non-uniformities and the related damaging effects. The best results were obtained when the FE-DBD was employed in the pulsed mode with pulse durations below 30-100 ns, resulting in sufficient uniformity and the possibility of non-damaging direct plasma treatment of living tissue (Ayan et al., 2009). Fridman et al. (Fridman et al., 2006) investigated human tissue sterilization by subjecting bacteria collected from cadaver skin containing *Staphylococcus*, *Streptococcus* and yeast to their FE-DBD. The authors observed that sterilization generally occurred within 4 seconds while in some cases a 6 second plasma treatment was found to be necessary. To examine whether living tissue remains intact after FE-DBD treatment, cadaver tissue was plasma-treated for up to 5 minutes showing no visible or microscopic changes in the tissue (Fridman et al., 2006). Subsequently, an animal model (SKH1 hairless mouse) was subjected to the plasma with varying doses to determine the damaging dose. First, an animal was treated at what was deemed to be a damaging dose based on trials with cadaver skin tissue (Fridman, 2008). Once the dose where the damage was visible was determined, a new animal was treated at a lower dose. If no damage is observed at that dose, two more animals were treated and if no damage occurred in all three cases, the dose was deemed "maximum acceptable dose". Once this maximum dose was determined, three animals were treated at that dose and left alive under close observation for 2 weeks. These tests have shown that the animals remain fine after a reasonably high plasma dose. Following the investigation in mice, a similar investigation was carried out on pigs, achieving the same results. Based on these findings, the authors concluded that atmospheric pressure non-thermal plasmas can thus be an efficient tool for the sterilization of living tissue. This conclusion opens interesting perspectives for non-thermal plasma applications in medicine, including pre-surgical patient treatment, sterilization of wounds and burns as well as treatment of internal organs.

4. Conclusions

During the last decades, the plasma community has witnessed a burst of research activity on the germicidal properties of both low pressure as well as atmospheric pressure non-thermal plasmas. While vacuum-based plasma sterilization is an already well-established technology, the use of atmospheric pressure cold plasmas for the inactivation of bacteria is a relatively recent event. As a result, there are still a lot of issues in atmospheric pressure plasma sterilization that need more in-depth investigations. For example, there is still no complete understanding of the biological pathways that cold atmospheric pressure plasmas induce in cells and tissues during treatment. Although preliminary results are very promising, a lot of work requiring collaborative efforts between plasma scientists, microbiologists and biochemists remains to be done before plasma can establish itself as a technique being routinely and effectively used for sterilization purposes. Despite all these challenges, non-thermal plasmas have undoubtedly great potential as a novel method for low temperature sterilization. Due to the growing amount of information and expertise on this subject, it seems to be most likely that real life applications of non-thermal plasmas for sterilization purposes will become a reality in the near future.

5. References

Ashman, L. E. & Menashi, W. P. 1972. *Treatment of surfaces with low pressure plasmas.*

Ayan, H., Fridman, G., Staack, D., Gutsol, A. F., Vasilets, V. N., Fridman, A. A. & Friedman, G. 2009. Heating Effect of Dielectric Barrier Discharges for Direct Medical Treatment. *IEEE Transactions on Plasma Science,* 37, 113-120.

Banerjee, A., Watson, T. F. & Kidd, E. A. M. 2000. Dentine caries excavation: a review of current clinical techniques. *British Dental Journal,* 188, 476-482.

Ben Gadri, R., Roth, J. R., Montie, T. C., Kelly-Wintenberg, K., Tsai, P. P. Y., Helfritch, D. J., Feldman, P., Sherman, D. M., Karakaya, F. & Chen, Z. Y. 2000. Sterilization and plasma processing of room temperature surfaces with a one atmosphere uniform glow discharge plasma (OAUGDP). *Surface & Coatings Technology,* 131, 528-542.

Birmingham, J. G. 2004. Mechanisms of bacterial spore deactivation using ambient pressure nonthermal discharges. *IEEE Transactions on Plasma Science,* 32, 1526-1531.

Bithell, R. M. 1982. *Package and sterilizing process for same.*

Bogaerts, A., Neyts, E., Gijbels, R. & van der Mullen, J. 2002. Gas discharge plasmas and their applications. *Spectrochimica Acta Part B-Atomic Spectroscopy,* 57, 609-658.

Bol'shakov, A. A., Cruden, B. A., Mogul, R., Rao, M. V. V. S., Sharma, S. P., Khare, B. N. & Meyyappan, M. 2004. Radio-frequency oxygen plasma as a sterilization source. *Aiaa Journal,* 42, 823-832.

Borcia, G., Anderson, C. A. & Brown, N. M. D. 2006. Surface treatment of natural and synthetic textiles using a dielectric barrier discharge. *Surface & Coatings Technology,* 201, 3074-3081.

Boscariol, M. R., Moreira, A. J., Mansano, R. D., Kikuchi, I. S. & Pinto, T. J. A. 2008. Sterilization by pure oxygen plasma and by oxygen-hydrogen peroxide plasma: An efficacy study. *International Journal of Pharmaceutics,* 353, 170-175.

Boudam, M. K., Moisan, M., Saoudi, B., Popovici, C., Gherardi, N. & Massines, F. 2006. Bacterial spore inactivation by atmospheric-pressure plasmas in the presence or absence of UV photons as obtained with the same gas mixture. *Journal of Physics D-Applied Physics,* 39, 3494-3507.

Bruce, R. L., Lin, T., Phaneuf, R. J., Oehrlein, G. S., Bell, W., Long, B. & Willson, C. G. 2010. Molecular structure effects on dry etching behavior of Si-containing resists in oxygen plasma. *Journal of Vacuum Science & Technology B,* 28, 751-757.

Cariou-Travers, S. & Darbord, J. C. 2001. Validation of plasma sterilization - The case of Sterrad. *Vide-Science Technique et Applications,* 56, 34-46.

Chau, T. T., Kao, K. C., Blank, G. & Madrid, F. 1996. Microwave plasmas for low-temperature dry sterilization. *Biomaterials,* 17, 1273-1277.

Chiang, M. H., Wu, J. Y., Li, Y. H., Wu, J. S., Chen, S. H. & Chang, C. L. 2010. Inactivation of E. coli and B. subtilis by a parallel-plate dielectric barrier discharge jet. *Surface & Coatings Technology,* 204, 3729-3737.

Choi, J. H., Han, I., Baik, H. K., Lee, M. H., Han, D. W., Park, J. C., Lee, I. S., Song, K. M. & Lim, Y. S. 2006. Analysis of sterilization effect by pulsed dielectric barrier discharge. *Journal of Electrostatics,* 64, 17-22.

Cvelbar, U., Vujosevic, D., Vratnica, Z. & Mozetic, M. 2006. The influence of substrate material on bacteria sterilization in an oxygen plasma glow discharge. *Journal of Physics D-Applied Physics,* 39, 3487-3493.

Daeschlein, G., von Woedtke, T., Kindel, E., Brandenburg, R., Weltmann, K. D. & Junger, M. 2010. Antibacterial Activity of an Atmospheric Pressure Plasma Jet Against Relevant Wound Pathogens in vitro on a Simulated Wound Environment. *Plasma Processes and Polymers,* 7, 224-230.

De Geyter, N., Morent, R., Gengembre, L., Leys, C., Payen, E., Van Vlierberghe, S. & Schacht, E. 2008. Increasing the Hydrophobicity of a PP Film Using a Helium/CF 4 DBD Treatment at Atmospheric Pressure. *Plasma Chemistry and Plasma Processing,* 28, 289-298.

De Geyter, N., Morent, R., Van Vlierberghe, S., Dubruel, P., Leys, C., Gengembre, L., Schacht, E. & Payen, E. 2009. Deposition of polymethyl methacrylate on polypropylene substrates using an atmospheric pressure dielectric barrier discharge. *Progress in Organic Coatings,* 64, 230-237.

Denes, F. S. & Manolache, S. 2004. Macromolecular plasma-chemistry: an emerging field of polymer science. *Progress in Polymer Science,* 29, 815-885.

Eto, H., Ono, Y., Ogino, A. & Nagatsu, M. 2008. Low-temperature internal sterilization of medical plastic tubes using a linear dielectric barrier discharge. *Plasma Processes and Polymers,* 5, 269-274.

Fraser, S. J., Gillette, R. B. & Olson, R. L. 1976. *Sterilizing process and apparatus utilizing gas plasma.*

Fridman, A. 2008. Plasma Biology and Plasma Medicine. *Plasma Chemistry.* New York: Cambridge University Press.

Fridman, G., Brooks, A. D., Balasubramanian, M., Fridman, A., Gutsol, A., Vasilets, V. N., Ayan, H. & Friedman, G. 2007. Comparison of direct and indirect effects of non-thermal atmospheric-pressure plasma on bacteria. *Plasma Processes and Polymers,* 4, 370-375.

Fridman, G., Friedman, G., Gutsol, A., Shekhter, A. B., Vasilets, V. N. & Fridman, A. 2008. Applied plasma medicine. *Plasma Processes and Polymers,* 5, 503-533.

Fridman, G., Peddinghaus, M., Ayan, H., Fridman, A., Balasubramanian, M., Gutsol, A., Brooks, A. & Friedman, G. 2006. Blood coagulation and living tissue sterilization by floating-electrode dielectric barrier discharge in air. *Plasma Chemistry and Plasma Processing,* 26, 425-442.

Gopal, N. G. S. 1978. Radiation Sterilization of Pharmaceuticals and Polymers. *Radiation Physics and Chemistry,* 12, 35-50.

Goree, J., Liu, B. & Drake, D. 2006a. Gas flow dependence for plasma-needle disinfection of S-mutans bacteria. *Journal of Physics D-Applied Physics,* 39, 3479-3486.

Goree, J., Liu, B., Drake, D. & Stoffels, E. 2006b. Killing of S-mutans bacteria using a plasma needle at atmospheric pressure. *IEEE Transactions on Plasma Science,* 34, 1317-1324.

Gut Boucher, R. M. 1980. *Seeded gas plasma sterilization method.*

Hahnel, M., von Woedtke, T. & Weltmann, K. D. 2010. Influence of the Air Humidity on the Reduction of Bacillus Spores in a Defined Environment at Atmospheric Pressure Using a Dielectric Barrier Surface Discharge. *Plasma Processes and Polymers,* 7, 244-249.

Heise, M., Neff, W., Franken, O., Muranyi, P. & Wunderlich, J. 2004. Sterilization of polymer foils with dielectric barrier discharges at atmospheric pressure. *Plasmas and Polymers,* 9, 23-33.

Henn, G. G., Birkinshaw, C., Buggy, M. & Jones, E. 1996. A comparison of the effects of gamma-irradiation and ethylene oxide sterilization on the properties of compression moulded poly-d,l-lactide. *Journal of Materials Science-Materials in Medicine,* 7, 591-595.

Herrmann, H. W., Henins, I., Park, J. & Selwyn, G. S. 1999. Decontamination of chemical and biological warfare, (CBW) agents using an atmospheric pressure plasma jet (APPJ). *Physics of Plasmas,* 6, 2284-2289.

Huang, C., Yu, Q. S., Hsieh, F. H. & Duan, Y. X. 2007. Bacterial deactivation using a low temperature argon atmospheric plasma brush with oxygen addition. *Plasma Processes and Polymers,* 4, 77-87.

Hury, S., Vidal, D. R., Desor, F., Pelletier, J. & Lagarde, T. 1998. A parametric study of the destruction efficiency of Bacillus spores in low pressure oxygen-based plasmas. *Letters in Applied Microbiology,* 26, 417-421.

Ikawa, S., Kitano, K. & Hamaguchi, S. 2010. Effects of pH on Bacterial Inactivation in Aqueous Solutions due to Low-Temperature Atmospheric Pressure Plasma Application. *Plasma Processes and Polymers,* 7, 33-42.

Ishigaki, I. & Yoshii, F. 1992. Radiation Effects on Polymer Materials in Radiation Sterilization of Medical Supplies. *Radiation Physics and Chemistry,* 39, 527-533.

Jacobs, P. T. & Lin, S. M. 1987. *Hydrogen peroxide plasma sterilization system.*

Jeong, J. Y., Babayan, S. E., Tu, V. J., Park, J., Henins, I., Hicks, R. F. & Selwyn, G. S. 1998. Etching materials with an atmospheric-pressure plasma jet. *Plasma Sources Science & Technology,* 7, 282-285.

Jiang, C. Q., Chen, M. T., Gorur, A., Schaudinn, C., Jaramillo, D. E., Costerton, J. W., Sedghizadeh, P. P., Vernier, P. T. & Gundersen, M. A. 2009. Nanosecond Pulsed Plasma Dental Probe. *Plasma Processes and Polymers,* 6, 479-483.

Kalghatgi, S., Friedman, G., Fridman, A. & Clyne, A. M. 2010. Endothelial Cell Proliferation is Enhanced by Low Dose Non-Thermal Plasma Through Fibroblast Growth Factor-2 Release. *Annals of Biomedical Engineering,* 38, 748-757.

Kalghatgi, S. U., Fridman, G., Cooper, M., Nagaraj, G., Peddinghaus, M., Balasubramanian, M., Vasilets, V. N., Gutsol, A. F., Fridman, A. & Friedman, G. 2007. Mechanism of blood coagulation by nonthermal atmospheric pressure dielectric barrier discharge plasma. *IEEE Transactions on Plasma Science,* 35, 1559-1566.

Kelly-Wintenberg, K., Hodge, A., Montie, T. C., Deleanu, L., Sherman, D., Roth, J. R., Tsai, P. & Wadsworth, L. 1999. Use of a one atmosphere uniform glow discharge plasma to kill a broad spectrum of microorganisms. *Journal of Vacuum Science & Technology A-Vacuum Surfaces and Films,* 17, 1539-1544.

Kelly-Wintenberg, K., Montie, T. C., Brickman, C., Roth, J. R., Carr, A. K., Sorge, K., Wadsworth, L. C. & Tsai, P. P. Y. 1998. Room temperature sterilization of surfaces and fabrics with a One Atmosphere Uniform Glow Discharge Plasma. *Journal of Industrial Microbiology & Biotechnology,* 20, 69-74.

Kim, S. J., Chung, T. H., Bae, S. H. & Leem, S. H. 2009. Characterization of Atmospheric Pressure Microplasma Jet Source and its Application to Bacterial Inactivation. *Plasma Processes and Polymers,* 6, 676-685.

Kogelschatz, U. 2003. Dielectric-barrier discharges: Their history, discharge physics, and industrial applications. *Plasma Chemistry and Plasma Processing,* 23, 1-46.

Kogelschatz, U., Eliasson, B. & Egli, W. 1997. Dielectric-barrier discharges. Principle and applications. *Journal de Physique IV,* 7, 47-66.

Kong, M. G., Kroesen, G., Morfill, G., Nosenko, T., Shimizu, T., van Dijk, J. & Zimmermann, J. L. 2009. Plasma medicine: an introductory review. *New Journal of Physics,* 11.

Kostov, K. G., Rocha, V., Koga-Ito, C. Y., Matos, B. M., Algatti, M. A., Honda, R. Y., Kayama, M. E. & Mota, R. P. 2010. Bacterial sterilization by a dielectric barrier discharge (DBD) in air. *Surface & Coatings Technology,* 204, 2954-2959.

Kuzmichev, A. I., Soloshenko, I. A., Tsiolko, V. V., Kryzhanovsky, V. I., Bazhenov, V. Y., Mikhno, I. L. & Khomich, V. A. Year. Feature of sterilization by different type of atmopsheric pressure discharges. *In:* 7th International Symposium on High Pressure Low Temperature Plasma Chemistry - Hakone VII, 2001 2000 Greifswald (Germany). 402-406.

Kylian, O. & Rossi, F. 2009. Sterilization and decontamination of medical instruments by low-pressure plasma discharges: application of Ar/O-2/N-2 ternary mixture. *Journal of Physics D-Applied Physics,* 42.

Langmuir, I. 1928. Oscillations in ionized gases. *Proceedings of the National Academy of Sciences of the United States of America,* 14, 627-637.

Laroussi, M. 1996. Sterilization of contaminated matter with an atmospheric pressure plasma. *IEEE Transactions on Plasma Science,* 24, 1188-1191.

Laroussi, M. 2002. Nonthermal decontamination of biological media by atmospheric-pressure plasmas: Review, analysis, and prospects. *IEEE Transactions on Plasma Science,* 30, 1409-1415.

Laroussi, M. 2005. Low temperature plasma-based sterilization: Overview and state-of-the-art. *Plasma Processes and Polymers,* 2, 391-400.

Laroussi, M. 2009. Low-Temperature Plasmas for Medicine? *IEEE Transactions on Plasma Science,* 37, 714-725.

Laroussi, M., Alexeff, I. & Kang, W. L. 2000. Biological decontamination by nonthermal plasmas. *IEEE Transactions on Plasma Science,* 28, 184-188.

Laroussi, M. & Leipold, F. 2004. Evaluation of the roles of reactive species, heat, and UV radiation in the inactivation of bacterial cells by air plasmas at atmospheric pressure. *International Journal of Mass Spectrometry,* 233, 81-86.

Laroussi, M., Sayler, G. S., Glascock, B. B., McCurdy, B., Pearce, M. E., Bright, N. G. & Malott, C. M. 1999. Images of biological samples undergoing sterilization by a glow discharge at atmospheric pressure. *IEEE Transactions on Plasma Science,* 27, 34-35.

Laroussi, M., Tendero, C., Lu, X., Alla, S. & Hynes, W. L. 2006. Inactivation of bacteria by the plasma pencil. *Plasma Processes and Polymers,* 3, 470-473.

Lee, K. Y., Park, B. J., Lee, D. H., Lee, I. S., Hyun, S. O., Chung, K. H. & Park, J. C. 2005. Sterilization of Escherichia coli and MRSA using microwave-induced argon plasma at atmospheric pressure. *Surface & Coatings Technology,* 193, 35-38.

Liu, F. X., Sun, P., Bai, N., Tian, Y., Zhou, H. X., Wei, S. C., Zhou, Y. H., Zhang, J., Zhu, W. D., Becker, K. & Fang, J. 2010. Inactivation of Bacteria in an Aqueous Environment by a Direct-Current, Cold-Atmospheric-Pressure Air Plasma Microjet. *Plasma Processes and Polymers,* 7, 231-236.

Liu, H., Chen, J., Yang, L. & Zhou, Y. 2008. Long-distance oxygen plasma sterilization: Effects and mechanisms. *Applied Surface Science,* 254, 1815-1821.

Liu, H. X. & Chen, J. R. 2008. Analysis of surface sterilization and properties of medical poly (tetrafluoroethylene) in remote argon plasma. *IEEE Transactions on Plasma Science,* 36, 230-236.

Lu, X. & Laroussi, M. 2006. Dynamics of an atmospheric pressure plasma plume generated by submicrosecond voltage pulses. *Journal of Applied Physics,* 100.

Lu, X. P., Cao, Y. G., Yang, P., Xiong, Q., Xiong, Z. L., Xian, Y. B. & Pan, Y. 2009. An RC Plasma Device for Sterilization of Root Canal of Teeth. *IEEE Transactions on Plasma Science,* 37, 668-673.

Maruyama, T., Narukage, T., Onuki, R. & Fujiwara, N. 2010. High-aspect-ratio deep Si etching in SF6/O-2 plasma. I. Characteristics of radical reactions with high-aspect-ratio patterns. *Journal of Vacuum Science & Technology B,* 28, 854-861.

Mendis, D. A., Rosenberg, M. & Azam, F. 2000. A note on the possible electrostatic disruption of bacteria. *IEEE Transactions on Plasma Science,* 28, 1304-1306.

Moisan, M., Barbeau, J., Crevier, M. C., Pelletier, J., Philip, N. & Saoudi, B. 2002. Plasma sterilization. Methods mechanisms. *Pure and Applied Chemistry,* 74, 349-358.

Moisan, M., Barbeau, J., Moreau, S., Pelletier, J., Tabrizian, M. & Yahia, L. H. 2001. Low-temperature sterilization using gas plasmas: a review of the experiments and an analysis of the inactivation mechanisms. *International Journal of Pharmaceutics,* 226, 1-21.

Montie, T. C., Kelly-Wintenberg, K. & Roth, J. R. 2000. An overview of research using the one atmosphere uniform glow discharge plasma (OAUGDP) for sterilization of surfaces and materials. *IEEE Transactions on Plasma Science,* 28, 41-50.

Moreau, S., Moisan, M., Tabrizian, M., Barbeau, J., Pelletier, J., Ricard, A. & Yahia, L. 2000. Using the flowing afterglow of a plasma to inactivate Bacillus subtilis spores: Influence of the operating conditions. *Journal of Applied Physics,* 88, 1166-1174.

Morent, R., De Geyter, N., Jacobs, T., Van Vlierberghe, S., Dubruel, P., Leys, C. & Schacht, E. 2009a. Plasma-Polymerization of HMDSO Using an Atmospheric Pressure Dielectric Barrier Discharge. *Plasma Processes and Polymers,* 6, S537-S542.

Morent, R., De Geyter, N., Van Vlierberghe, S., Dubruel, P., Leys, C. & Schacht, E. 2009b. Organic-inorganic behaviour of HMDSO films plasma-polymerized at atmospheric pressure. *Surface & Coatings Technology,* 203, 1366-1372.

Nagatsu, M., Terashita, F. & Koide, Y. 2003. Low-temperature sterilization with surface-wave-excited oxygen plasma. *Japanese Journal of Applied Physics Part 2-Letters & Express Letters,* 42, L856-L859.

Nelson, C. L. & Berger, T. J. 1989. Inactivation of Microorganisms by Oxygen Gas Plasma. *Current Microbiology,* 18, 275-276.

Nie, Q. Y., Cao, Z., Ren, C. S., Wang, D. Z. & Kong, M. G. 2009. A two-dimensional cold atmospheric plasma jet array for uniform treatment of large-area surfaces for plasma medicine. *New Journal of Physics,* 11.

Park, B. J., Lee, D. H., Park, J. C., Lee, I. S., Lee, K. Y., Hyun, S. O., Chun, M. S. & Chung, K. H. 2003. Sterilization using a microwave-induced argon plasma system at atmospheric pressure. *Physics of Plasmas,* 10, 4539-4544.

Park, J., Henins, I., Herrmann, H. W., Selwyn, G. S., Jeong, J. Y., Hicks, R. F., Shim, D. & Chang, C. S. 2000. An atmospheric pressure plasma source. *Applied Physics Letters,* 76, 288-290.

Philip, N., Saoudi, B., Crevier, M. C., Moisan, M., Barbeau, J. & Pelletier, J. 2002. The respective roles of UV photons and oxygen atoms in plasma sterilization at reduced gas pressure: The case of N-2-O-2 mixtures. *IEEE Transactions on Plasma Science,* 30, 1429-1436.

Pointu, A. M., Ricard, A., Odic, E. & Ganciu, M. 2008. Nitrogen atmospheric pressure post discharges for surface biological decontamination inside small diameter tubes. *Plasma Processes and Polymers*, 5, 559-568.

Purevdorj, D., Igura, N., Ariyada, O. & Hayakawa, I. 2003. Effect of feed gas composition of gas discharge plasmas on Bacillus pumilus spore mortality. *Letters in Applied Microbiology*, 37, 31-34.

Ratner, B. D., Chilkoti, A. & Lopez, G. P. 1990. Plasma Deposition and Treatment for Biomaterial Applications. *In:* D'AGOSTINO, R. (ed.) *Plasma Deposition, Treatment, and Etching of Polymers.* San Diego: Academic Press, Inc.

Richardson, J. P., Dyer, F. F., Dobbs, F. C., Alexeff, I. & Laroussi, M. Year. On the use of the resistive barrier discharge to kill bacteria: Recent results. *In:* 27th IEEE International Conference on Plasma Science - ICOPS2000, 2000 2000 New Orleans (USA). 109-109.

Rossi, F., Kylian, O. & Hasiwa, M. 2006. Decontamination of surfaces by low pressure plasma discharges. *Plasma Processes and Polymers*, 3, 431-442.

Rossi, F., Kylian, O., Rauscher, H., Gilliland, D. & Sirghi, L. 2008. Use of a low-pressure plasma discharge for the decontamination and sterilization of medical devices. *Pure and Applied Chemistry*, 80, 1939-1951.

Roth, J. R., Sherman, D. M., Ben Gadri, R., Karakaya, F., Chen, Z. Y., Montie, T. C., Kelly-Wintenberg, K. & Tsai, P. P. Y. 2000. A remote exposure reactor (RER) for plasma processing and sterilization by plasma active species at one atmosphere. *IEEE Transactions on Plasma Science*, 28, 56-63.

Rutala, W. A., Gergen, M. F. & Weber, D. J. 1998. Comparative evaluation of the sporicidal activity of new low-temperature sterilization technologies: Ethylene oxide, 2 plasma sterilization systems, and liquid peracetic acid. *American Journal of Infection Control*, 26, 393-398.

Sato, T., Furuya, O., Ikeda, K. & Nakatani, T. 2008. Generation and transportation mechanisms of chemically active species by dielectric barrier discharge in a tube for catheter sterilization. *Plasma Processes and Polymers*, 5, 606-614.

Schutze, A., Jeong, J. Y., Babayan, S. E., Park, J., Selwyn, G. S. & Hicks, R. F. 1998. The atmospheric-pressure plasma jet: A review and comparison to other plasma sources. *IEEE Transactions on Plasma Science*, 26, 1685-1694.

Shimizu, T., Nosenko, T., Morfill, G. E., Sato, T., Schmidt, H. U. & Urayama, T. 2010. Characterization of Low-Temperature Microwave Plasma Treatment With and Without UV Light for Disinfection. *Plasma Processes and Polymers*, 7, 288-293.

Shimizu, T., Steffes, B., Pompl, R., Jamitzky, F., Bunk, W., Ramrath, K., Georgi, M., Stolz, W., Schmidt, H. U., Urayama, T., Fujii, S. & Morfill, G. E. 2008. Characterization of microwave plasma torch for decontamination. *Plasma Processes and Polymers*, 5, 577-582.

Singh, M. K., Ogino, A. & Nagatsu, M. 2009. Inactivation factors of spore-forming bacteria using low-pressure microwave plasmas in an N-2 and O-2 gas mixture. *New Journal of Physics*, 11.

Sladek, R. E. J., Baede, T. A. & Stoffels, E. 2006. Plasma-needle treatment of substrates with respect to wettability and growth of Escherichia coli and Streptococcus mutans. *IEEE Transactions on Plasma Science,* 34, 1325-1330.

Sladek, R. E. J. & Stoffels, E. 2005. Deactivation of Escherichia coli by the plasma needle. *Journal of Physics D-Applied Physics,* 38, 1716-1721.

Sladek, R. E. J., Stoffels, E., Walraven, R., Tielbeek, P. J. A. & Koolhoven, R. A. 2004. Plasma treatment of dental cavities: A feasibility study. *IEEE Transactions on Plasma Science,* 32, 1540-1543.

Stoffels, E. 2007. "Tissue processing" with atmospheric plasmas. *Contributions to Plasma Physics,* 47, 40-48.

Stoffels, E., Flikweert, A. J., Stoffels, W. W. & Kroesen, G. M. W. 2002. Plasma needle: a non-destructive atmospheric plasma source for fine surface treatment of (bio)materials. *Plasma Sources Science & Technology,* 11, 383-388.

Stoffels, E., Kieft, I. E. & Sladek, R. E. J. 2003. Superficial treatment of mammalian cells using plasma needle. *Journal of Physics D-Applied Physics,* 36, 2908-2913.

Stoffels, E., Kieft, I. E., Sladek, R. E. J., van den Bedem, L. J. M., van der Laan, E. P. & Steinbuch, M. 2006. Plasma needle for in vivo medical treatment: recent developments and perspectives. *Plasma Sources Science & Technology,* 15, S169-S180.

Stoffels, E., Sakiyama, Y. & Graves, D. B. 2008. Cold atmospheric plasma: Charged species and their interactions with cells and tissues. *IEEE Transactions on Plasma Science,* 36, 1441-1457.

Trompeter, F. J., Neff, W. J., Franken, O., Heise, M., Neiger, M., Liu, S. H., Pietsch, G. J. & Saveljew, A. B. 2002. Reduction of Bacillus Subtilis and Aspergillus Niger spores using nonthermal atmospheric gas discharges. *IEEE Transactions on Plasma Science,* 30, 1416-1423.

Vandamme, M., Robert, E., Pesnel, S., Barbosa, E., Dozias, S., Sobilo, J., Lerondel, S., Le Pape, A. & Pouvesle, J. M. 2010. Antitumor Effect of Plasma Treatment on U87 Glioma Xenografts: Preliminary Results. *Plasma Processes and Polymers,* 7, 264-273.

Vassal, S., Favennec, L., Ballet, J. J. & Brasseur, P. 1998. Hydrogen peroxide gas plasma sterilization is effective against Cryptosporidium parvum oocysts. *American Journal of Infection Control,* 26, 136-138.

Vicoveanu, D., Popescu, S., Ohtsu, Y. & Fujita, H. 2008. Competing inactivation agents for bacterial spares in radio-frequency oxygen plasmas. *Plasma Processes and Polymers,* 5, 350-358.

Villeger, S., Cousty, S., Ricard, A. & Sixou, M. 2003. Sterilization of E-coli bacterium in a flowing N-2-O-2 post-discharge reactor. *Journal of Physics D-Applied Physics,* 36, L60-L62.

Villeger, S., Sarrette, J. P. & Ricard, A. 2005. Synergy between N and O atom action and substrate surface temperature in a sterilization process using a flowing N-2-O-2 microwave post discharge. *Plasma Processes and Polymers,* 2, 709-714.

Yamamoto, M., Nishioka, M. & Sadakata, M. Year. Sterilization using a corona discharge with H2O2 droplets and examination of effective species. *In:* 15th International Symposium on Plasma Chemistry, 2001 2001 Orleans (France). 743-750.

Yang, L. Q., Chen, J. R. & Gao, J. L. 2009. Low temperature argon plasma sterilization effect on Pseudomonas aeruginosa and its mechanisms. *Journal of Electrostatics,* 67, 646-651.

Yasuda, H., Hashimoto, M., Rahman, M. M., Takashima, K. & Mizuno, A. 2008. States of biological components in bacteria and bacteriophages during inactivation by atmospheric dielectric barrier discharges. *Plasma Processes and Polymers,* 5, 615-621.

3

Photocrosslinkable Polymers for Biomedical Applications

P. Ferreira, J. F. J. Coelho, J. F. Almeida and M. H. Gil
Chemical Engineering Department, University of Coimbra
Portugal

1. Introduction

Photopolymerization techniques provide a number of economic advantages over the usual thermal techniques. These include: rapid cure reaction, low energy requirements, use of room temperature and solvent free formulations as well as low cost. Light beams are used to start the photochemical reactions in organic materials (monomers, oligomers, polymers) to form a new polymeric system This technique allows us to prepare materials with several applications in industry (UV curable inks, printing plates and adhesives, among others). Photopolymerization has also been used in electronic materials, optical materials, membranes, coatings and surface modifications. The efficiency of the polymerization reaction is dependent on the monomers, the photoinitiator and the beam wavelength.

More recently, this technique has been used in the preparation of biomaterials with applications in important areas as tissue engineering, (Nguyen & West, 2002), biosensors, (Alves et al., 2009), development of drug delivery systems (Rydhholm et al., 2007) dental restorations in situ (Gatti et al. 2007)) and surface modifications to control the materials cell adhesion (Alves et al., 2011). Photopolymerizable polymers have found numerous applications in the field of tissue engineering for the engineering of tissues as bone, cartilage and liver (Ifkovits & Burdick, 2007) as they may be photopolymerized in vivo and in vitro.

Here we will report some of the literature scientific reports in this field.

Ortega and co-workers (2008) showed that the photopolymerization kinetics as well as the resulting structure of the methacrylate based structures are influenced by the monomers and oligomers properties, the reaction conditions, e.g. light intensity, reaction temperature and type of photoinitiator.

Gatti et al. (2007) referred that photopolymers have been widely used in several dentistry applications. Different monomers have been used for this purpose. Gatti et al. (2007) prepared and characterized copolymers obtained from bisphenylglycidyl dimethacrylate, triethylene glycol dimethacrylate and urethane dimethacrylate. These copolymers were used to obtain dentistry resins. The kinetic parameters of the reaction were evaluated by using photocalorimetry

As it is well known, hydrogels are three-dimensional, hydrophilic, polymeric networks capable of imbibing large amounts of water or biological fluids. They represent an important class of materials to be applied in biotechnology and medicine. These networks have been used as membranes for separating solutes, wound dressings, delivery systems for gene therapy and protein controlled-released systems. Hydrogels have also been applied as bioadhesives, for immobilization of enzymes and cells and in tissue engineering. These photocrosslinked polymers can be obtained either from natural polymers (eg. hyaluronic acid) or from synthetic monomers in the presence of a photoinitiator, using visible or ultraviolet light (Nguyen & West, 2002).

Tai et al. (2009) prepared and characterized photocrosslinked hydrogels from synthetic monomers to be used as advanced injectable biomaterials. They observed that the PEGMEMA-PPGMA-EGDMA copolymers, with both thermoresponsive and photocrosslinkable properties, have excellent mechanical properties above the LCST. They suggested that the biodegradability of these gels could be increased by copolymerization with biodegradable blocks.

Other authors (Seiffert et al., 2007) prepared hydrogels by crosslinking a dimethylmaleimide functionalized polyacrylamide. They observed that this method could give a very efficient method to synthesize hydrogels in a selective and controlled manner.

Tae Il Son group developed a visible light-crosslinkable porcine gelatine containing furfuryl groups by using Rose Bengal (4,5,6,7-tetrachloro-2',4',5',7'-tetraiodofluorescein) as a visible light sensitizer. These authors referred that the material could be used in the dental field as well as a visible light induced crossslinkable bioselant.

Schuster and co-workers (2009) developed gelatine based photopolymers for bone replacement materials. For this purpose, as a first step, they prepared different methacrylate based gelatine derivatives by reaction of this polymer with glycidylmethacrylate and other acrylate monomers. In this way, they obtained polymerizable gelatin that was polymerized with a polyethyleneglycol monomethacrylate comonomer. They where then, able to prepare cellular structures by using stereolithography.

Nichol and colleagues (2010) prepared a photopolymerizable gelatine methacrylate for tissue engineering applications. They modified gelatine with methacrylic anhydride, which was subsequently photopolymerized with UV irradiation, in the presence of Irgacure 2959. These authors suggested that these hydrogels could be applied in microscale applications to create endothelial-lined vessels within engineered tissues.

Hu and co-workers (2010) used a carboxymethylated chitosan modified with 4-nitrocinnamate acid to obtain a photopolymerizable derivative without initiator. They were able to prepare a gel with good mechanical properties that was efficiently used as a matrix in a drug delivery system.

Although the extension of described works, the photopolymerization/photocrosslinkage are processes which are still being studied and therefore explored by many researchers. In this chapter, we wish to report some of the highlights of our work, in this field, still on course in our research group.

2. Photoinitiators

The photocrosslinking technology by using ultraviolet (UV) or visible light has been used extensively in several applications including several types of coatings and biomedical applications. When this technology is used in combination with biodegradable polymers very interesting solutions can be found for drug delivery and tissue engineering applications. The photoinitiators are one of most important compounds used in the formulation due to its influence on different reaction parameters. The chemical nature of the photoinitiator determines the reaction rate, the spectral sensitivity (wavelength of absorption), the light resistance and the stability of the materials under storage conditions.

In order to obtain crosslinked polymers, it is necessary to generate free radicals in the system that will induce a free radical chain polymerization of monomers and oligomers. Both have reactive functional groups that can be activated under the presence of reactive radicals, resulting in the formation of crosslinked structures (Corrales et al., 2003). In the mechanism involved in the process we can consider three main reactions: initiation, propagation and termination. Photoinitiators have an essential role in this process, since they are excited under UV radiation leading to the formation of the active radicals that start the polymerization mechanism (initiation). The crosslinking can occur by the reaction of the functional groups that exist in the monomer or polymer structure, which results in a direct intermolecular crosslinking (Figure 1).

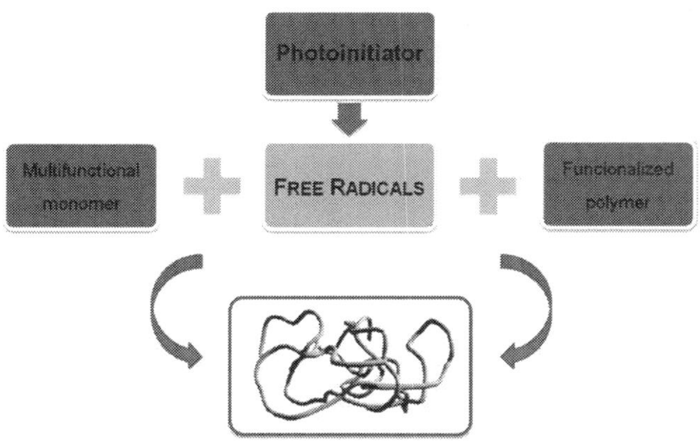

Fig. 1. Representation of the photopolymerization/photocrosslinking processes (Adapted from Decker, 2002).

The crosslinking density plays a critical role in the performance of the biomaterial since it controls properties including permeability, degradation, thermal and mechanic and water uptake (Martens et al., 2003). The use of the proper photoinitiator allows the fine tuning of the reaction rate and therefore the control of the density of crosslinking.

We can consider the existence of two basic types of photoinitiators (Allen et al., 1999): Type I, and Type II. Type I photoinitiators when exposed to UV radiation suffer a fragmentation process that origins the formation of the active radicals with the capacity to start the radical polymerization. Examples of such compounds are the acetophenone derivatives and the α-hidroxyalkyl phenones. The α- hydroxyalkylphenones, as for example 4-(2-hydroxyethylethoxy)-phenyl-(2-hydroxy-2-methyl propyl) ketone (Irgacure® 2959, Ciba) are extremely reactive and present a high thermal stability. Once irradiated, benzoyl and alkyl radicals are formed and although both radicals are reactive to initiate the polymerization, the benzoyl presents higher reactivity.

Type II photoinitators require the presence of molecules, in the system, that suffer a primary process of hydrogen abstraction. These molecules are often referred as co-initiators and are usually tertiary amines. The reaction starts with the formation of the intermediary species resulting from the interaction between the amine and the photoinitiator carbonyl group. The

process continues with an electron and a hydrogen transfer resulting in the radical formation.
When biomedical applications are concerned, the biocompatibility of the photoinitiator is a critical issue to be considered. Williams and co-authors have studied the biocompatibility of the three different photoinitiators (2-hidroxy-1-[4-(2-hidroxyethoxy)phenyl]-2-methyl-1-propanone (Irgacure® 2959); 1-hidroxycyclohexyl-1-phenyl ketone (Irgacure® 184) and 2,2-dimethoxy-2-phenylacetophenone (Irgacure® 651)) commonly used in the preparation of biomaterials using six cellular lines (Williams et al., 2005). Their results revealed that different cell types react differently to the same concentrations of the same photoinitiator. Among the three compounds tested, Irgacure® 2959 presented the better results since very high cell tolerance (in all cell lines) was observed for a broad range of photoinitiator concentrations.

3. Biomedical applications

The UV irradiation is frequently used in the area of biomaterials as a strategy to modify both surface and bulk properties of polymers. These modifications allow us to improve some of their assets such as hemo and biocompatibility. It is also possible, by using radiation, to prepare crosslinked systems that may be used to encapsulate cells (Cruise et al., 1999; Hill et al., 1997; Li et al., 2006), proteins (Leach et al., 2005) or other compounds to be controlled delivered (Vieira et al., 2008; Tripodo et al., 2005).
In the following sections a literature review in some of the possible applications of photocrosslikable polymers will be presented. Also, some examples of some of the work that has been done in our own research group will be given.

3.1 Bioadhesives

Primary wound healing of a plan-to-plan oriented scar formation is usually accomplished by hand sewing or stapling the corresponding layers of each side of the incision (Sheikh et al., 2000). However, both methods have been associated to wound infection and granule formation due to their degradation in the organism. They also present other disadvantages, such as the need to be removed, in most cases and the pain associated with their use.
Topical skin adhesives are increasingly being used by health professionals to replace sutures, staples and adhesive strips for wound closure. The use of adhesives provides several advantages that include: rapid application, unnecessary administration of anesthetics, no trauma is induced to tissues, less pain, unnecessary sutures or staples removal and improved cosmetic results.
Tissue adhesives may also be used as delivery systems and can be engineered for slow, localized release of bioactive molecules (Spicer & Mikos, 2010), such as pain treatment drugs or antibiotics (Fujimoto et al., 1997). They can be used as vehicles to growth factors (Catelas et al., 2008), and cell lines to assist on healing, namely, in poorly healing tissues like cartilage (Hoemann et al., 2005). Very recently, Spicer & Mikos (2010) reported several studies concerning the entrapment of drugs and growth factor in fibrin gels. Entrapment of such bioactive compounds was achieved by simply mixing the components before crosslink of the fibrinogen. At the end of the process a fibrin gel containing a bioactive molecule was obtained (Figure 2). The authors concluded that controlled delivery of drugs or factors by this method was in fact possible, and that release kinetics could be tailored through composition, affinity and covalent linkage between the bioactive molecules and fibrin.

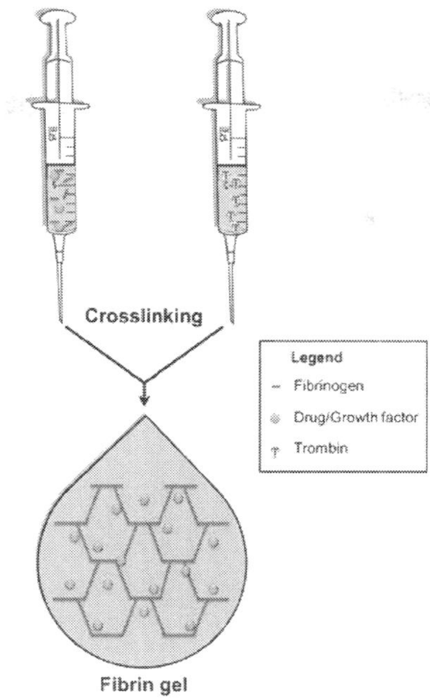

Fig. 2. Fibrin gel preparation and drug/growth factor entrapment. (Adapted from Spicer and Mikos, 2010).

Regardless their nature, surgical adhesives must obey some clinical requirements. They must hold the two sides of the tissue together, until it is no longer necessary, and then they should be degraded to biocompatible products (Lipatova, 1986). Also, an adhesive would ideally present the ability to cure in a moist environment.

Among the adhesives available on the market, the most applied are the ones based either on fibrin (Silver et al., 1995; Dunn & Goa, 1999) or cyanoacrylates (Leahey et al., 1993; King & Kinney, 1999). Both classes present some advantages as well as some disadvantages. Although fibrin glues contribute efficiently to hemorrhage control at bleeding wounds, their application is limited by their possible immunogenicity and risk of blood transmission diseases such as HIV and BSE. On the other hand, cyanoacrylates present a fast curing rate and a very strong adhesion to tissues but have been reported to degrade in aqueous media to produce formaldehyde, which causes inflammation and has got carcinogenicity potential.

Considering the described limitations, other options are now being considered, and among synthetic materials, urethane-based adhesives have been considered to be quite promising for this application. However, although several studies have already been conducted by other authors (Lipatova, 1986; Sheikh et al., 2000) and also by our research group in trying to develop urethane pre-polymers to be applied as bioadhesives (Ferreira et al., 2007, 2008a), these have proved that despite the good adhesion results, the curing time is too long to face surgical demands. UV curable adhesives offer major advantages compared to pre-polymers systems, such as fast-curing rate, control of the polymerization heat evolution and are ideal for application to weakened and diseased tissue (Benson, 2002).

The photopolymerization and photocrosslinkage of polymers intending the preparation of bioadhesives has been largely developed during the second half of the 20th century. Throughout this period, several works translated into patents and scientific papers were published focusing on the development of various aspects of photopolymerization. Among them, new UV radiation sources, functionalized monomers and oligomers as well as new technologies for preparation of particles stand out (Moon et al., 2005).

A biological adhesive must present a combination of biocompatibility, performance and effectiveness. It should also present a fast curing rate when in contact with the living tissues. UV curable adhesives offer major advantages, such as fast-curing rate, control of the polymerization heat evolution, superior control over the final properties of the material and are ideal for application to weakened and diseased tissue (Benson, 2002). Another great advantage of such UV sensitive systems is allowing the adhesive to cure almost instantaneously, however selectively, in strongly illuminated areas such as the operating rooms (Decker, 2002).

Kao et al. (1997) have synthesized UV irradiation curable bioadhesives based on *N*-vinylpyrrolidone. The obtained results showed that these adhesives presented suitable adhesive strength. However, the UV induced setting time was of approximately 3 min which is a value that should be improved when surgical applications are concerned. A few years later, Ono and co-workers developed another photocrosslinkable adhesive based on chitosan. Its UV sensitivity and consequent crosslinking was dependent on azide groups that were introduced to the chitosan molecules. In vivo tests were conducted to evaluate its efficacy as well as the organism response (Ono et al., 2001). The final results showed that, 30 days after the surgical procedure, the adhesive was still present at implantation site surrounded by fibrous tissue. Also, inflammatory cells were observed around the material.

Since then, some work has been published describing attempts to develop a bioadhesive based on photosensitive polymers (Ho & Young, 2006; Grinstaff, 2007; Brigham et al., 2009). As an example, in our research group, Ferreira and co-workers (2008b) developed a photocrosslinkable biodegradable bioadhesive based on polycaprolactone (PCL). PCL is a semi-crystalline linear biodegradable aliphatic polyester that has been used in several medical applications already approved by the US Food and Drug Administration. Its structure presents several aliphatic ester linkages (Figure 3) that can undergo hydrolysis and its products of degradation are either metabolized by being included in the tricarboxylic acid cycle or eliminated by renal secretion.

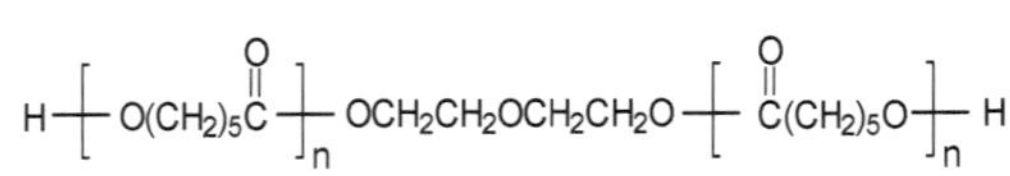

Fig. 3. Chemical structure of PCL.

The authors modified the polymer with 2-isocyanatoethylmethacrylate (IEMA) to form a macromer that was crosslinked via UV irradiation using Irgacure® 2959 by CIBA as the photoinitiating agent. Results showed that after 60s of irradiation the curing of the polymer was complete and membranes were obtained. The resultant films were then characterized by several techniques that included swelling evaluation, thermal characterization, surface energy determination, electronic microscopy, biodegradation in human plasma and haemocompatibility (haemolysis and thrombogenicity). In a global appreciation, it was concluded that the obtained membranes presented a porous morphology and that biodegradation occurred although in a slow rate (10% of weight loss after 6 weeks). Also, the material was haemocompatible (no significant value of haemolyisis was measured) and presented thrombogenic character (which would contribute to control wound bleeding). Finally, the adhesive was also able to promote efficient adhesion between the aminated substrates (gelatin was used as a model material), since during the binding strength tests, the gelatin pieces broke without compromising the glued section. The adhesive was posteriorly tested in vivo using Wistar rats, in two organs (skin and liver) and it proved to be efficient in keeping the glued surfaces together (even in moisture conditions) for the entire experimental protocol. After this period, the animals were euthanized and histological study of these organs was performed (hematoxylin & eosin coloration technique). No signs of necrosis or inflammation were detected in any of the target organs. Figure 4 presents a scheme summarizing the steps involved in this study.

3.2 Drug delivery systems

Drug delivery systems aim to control and sustain the distribution of drugs to attain optimal therapeutic efficiency. The earliest drug delivery systems were introduced in the 1970s and were based on poly(lactic acid). Nowadays, polymers are still the most used materials in this field of research mainly because of their ease of processing and also because of the possibility of researchers to control both their physical and chemical properties.

3.2.1 Ophthalmology

Recently, significant advances have been made in optimizing the delivery of drugs to target tissues within the eye and in maintaining effective drug doses within those tissues (Geroski & Edelhauser, 2000). However, and despite all efforts, conventional ocular therapy for the treatment of acute and chronic diseases makes use of topical appliance of eye drops. This type of therapeutics represents nearly 90% of the marketed formulations. Still, this kind of appliance has a limited efficacy that is due to several factors, namely lacrimation, tear drainage and turnover, and the composition of the precorneal tear film itself.

One of the major limiting factors for drug absorption from the lachrymal fluid into the anterior chamber, after eye drop administration, is the low permeability of the corneal epithelium that results in a very low (around 5%) drug absorption by the cornea. The corneal epithelium consists of approximately five to seven cell layers (Figure 5) which make it a strong barrier to drug permeation.

The remaining amount of drug flows with tears through the upper and lower canonically into the nasolachrymal ducts and consequently may cause unwanted systemic side effects (Ali & Lehmussaari, 2006). The self-protective mechanisms of the eye, such as rapid tear turnover, limit the absorption of the instilled drug in the eye. In addition, application of ophthalmic drugs as drops results in rapid variation in drug delivery rates to the cornea that limits the efficacy of therapeutic systems.

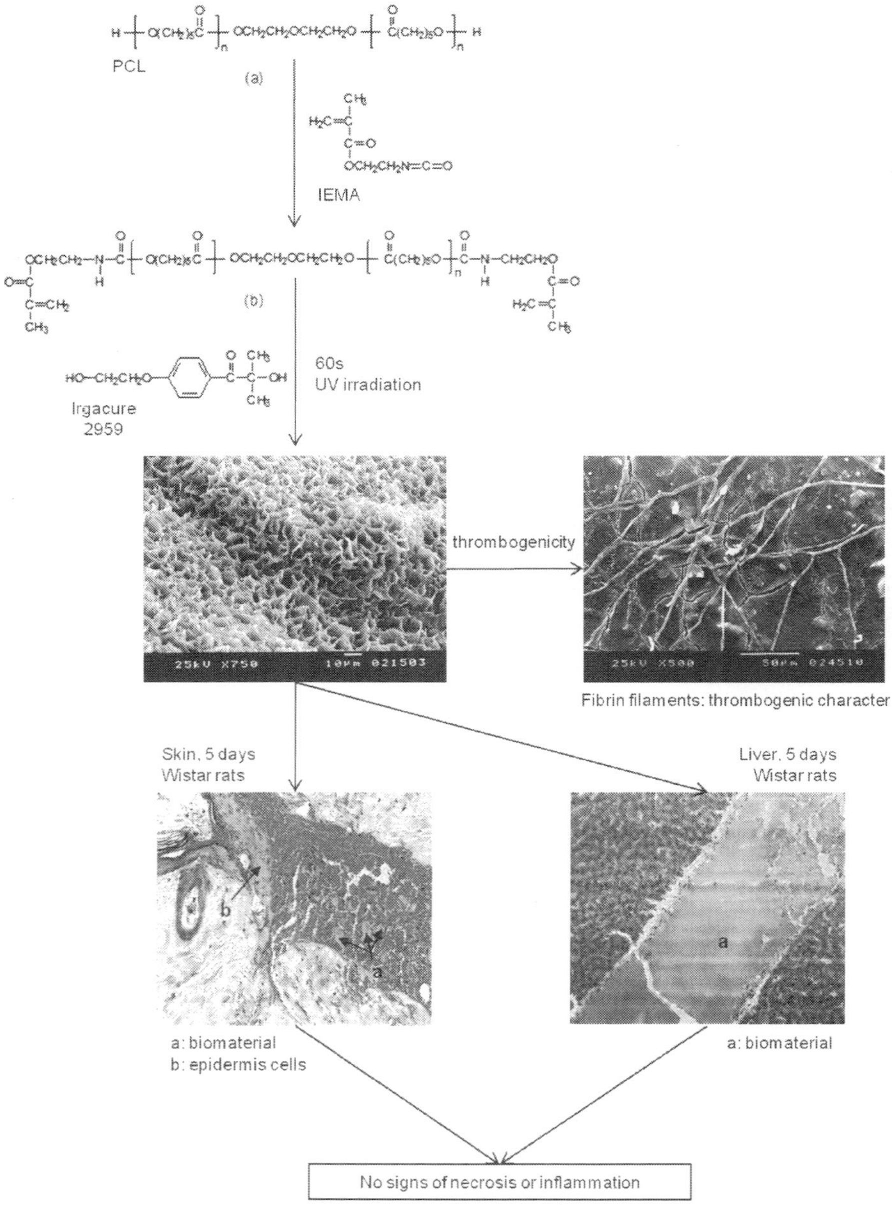

Fig. 4. Summary of the development and characterization of a UV curable PCL based bioadhesive.

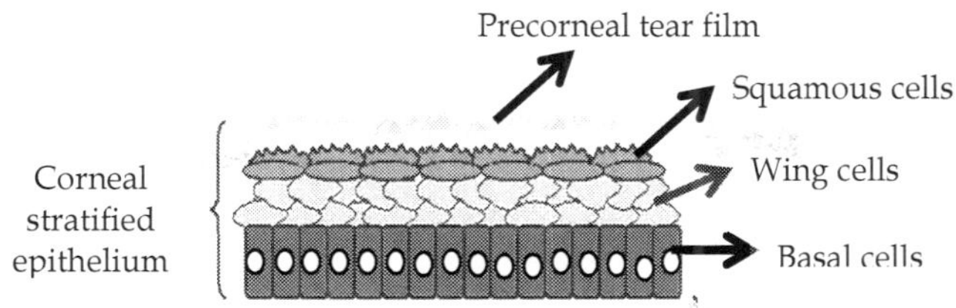

Fig. 5. Diagram showing the various layers of the corneal epithelium.

In order to improve the patient compliance for delivering the medications there is the need for finding some new implantable devices which could deliver the drugs in a long-lasting controlled manner. Using this strategy, the drug loss associated with systemic absorption would be minimized, and the resident time of the drug in the tear film increased (Ludwig, 2005). An alternative approach to optimize ophthalmic drug delivery is the adaptation of bioadhesive systems (Vasir et al., 2003), namely mucoadhesive ones, which have been proved to be successful in oral applications (Bernkop-Schnürch, 2005).
Initially, intraocular implants aimed to achieve controlled and long lasting drug delivery for patients with glaucoma, proliferative vitroretinopathy, cytomegalovirus retinitis, endophtalmitis, and posterior capsule opacification. Nowadays, new ambitions rely on the development of new drug delivery systems namely therapeutic targeting of retinal degenerative diseases and angiogenic reactions which lead to blindness (Bourges et al., 2006). These systems are prepared using different kinds of biodegradable or non-biodegradable polymers and can present several shapes: sheet, pellet, disc, rod, or plug (Figure 6).

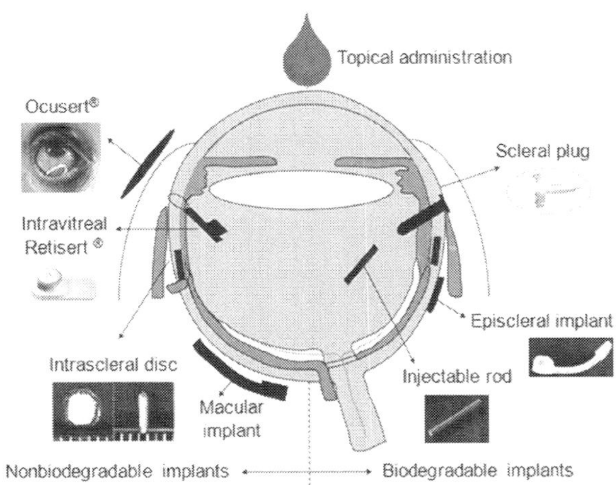

Fig. 6. Routes of ocular drug delivery. (Adapted from Short, 2008).

Among non-biodegradable implants, the best documented are based on polyvinyl alcohol (PVA)-ethylene vinyl acetate (EVA) (Okabe et al., 2003) and polysulfone (under the form of capillary fibers; Rahimy et al., 1994) Although both systems proved to efficiently control drug delivery for a long period of time, they present the disadvantage of being surgically removed once the entire amount of drug has been released (Bourges et al., 2006). In order of overcoming this limitation biodegradable systems have been prepared based on several different polymers, namely: poly(lactic-co-glycolic acid) (Yasukawa et al., 2005); polycaprolactone (Shi et al., 2005); polyanhydrides (Leong et al., 1986) and poly(ortho esters) (Heller, 2005).

In our research group, a starch-based polymer with urethane linkages to be used as a controlled drug delivery system for biomedical applications was developed (Vieira et al., 2008). Hydroxyl groups present on starch were modified with 2-isocyanatoethyl methacrylate (IEMA) in order to obtain a polymer containing carbon–carbon double bonds. This modified starch was then used to prepare films by UV irradiation using Irgacure® 2959 (CIBA) as the photoinitiator.

The obtained films were characterized by several techniques and some parameters were evaluated. The swelling capacity in artificial lachrymal fluid (performed both at room temperature and physiological temperature), was determined and even though some hydroxyl groups of starch were modified, it was observed that polymeric matrix remained hydrophilic. The in vitro biodegradation in artificial lachrymal fluid supplemented with lysozyme was also studied for 6 weeks and it was verified that biodegradation of the samples remained almost constant during experimentation time. Scanning electronic microscopy (SEM) was used to characterize the morphology of the materials immediately after synthesis and after biodegradation and it was possible to visualize pore size increasing due to the degradation process. Since the main goal of this work was to develop a controlled drug delivery system for ophthalmic application, timolol maleate and sodium flurbiprofen were immobilized by adsorption inside the polymeric matrix and their in vitro release profiles were followed spectroscopically (for 10 days). As general conclusions, one can mention that it was possible to verify that the drugs' incorporation into the polymer matrix was mainly controlled by the swelling behavior of the polymer, rather than the different characteristics of each tested drug. Also, drug release studies proved that incorporation of the each drug resulted in a different diffusional behavior. Timolol revealed to be a Case II diffusional anomalous process, whereas flurbiprofen diffusion presented a typical Fickian release pattern. However, the main driving force of the release pattern in both cases appears to be diffusion of the drugs from the polymeric matrices. Figure 7 presents a scheme summarizing the steps involved in this study.

3.2.2 Responsive hydrogels for dermatologic applications

Human skin is an easily accessible surface for drug delivery and covers a surface of approximately $2m^2$ in a young adult. Also, it receives about one-third of the blood circulating through the body. For these reasons, transdermal drug delivery (Figure 8) represents an attractive alternative to oral delivery of drugs as well as to hypodermic injection since is a non-invasive technique and can be self-administered.

The first transdermal drug delivery system was approved by the FDA in 1979 and consisted in a patch with a 3 days release of scopolamine (an alkaloid used in the treatment of nausea and motion sickness). During following years, many systems were developed and some of them remain until now as real best-sellers (Prausnitz and Langer, 2008). Among them, nicotine patches are probably the more broadly used. Other systems available on the market include the ones containing: fentanyl (a synthetic narcotic analgesic), lidocaine (a local anesthetic) and hormones (either for contraception or hormone replacement). In fact, transdermal patches are so largely used nowadays, that it is estimated that more than one billion are currently manufactured each year.

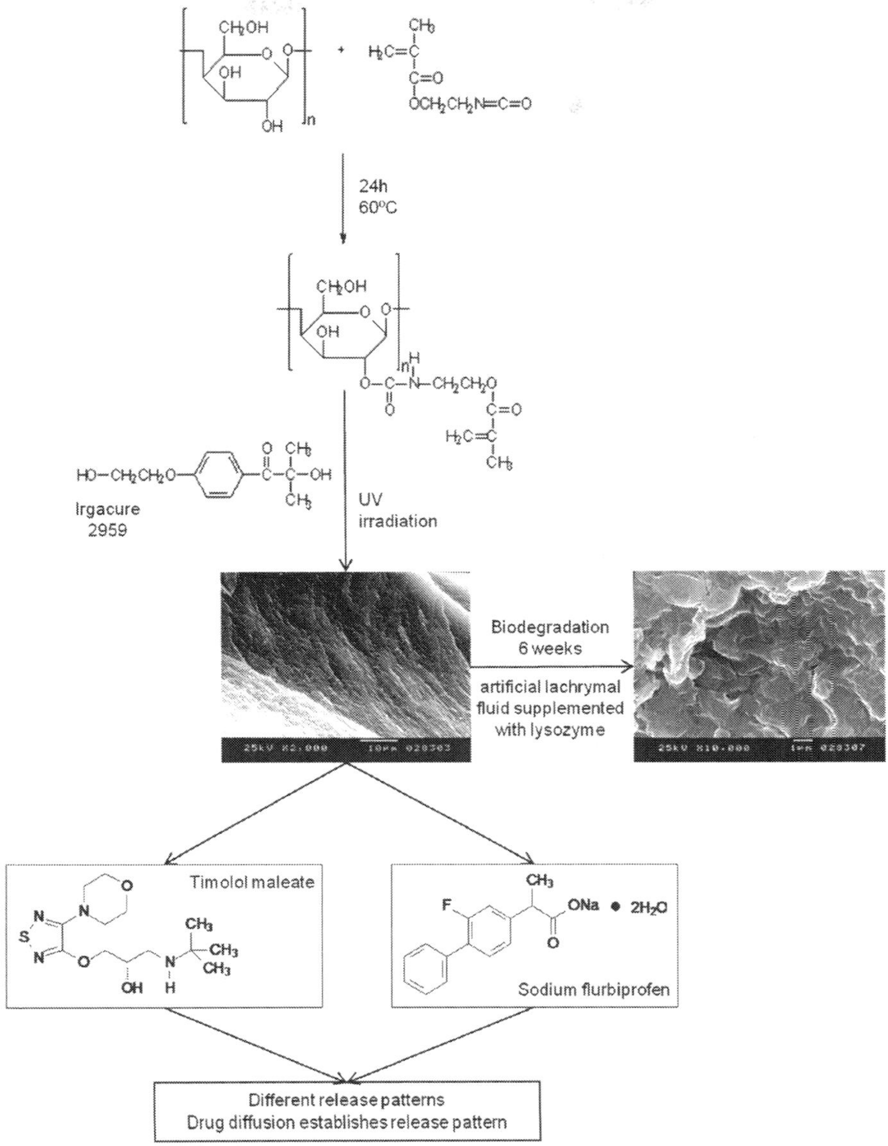

Fig. 7. Summary of the development and characterization of a UV curable starch based drug delivery system.

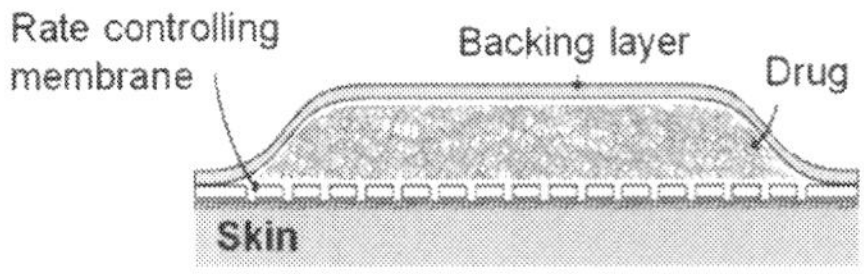

Fig. 8. Scheme of a transdermal drug delivery system.

Among the systems designed for drug release, the ones based on hydrogels are receiving most of the current attention. Hydrogels used for this purpose are usually prepared outside the organism and impregnated with drugs before placement of the system in the body. Several methods are available to achieve crosslinking of the matrices, namely UV photopolymerization and various chemical cross-linking techniques (Hoare and Kohane, 2008).

Hydrogels are materials that, when placed in aqueous medium absorb and retain large amounts of water without dissolving in the solution (Hennink and van Nostrum, 2002; Hatice Kaplan, 2005). In the polymeric structure of hydrogels, the hydrophilic parts of gels tend to be highly hydrated in the aqueous environment triggering the big water uptake that characterizes these structures (Coviello et al., 2007). Because of their properties, namely hydrophilicity and biocompatibility, hydrogels have been a subject of interest in different areas especially in the preparation of drug delivery systems (DDS) (Hoffman, 2002; Ulbrich, 1995).

Both natural and synthetic polymers can be used to prepare hydrogels. Natural-based hydrogels lack mechanical strength and may contain pathogens that induce immune or inflammatory host responses. However, they simultaneously present some advantages such as their biodegradability, biocompatibility and biologically recognizable moieties that are compatible with cellular activities Synthetic hydrogels, on the other hand, do not possess these inherent bioactive properties and are often modified in order to improve their bioactivity (Bajpai et al., 2008).

Although the variety of hydrogels already used as DDS, a great interest in this field of research still exists mainly in the development of gels that present a phase transition that responds to changes in external conditions. The most important systems from biomedical point of view are those sensitive to temperature and/or pH of the surroundings. These materials are known as "stimuli-responsive" or "smart" gels and can undergo abrupt volume changes in response to small changes in environmental parameters. Their ability to swell or deswell according to external conditions, leads to a drug release profile that varies with the same specific parameters (Figure 9).

Among stimuli responsive hydrogels, we will be focusing on the ones sensitive to temperature. These materials are prepared using polymers in carefully chosen in order to achieve a delicate balance between hydrophilic and hydrophobic groups. The most extensively studied temperature-sensitive polymer is poly(N-isopropylacrylamide) or PNIPAAm which consists on a non-biodegradable polymer (Figure 10).

PNIPAAm shows a lower critical solution temperature (LCST) at approximately 32°C which means that is soluble in water below this temperature but precipitates rapidly when temperature is raised above 32°C. This means that crosslinked gels prepared using these polymers suffer an abrupt change in their volume when temperature value varies above or below the LCST (Satish et al., 2006). In fact, these materials expand and swell when cooled below the LCST, and shrink and collapse when heated above the LCST. As a consequence, drug release profile undergoes the same variations patterns.

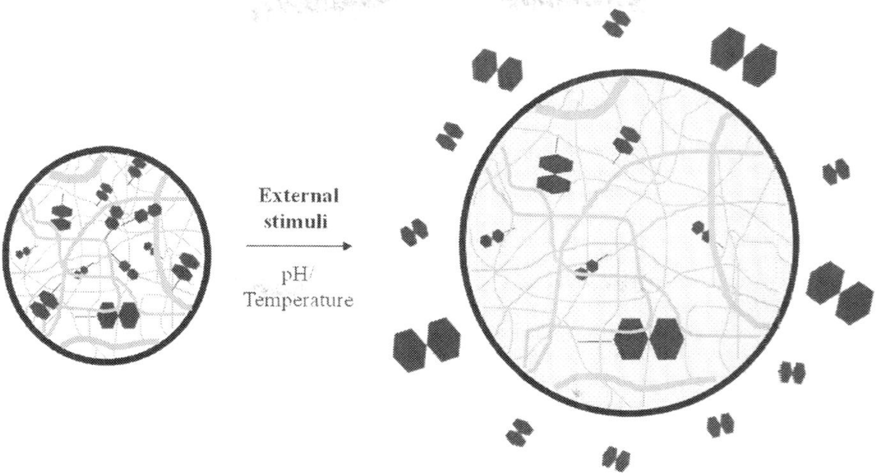

Fig. 9. Schematic representation of the on-off release from an intelligent stimuli-responsive hydrogel designed for drug release.

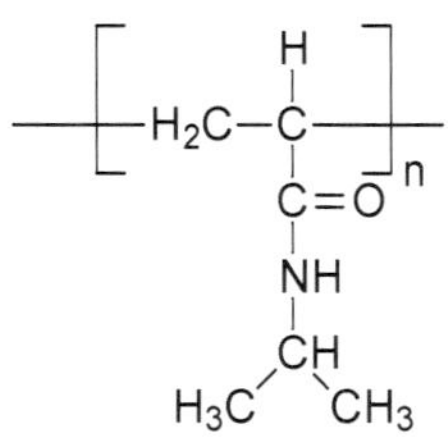

Fig. 10. Chemical structure of PNIPAAm.

Several works have been reported using crosslinked gels based on PNIPAAm starting with Tanaka (1981). Later, this same polymer was used to develop materials to be applied as biomaterials (Dong and Hoffman, 1990). These authors recognized its potential to entrap enzymes or cells and regulate their activity by manipulating swelling/deswelling of the hydrogel (Dong and Hoffman, 1986; 1987). They also studied the possibility or delivering drugs or removing toxins by such hydrogels when controlling external stimuli (Dong and Hoffman, 1991; Park and Hoffman, 1992). Since then, PNIPAAm hydrogels have been prepared under several forms and for various purposes. Vernon and co-workers synthesized gels with entrapped cells to be used as artificial organs (Vernon et al., 2000). A few years later, Dubé and co-workers (Dubé et al., 2002) prepared drug carriers for tumoral cells by synthesizing folate-PNIPAAm conjugates that were fluorescently labeled. They evaluated the targeting specificity of this complex by measuring its cellular uptake. They also conducted direct competition experiments with free folate and demonstrated that the PNIPAAm-folate conjugates effectively target the cells even at folate concentration above normal serum levels. PNIPAAm nanoparticles have also been prepared and their potential applications in biotechnology and in medicine evaluated. Koňák and colleagues (2007) prepared thermoresponsive nanoparticles by heating PNIPAAm solutions with low surfactant additions above the LCST. More recently the preparation of a poly(*N*-isopropylacrylamide)-co-poly(ethylene glycol) (PNIPAAm–PEG) injectable scaffold platform for the repair of spinal cord injury (SCI) was reported (Comolli et al., 2009). The authors stated that this scaffold allows cell attachment, provides mechanical support and allows a sustained release of neurotrophins (growth factors that induce the survival, development, and function of neurons).

Another approach on the synthesis of crosslinkable hydrogels is grafting of PNIPAAm linear chains onto natural polymers (Hoare and Kohane, 2008). As an example, temperature-sensitive injectable gels were prepared by grafting amino-terminated semi-telechelic PNIPAAm onto hyaluronic acid (HA) backbones (Ha et al., 2006). Riboflavin was entrapped in the resulting gel and in vitro tests results showed a more sustained release behavior when the grafting yield of PNIPAAm onto the HA backbone was increased. Another example is the work performed by Bae and co-workers (2006). These authors prepared two types of injectable systems using thermosensitive chitosan (chitosan grafted with PNIPAAm): a hydrogel and microparticles-embedded hydrogel. Both systems were developed as drug carriers for controlled release of 5-fluorouracil (5-FU). The results from this study showed that 5-FU release profile from microparticles-embedded hydrogel reduced the burst effect from the beginning of each initial stage. Therefore, the authors suggest that this combined system could be used as an injectable drug carrier for local drug delivery.

PNIPAAm networks interpenetrated in alginate-Ca^{2+} networks were synthesized and the release of bovine serum albumin (BSA) from the hydrogels was evaluated by Moura and co-workers (2008). The authors concluded that the amount and rate of BSA release could be tailored by the tuning up of the PNIPAAm and/or alginate quantity in the hydrogel and by the control of temperature.

Recently a combination of biodegradable microspheres with a PNIPAAm hydrogel was prepared by Yang and colleagues (2011). They studied the release of BSA from the system and concluded that controlled release of BSA encapsulated in the microspheres embebbed in PNIPAAm scaffold was better controlled than when encapsulated in the hydrogel alone.

Temperature-sensitive hydrogels can also be useful for topical delivery of drugs to skin or mucous membranes such as the nose or the eyes. Although the temperature of such surfaces is slightly below 37°C, its value is still above ambient temperature which means that it would be possible to deliver a drug through a thermo-responsive polymer.

One example of such application is the work developed by Almeida and co-workers (2010) at our laboratory during which, graft polymer hydrogels based on dextran and N-isopropylacrylamide (NIPAAm) were prepared and characterized. For that purpose, dextran was firstly modified in order to incorporate carbon-carbon double bonds and then NIPAAm was added to the modified polymer. The resultant material (dextran-grafted-PNIPAAm) was obtained by crosslinking using UV irradiation in the presence of the photoinitiating agent Irgacure® 2959 by CIBA. The drug Ondansetron® (an antiemetic used to treat nausea and vomiting, frequently following chemotherapy, Figure 11) was entrapped in the final system and its release profile was determined at 25 and 37°C. The authors concluded that controlled release of the drug occurred for at least one week and that temperature influenced drug release pattern.

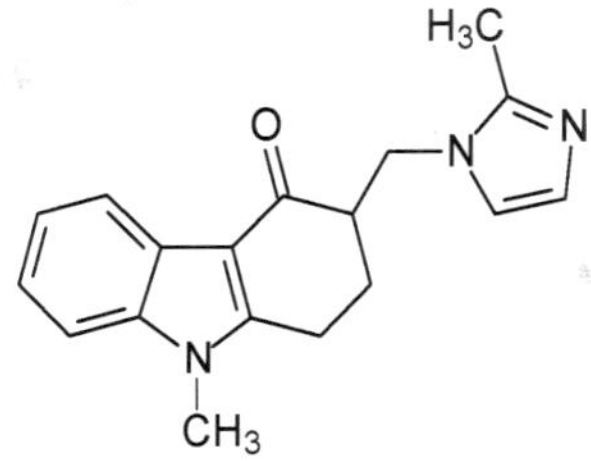

Fig. 11. Chemical structure of Ondansetron®.

These results are extremely important as they show that these systems can be adjusted to have different transition temperatures according to the applications needed giving them a wide range of use.

4. Conclusions

Photocrosslinked polymers may be very useful for biomedical applications.
The use of photopolymerization is advantageous in comparison with other conventional crosslinking methods, since we can obtain biomaterials in situ and in a minimally invasive manner.
The photopolymerizable polymers based either in natural (starch, chitosan and dextran) or synthetic polymers (polycaprolactone), were used for the development of biomaterials, mainly hydrogels.
These materials were applied in the development of bioadhesives, drug delivery systems for ophthalmology and wound dressings.
The results of our research indicate that the systems are suitable for medical applications and make feasible innovative strategies for photocrosslinked polymers in clinical use.

5. References

Ali, Y. & Lehmussaari, K., (2006). Industrial perspective in ocular drug delivery. *Advanced Drug Delivery Reviews*, Vol.58, No.11, (November 2006), pp. 1258–1268, ISSN 0169-409X

Allen, N. S.; Marin, M. C.; Edge, M.; Davies, D. W.; Garrett, J.; Jones, F.; Navaratnam, S. & Parsons, B. J. (1999). Photochemistry and photoinduced chemical crosslinking activity of type I & II co-reactive photoinitiators in acrylated prepolymers. *Journal of Photochemistry and Photobiology A*, Vol. 126, No. 1, (September 1999), pp.135-149, ISSN 1010-6030

Alves, P. , Pinto, S.; Kaiser, J.-P.; Bruinink, A.; Sousa, H. C. & Gil, M. H. (2011). Surface grafting of a thermoplastic polyurethane with methacrylic acid by previous plasma surface activation and by ultraviolet irradiation to reduce cell adhesion. *Colloids and Surfaces B: Biointerfaces*, Vol.82, No.2, (February 2011), pp. 371-377, ISSN 1873-4367

Alves, P.; Coelho, J.F.J.; Haack, J.; Rota, A.; Bruinink, A. & Gil, M.H. (2009). Surface modification and characterization of thermoplastic polyurethane. *European Polymer Journal,* Vol.45, No.5, (May 2009), pp. 1412-1419, ISSN 0014-3057

Bae, J. W.; Go, D. H.; Park, K. D. & Lee, S. J. (2006). Thermosensitive Chitosan as an Injectable Carrier for Local Drug Delivery. *Macromolecular Research,* Vol.14, No.4, (2006), pp. 461-465, ISSN 1598-5032

Bajpai, A. K.; Shukla, S. K.; Bhanu, S. & Kankane, S. (2008). Responsive polymers in controlled drug delivery. *Progress in Polymer Science,* Vol.33, No.11, (November 2008), pp. 1088-1118, ISSN 0079-6700

Benson, R. S. (2002). Use of radiation in biomaterials science. *Nuclear Instruments and Methods in Physics Research Section B: Beam Interactions with Materials and Atoms,* Vol.191, No.1-4, (May, 2002), pp. 752–757, ISSN 0168-9002

Bernkop-Schnürch, A. (2005). Mucoadhesive systems in oral drug delivery. *Drug Discovery Today: Technologies,* Vol.2, No.1, (Spring 2005) pp. 83–87, ISSN 1740-6749

Bourges, J. L.; Bloquel, C.; Thomas, A.; Froussart, F.; Bochot, A.; Azan, F.; Gurny, R.; BenEzra, D. & Behar-Cohen, F. (2006). Intraocular implants for extended drug delivery: Therapeutic applications. *Advanced Drug Delivery Reviews,* Vol.58, No.11, (November 2006), pp. 1182-1202, ISSN 0169-409X

Brigham, M. D.; Bick, A.; Lo, E.; Bendali, A.; Burdick, J. A. & Khademhosseini, A. (2009). Mechanically robust and bioadhesive collagen and photocrosslinkable hyaluronic acid semi-interpenetrating networks. *Tissue Engineering Part A,* Vol.15, No.7, (July 2009), pp. 1645-1653, ISSN 1937-3341

Catelas, J. F. D. & Helgerson, S. (2008). Controlled release of bioactive transforming growth factor beta-1 from fibrin gels in vitro. *Tissue Engineering Part C: Methods,* Vol.14, No.2 (June 2008), pp. 119–128, ISSN 1937-3384

Comolli, N.; Neuhuber, B.; Fischer, I. & Lowman, A. (2009). In vitro analysis of PNIPAAm–PEG, a novel, injectable scaffold for spinal cord repair. *Acta Biomaterialia,* Vol.5, No.4, (May 2009), pp. 1046-1055, ISSN 1742-7061

Corrales, T.; Catalina, F.; Peinado, C. & Allen, N. S. (2003). Free radical macrophotoinitiators: an overview on recent advances. *Journal of Photochemistry and Photobiology A: Chemistry,* Vol.159, No.2, (July 2003), pp. 103-114, ISSN 1010-6030

Cruise, G. M.; Hegre, O. D.; Lamberti, F. V.; Hager, S. R.; Hill, R.; Scharp, D. S. & Hubbell, J. A. (1999). In vitro and in vivo performance of porcine islets encapsulated in interfacially photopolymerized poly(ethylene glycol) diacrylate membranes. *Cell Transplantation* Vol.8, No.3, (May-June 1999), pp. 293-306, ISSN 0963-6897

Decker, C. (2002). Kinetic Study and New Applications of UV Radiation Curing. *Macromolecular Rapid Communications,* Vol.23, No.18, (January 2003), pp. 1067-1093, ISSN 1521-3927

Dunn, C. J. & Goa, K. L. (1999). Fibrin sealant. A review of its use in surgery and endoscopy. *Drugs,* Vol.58, No.5, (November, 1999), pp. 863–886, ISSN 0012-6667

Ferreira, P.; Coelho, J. F. J. & Gil, M. H. (2088b). Development of a new photocrosslinkable biodegradable bioadhesive. *International Journal of Pharmaceutics,* Vol.352, No.1-2, (March 2008), pp. 172-181, ISSN 0378-5173

Ferreira, P.; Coelho, J. F. J.; Pereira, R.; Silva, António F. M. & Gil, M. H. (2007). Synthesis and characterization of polyethylene glycol pre-polymer to be applied as bioadhesive. *Journal of Applied Polymer Science*, Vol.105, No.2, (July 2007), pp. 593-601, ISSN 1097-4628

Ferreira, P.; Silva, António F. M.; Pinto, M. I. & Gil, M. H. (2008a). Development of a biodegradable bioadhesive containing urethane groups. *Journal Materials Science: Materials in Medicine*, Vol.19, No.1, (January 2008), pp. 111-120, ISSN 0957-4530

Fujimoto, K.;Yamamura, K.; Osada, T.; Hayashi, T.; Nabeshima, T.; Matsushita, M.; Nishikimi, N.; Sakurai, T. & Nimura, Y. (1997). Subcutaneous tissue distribution of vancomycin from a fibrin glue/Dacron graft carrier. *Journal of Biomedical Materials Research*, Vo.36, No.4, (September 1997), pp. 564–567, ISSN 1549-3296

Gatti, A.; Rastelli, A. N. S.; Ribeiro, S. J. L.; Messaddeq, Y. & Bagnato, V. S. (2007). Polymerization of photocurable commercial dental methacrylate-based composites. *Journal of Thermal Analysis and Calorimetry*, Vol.3, No.3, (March 2007), 631-634), ISSN 1388-6150

Geroski, D. H. & Edelhauser, H. F. (2000). Drug Delivery for Posterior Segment Eye Disease. *Investigative Ophthalmology & Visual Science*, Vol.41, No.5, (April 2000), pp. 961-964, ISSN 0146-0404

Grinstaff, M. W. (2007). Designing hydrogel adhesives for corneal wound repair. *Biomaterials*, Vol.28, No.35, (December 2007), pp. 5205-5214, ISSN 0142-9612

Ha, D. I.; Lee, S. B.; Chong, M. S.; Lee, Y. M.; Kim, S. Y. & Park, Y. H. (2006). Preparation of Thermo-Responsive and Injectable Hydrogels Based on Hyaluronic Acid and Poly(N-isopropylacrylamide) and Their Drug Release Behaviors. *Macromolecular Research*, Vol.14, No.1, (2006), pp. 87-93, ISSN 1598-5032

Heller, J. (2005). Ocular delivery using poly(ortho esters). *Advanced Drug Delivery Reviews*, Vol.57, No.14, (December 2005), pp. 2053–2062, ISSN 0169-409X

Hill, R. S.; Cruise, G. M.; Hager, S. R.; Lamberti, F. V.; Yu, X.; Garufis, C. L.; Yu, Y.; Mundwiler, K. E.; Cole, J. F.; Hubbell, J. A.; Hegre, O. D. & Scharp, D. W. (1997). Immunoisolation of adult porcine islets for the treatment of diabetes mellitus. The use of photopolymerizable polyethylene glycol in the conformal coating of mass-isolated porcine islets. *Annals of the New York Academy of Sciences*, Vol.831, No.1, (December 1997), pp. 332-343, ISSN 1749-6632

Hoare, T. R. & Kohane, D. S. (2008). Hydrogels in drug delivery: Progress and challenges. *Polymer*, Vol.49, No.8, (April 2008), pp. 1993-2007, ISSN 0032-3861

Hoemann, C. D.; Sun, J.; Légaré, A.; McKee, M.D., Buschmann, M. D. (2005). Tissue engineering of cartilage using an injectable and adhesive chitosan based cell-delivery vehicle. *Osteoarthritic and Cartilage*, Vol.13, No.4, (April 2005), pp. 318–329, ISSN 1063-4584

Hu, R.; Chen. Y.-Y. & Zhang, L.-M. (2010). Synthesis and characterization of in situ photogelable polysaccharide derivative for drug delivery. *International Journal of Pharmaceutics*, Vol.393, No.1-2, (June 2010), pp. 96-103, ISSN 0378-5173

Ifkovits, Jamie I. & Burdick, Jason A. (2007). Photopolymerizable and Degradable Biomaterials for Tissue Engineering Applications. *Tissue Engineering*, Vol.13, No.10, (October 2007), pp. 2369-2385, ISSN 1937-3341

IUPAC. (1996). Compendium of Chemical Therminology. *Pure and Applied Chemistry*, Vol. 68, No. 12, pp. 2223-2286, ISSN 0033-4545

Kao, F.; Manivannan, G. & Sawan, S. (1997). UV curable bio-adhesives: Copolymers of N-vinyl pyrrolidone. *Journal of Biomedical Materials Research Part B: Applied Biomaterials*, Vol.38, No.3, (Autumn 1997), pp. 191-196, ISSN 1552-4973

King, M. E. & Kinney, A. Y. (1999). Tissue adhesives: a new method of wound repair. *Nurse Practitioner*, Vol.24, No. 10, (October 1999), pp. 66, 69–70, 73-74, ISSN 0361-1817

Koňák, Č.; Pánek, J. & Hrubý, M. (2007). Thermoresponsive polymeric nanoparticles stabilized by surfactants. *Colloid and Polymer Science*, Vol.285, No.13, (October 2007), pp. 1433–1439, ISSN 0303-402X

Leach, J. B. & Schmidt, C. E. (2005). Characterization of protein release from photocrosslinkable hyaluronic acid-polyethylene glycol hydrogel tissue engineering scaffolds. *Biomaterials*, Vol.26, No2, (January 2005), pp. 125-135, ISSN 0142-9612

Leahey, A. B.; Gottsch, J. D. & Stark, W. J. (1993). Clinical experience with *N*-butyl cyanoacrylate (Nexacryl®) tissue adhesive. *Ophthalmology*, Vol.100, No.2, (February 1993), pp. 173–180, ISSN 0161-6420

Leong, K. W.; D'Amore, P. D.; Marletta, M.,& Langer, R. (1986). Bioerodible polyanhydrides as drug-carrier matrices. II. Biocompatibility and chemical reactivity. *Journal of Biomedical Materials Research*, Vol.20, No.1, (January 1986), pp. 51-64, ISSN 1552-4965

Li, Q.; Wang, J.; Shahani, S.; Sun, D. D.; Sharma, B.; Elisseeff, J. H. & Leong, K. W. (2006). Biodegradable and photocrosslinkable polyphosphoester hydrogel. *Biomaterials*, Vol.27, No.7, (March 2006), pp. 1027-1034, ISSN 0142-9612

Lipatova, T. E. (1986). Medical polymer adhesives. *Advances in Polymer Science*, Vol.79, (January 2006), pp. 65–93, ISSN 1436-5030

Ludwig, A. (2005). The use of mucoadhesive polymers in ocular drug delivery. *Advanced Drug Delivery Reviews*, Vol.57, No., (November 2005), pp. 1595–1639, ISSN 0169-409X

Martens, P.J.; Bryant, S.J. & Anseth, K.S. (2003). Tailoring the degradation of hydrogels formed from multivinyl poly(ethylene glycol) and poly(vinyl alcohol) macromers for cartilage tissue engineering. *Biomacromolecules*, Vol. 4, (March 2003), pp. 283-292, ISSN 1525-7797

Moon, J. H.; Shul, Y. G.; Han, H. S.; Hong, S. Y.; Choi, Y. S. & Kim, H. T. (2005). A study on UV-curable adhesives for optical pick-up: I. Photo-initiator effects. *International Journal of Adhesion and Adhesives*, Vol.25, No.4, (August, 2005), pp. 301-312, ISSN 0143-7496

Moura, M. R.; Aouada, F. A.; Favaro, S. L.; Radovanovic, E.; Rubira, A. F. &. Muniz, E. C. (2009). Release of BSA from porous matrices constituted of alginate–Ca^{2+} and PNIPAAm-interpenetrated networks. *Materials Science and Engineering: C*, Vol.29, No.8, (October 2009), pp. 2319-2325, ISSN 0928-4931

Nguyen, K.T. & West, J. L. (2002). Photopolymerizable hydrogels for tissue engineering applications. *Biomaterials*, Vol.23, No.22, (November 2002), pp. 4307-4314, ISSN 0142-9612

Nichol, J. W.; Koshy, S. T.; Bae, H.; Hwang, C. M.; Yamanlar, S. & Khademhosseini, A. (2010). Cell-laden microengineered gelatin methacrylate hydrogels. *Biomaterials*, Vol.31, No.21, (July 2010), pp. 5536-5544, ISSN 0142-9612

Okabe, K.; Kimura, H.; Okabe, J.; Kato, A.; Kunou, N. & Ogura, Y. (2003). Intraocular tissue distribution of betamethasone after intrascleral administration using a non-biodegradable sustained drug delivery device. *Investigative Ophthalmology & Visual Science,* Vol.44, No.6, (June 2003), pp. 2702–2707, ISSN 0146-0404

Ono, K.; Ishihara, M; Ozeki, Y.; Deguchi, H.; Sato, M.; Saito, Y.; Yura, H.; Sato, M.; Kikuchi, M.; Kurita, A. & Maehara, T. (2001). Experimental evaluation of photocrosslinkable chitosan as a biologic adhesive with surgical applications. *Surgery,* Vol.130, No.5, (November 2001), pp. 844-850, ISSN 0039-6060

Ortega, A. M.; Kaspzak, S. E.; Yakacki, C. M.; Diani, J.; Greenberg, A. R. & Gall, K. (2008). Structure-Property Relationships in Photopolymerizable Polymer Networks : Effect of Composition on the Crosslinked Structure and Resulting Thermomechanical Properties of a (Meth)acrylate-Based System. *Journal of Applied Polymer Science,* Vol.110, No.3, (2008), pp. 1559-1572, ISSN 0021-8995

Prausnitzl, M. R. & Langer, R. (2008). Transdermal drug delivery. *Nature Biotechnology,* Vol.26, No.11, (November 2008), pp. 1261–1268, ISSN 1087-0156

Rahimy, M. H.; Peyman, G. A.; Chin, S. Y.; Golshani, R.; Aras, C., Borhani, H. & Thompson, H. (1994). Polysulfone capillary fiber for intraocular drug delivery: in vitro and in vivo evaluations. *Journal of Drug Targeting,* Vol.2,m No.4, (1994), pp. 289–298, ISSN 1061-186X

Rydhholm, A. E.; Sirish, K; Reddy, Anseth, K. S.; Bowman, C. N. (2007). Development and Characterization of Degradable Thiol-Allyl Ether Photopolymers. *Polymer,* Vol.48, No.15, (August 2007), pp. 4589-4600, ISSN 0032-3861

Satish, C. S.; Satish, K. P. & Shivakumar, H. G. (2006). Hydrogels as controlled drug delivery systems: Synthesis, crosslinking, water and drug transport mechanism. Indian *Journal of Pharmaceutical Sciences,* Vol.68, No.2, (April 2006), pp. 133-140, ISSN 0250-474X

Schuster, M.; Yurecek, C.; Weigel, G., Saf, R., Stampfl, J., Varga, F. & Liska, R. (2009). *Journal of Polymer Science Part A: Polymer Chemistry,* Vol.47, No.24, (December 2009), pp. 7078-7089, ISSN 0887-624X

Seiffert, S.; Oppermann W. & Saalwachter, K. (2007). Hydrogel formation by photocrosslinking of dimethylmaleimide functionalized polyacrylamide. *Polymer,* Vol.48, No.19, (September 2007), pp. 5599-5611, ISSN 0032-3861

Sheikh, N.; Katbab, A. A. & Mirzadeh, H. (2000). Isocyanate-terminated urethane prepolymer as bioadhesive base material: synthesis and characterization. *International Journal of Adhesion and Adhesives,* Vol.20, No.4, (August 2000), pp. 299-304, ISSN 0143-7496

Shi, W.; Liu, T.; Xie, L. & Wang, S. (2005). FK506 in a biodegradable glycolide-co-clatide-co-caprolactone polymer for prolongation of corneal allograft survival. *Current Eye Research,* Vol.30, No.11, (November 2005), pp. 969–976, ISSN 0271-3683

Short, B. G. (2008). Safety Evaluation of Ocular Drug Delivery Formulations: Techniques and Practical Considerations. *Toxicologic Pathology,* Vol.36, No.1, (January 2008), pp. 49-62, ISSN 0192-6233

Silver, F. H.; Wang, M. & Pins, G. D. (1995). Preparation and use of fibrin glue in surgery. *Biomaterials,* Vol.16, No.12, (August 1995), pp. 891–903, ISSN 0142-9612

Son, T. I.; Sakuragi, M.; Takahashi, S.; Obuse, S.; Kang, J.; Fujishiro, M.; Matsushita, H.; Gong, J.; Shimizu, S.; Tajima, Y.; Yoshida, Y.; Suzuki, K.; Yamamoto, T.; Nakamura,

M. & Ito Y. (2010) Visible light-induced crosslinkable gelatin. *Acta Biomaterialia,* Vol.6, No.10, (October 2010), pp. 4005-4010, ISSN 1742-7061

Spicer, P. P. & Mikos, A. G. (2010).Fibrin glue as a drug delivery system. *Journal of Controlled Release*, Vol.148, No.1, (November 2010), pp. 49-55, ISSN 0168-3659

Tai, H.; Takae, D. H. S.; Wang, W.; Vermonden, T.; Hennink, W. E.; Stayon, P. S.; Hoffman, A. S.; Endruweit, A.; Alexander, C.; Howdle, T. M.; Shakesheff, K. M. (2009). Thermoresponsive and Photocrosslinkable PEGMEMA-PPGMA-EGDMA Copolymers from a One-Step ATRP Synthesis. *Biomacromolecules,* Vol.10, No.4 , (February 2009), pp. 2895-2903, ISSN 1525-7797

Tripodo, G.; Pitarresi, G.; Palumbo, F. S.; Craparo, E. F. & Giammona, G. (2005). UV-photocrosslinking of inulin derivatives to produce hydrogels for drug delivery application. *Macromolecular Bioscience,* Vol.5, No.11, (November 2005), pp. 1074-1084, ISSN 1616-5195

Vasir, J. K.; Tambwekar, K. & Garg, S. (2003). Bioadhesive microspheres as a controlled drug delivery system. *International Journal of Pharmaceutics,* Vol.255, No.1-2, (April, 2003), pp. 13–32, ISSN 0378-5173

Vieira, A. P.; Ferreira, P.; Coelho, J. F. J. & Gil, M. H. (2008). Photocrosslinkable starch based polymers for ophthalmologic drug delivery. *International Journal of Biological Macromolecules,* Vol.43, No.4, (November 2008), pp. 325-332, ISSN 0141-8130

Williams, C. G.; Malik, A.; Kim, T. K.; Manson, P. & Elisseeff, J. (2005). Variable cytocompatibility of six cell lines with photoinitiators used for polymerizing hydrogels and cell encapsulation. *Biomaterials,* Vol.26, No.11, (April 2005), pp. 1211-1218, ISSN 0142-9612

Yang, J.; Huo, D. Q.; Hou, C. J.; Zhang, G. P.; Yang, L. M.; Zhang, Y. C.; Le Dong, J. & Li, J. (2011). Fabrication of Degradable Microsphere/PNIPAAm Hydrogel Combination Systems for Protein Delivery. *Advanced Materials Research,* Vol.160-162, (2011), pp. 1072-1076, ISSN 1022-6680

Yasukawa, T.; Ogura, Y.; Sakurai, E.; Tabata, Y. & Kimura, H. (2005). Intraocular sustained drug delivery using implantable polymeric devices. *Advanced Drug Delivery Reviews,* Vol. 57, No.14, (December 2005), pp. 2033–2046, ISSN 0169-409X

Young, A. M. & Ho, S. M. (2008). Drug release from injectable biodegradable polymeric adhesives for bone repair. *Journal of Controlled Release,* Vol.127, No.2, (April 2008), pp.162-172, ISSN 0168-3659

4

Hydroxyapatite-Based Materials: Synthesis and Characterization

Eric M. Rivera-Muñoz
Centro de Física Aplicada y Tecnología Avanzada, Universidad Nacional Autónoma de México, México

1. Introduction

The use of foreign materials to be used as implants within or outside the human body is not new. There are reports of more than 2000 years old which indicate the replacement of bone material in order to repair seriously damaged tissues. In the mid-nineteenth century it was attempted to repair human body parts using the materials available according to the technological advance of the time, unfortunately, these materials were mainly based on copper or bronze, suffering severe corrosion within the human organism's environment, and causing infections that also endangered the lives of patients. For this reason the prostheses used were basically external. Over the years (the late nineteenth and early twentieth century) were made several attempts to use different materials such as gold, glass and new alloys with better results.

Advances in polymer chemistry and the development of new alloys in modern metallurgy during the second half of the twentieth century gave rise to a variety of materials for reconstruction and replacement of some tissues inside and outside the human body. In the case of ceramic materials, the development of modern technologies has led to new materials with chemical, physical and mechanical properties that make them an excellent choice for applications in dental and orthopedic implants.

There are many ways to define a biomaterial, which has not been easy given the breadth of the term. In the European Society for Biomaterials Consensus Conference in 1986, was given the following definition: "Biomaterial is a material or substance, whether used alone or in making a medical device designed to interact with human tissues to monitor body functions or to treat pathological conditions of the same" (Mattox, 1992; Ravaglioli & Krajewski, 1992). A synonym for this is "biomedical material".

All definitions include the word "material", which usually indicates a solid consistency substance used to manufacture an object, which may consist of living or nonliving materials. If the material is alive, then is called "graft" and those non-living, placed inside the body, are called "implants". With a more limited meaning, the so-called "prostheses" can be considered as "endoprostheses", if they are contained entirely within the body, or "exo-prosthesis"(or "external prosthesis") if they are completely out.

In other hand, the "biocompatibility" of a biomaterial is defined as their ability to successfully fulfill a specific application, with an appropriate response of the host. That is, the biocompatibility means more than the fact that a material is not harmful in the body; it also includes local interactions of the material and surrounding tissue in both directions. That is, it is vitally important, both the effect of the material on the living tissues as the effect of them on the former one (Hench, 1991).

A material is "not biocompatible" if it is toxic and/or if cause the death of surrounding tissue.

A biocompatible material may be considered "inert" if there is no reaction with tissue and the material is stable for indefinite periods of time (the only answer may be the formation of a fibrous layer around the implant), "bioactive" if there specific interactions with surrounding tissue, "bioabsorbable" if it dissolves into the body through a cellular activity and the vacant space is then filled with tissue, and finally "biodegradable"if the material fails gradually due to biological or specific biochemical activity (Hench 1991; Ravaglioli & Krajewski, 1992).

In general, different types of biomaterials are classified according to their nature and application; polymeric materials are used when complex shapes are required or require high flexibility; metals are used when the implant is subject to high mechanical loads. The applications of ceramics have taken great importance due to its high biocompatibility, corrosion resistance and primarily because the bone tissue is composed largely of mineral phases, which makes them an important option for replacement of bone or to promote regeneration of it. Composite materials are used to improve the interaction between the tissue and the implant (mainly metallic) at the interface (Lemons, 1986; Mattox, 1992; Park, 1984).

The current status of biomaterials is clearly in a state of rapid change, which provide a wide range of opportunities for both conventional materials as well as for the new materials developments (such as in nanotechnology, for example), and improvements in these areas are needed day by day, therefore which not only justified but also they requires the development of new technology in the production of those biomaterials.

While basic research in materials science and engineering, plus physics and chemistry involved in it is of vital importance, we can not ignore the economic aspect of these developments at the moment of entering the market.

It is very difficult to do a count on total sales worldwide biomaterials; however, one could refer to information published by Millennium Research Group on its website in 2002. Considering only the market for orthopedic biomaterials, according to this company was worth US$ 930 million in 2001 only in the United States, anticipating a growth rate of 25.7% annually over the next five years, increasing the value of that market up to a level of US$ 3700 million in 2006 (Millennium Research Group [MRG], 2002).

In a latest study conducted by MarketsandMarkets Research (MarketsandMarkets Research, 2010), called Global Biomaterial Market (2010-2015), has been reported that currently the biomaterials market has crossed the US$ 28 billion worldwide. This study indicates that the total global biomaterials market is expected to be worth US$ 58.1 billion by 2014, growing at a Compound Annual Growth Rate (CAGR) of 15 % from 2009 to 2014. It also indicates that the U.S. market is the largest geographical segment for biomaterials; and is expected to be worth US$ 22.8 billion by 2014 with a CAGR of 13.6% from 2009 to 2014. Europe is the second largest segment and is expected to reach US$ 17.7 billion by 2014 with a CAGR of 14.6% and the Asian market size is estimated to increase at the highest CAGR of 18.2% in the same period. They mention that improvement in fabrication technology and new product development at competitive prices will be the key to future market growth.

Taking into account the above it is clear that the market opportunities for new developments in the area of biomaterials are very promising, there is no doubt that the production of items and medical devices worldwide is growing rapidly, coupled with this is the fact that this is a highly competitive industry and has a relationship of high cost - low volume, reasons why it is important to develop new technologies to production, because given their high costs are often far from the reach of those most in need.

The manufacture of biomaterials and devices depends on both the application and the availability of raw materials, so if one that manufactures has the potential to provide raw materials and generate the appropriate technology, their production costs, and hence the consumer price, will be decrease.

An important fact to note is that biomedical engineering has enormous potential of development, and that to achieve significant progress is not always necessary to have a dominant technological position because, in many cases, innovation comes from the improvement and integration of already existing technologies.

Among the areas with greatest potential for development are found Bioceramics and Biomechanics, as well as Nano-biotechnology, Microsystems and Micro-Robotics, Biomedical Imaging, Bioinformatics, Medical Instrumentation and Telemedicine.

Given the broad scope in terms of existing types of biomaterials, in this chapter we focus only in the case of bioceramics and more specifically in the case of calcium phosphates, in their characteristics, their importance and methods of synthesis, as well as the various applications that take place at this time.

This chapter will show different progress made by our research group in the area; from the discussion on different methods of synthesis of calcium phosphates (particularly hydroxyapatite), using in some cases unconventional sources as precursors (such as eggshells, for example) as well as the obtaining of nanoparticles and other nanostructures of hydroxyapatite. Also the obtention of shaped articles made from hydroxyapatite-based composite materials with different forms to be used in the manufacture of artificial prosthesis and replacement of bone tissue as well as improvements in their mechanical properties will be shown.

2. Bone tissue

Bone is specialized tissue that characterizes vertebrates. Bones and teeth are living organisms made up of minerals and tissues, the latter consist of cells, fatty substances, natural polymers (such as polysaccharides, collagen and polyphosphates) and other substances. While the properties of bone tissue, and the proportions of the substances that form them, vary according to different parts of the skeleton, we can consider that contain about two thirds of his weight of inorganic material and a third of organic material in average. So, bone tissue is composed of a mineral phase that occupies about 69% of its total weight, about 9% water and about 22% of an organic matrix, which consists, in turn, mainly of collagen (90-96%).

The mineral phase is composed mainly of microscopic crystals of calcium phosphates, in which the hydroxyapatite (HAp), whose chemical formula is $Ca_{10}(PO_4)_6(OH)_2$, is the most important. Other mineral phases that are present in bone are dicalcium phosphate ($Ca_2P_2O_7$), dibasic calcium phosphate (DCP, $CaHPO_4$), tricalcium phosphate (TCP, $Ca_3(PO_4)_2$) and some amorphous phases of calcium phosphate. There are also other ions such as citrate ($C_6H_5O_7^{4-}$), carbonate (CO_3^{2-}), fluoride (F^-) and hydroxyl ions (OH^-), which can lead to subtle differences in bone microstructure. Finally, there are also some impurities such as magnesium and sodium, traces of chlorine and iron (Park, 1984).

Only both the HAp as well as the DCP are the calcium phosphate phases that are chemically stable at the temperature and pH of the human body (37 ° C and about 7, respectively) (Neuman & Neuman, 1958).
From a biological standpoint, the bones are defined as connective tissue and their function as a structural component of the human body are well known, serves to support, protect delicate parts and organs and provides a connection between the muscles, allowing movement.
From the standpoint of Materials Science, bone tissue is classified as a "composite", in which the mineral phase supports almost all the mechanical loads and the organic phase (collagen) serves as a binding material, also absorbs impacts, providing flexibility to the bone (Miller & Wray, 1971; Natali & Meroi, 1989).
In terms of the microstructure of the mineral phase, the bone can be classified as cancellous (or spongy) or as cortical, resulting in different mechanical properties.
The process of mineralization of bone tissue is very complex and remains largely unknown. The main constituents of the inorganic salts that make bone tissue are present, in the form of aqueous solutions, in the physiological fluid (blood plasma or extracellular fluid) comming from the blood vessels vascularized bone tissue. Under a chemical analysis, the bone has large amounts of complex groups of cations and anions, such as Ca^{2+}, PO_4^{3-} and CO_3^{2-}; other ions present in lesser amounts are Mg^{2+}, Fe^{2+}, F^- y Cl^-. Due at the cellular exchange, are also found small traces of Na^+ and K^+, ascorbic acid, citric acid and polysaccharides, as well as some heavy atoms, such as Ba^{2+}, Sr^{2+} y Pb^{2+} (Ravaglioli & Krajewski, 1992).
The phosphorus and calcium ions promote the formation of salts, primarily amorphous hydroxyapatite and calcium triphosphate, which are dispersed within the organic phase, while once crystallized, the inorganic phase is practically hydroxyapatite, which provides the mechanical features of the bones previously mentioned. Because of this, it is obvious the study of ceramics as potential bone substitutes, and in particular calcium phosphates such as hydroxyapatite.

3. Hydroxyapatite

The term "apatite"applies to a group of compounds (not only at calcium phosphates) with a general formula in the form $M_{10}(XO_4)_6Z_2$, where M^{2+} is a metal and species XO_4^{3-} and Z^- are anions. The particular name of each apatite depends on the elements or radicals M, X and Z. In these terms, hydroxyapatite (HAp) has the molecular structure of apatite, where M is calcium (Ca^{2+}), X is phosphorus (P^{5+}) and Z is the hydroxyl radical (OH^-). This is known as stoichiometric hydroxyapatite and its atomic ratio Ca/P is 1.67. Its chemical formula is $Ca_{10}(PO_4)_6(OH)_2$, with 39% by weight of Ca, 18.5% P and 3.38% of OH.
Hydroxyapatite crystallizes in a hexagonal system, although with some exception in a monoclinic system (Elliot et al., 1973; Kay et al., 1964). The system belongs to the hexagonal space group $P6_3/m$, with hexagonal rotational symmetry and a reflection plane and with cell parameters of a=b=9.418 Å y c=6.884 Å. Figure 1 shows the unit cell of hydroxyapatite.
HAp structure is formed by a tetrahedral arrangement of phosphate (PO_4^{3-}), which constitute the "skeleton" of the unit cell. Two of the oxygens are aligned with the c axis and the other two are in a horizontal plane. Within the unit cell, phosphates are divided into two layers, with heights of 1/4 and 3/4, respectively, resulting in the formation of two types of channels along the c axis, denoted by A and B.

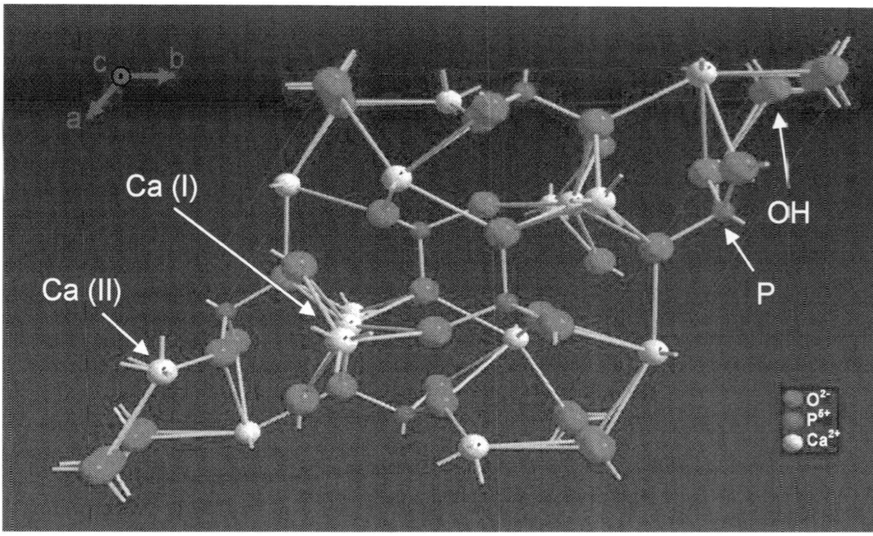

Fig. 1. Crystalline structure of hydroxyapatite.

The walls of channels A type are occupied by oxygen atoms of phosphate group and calcium ions, called calcium ions type II [Ca (II)], consisting of two equilateral triangles rotated 60 degrees relative to each other, at the heights of 1/4 and 3/4, respectively. Type B channels are occupied by other ions of calcium, called calcium ions type I [Ca (I)]. In each cell there are two such channels, each of which contains two calcium ions at heights 0 and 1/2. In the stoichiometric HAp, the centers of the channels type A are occupied by OH radicals, with alternating orientations.

The monoclinic form of HAp is more ordered and thermodynamically stable and is formed at high temperatures, but have never had evidence of its presence in calcified tissues.

Despite being taken to the stoichiometric hydroxyapatite as a model, it is noteworthy that hydroxyapatites produced biologically are much more complicated, they are not stoichiometric, have an atomic ratio Ca/P <1.67 and does not contain only ions and radicals of the HAp but also traces of CO_3, Mg, Na, F and Cl. These amounts vary according at the specific type of tissue, which is related to the properties and bioactivity of it.

One aspect that is important to note is that, the closer the value of Ca/P to 1.67, the greater the stability of the material inside the human body as they tend to be inert, and on the other hand, if this value decreases (deficient HAp), the better the bioactivity.

Another aspect we must consider is the degree of crystallinity. It has been observed that the crystallinity in the tissues for the tooth enamel is very high, while in the cases corresponding to dentin and bone, it is very poor. This means that the reactivity depends on the degree of crystallinity, since the reactivity in dentin and bone is higher than in tooth enamel.

In order to manufacture articles made of hydroxyapatite, it is necessary to take into account, besides the above, that differences in structure and composition of apatites also depend on the different processing techniques, as well as temperature and atmosphere in which are made.

3.1 Quick review on synthesis methods

Different methods of preparation of HAp have been reported (Khon & Ducheyne, 1991; Park, 1984; Ravaglioli & Krajewski, 1992; Yoshimura & Suda, 1994), which may be classified as follows:

i. Solid state synthesis at high temperatures.
ii. Synthesis in aqueous phase.
iii. Hydrothermal methods.
iv. Growth from molten salts.
v. Growth in gels.

Have also been reported other methods, including synthesis by alkoxides, sol-gel and chemical methods, and several procedures for obtaining coatings on various substrates, such as electrochemical deposition, plasma spray methods, etc (Chae et al., 1992; Dhert et al., 1991; Ducheyne et al., 1990).

The solid state synthesis at high temperatures has been generally used for processing ceramic powders and to study the stability of the phases.

Within the aqueous phase synthesis can found hydrolysis, acid-base reactions, in vitro culture, etc. For example, hydrolysis of brushite (DCPD , $CaHPO_4 \bullet 2H_2O$) at temperatures between 40 and 60 °C and at pH of about 8 .(Monma & Kamiya, 1987), or TCP hydrolysis under similar conditions, produce HAp powder. Another method of synthesis of HAp in aqueous phase includes ultrasonic acceleration of the reaction.

With regard to hydrothermal methods, they allow the preparation of well-crystallized powders with homogeneous composition, uniform and easily sintered. This is due to the effects of high temperatures and pressures that are applied to the aqueous solutions ($T > 100°C$, $P > 1$ atm) (Yoshimura & Suda, 1994).

The method of growth from molten salts has been used for the preparation of HAp monocrystals. These crystals grow from the molten phase (with a given composition) at high temperatures, but are severely deformed due to high temperature gradients that occur during growth.

The growth in gels is produced by immersing these in an aqueous system containing Ca^{2+} and PO_4^{3-} ions. The conditions under which it makes are similar to the physiological environment (pH close to 7 and temperatures around 37 °C), although there are reports in which they have used lower or higher temperatures (60 °C) (Castaño et al., 1996; Li, 1992, 1993; Rivera et al., 1997; Rivera-Muñoz et al., 2001, 2011)

Since wet chemistry methods are relatively easy to drive, HAp is synthesized by them often. In particular, since the reactions occur in any living being in aqueous solutions and at low temperatures, many experiments in the preparation of HAp have been performed to investigate the mechanisms of formation of calcium phosphates in vitro and in vivo.

3.2 Applications

Among the main areas of application of calcium phosphates, and particularly the HAp, we have all areas of orthopaedics and orthodontics, where they have to replace, partially or totally, parts of bone tissue.

In the first place we have the applications as filling material for bone. This is where there is greater application mainly because it is not necessary that the material supports high mechanical loads. The idea is to create physicochemical links, between ceramic and surrounding bone tissue, promoting their integration and growth of new tissue (Oonishi, 1991, 1992).

Another factor to consider is the phenomenon called osteoconductive, which occurs in materials with high affinity with bone tissue, which promote the formation of new tissue, but are also capable of directing their growth, depending on the structure they have. It is known that these materials should have high porosity (the order of hundreds of microns) to allow the development of bone within and across them. This property has been used both for filling bone as well as for cement with additives of HAp particles (Castaldini & Cavallini, 1985; denHollander et al., 1991).

Another important application is as a coating of metallic prostheses, which is done to give at the tissues a better suited and recognizable surface, given their characteristics and biocompatibility. Currently it has being working to improve the different techniques to achieve coatings with adequate stoichiometry and thickness. Among these techniques can find: physical and chemical deposition, elecro-deposition, radiation treatments on surfaces, plasma spray, electrophoresis, etc. (Ducheyne et al., 1990; Sendax, 1992; Yoshimura & Suda, 1994).

Due to the reduced of both stability and bioactivity of HAp, a large number of applications have being developed in the field of maxillofacial surgery (Block & Kent, 1992; Jarcho, 1992; Kay, 1992; Trager et al., 1992). Although due to their reduced mechanical properties is primarily used in coatings for dental prostheses and metal plates, for the reconstruction of some cranial bones.

In all cases, these materials provide a surface suitable for cell adhesion, which by enzymatic action remains in a long term.

The in vivo behavior of calcium phosphate implants depends on several factors, among which the most important are the Ca/P ratio, the crystal structure and porosity. The physiological environment may also have a decisive influence on the biological response.

In the case of porous ceramics made of hydroxyapatite, implants are surrounded by connective tissue and osteoids, developing a network structure accompanied by some degree of collapse around the ceramic, unless osseointegration takes place at the implant site (Ravaglioli & Krajewski, 1992).

One of the most important aspects in the application of these materials is the interaction that may exist at the interface with living tissues, both in terms of toxicity, such as dissolution and the active roles that promote the formation of new bone (Ravaglioli & Krajewski, 1992; Park, 1984; Williams, 1991, 1994).

The development of new ceramics today must take into account the compromise between the above aspects, trying to improve the mechanical properties for a better performance of the implants in vivo, and also controlling the level of interaction between the material and surrounding tissue (Hench, 1991).

Taking into account that the devices manufactured with hydroxyapatite for biomedical applications have to withstand mechanical stress, friction and consequently wear, it is necessary to study their mechanical properties as well as its thermal behavior.

Some studies reported that the stoichiometry of HAp plays an important role in the mechanical properties; obtaining better results when the Ca/P ratio is between 1.60 and 1.67. In these studies it reported also that the mechanical strength decreases when the grain size exceeds the 2 microns (Royer, 1993).

Another important aspect is that these properties should be taken into account, both for the synthesis of HAp, as for processing. For this reason, become of vital importance the control of morphology and microstructure during the synthesis process of HAp, as well as the control of manufacture process of parts or objects with mechanical properties suitable for biomedical applications.

4. Some experimental experiences

Different methods of synthesis of hydroxyapatite have been used by our research group. In some cases innovations have been achieved by improving and integrating existing technologies.
As examples, we mention the following:

4.1 Synthesis of hydroxyapatite nanoparticles on silica gels

The method is based on the immersion of silica gels in an aqueous system containing Ca^{2+} and PO_4^{3-} ions. The conditions under which it takes place are similar to the physiological environment (pH close to 7 and temperatures around 37 °C) (Castaño et al., 1996; Li, 1992, 1993).
Silica gels were obtained by the standard method of hydrolysis and condensation of Tetraethyl Orthosilicate (TEOS) in an acidic environment and using different chemical additives for surface modification and control the contraction of the gels during drying process (Rivera et al., 1997; Rivera-Muñoz et al., 2001, 2011).
Chemical additives that were used are monoethylene glycol (MEG), diethylene glycol (DEG) and glycerin. An important aspect is that the catalyst was chosen by considering the application of those gels, i.e. it was used hydrofluoric acid (HF) since the fluoride ion replaces some of the OH^- radicals in the crystal structure of hydroxyapatite, where their positions are not very stable, but since the fluoride ion occupies fixed positions, its chemical stability increases. Besides, it was found that the time of gelation decreases considerably, being the order of minutes, which benefits at the method of synthesis. It is also known that the particle size and pore size is very uniform when the process is carried out under acidic conditions.
Thus, a solution was prepared as a basis for the synthesis of all the gels, dissolved 7 ml of TEOS (Aldrich Chemical Co., analytical grade) in 11 ml of ethanol (EtOH) (Baker Analyzed, reagent grade) and 1.5 ml distilled water under stirring. In this manner, the resulting solution has a composition TEOS: H2O: EtOH of 1:4:6. At this point, start the hydrolysis reaction and to accelerate the process was added 2 ml of hydrofluoric acid (HF) (Baker Analyzed, reagent grade) to 40% by weight and the additive. Under these conditions, the gelation occurs in about 7 minutes.
In addition, different chemical additives monoethylene glycol (MEG, J. T. Baker), diethylene glycol (DEG, Fluka) and glycerin (J. T. Baker, 99.8%) were used. The optimal concentrations correspond to 35 vol% MEG, 35 vol% DEG and 10 vol% glycerine with respect to the ethanol. After one week of slow drying, silica gels were obtained.
It is noteworthy that the whole process was carried out at room temperature, which has implications for energy savings.
After the drying process of silica gels, Simulated Body Fluid (SBF) was prepared by dissolving NaCl, $NaHCO_3$, KCl, K_2HPO_4, $MgCl_2{\bullet}6H_2O$, $CaCl_2{\bullet}2H_2O$ and Na_2SO_4 in deionized water and finally it has ion concentrations nearly equal to those in human blood plasma (Rivera et al., 1997; Rivera-Muñoz et al., 2001, 2011). The growth of hydroxyapatite nanoparticles was promoted by immersing small specimens of silica gels in the SBF at 37°C for six weeks. The SBF was replaced every week to keep constant the Ca^{2+} and P^{+5} ion concentrations.
Samples obtained by this method were characterized to confirm the presence of HAp. Representative results of Energy Dispersive Spectroscopy (EDS), Fourier Transform Infra

red Spectroscopy (FTIR) and X-ray Diffraction (XRD) techniques are showed in Figures 2, 3 and 4, respectively.

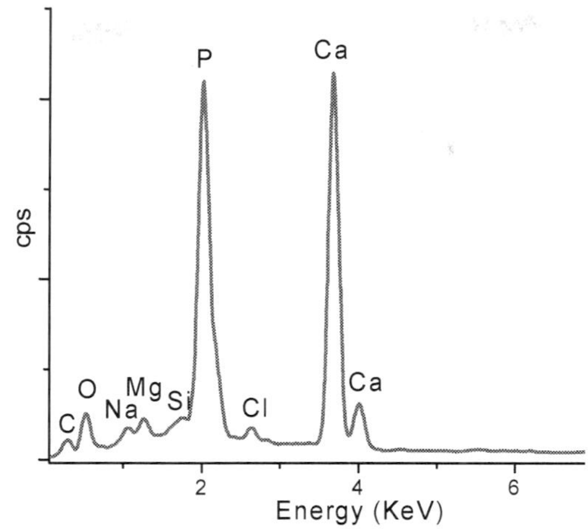

Fig. 2. Determination of the chemical species present in the samples by elemental analysis using energy dispersion spectroscopy (EDS).

Elementary analysis (EDS) results show an average Ca/P atomic ratio of 1.6 and it can be observed the presence of other elementary components in a smaller scale.
A typical Infra Red spectroscopy (FTIR) analysis result is showed in figure 3. Bands at 560–640, 963 and 1028 to 1110 cm^{-1}, correspond to the phosphate group (PO_4^{3-}), and the band at

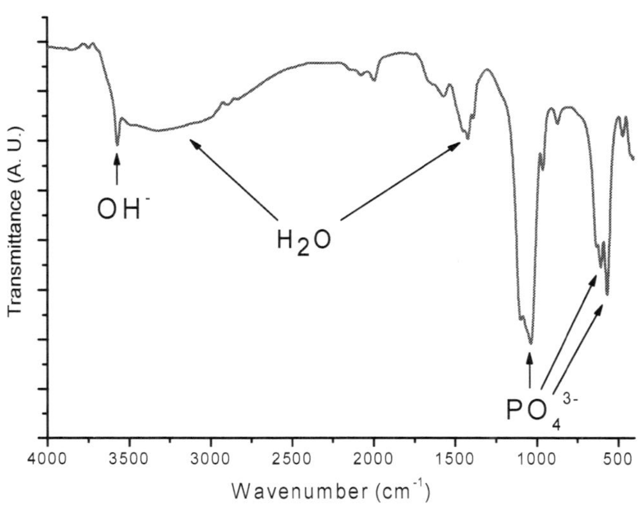

Fig. 3. FTIR spectrum of a sample of silica gel with glycerin extracted from PHS after six weeks. It shows the identification of characteristic bands corresponding to hydroxyapatite.

3572 cm^{-1} corresponds to structural OH^- group; these are typical bands corresponding to the HAp spectrum. These assignments are in agreement with those reported in literature for that phase (Panda et al., 2003).
Figure 4 corresponds to an X - ray powder diffractogram, taken to a sample of silica gel extracted from SBF after six weeks. Reflections corresponding to hydroxyapatite structure are showed and they have been identified by the PDF (JCPDS) file # 09-0432; it also appears a broad peak due to the typical sign of an amorphous material (the silica gel) at an angle 2θ about 22°.

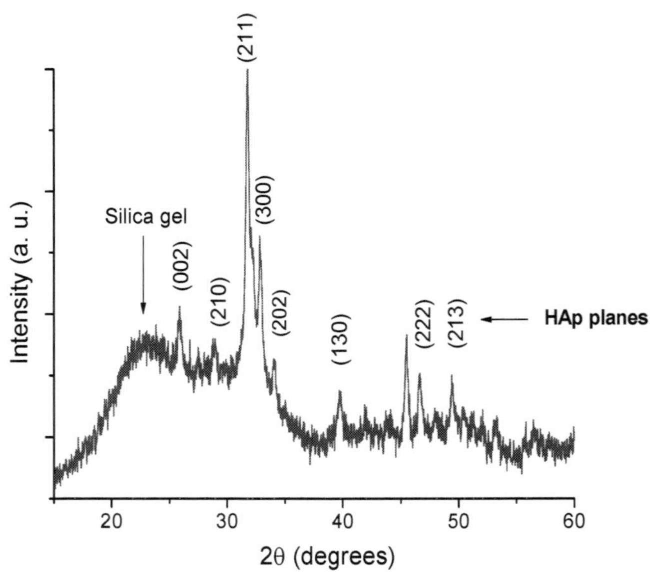

Fig. 4. X-ray diffraction pattern of a silica gel sample removed from PHS after six weeks. It shows the identification of crystalline HAp reflections.

Thus, the results of EDS, FTIR and XRD techniques confirm the presence of hydroxyapatite on the surface of silica gels.
Scanning Electron Micrograph of the surface of silica gel taken after six weeks of soaking into Simulated Body Fluid at 37 °C is showed in figure 5. As it can be observed, HAp nanoparticles grow on the surface of the gel. Those nanoparticles present a spherical-like shape with an average diameter of 800 nm. They can also be observed a few crystals of NaCl and the surface of silica gels.
A more detailed image, as in Fig. 6, shows that those particles are not compact spheres but formed by smaller particles. Thus, the particle size must be adjusted depending on the scale and resolution of the measure instrument. This is an important feature, typical of the structures with fractal geometry.
The presence of those HAp nanoparticles over the surface of silica gels can be explained as follows: it carries out a process of heterogeneous nucleation due to the large surface

area of silica gel as well as abundant and dispersed nucleating centers in the SBF due to the dissolved salts; this process occurs mainly in the liquid and to a lesser extent on the gel surface and this could be attributed to the presence of chemical additives used in the sol-gel process since they affect the liquid-to-solid interface by reducing the interfacial energy as well as stabilizing the gel structure (Brice, 1973; Brinker & Scherer, 1990).

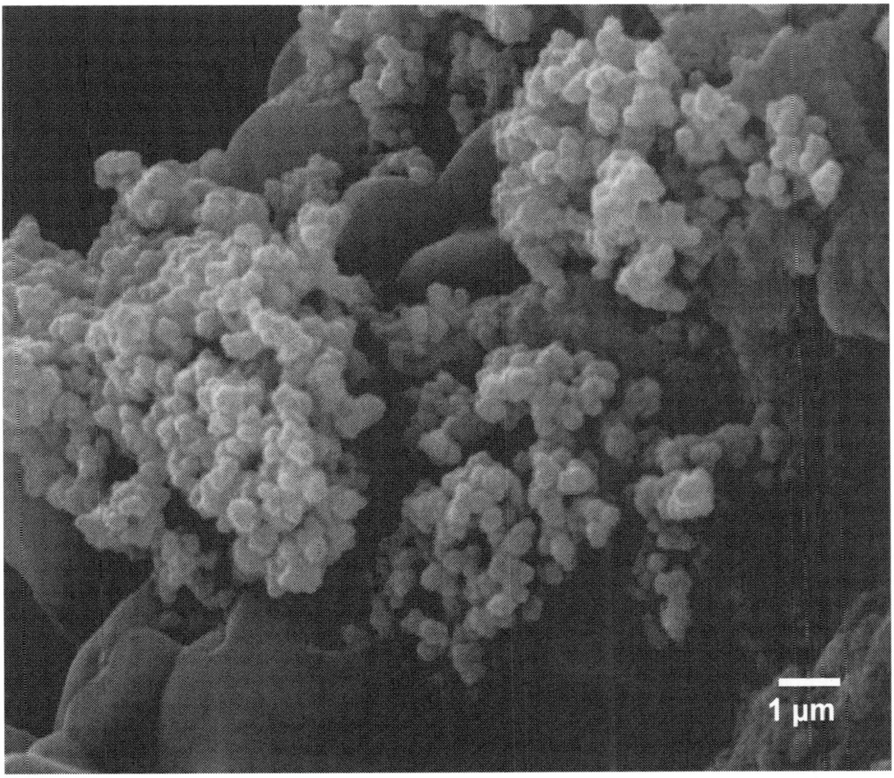

Fig. 5. SEM micrograph of HAp nanoparticles grown on the surface of silica gels.

Finally, the growth of HAp nanoparticles could be carried through a diffusion limited aggregation process (DLA).
In summary, the size and morphology of HAp nanoparticles can be controlled by using chemical additives during the process of obtaining silica gels, as these modify the surface energy of the system, resulting in the nucleation of HAp into the SBF, while growth occurs on the surface of silica gels.
Moreover, since many applications of biomaterials depend, among other factors, of the control of morphology, this work may lead to a wide range of applications in modern biotechnology processes.

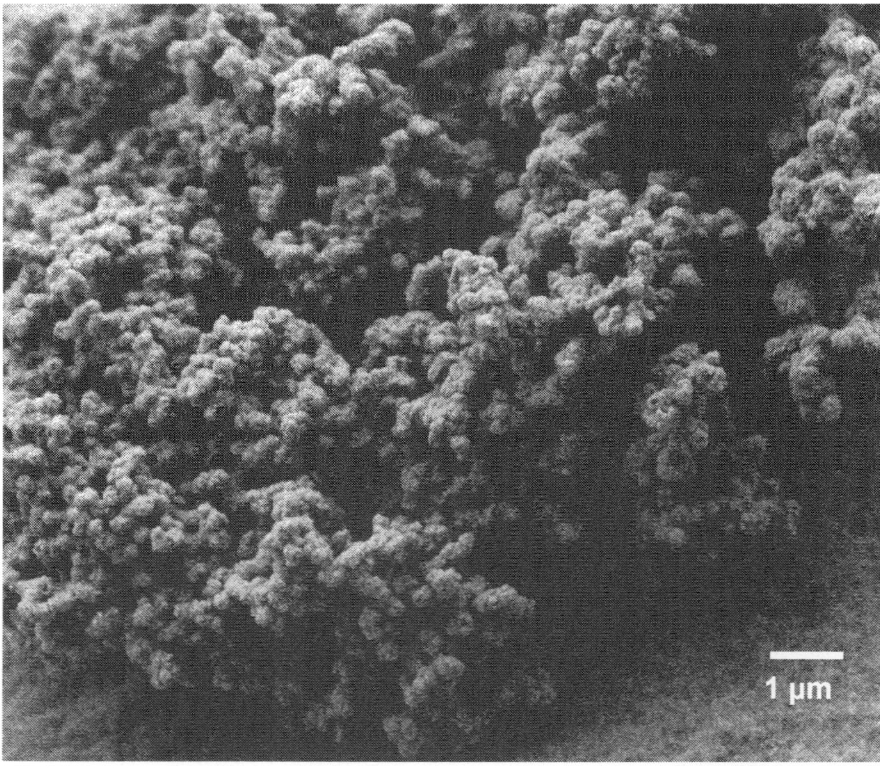

Fig. 6. SEM micrograph of HAp nanoparticles. There is evidence of a texture at an even smaller scale.

4.2 Synthesis of hydroxyapatite from eggshell

An important aspect in the development of methods of synthesis of hydroxyapatite is the use of raw materials from unconventional sources. Here, it is reported the use of eggshells as a calcium source for the synthesis of HAp.

It is estimated that the world's egg production was approximately 6.37×10^7 tons in 2010 (Global poultry trends, 2010). Taking into account that the shell occupies about 11% of the weight of each egg, the amount of eggshells produced in the world in the last year ascends to about 7×10^6 ton.

This material is basically useless after the production of eggs and egg derivatives. Moreover, in many cases, once the egg is used, manufacturers store waste and are then discarded so that it contributes to environmental pollution due to microbial action as a result of the decomposition of organic compounds present in these wastes.

In the best case scenario, the eggshells are used as part of the diet of some animals (chickens) or as fertilizer, although in these cases the benefits are scarce.

This underscores the importance of using these eggshells as a calcium source for the obtention of a useful material, giving an added value to both the material obtained, as well as to the waste coming from human daily activity.
As mentioned, eggshells represent the 11% of the total weight of the egg and it is composed by crystals of calcium carbonate (94%), organic matter (4%), calcium phosphate (1%) and magnesium carbonate (1%).
Figure 7 (a) corresponds to a Scanning Electron Micrograph of the cross section of an eggshell. It shows the spatial arrangement of crystals of calcium carbonate ($CaCO_3$) and its size. It is also noted, in figure 7 (b), that these crystals grow with a preferential crystal orientation in the direction corresponding to the c axis of the unit cell of $CaCO_3$, perpendicular to the surface of the shell; this is because the structure is more stable mechanically in that direction.

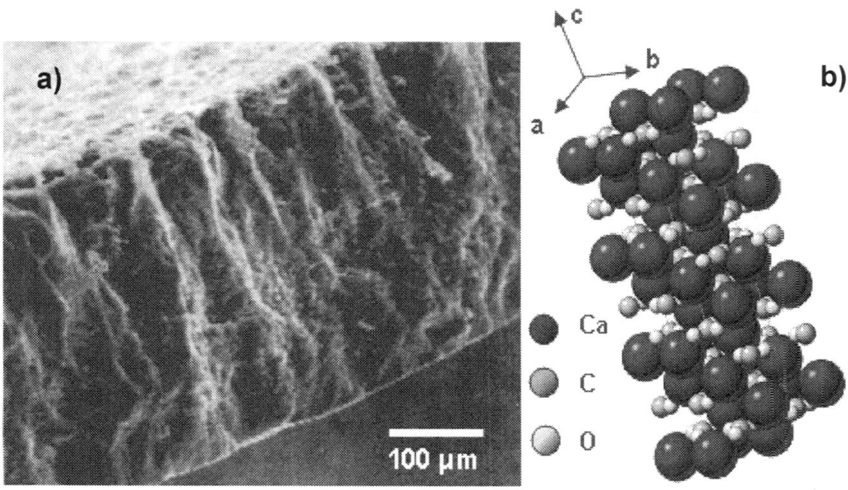

Fig. 7. a) SEM image of the cross section of an eggshell. b) Unit cell of $CaCO_3$

The synthesis method is described in previous works (Rivera et al., 1999; Rivera-Muñoz et al., 2003) and can be summarized as follows: after collecting and mechanically cleaned eggshells, they were subjected to a heat treatment in two stages: the first consisted of heating at a rate of 5 °C per minute to reach a temperature of 450 °C, maintained for 2 hours. At this stage eliminates the organic phase that could be present in the sample. The second stage consisted of heating the samples to reach 900 °C at a rate of 0.5 °C per minute and maintaining this temperature for 2 hours. At this temperature the calcium carbonate transform into calcium oxide through the freeing carbon dioxide according to the following equation:

$$CaCO_3 \rightarrow CaO + CO_2 \tag{1}$$

This was confirmed by X - ray Diffraction analysis (DRX).
The concentration of reagents was calculated taking into account that the Ca/P in the stoichiometric hydroxyapatite is 1.67, so the CaO was transformed into HAp by reaction

with tricalcium phosphate (TCP, $Ca_3(PO_4)_2$). The reaction was carried out at 1100 °C for 3 hours in a moist atmosphere using different heating rates to have control of the species obtained.

In the first place, when the calcium oxide is mixed with water, a reaction between CaO and H_2O takes place to obtain $Ca(OH)_2$. Therefore, this phase is present as initial reactant, as well as during reaction and then hydroxyapatite can be obtained according to the following equation:

$$3Ca_3(PO_4)_2 + Ca(OH)_2 \rightarrow Ca_{10}(PO_4)_6(OH)_2 \quad (2)$$

At end of process, HAp is obtained and small amounts of monetite ($CaHPO_4$) and unreacted CaO. This was confirmed by performing X - ray Diffraction analysis (DRX).The relative amount of HAp obtained can be controlled depending on the heating rate during heat treatment and the presence of monetite as an impurity can be explained by the simultaneous occurrence of the following reactions:

$$6CaHPO_4 + 4CaO \rightarrow Ca_{10}(PO_4)_6(OH)_2 + 2H_2O \quad (3)$$

$$6CaHPO_4 + 4Ca(OH)_2 \rightarrow Ca_{10}(PO_4)_6(OH)_2 + 6H_2O \quad (4)$$

In summary, it is possible to obtain hidroxyapatite from eggshell as unconventional source of raw material. It is also possible to control the relative amount of different calcium phosphate species by controlling the heating rate during the reaction.

Finally, it is important to highlight the fact that it was used a waste material to produce a useful material with great potential for the biomedical industry, adding a high value to the process described and a valuable alternative, both in egg product-derived industry (in waste management and also by reducing environmental pollution), as well as in the industry of biomaterials.

4.3 Molding of objects with different shapes and improvement of their mechanical properties

As previously mentioned, in addition to the development and improvement of different methods of synthesis of hydroxyapatite, is important to develop new processing methods to obtain HAp-based objects with specific shapes for use as potential bone tissue substitutes or in the manufacturing of prostheses.

In addition, once shaped, these objects must have adequate mechanical strength according to the appropriate application, so that it becomes necessary to develop innovative technologies for improving their mechanical properties.

There are different methods in the processing of ceramics, which can be divided in general into three stages: a mixing step, a step of cold-molding and consolidation phase. Within the cold-molding step it can be include pressure molding, slip casting, electrophoresis, extrusion and injection, among others.

One method, called "gelcasting", has been developed to obtain objects with almost any geometry when working at low temperatures and high load of solids (up to 60%), with low amounts of solvents and polymers (Omatete et al., 1991).

The gelcasting method is based on the synthesis of ideas from the traditional processing of ceramics and polymer chemistry. The basis of the process is the use of a monomeric solution, which can be polymerized *in-situ* to form a strong crosslinked structure in the form of gel, the monomeric solution provides a low viscosity vehicle which supports the ceramic powders and allows their handling. The crosslinking provides a mechanism for permanent immobilization of the ceramic mixture into the desired shape after being poured into a mold. Because the vehicle consisting of monomer solution to form the gel contains only 10 to 20% by weight of polymer, the solvent can be easily removed from the structure through a drying process and the crosslinked polymer can not migrate with him. The part corresponding to polymer can then be removed by burning at temperatures between 400 and 900 °C, depending on the product used, and finally, the obtained green body is subjected to sintering and densification process by various heat treatments.

Gelcasting method has several advantages over the traditional (such as slipcasting): the process is faster in green body formation, the polymerization can be performed *in situ*, the molds used may be metal, glass, plastic or wax and need not be scrupulously cleaned before reuse, and finally, the green body obtained is consistent enough to be easily handled.

The essential components of gelcasting method are: ceramic powders, organic monomers, a polymerization initiator, a dispersant and a solvent. With ceramic powders, solvent, dispersant and the binder is prepared a mixture of liquid consistency. The binder usually consists of organic monomers, the initiator or catalyst is added to the mixture before the molding stage. Then the mixture is poured into the mold and it takes place the gelation process, after which the ceramic keeps the final shape. At this point is obtained a green body and the solvent is removed by drying. The plastifier is then burned and finally the ceramic is subjected to a process of densification by thermal treatment.

The principal modifications to the gelcasting method, which led to the "modified gelcasting process", reported by our research group (Rivera-Muñoz et al., 2001b, 2003, 2007) consists of: 1) The use of polymers to form an interpenetrated network, that supports HAp ceramic particles and takes the form of the mold, and 2) The introduction of a pore-forming agent to promote controlled porosity, without changing the structural characteristics of the finally molded article.

Modified gelcasting process (MGCP), described in previous works (Rivera-Muñoz et al., 2001b, 2003, 2007) can be summarized in figure 8.

As shown in figure 9, it can be molded objects with almost any kind of shape through this method. In fact, we have previously reported the production of porous HAp spheres for use as prosthetic eyeball (Rivera-Muñoz et al., 2001b).

Once obtained porous HAp objects, molded with different shapes, as mentioned in section 3.2., it is vitally important to have control of manufacture processes of parts or objects so they have mechanical properties suitable for biomedical applications.

According to the previously mentioned, from the standpoint of Materials Science, bone tissue is classified as a "composite material", in which the mineral phase supports almost all the mechanical loads and the organic phase (collagen) serves as a binding material, also absorbs impacts, providing flexibility to the bone. So we introduce an organic phase to the system to mimic the conformation of actual bone tissue.

With the inclusion of the second phase was obtained an organic-inorganic composite material in which the inorganic part form a porous structure (made of HAp), while the organic phase is chemically attached to it, forming a flexible matrix.

Figure 10 corresponds to a SEM micrograph of a porous sample, made of HAp through the MGC process. Micro (and interconnected) porosity can be observed, as well as the sintered HAp particles used to obtain the molded object.

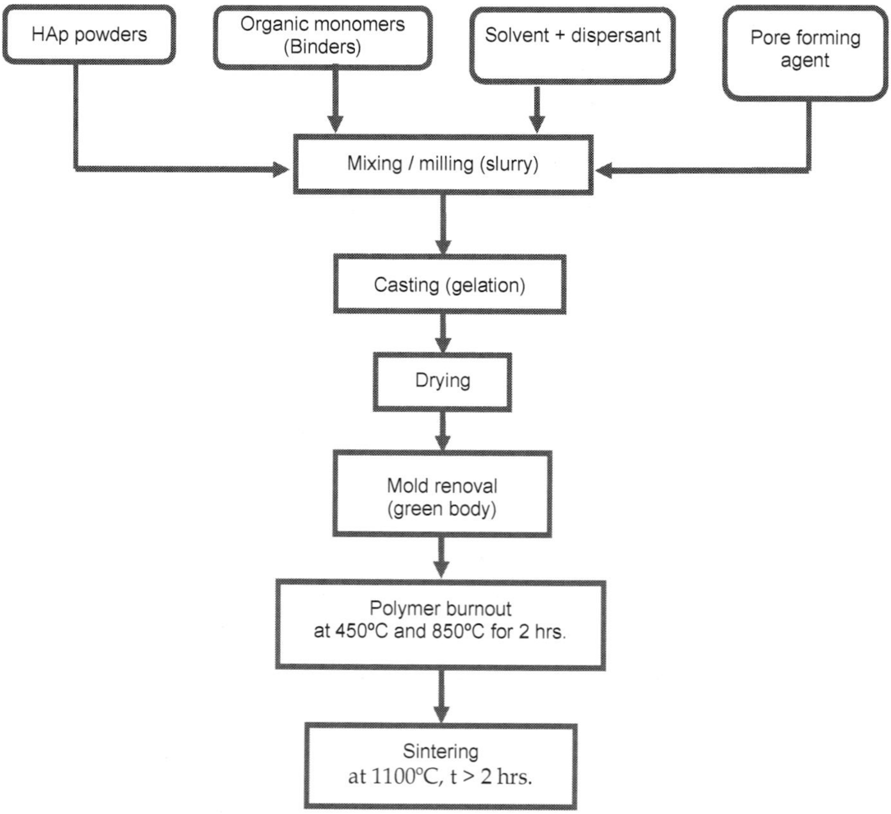

Fig. 8. Modified Gelcasting Process (MGCP) to produce controlled pore size HAp objects.

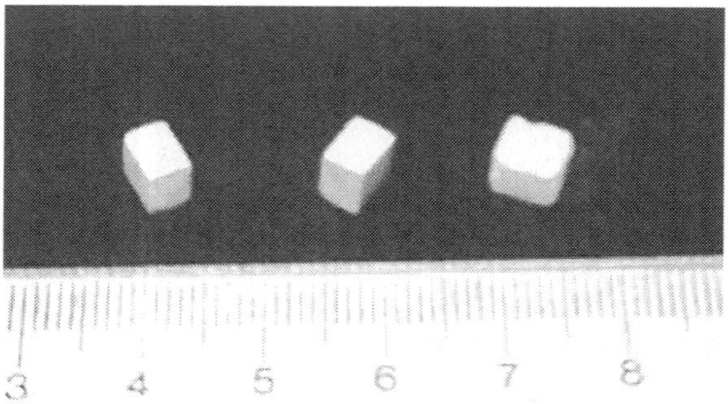

Fig. 9. Molded objects of porous HAp obtained by MGCP (Scale in cm).

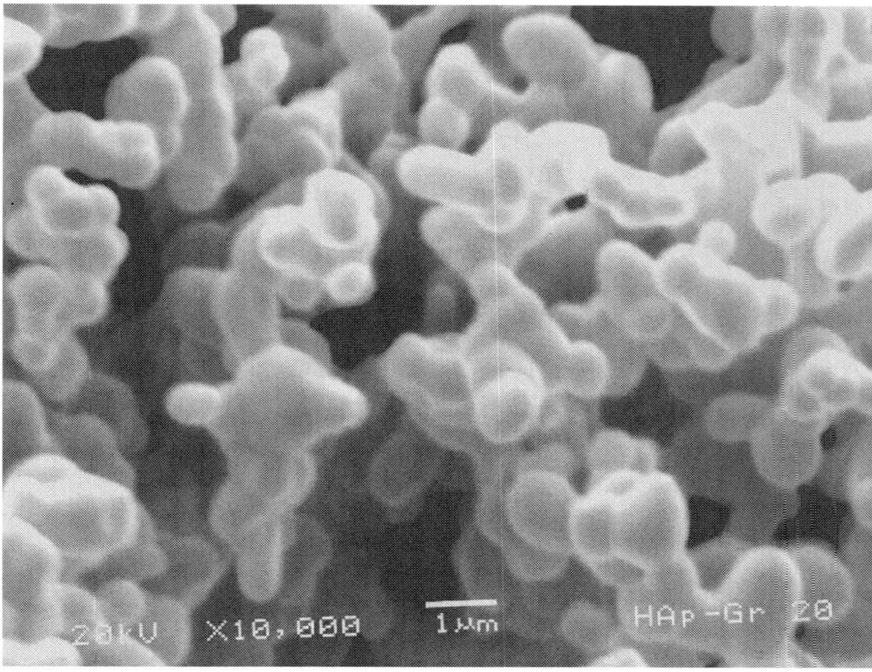

Fig. 10. Scanning Electron Micrograph of a porous sample, made from HAp powders through the Modified Gelcasting Process.

Gelatin was used as the organic phase, primarly because of its similarity to the structure and chemical composition of collagen (as derived from the latter), also due to its ease of handling and processing and, finally, because it is economically affordable.

Figure 11 shows a SEM micrograph of a sample taken after addition of the organic phase. It is observed the integration of the two phases to form an organic-inorganic composite material based on hydroxyapatite.

It is noteworthy that the inorganic structure formed by interconnected pores is connected to one another through the organic phase, showing a cellular-type structure, as in the case of a Voronoi foam, where there are interconnected pores of different sizes in three dimensions.

Once obtained the composite material, it was carried out mechanical testing in compression to study the mechanical behavior of the samples. It was found that the presence of the organic phase significantly improve the compressive strength of the samples. The improvement in these properties was of two orders of magnitude, which indicates a synergistic behavior between the two phases.

Moreover, Figure 12 shows a graph of stress-strain corresponding to a typical result of mechanical compression test performed on composite materials. It notes that the behavior is consistent with a typical non-linear elastic behavior showed by cellular materials and agrees completely with the observations of SEM images showed in figure 11.

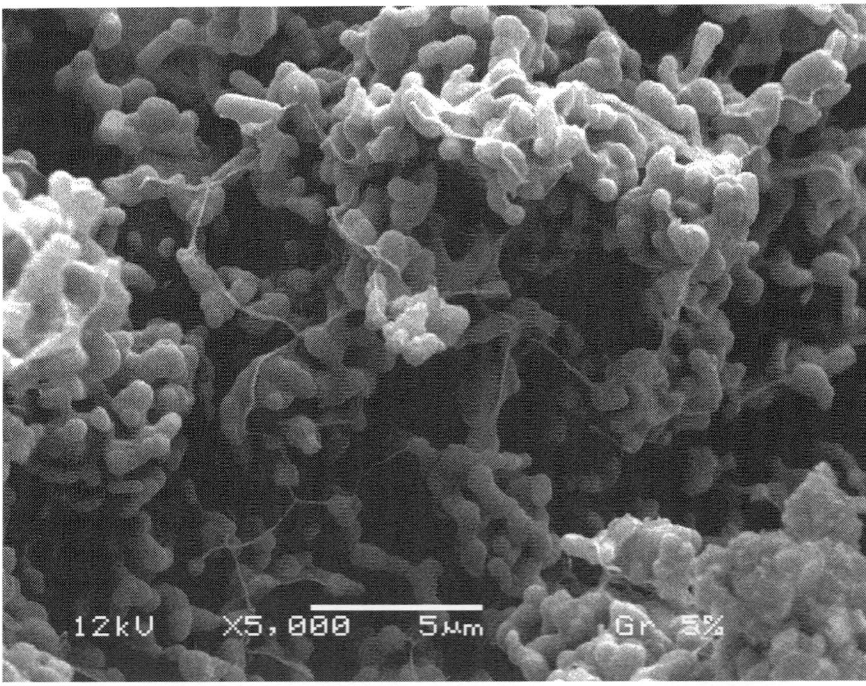

Fig. 11. Scanning Electron Micrograph of a HAp-based, organic-inorganic composite material.

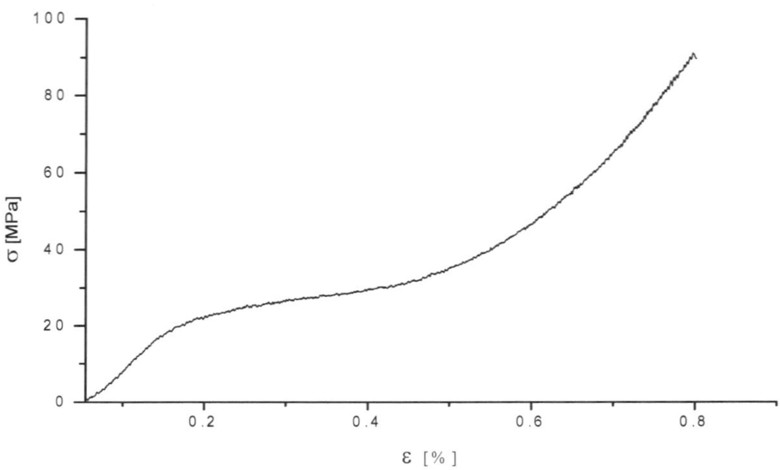

Fig. 12. Typical non-linear elastic behavior of HAp-based, organic-inorganic composites.

Mechanical characterization was performed on samples after MGCP as well as on composite samples with different gelatin concentrations. A dramatic improvement of two magnitude order in compressive strength can be observed in figure 13.

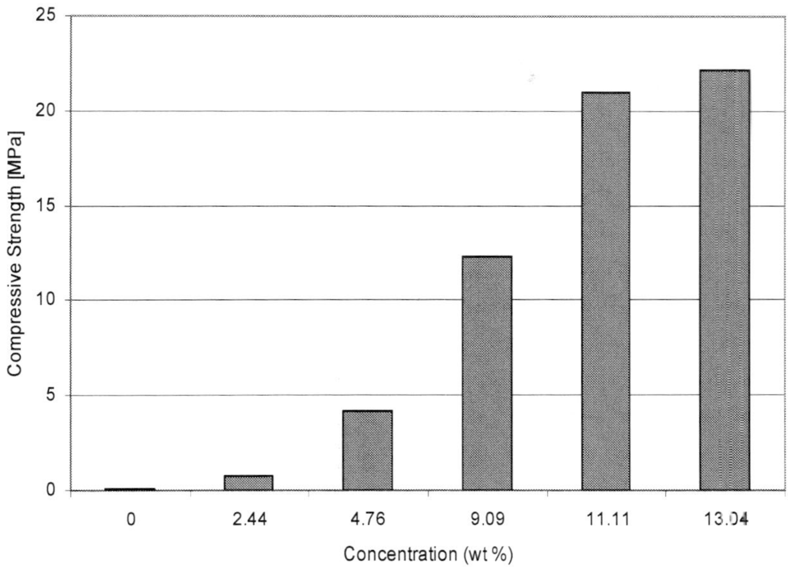

Fig. 13. Improvement of compressive strength with organic phase concentration.

In fact, compressive strength increases with increasing the concentration of the organic phase up to a maximum limit. At that point, the mechanical strength of the composite material is almost 200 times greater than that of the porous material obtained through the MGCP, in which no was added the organic phase. This again is due to a synergistic behavior between the two phases, as occurs in natural bone tissue.

Finally, given some published results on the mechanical strength of natural bone samples, performed under the same conditions as in our samples, we observed: The values reported by Ravaglioli & Krajewski (Ravaglioli & Krajewski, 1992) are: for the compressive strength of trabecular or cancellous bone, of 5.62 ± 2.37 MPa, for cancellous-cortical bone of 15.1 ± 12.6 MPa, while for the cortical bone of 171.67 ± 17.53 MPa. In the case of our samples, they showed a maximum compressive strength of 22.2 ± 5.9 MPa, ie about four times higher than for the trabecular bone and in the same order than the cancellous-cortical bone.

This is a remarkable result, since it opens the door to important applications because we are at a point where it is possible the manufacture of hydroxyapatite-based porous objets, with different shapes using an innovation developed by our group, besides the control, to a large extent, of its mechanical properties. Moreover, the results show that both the structure and mechanical behavior of these composites resemble, to some extent, to the natural bone tissue.

5. Summary

Hydroxyapatite nanoparticles were synthesized on silica gel using various chemical additives introduced during the sol-gel process. Chemical additives used affect the solid-to-liquid interface by reducing the interfacial energy and by stabilizing the structure of the gel. This suggests that the nucleation of hydroxyapatite occurs mainly in the SBF and that growth occurs through a diffusion limited aggregation process (DLA) on the surface of silica gel. By modifying the concentration and type of additive is possible to control both the morphology and the size of the nanoparticles. It was found that these particles show spherical-like shapes, always within the nanometric scale and through smaller-scale observations, shows that consist of even smaller particles, suggesting a fractal-like behavior.

Since many applications of biomaterials depends, among other factors, of the control of morphology, this work may lead to a wide range of applications in modern biotechnology processes, as in the area of dentistry, orthopedics etc., and which highlights the originality of this method, developed in our labs.

In other hand, hydroxyapatite was synthesized successfully by solid state reactions and high temperatures, using eggshells as a calcium source. It was established the optimum conditions for obtaining that calcium phosphate, such as concentration of reagents, reaction temperatures and times, as well as appropriate heating rates in the thermal treatments.

It is important to highlight the fact that it was used a waste material to produce a useful material with great potential for the biomedical industry, adding a high value to the process described and a valuable alternative, both in egg product-derived industry (in waste management and also by reducing environmental pollution), as well as in the industry of biomaterials.

Finally, it was established a procedure for obtaining organic-inorganic composites based on hydroxyapatite with controlled porosity and adequate mechanical strength for use in the manufacture of bioceramics. This innovation was the result of the modification of an existing technology which has been applied to other materials. It was integrated an organic phase so that the composite material obtained has characteristics similar to natural bone tissue: is composed of an inorganic phase consisting of a three-dimensional interconnected pore structure (which supports most of the mechanical loads) embedded in an organic matrix (which gives flexibility to the structure and which also absorbs mechanical energy), showing a synergistic behavior between both phases.

In summary, it has been shown different progress made by our research group in the area of bioceramics; from the discussion on different methods of synthesis of hydroxyapatite, using in some cases unconventional sources as precursors (such as eggshells) as well as the obtaining of nanoparticles of hydroxyapatite. Also the obtention of shaped articles with different forms, made from hydroxyapatite-based composite materials, to be used in the manufacture of artificial prosthesis and replacement of bone tissue as well as improvements in their mechanical properties.

Also important is the fact that any improvement, innovation or development in the area of biomaterials has a positive impact, both from the standpoint of basic science and from the point of view of biomedical applications. That is, there are many beneficiaries: those who are involved in basic science, those who are engaged to research in biotechnology or biomedical engineering, but also the industry and ultimately the greatest beneficiaries will be patients who will be the ones that wear these materials.

6. Acknowledgment

Author wants to thank Dr. Beatríz Millán Malo for technical assistance in X-ray Diffractiometry, M. Q. Alicia del Real López for technical assistance in Scanning Electron Microscopy and Dr. Genoveva Hernández Padrón for technical assistance in Infrared Spectroscopy. Also acknowledges the help of Claudia Medina Ríos and Alejandra Cortez Pérez, students of Biotechnology at the Universidad Autónoma de Querétaro, México. Finally, author thanks the financial support of Project DGAPA-UNAM PAPIITIN107311-3.

7. References

Block, M.S. & Kent, J.N. (1992). "Prospective review of integral implants", In: *The dental clinics of north america, Hydroxyapatite-coated implants,* Vol. 36, No. 1. V.I. Sendax (Ed.), W.B. Saunders Co., Philadelphia, USA.

Brice, C. (1973). *The growth of crystals from liquids, Selected Topics in Solid State Physics,* Vol. XII. North-Holland Publishing Co., USA.

Brinker, C. J. & Scherer, G. W. (1990). *Sol-Gel Science: The Physics and Chemistry of Sol-Gel Processing,* Academic Press, Boston, USA.

Castaldini, A. & Cavallini, A. (1985). "Setting properties of bone cement with added synthetic hydroxyapatite", *Biomaterials,* 6, 50-56.

Castaño, V.M., Suárez, D., Rivera, E., Estévez, M. and Hernández, J.C. (1996). "Growth of hydroxyapatite on silica gels", *Ceram. Trans.,* 53, 49-56.

Chae, J.C., Collier, J.P., Mayor, M.B., Suprenant, V.A. and Dauphinais, L.A. (1992). "Enhanced ingrowth of porous-coated cocr implants plasma-sprayed with ticalcium phosphate", *J. Biomed. Mater. Res.,* 26, 93-101.

den Hollander, W., Patka, P., Klein, C.P.A.T. and Heidendal, G.A.K. (1991). "Macroporous calcium phosphate ceramics for bone substitution: a tracer study on biodegradation with ^{45}Ca tracer", *Biomaterials,* 12, 569-573.

Dhert, W.J.A., Klein, C.P.A.T., Wolke, J.G.C., van der Velde, E.A. and deGroot, K. (1991). "A mechanical investigation of fluorapatite, magnesium whitlockite and hydroxyapatite plasma-sprayed coatings in goats", *J. of Biomed. Mat. Res.,* 25, 1183-1200.

Ducheyne, P., Beight, J., Cuckler, J., Evans, B. and Radin, S. (1990). "Effect of calcium phosphate coating characteristics on early post-operative bone tissue ingrowth", *Bimaterials,* 11, 531-540.

Elliot, J.C., Mackie, P.E. and Young, R.A. (1973). "Monoclinic hydroxyapatite", *Science,* 180: 1055-1057.

Global poultry trends, 2010 (2010), *The poultry site,* www.thepoultrysite.com

Hench, L.L. (1991). Bioceramics; from concept to clinic. *J. Am. Ceram. Soc.,* 74: 1487-1510.

Jarcho, M. (1992). "Retrospective Analysis of hydroxyapatite development for oral implant applications", In: *The dental clinics of north america, Hydroxyapatite-coated implants,* Vol. 36, No. 1. V.I. Sendax (Ed.), W.B. Saunders Co., Philadelphia, USA.

Kay, J.F. (1992). "Calcium phosphate coatings for dental implants: Current status and future potential", In: *The dental clinics of north america, Hydroxyapatite-coated implants,* Vol. 36, No. 1. V.I. Sendax (Ed.), W.B. Saunders Co., Philadelphia, USA.

Kay, M.I., Young, R.A. and Posner, A.S. (1964). "Crystal structure of hydroxyapatite", *Nature* 204: 1050.

Kohn, D.H. & Ducheyne, P. (1991). "Materials for bone and joint replacement" In: *Materials Science and Technology. A comprehensive Treatment., Medical and Dental Materials,* Vol.14. R.W. Cahn, P. Haasen, E.J. Kramer, D.F. Williams (Eds.) VCH, USA.

Lemons, J.E. (1986). "General Characteristics and Clasifications of Implant Material" In: *Pesrpectives on Biomaterials, Materials Science Monographs.* No. 33. O.C. Lin & E.Y.S. Cho, (Eds.). Elsevier, Amsterdam.

Li, P., Ohtsuki, C., Kokubo, T., Nakanishi, K. and Soga, N. (1992). "Apatite formation induced by silica gel in a simulated body fluid", *J. Am. Ceram. Soc.,* 75 {8}, 2094-2097.

Li, P., Ohtsuki, C., Kokubo, T., Nakanishi, K., Soga, N., Nakamura, T., and Yamamuro, T. (1993). "Process of formation of bone-like apatite layer on silica gel", *J. of Mat. Sc. Med.,* 4, 127-13.

Mattox, K. (1992). "The Global Biomaterials Market Where Hard Tissue Biomaterials Fit In" In: *BIOMATERIALS - Hard Tissue Repair and Replacement.* Vol. 3, D. Muster, (Ed.), Elsevier, Amsterdam.

MerketsandMarkets (2010), Global Biomaterial Market (2010 - 2015) http://www.marketsandmarkets.com/Market-Reports/biomaterials-market-report-131.html

Millennium Research Group (2002). "U.S. Markets for Orthopedic Biomaterials 2002", http://mrg.net

Miller, A. & Wray, J.S. (1971). Molecular packing in collagen, *Nature,* 230: 437-439.

Monma, H. & Kamiya, T. (1987). "Preparation of hydroxyapatite by the hidrolysis of brushite", *J. of Mat. Sci.,* 22, 4247-4250.

Natali, A.N. & Meroi, E.A. (1989). "A review of the biomechanical properties of bone as biomaterial", *Biomaterials,* 11: 266-276.

Neuman, W.F. & Neuman, M.W. (1958). *The chemical dynamics of bone mineral.,* The University of Chicago Press., Chicago.

Omatete, O.O., Janney, M.A. and Strehlow, R.A. (1991). "Gelcasting - A new ceramic forming process", *Ceram. Bull.,* 70: 10, 1641-1649.

Oonishi, H. (1991). "Orthopaedic applications of hydroxyapatite", *Biomaterials,* 12, 171-178.

Oonishi, H. (1992). "Development and application of bioceramics in orthopaedic surgery" In: *BIOMATERIALS - Hard Tissue Repair and Replacement.* Vol. 3. D. Muster (Ed.), Elsevier, Amsterdam.

Panda, R. N., Hsieh, M. F., Chung, R. J. and Chin, T. S. (2003). "FTIR, XRD, SEM and solid state NMR investigations of carbonate-containing hydroxyapatite nanoparticles synthesized by hydroxide-gel technique" *J. Phys. Chem. Solids*. 64, 193-199.

Park, J.B. (1984). *Biomaterials Science and Engineering*, Plenum Press, New York, USA.

Ravaglioli, A. & Krajewski, A. (1992). *Bioceramics; Materials Properties and Applications*, Chapman & Hall, London.

Rivera, E., Bonilla, M., Hernández, R., Rodríguez, R. and Castaño, V.M. (1997). "Effect of chemical additives on the growth of hydroxyapatite on silica gels", *Journal of Materials Synthesis and Processing*, 5, 2, 153-167.

Rivera, E., Brostow, W., Díaz, J. R., Araiza, M., Rodríguez, R., Hernández, R. and Castaño, V.M. (1999). "Synthesis of hydroxiapatite from eggshell", *Materials Letters*, Vol. 41 (3) 128 - 134.

Rivera-Muñoz E., Brostow, W. Rodríguez, R. and Castaño, V.M. (2001). "Growth of hydroxyapatite on silica gels in the presence of organic additives: kinetics and mechanism" *Mat. Res. Innovat.* 4: 222–230

Rivera-Muñoz E., Velazquez R. and P. Muñoz-Álvarez (2007) "Mechanical characterization of hydroxyapatite-based, organic-inorganic composites", *Materials Science Forum*, Vol. 539-543: 583-588.

Rivera-Muñoz E., Velazquez R. and Rodriguez R. (2003) "Improvement in mechanical properties of hydroxyapatite objects with controlled porosity made by modified gelcasting process", *Materials Science Forum*, Vol. 426-432: 4489-4494.

Rivera-Muñoz, E. M., Huirache-Acuña, R., Velázquez, R., Alonso-Núñez, G. and Eguía-Eguía, S. (2011). "Growth of Hydroxyapatite Nanoparticles on Silica Gels", *Journal of Nanoscience and Nanotechnology*, Vol. 11, No. 6, 5592 - 5598

Rivera-Muñoz, E., Curiel, R. and Rodríguez, R. (2003). "Selectivity in the hydroxyapatite synthesis from eggshell using different thermal treatments", *Materials Research Innovations*, Vol. 7, 85-90.

Rivera-Muñoz, E., Díaz, J. R., Rodríguez, R., Brostow, W. and Castaño, V.M. (2001). "Hydroxyapatite spheres with controlled porosity for eye ball prosthesys: processing and characterization", *Journal of Meterials Science: Materials In Medicine*, 12, 305-311

Royer, A., Vigure, J.C., Heughebaert, M. and Heughebaert, J.C. (1993). "Stoichimetry of hydroxyapatite: influence of flexural strength", *J. Mater. Sci.: Materials in Medicine.*, 4: 76-82.

Sendax, V.I. (1992). "Postscript: Hydroxyapatite-coated implants", In: *The dental clinics of north america, Hydroxyapatite-coated implants*, Vol. 36, No. 1. V.I. Sendax, (Ed.), W.B. Saunders Co., Philadelphia, USA.

Trager, T., Matrai, J., Gyorgy, J. and Szabo, G. (1992). "Ceramics for dental and maxillo-facial use", In: *BIOMATERIALS - Hard Tissue Repair and Replacement*. Vol. 3. D. Muster (Ed.), Elsevier, Amsterdam.

Williams, D.F. (1991). "Biofunctionality and Biocompatibility" In: *Materials Science and Technology. A comprehensive Treatment., Medical and Dental Materials*, Vol.14. R.W. Cahn, P. Haasen, E.J. Kramer, (Eds.), D.F. Williams, vol. (Ed.) VCH, USA.

Williams, D.F. (1994). "The Science and Applications of Biomaterials", *Adv. Mater. Tech. Monitor,* Vol 1, No. 2.

Yoshimura, M. & Suda, H. (1994). "Hydrothermal processing of hydroxyapatite: Past, present, and future", In: *Hydroxyapatite and Related Materials,* P.W. Brown, B. Constantz (Eds.), CRC Press, Boca Raton.

5

Non Thermal Plasma Sources of Production of Active Species for Biomedical Uses: Analyses, Optimization and Prospect

M. Yousfi, N. Merbahi, J. P. Sarrette, O. Eichwald, A. Ricard, J.P. Gardou, O. Ducasse and M. Benhenni
University of Toulouse, France

1. Introduction

Non thermal and low temperature plasmas in air or in another gas or gas mixtures at atmospheric pressure or at reduced pressure are very efficient sources of active species (radicals, excited species, charged particles, photons emission covering UV up to IR wavelength range, etc.). The case of reduced pressure plasmas where the gas is conditioned into a tight cell with no contact with ambient air can be very interesting for the treatments of more particularly inert material and also for in vitro plasma exposure when it is needed a well controlled gas composition and specific active species for instance without molecular oxygen in order to avoid oxidation processes. The atmospheric pressure plasma in comparison to the lower pressure cases, can be directly used in the ambient air without using any vacuum system and no gas feed but the nature of the active species are not well controlled because this includes many byproducts of the main molecules of air (N_2 and O_2) and also the byproducts of the low concentration species or impurities (H_2O, CO_2, NO_x, ozone, rare gases, etc.). Many applications can be fulfilled from such non thermal plasmas in for instance the domains of gas pollution control (see e.g. Penetrante 1993, Eichwald et al 1998, Dorai 2003, Kim 2004) or surface treatment (see e.g. Kunhardt 2008, Fang 2004 and Bhoj 2008), or plasma actuators (see e.g. Eichwald et al 1998, Moreau 2007). There are also the biomedical applications of low temperature plasmas concerning sterilization and decontamination (see e.g. Laroussi 2002, Villeger et al 2005, Pointu et al 2005, Sarrette et al 2010), engineering of tissues and biomaterial (see e.g. Sardella et al 2008, d'Agostino 2008, Desmet et al 2009) and more recently the field of plasma medicine (see e.g. Fridman et al 2008, Stoffels et al 2008, Morfill et al 2009, Lloyd et al 2010, Wetman et al 2010, Kim et al 2010).

In the sections following this introduction, an overview on several kinds of non thermal and low temperature plasma sources are given in section 2 with a specific emphasis on sources of active species used in our laboratory. Sections 3 and 4 are devoted to the characterization and the possible optimizations of these plasma sources of active species by using experimental diagnostics as well as the different discharge modeling tools experimentally validated and fed by basic data collected or determined in the case of the non thermal plasmas of our interest. In section 5, two illustrative examples of the use of active species at reduced and atmospheric pressure are shown in the field of biomedical applications.

2. Overview on different non thermal plasma sources

An overview on the main kinds of plasma sources that can be used more particularly for biomedical applications will be given in this section with a focus on the plasma sources used in our laboratory (http://www.laplace.univ-tlse.fr/groupes-de-recherche/plasmas-reactifs-hors-equilibre/)

2.1 Flowing afterglow discharge generated at reduced pressure by a microwave source for plasma remote sterilization

In the experimental setup developed in our laboratory for sterilization applications (see e.g. Villeger et al 2005, Ricard et al 2007, Sarrette et al 2010), the discharge is generated by a classical 2.45 GHz microwave surfatron cavity at powers up to 300 W. The microwave plasma is then launched using a gas flow through a small diameter tube up to a Pyrex treatment chamber of 15 cm diameter and 20 cm height. The gas flow could be varied up to 3 l/min and the gas pressure in the reactor is adjustable between 0.1 and 5 kPa by means of a throttle valve above the primary pump. Such conditioned gas at reduced pressure allows the use of different gas compositions as for instance pure N_2, and also gas mixtures such as Ar/N_2, H_2/N_2, or O_2/N_2 following the species required for the sterilization processes as for instance the atomic nitrogen whose the recombination at the surface of the bacteria (see support in Fig. 1a) plays a major role during the sterilization process. In fact, the reduced pressure has the advantage to avoid the volume recombination of atomic nitrogen in the flowing afterglow and also to need a low surfatron power.

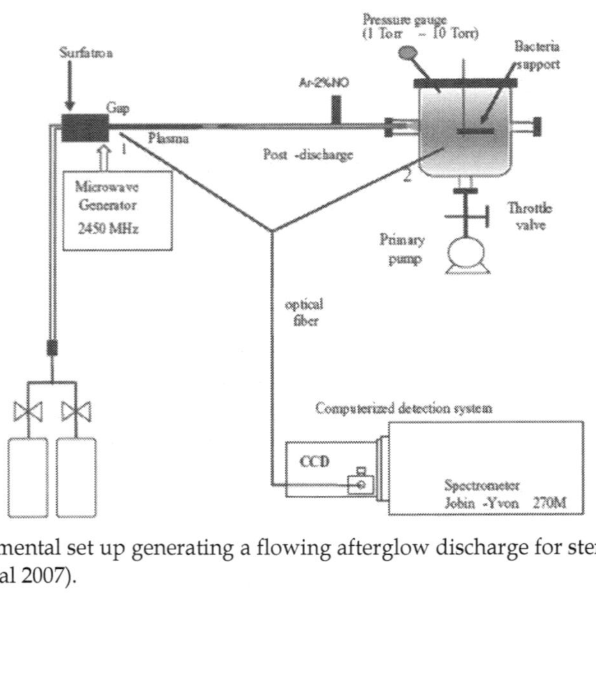

Fig. 1. a. Experimental set up generating a flowing afterglow discharge for sterilization (from Ricard et al 2007).

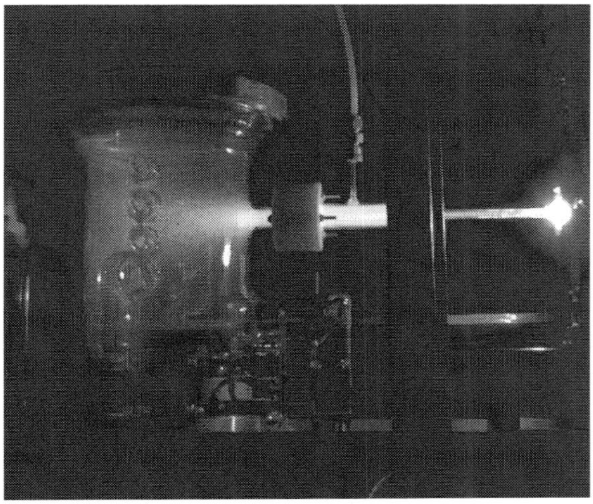

Fig. 1. b. View on the experimental setup generating flowing afterglow discharge (surfatron is on the right side and the treatment chamber on the left side)

2.2 DBD discharge using a mono-polar source

Dielectrics barriers discharges (DBD) are very well known since a long time with one or two electrodes recovered by the dielectric (Fig. 2). The role of the dielectric is to limit the current thus avoiding the gas spark or breakdown. Under such configuration, an alternating or pulsed power supply is generally used in the case of a quite low (a few mm) gap distance (see e.g. Eliasson 1998, Koslov 2005). Generally the DBD power supply is a bipolar source. The polarity inversion at the half period allows to the discharge, stopped by the charge accumulated on the dielectric, to start again. It is worth noting that a mono polar pulsed power was successfully tested in the literature (Liu et al 2001, Laroussi et al 2004) and in our laboratory (Panousis et al 2009). In the case of such a mono-polar power supply, the the discharge occurs alternatively during the increasing part of the pulsed voltage and is inversed during the decreasing one. It is shown that this mono polar system leads to better efficiency of the production of active species than a classical bipolar power supply.

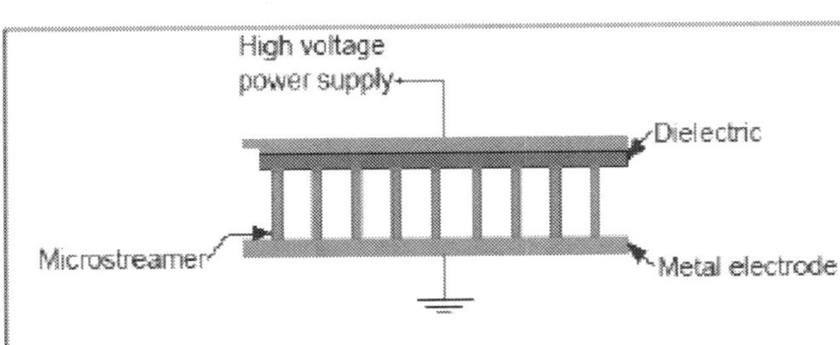

Fig. 2. Schematic view of a DBD discharge with a barrier dielectric on the upper electrode and a filamentary structure which is its usual morphology at atmospheric pressure

2.3 Volume corona discharges for mono and multi-tips

Corona discharges can be generated under many electrode configurations, provided one of which has a curved shape as a tip or a wire, etc. In the case of for instance a positive point-to-plane geometry under DC or pulsed power supply, the discharge can have either a mono-filamentary structure for DC power supply or a branching structure for pulsed power supply (see e.g. Merbahi 2008, Briels et al 2005). Fig. 3a displays the mono- filament and branching cases. The filamentary structure corresponds to a complex streamer dynamics that is analyzed largely in the literature showing that the active species are generated inside the ionized channels during both primary and secondary streamer developments (see e.g. Eichwald et al 2008). Furthermore in order to increase the efficiency of the production of active species it is better to use a multi-tip electrode configuration (Fig. 3b) where it is easy to see in Fig. 4, showing the instantaneous discharge current, that the peak of the corona current and therefore the dissipated power does not increase linearly with the number of the tips.

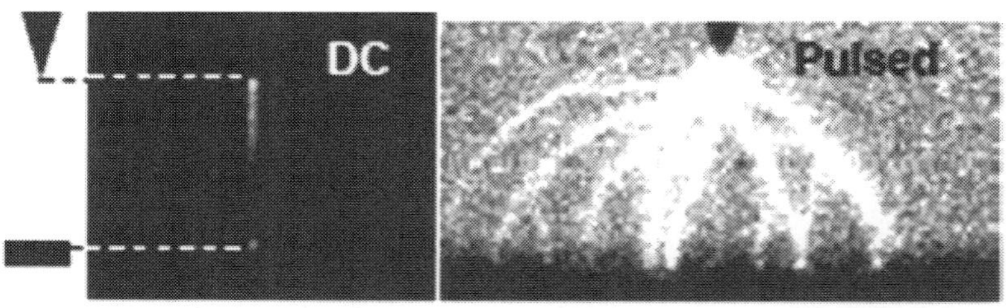

Fig. 3. a. Dc and pulsed corona discharge in a positive point-to-plane geometry (from Abahazem et al 2008)

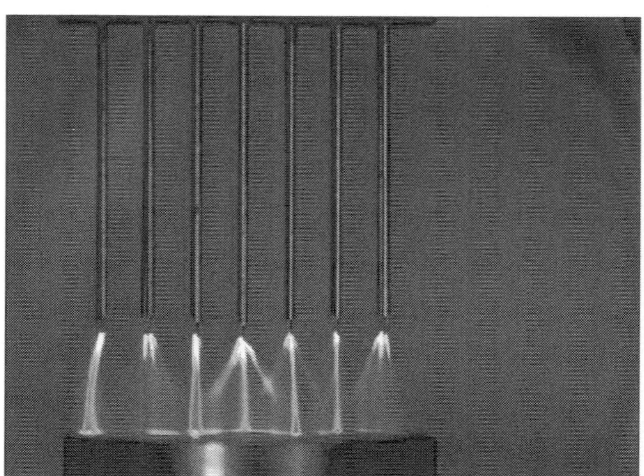

Fig. 3. b. View on a multi-tip pulsed corona discharge tested at LAPLACE-PRHE Laboratory.

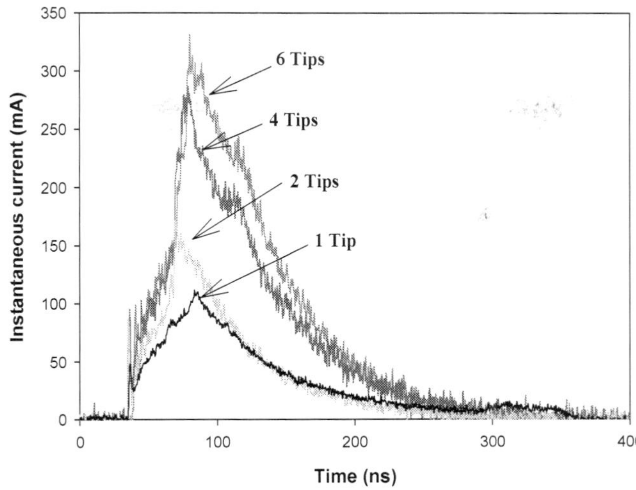

Fig. 4. Corona discharge current in the case of positive point to plane geometry as a function of time for different number of tips (when the number of tips is increased from 1 to 6, the peak current is increased only by a factor 3) from Abahazem et al 2011

2.4 Surface corona discharge

Surface discharges can be generated from many electrode configurations. A specific setup analyzed in our laboratory is displayed in Figs 5a, 5b and 5c (Gardou et al 2009). In such a case, both surface and volume discharges are present as displayed in Fig. 5c and also as already emphasized in the literature (see e.g. Allen et al 2004, Timatkov et al 2005).

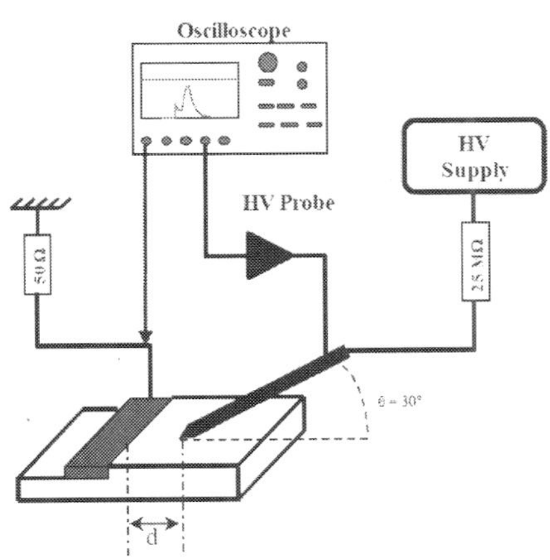

Fig. 5. a. Experimental setup of surface corona discharge with an inclination angle of 30° between the anodic needle and the dielectric surface (d being the gap separation between the tip of the needle and the cathode copper) from Merbahi et al 2011

However, the surface discharge is developed faster with a less energy consuming than its homologous in the volume because the main processes of the discharge propagation is the photo-emission from the dielectric in the case of the surface discharge (see e.g. Allen et al 2004) while it is the gas photo-ionization in the case of the volume discharge. As it is known the surface photo-emission requires less energy (2 or 3 eV) than the gas photo-ionization (e.g. 15.7 eV for N_2). This prefigures a better efficiency of active species production by the surface discharges in comparison to the classical corona volume discharge presented in sub section 2.3.

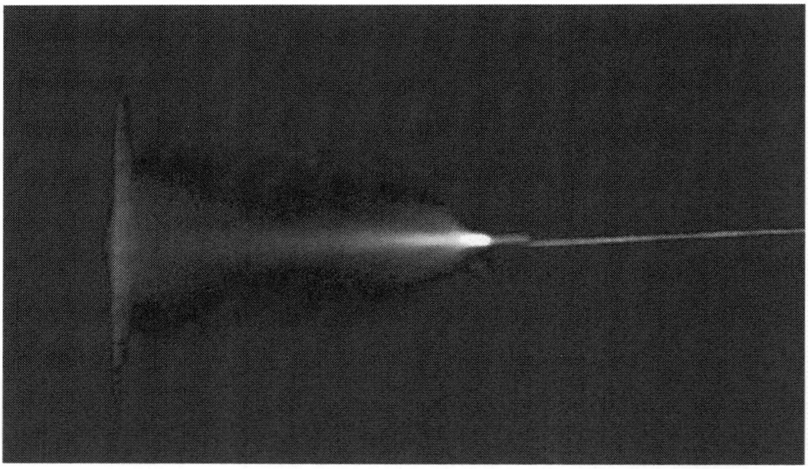

Fig. 5. b. Top view photograph of the corona surface discharge for radius tip ρ =50 µm, d = 13 mm, Uo = 11,5 kV, (cathode is on the left side, anodic point on the right side) in the case of PMMA insulator (from Gardou et al 2009).

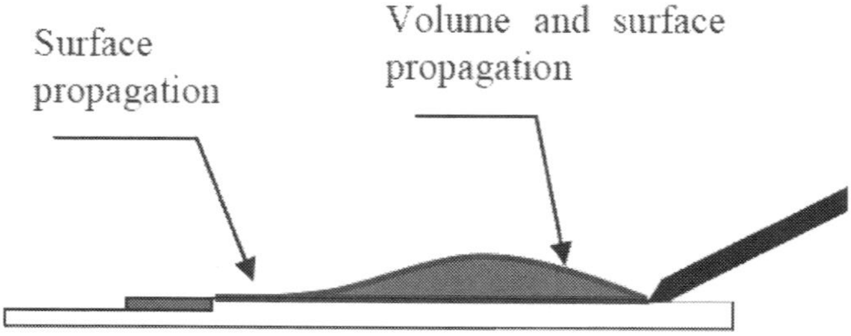

Fig. 5. c. Schematic cross section of the surface discharge in the case of PMMA insulator from (Gardou et al 2009).

2.5 Atmospheric pressure plasma jets

There are in the literature many devices developed to produce a low temperature plasma jet more particularly for biomedical uses as emphasized in for instance the review of Laroussi

2007. Plasma jet at atmospheric pressure allows a remote treatment very convenient for instance for in vivo treatment where it is dangerous to put the living tissue inside the zone of plasma generation. Plasma jet is also very interesting for biomaterial treatment more particularly when it is needed for instance to immerse the biomaterial in water for a treatment under hydrated form. There are many examples of plasma jet devices as for instance Plasma needle (Kieft 2005), plasma pencil (Laroussi 2005), plasma brush (Duan 2005) and other setups of plasma jets driven by various power supplies (DC or AC or RF and also micro-wave sources). Such plasma devices produce generally low temperature plasmas using various gas compositions and electrode configurations. In most cases, the plasma is launched outside the generation zone with the help of an external imposed continuous gas flow.

A specific low temperature plasma jet already used for the collagen treatment (Delaunay et al 2011) has been developed in our laboratory (see the patent of Merbahi et al 2011). The measured plasma temperature on the top of this specific plasma jet, that has a length of about 1 cm, does not exceed 27°C. This plasma jet shown in Fig. 6a is generated directly in the ambient air at atmospheric pressure and launched by itself without any external system of gas inlet feed that making it very easily transportable because there is neither gas bottle nor gas pumping (Merbahi et al 2011). It is generated by a specific corona discharge design giving a natural repetitive discharge current with a frequency of about 20 kHz under a high voltage power supply. Fig. 6b displays the instantaneous discharge current and the applied voltage that corresponds to a dissipated power of about 100 mW to generate the plasma jet. The UV-visible spectrum corresponding of the light emission of the top of the air plasma jet is displayed in Figs. 7ab. This shows the classical emission bands of Nitrogen such as the Second positive system (SPS) of $N_2(C^3\pi_u)_v \rightarrow N_2(B^3\pi_g)_{v'}$ from about 290 nm up to 440 nm corresponding to the different vibration states v and v'(for instance see the peaks at 315.93 nm, 337.13 nm, 357.69 nm, 375.54 nm and 380.49 nm). The first positive system (FPS) $N_2(B^3\pi_g) \rightarrow N_2\ (A^3\Sigma_u^+)$ which is apparent in the visible-near infrared (between about 600 nm up to 900 nm) range indicates this radiative way of the formation of metastable $N_2\ (A^3\Sigma_u^+)$ states. However, $N_2\ (A^3\Sigma_u^+)$ can be in turn quenched by the air species following several reactions given with their reaction rates (Herron, 1999):

$$N_2\ (A^3\Sigma_u^+) + O_2 \rightarrow \text{prod}\ (2.5\ 10^{-12}\ cm^3s^{-1})\ ;$$
$$N_2\ (A^3\Sigma_u^+) + O \rightarrow \text{prod}\ (2.5\ 10^{-11}\ cm^3s\text{-}1)\ ;$$
$$N_2\ (A^3\Sigma_u^+) + N \rightarrow \text{prod}\ (4.4\ 10^{-11}\ cm^3s^{-1})\ ;$$
$$N_2\ (A^3\Sigma_u^+) + NO \rightarrow N_2 + NO(A^2\Sigma^+)\ (6.4\ 10^{-11}\ cm^3s^{-1}),$$
$$N_2\ (A^3\Sigma_u^+) + H \rightarrow \text{prod}\ (2.1\ 10^{-10}\ cm^3s^{-1})\ ;$$
$$N_2\ (A^3\Sigma_u^+) + OH \rightarrow N_2 + OH(A^2\Sigma^+)\ (10^{-10}\ cm^3s^{-1})$$

The detection of the first negative system (FNS) of $N^+_2(B^2\ \Sigma_u^+) \rightarrow N+2(X^2\ \Sigma_g^+)$ around 390 nm is synonymous of high electron energies leading to the ion formation. However, concentration of positive nitrogen ion is probably very low due to the very small intensity of the FNS emission. There are also the oxygen emissions at for instance 759 nm coming from the band $O_2(b^1\Sigma^+_g\ v=0) \rightarrow O_2(X^3\Sigma^-_g, v=0)$ and the atomic line of the triplet state of O at 615 nm and 777.47 nm.

The NOγ bands due to the emission of $NO(A^2\Sigma^+)_v \rightarrow NO(X^2\ \pi)_{v'}$ synonymous of dissociation of molecular nitrogen and oxygen leading to NO formation, (usually observable in classical corona discharges in quasi-pure N_2) are not observable in our plasma jet ambient air between about 200 nm up to 290 nm due to the quenching of NOγ bands by the molecular oxygen following the reaction: $NO(A^2\Sigma^+) + O_2 \rightarrow NO(X^2\pi) + O_2$ (10^{-10} cm^{3}s-1) with a rate coefficient that is 1000 times higher than the $NO(A^2\Sigma^+)$ quenching by N_2 (10^{-13} cm^{3}s^{-1}).

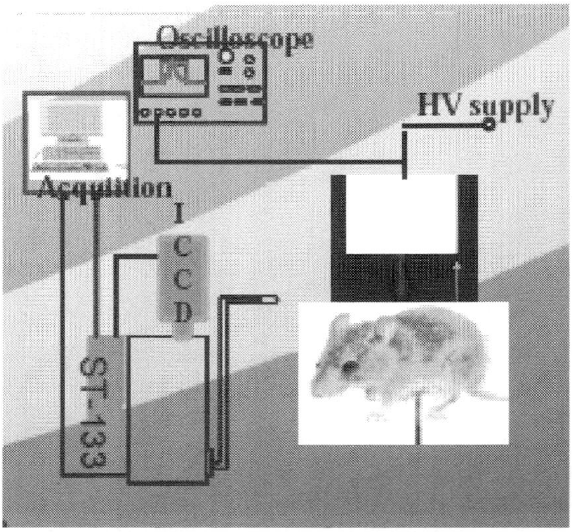

Fig. 6. a. Schematic view on the low temperature plasma jet generated in ambient and atmospheric pressure air.

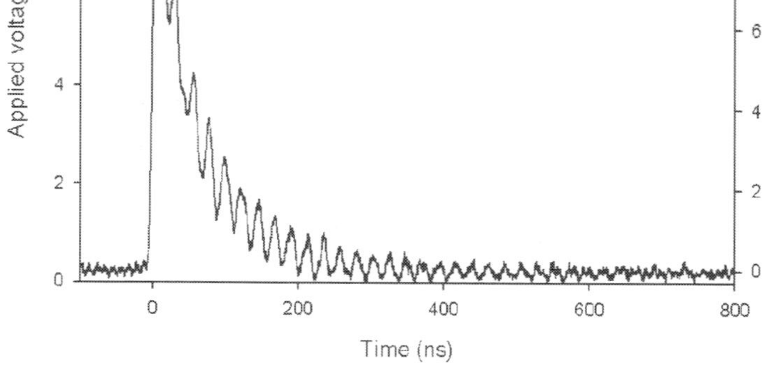

Fig. 6. b. Time evolution of the current of corona Discharge generating the plasma jet

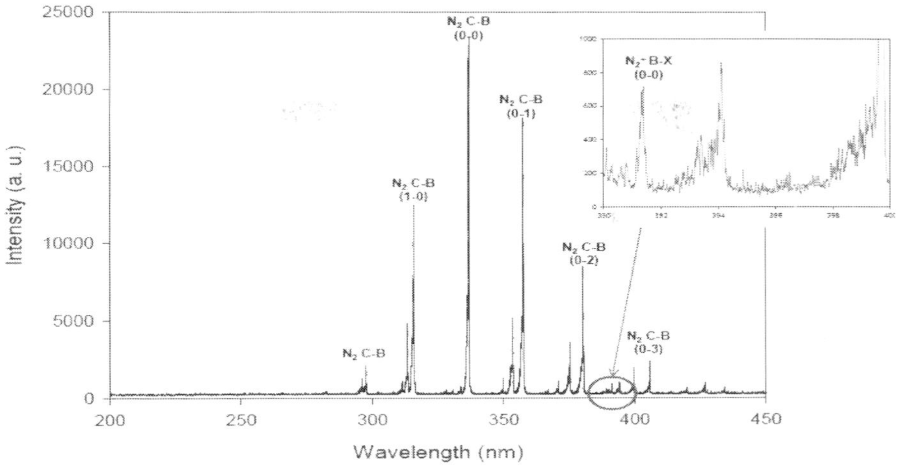

Fig. 7. a. UV-visible spectrum in the 200 nm-450 nm range collected in the top of the plasma jet.

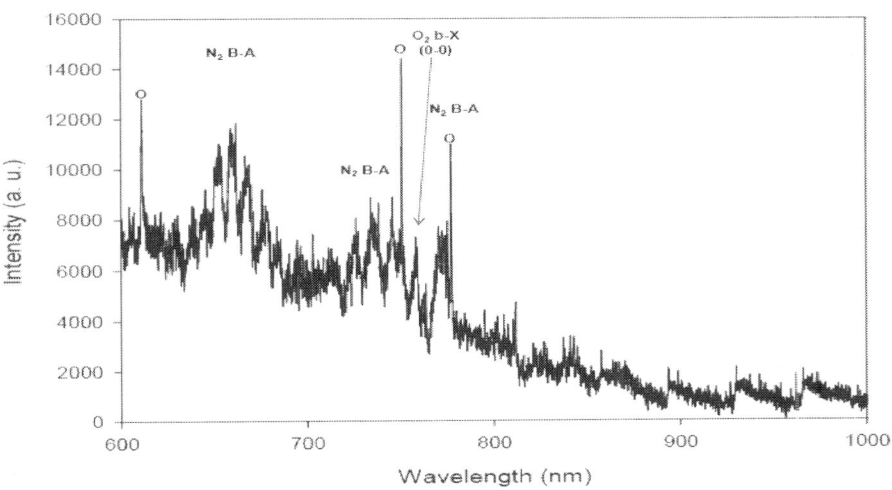

Fig. 7. b. UV-visible spectrum in the 600 nm-1000 nm range collected in the top of the plasma jet. NB: Between 450 nm up to 600 nm no significant emission has been observed.

The same remark is true for the $OH(A^2\Sigma^+) \rightarrow OH(X^2\pi_{3/2})$ emission bands between about 300 nm up to 320 nm coming from the dissociation of water vapor impurities present in ambient air and not observed due to the quenching by molecular oxygen following the reaction: $OH(A^2\Sigma^+) + O_2 \rightarrow OH(X^2\pi_{3/2}) + O_2$ with a rate coefficient that is roughly 10 times higher than the $OH(A^2\Sigma^+)$ quenching by N_2.

In fact, the absence of emissions of NOγ and OH(A-X) can also be attributed to the quenching of metastable state N_2 ($A^3\Sigma_u^+$) that contributes in complement of electron collisions to the formation of the upper states of these two emission bands.
This overview on plasma jet spectrum means that the excited species present on the top of the jet are at least those involved by the emission bands from $N_2(C_3\Pi_u)_v$, $N_2(B_3\Pi_g)_{v'}$, $O_2(b^1\Sigma^+_g$ v=0), N_2 ($A^3\Sigma_u^+$) and O* after electron collisions with O_2 and O. Due to the kinetics of formation of such excited species, it is obvious that we have also another metastable states of molecular nitrogen and oxygen, and also dissociation products of air such as the atomic nitrogen N and even the atomic hydrogen.
There are certainly another active species in the present ambient air plasma jet but they are not observable in the optical emission spectrum of Figs. 7ab due to mainly the quenching processes or to emission outside the present wavelength range (for instance specific atomic lines of nitrogen are in the VUV range less 200 nm and in the IR above 1000 nm).

3. Diagnostic tools for analysis and identification of active species

Dielectric barriers and Corona discharges generating non thermal plasmas in air or in other gas or gas mixtures at atmospheric pressure usually develop following streamer discharges having a thin filamentary structure (a few tens of μm wide) which propagates during a short time scale (a few tens of ns). A steady state glow discharge with a diffuse structure results at atmospheric pressure only from specific operating conditions (as e.g. a given frequency of the power supply and/or a chosen nature of the used dielectric and/or a specific gas composition: see e.g. Kelly-Wintenberg et al 1998).
Due to their short time and space scales, the streamer discharges are not easy to experimentally analyze and characterize in order to better know and to optimize these sources of active species. For these reasons, a large variety of plasma diagnostic tools covering optical, chemical and electrical methods are needed (see e.g. Creighton 1994, Ono et al 2005). These experimental tools can obviously be used for low temperature and non thermal plasmas generated at atmospheric pressure and also at reduced pressures. These experimental tools can be summarized as follows:

- OES (optical Emission spectroscopy) to detect radiative species with their temperature (see e.g. Ricard 2005, Zhao et al 2007)
- Absorption spectroscopy and FTIR (Fourier Transform Infra Red) spectral analysis to determine the species concentration (see e.g. Gorry et al 2007, Nair et al 2007)
- Laser spectroscopy such as LIF (Laser Induced Fluorescence) or TALIF (see e.g. Marchal et al 2010) to obtain the spatio-temporal evolution of the species concentration even at low proportion using CRDS (Cavity-Ring Down Spectroscopy)
- CARS (Coherent Anti-Stokes Raman Spectroscopy) for distribution of vibration molecules (see e.g. Oda et al 2006, Srivastava 2009, Stancu 2009)
- Image intensifier with CCD for spatial discharge structure analysis and streak camera for spatio-temporal analysis (see e.g. OCHKIN et al 1998, KEMPKENS et al 2000)
- Schilieren photography to visualize neutral gas variation and heat transfer from streamers to gas (see e.g. WINANDS et al 2006, Ohyama et al 2007)
- Mass spectroscopy to detect various ions and the stable radicals and neutrals, (see e.g Held et al 1999, EBELING et al 2000)
- Gas chromatography to analyze stable oxide evolution before and after gas treatment (see e.g. CASANOVAS et al 1992)

- Electric measurements (voltage and current) to analysis electric behavior and to deduce energy discharge consumption (see e.g. Abahazem et al 2008, Merbahi et al 2008), etc.

4. Modeling tools for optimization of the source of active species

4.1 Overview on the different models

On the other hand, plasma modeling is also required to better understand and to optimize the formation and the behavior of our sources of active species. Plasma modeling and simulations which are very complementary tools to the experimental ones have generally the following main goals:

- a better understanding of basic phenomena and processes
- a good prediction of the plasma properties from validated models
- a reliable tool to research the optimal operating conditions for the plasma devices

Non thermal plasma modeling can concern a large variety of processes and phenomena contributing to the formation of active species and occurring during the discharge development and also during the post discharge stage. There are in the literature a lot of research works already devoted to modeling and simulations of the discharges or post discharge stages. A recent review on plasma modeling can be found in the paper of Lee et al 2011. However plasma modeling is generally undertaken without considering the strong coupling between the different models of for example streamer dynamics, gas dynamics, chemical kinetics and electrical circuit as it is summarized in the flowchart of Fig. 8. In fact when the streamer discharges develop and propagate, a streamer dynamics model is required to describe the spatio-temporal evolution of the streamer characteristics both in the streamer head and channel. The electric circuit model can give the input data for the streamer dynamics model. In the ionized channel left behind the streamer, there are a complex gas dynamics (gas pressure waves with gas density and temperature variations) influenced more particularly by the relaxation of excited species (metastable and vibration) which play the role of an energy tank: this is described by the gas dynamics model including the relaxation of excited states, the Joule effect corresponding to the energy transferred from electrons to the gas and the momentum transfer from ion towards neutral gas (ionic wind). A chemical kinetics model is also needed to describe the complex and various plasma chemistry involving the different active species whose the evolutions are initially affected by the streamer development and then are durably influenced by the local gas dynamics (gas temperature and density variations: see e.g. see e.g. Eichwald et al 2002). As it is shown in the flowchart of Fig. 8, each model is directly linked to the basic data models and therefore absolutely needs at its input the most reliable basic data in order to have the most reliable results.

In fact in our case of non equilibrium discharge at atmospheric pressure, the results of plasma models are first very sensitive to a lot of mathematical and numerical choices, approximations and parameters as for example:

- the good choice of the physical model (e.g. 1rst order i.e. continuity equation with momentum transfer conservation equation, second order i.e. up to energy conservation equation, ..) with its corresponding approximations (local field or local energy approximations, …) (see e.g. Kanzari et al 1998)
- the good choice of the numerical scheme that have to take into account the strong coupling between transport, field and chemistry
- the numerical scheme is itself sensitive to the choice of criteria of stability and convergence, to boundary conditions, etc.

Results of plasma models are also very sensitive to the considered physical processes and phenomena and the associated basic data. If the aim of the plasma modeling is to have a quantitative description (not only a qualitative one) of our electrical discharge, it is necessary to obtain the various needed basic data with the best possible accuracy.

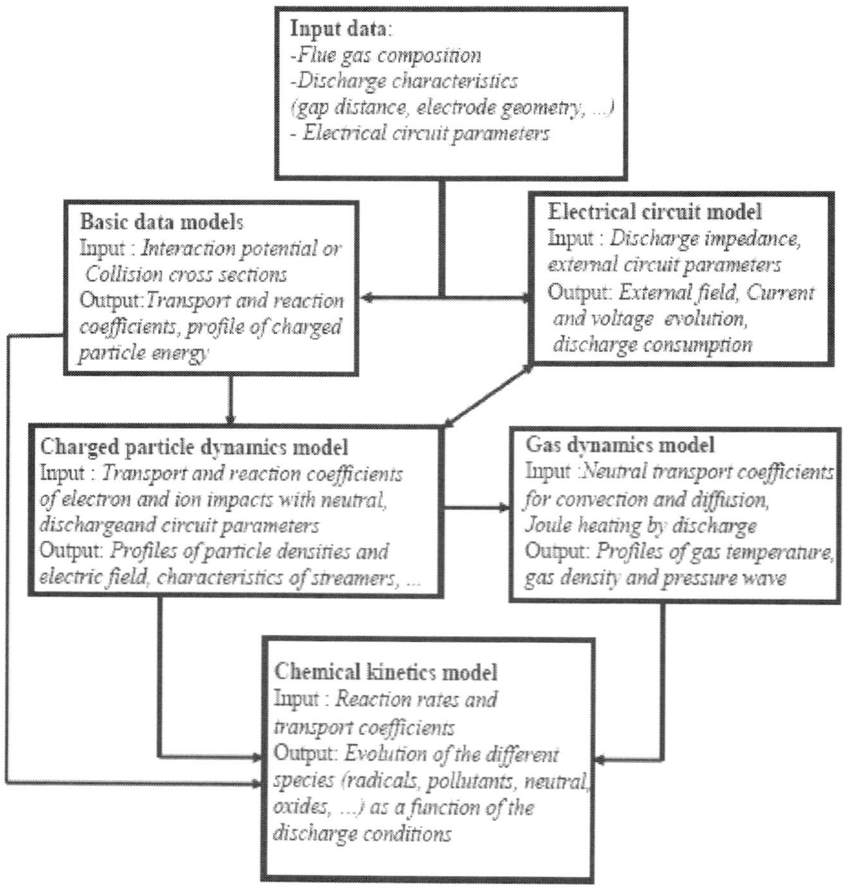

Fig. 8. Diagram showing the coupling between the different models which can be used to describe the electro-hydrodynamic and reaction kinetics phenomena and processes in the case of atmospheric pressure non thermal plasmas generated by corona or DBD discharges (Yousfi et al 2010)

4.2 Example of formation of specific active species in humid air discharge

In order to focus on the coupling of the different models previously evoked and the required corresponding basic data, let us consider the example of simplified reaction processes involved during the generation and the loss of radical O in humid air non equilibrium discharge. As atomic oxygen can be a major active species in many biomedical applications, it is often necessary to quantify it very precisely as a function of the different discharge operating parameters (gas composition, power supply, design of electrodes, etc.) during the spatio-temporal discharge development.

Atomic oxygen in a humid air discharge is first affected by the dissociative electron impacts on O_2 and H_2O. This means that the knowledge of electron energy distribution (EEDF) or the electron transport and reaction have to be known as a function of the space charge electric field distribution.

Atomic oxygen density depends on ion-ion recombination processes, followed by electron detachment and ion conversions. This means the ion energy distribution (IEDF) or the ion transport and reaction has also to be known as a function of the space charge electric field distribution.

Furthermore, the production and loss of atomic oxygen depends on the reactions with metastable states and also on the reactions between radicals (N, OH, O, etc.) and background gas. This means that the distribution of excited species and radicals initially created by electron impacts have also to be precisely quantified as a function of the space charge electric field.

The evoked reactions involving electrons, ions, excited species and radical are summarized in table 1.

1. Electron impacts:

$e + O_2$	$\rightarrow e + O + O(^1D)$
$e + O_2$	$\rightarrow 2e + O + O^+$
$e + O_2$	$\rightarrow O^- + O$
$e + H_2O$	$\rightarrow e + O(^1D) + H_2$
$e + H_2O$	$\rightarrow 2e + H_2^+ + O$
$O^+ + e$	$\rightarrow O$
$O_2^+ + e$	$\rightarrow O + O$
$H_2O^+ + e$	$\rightarrow H_2 + O$
$H_2O^+ + e$	$\rightarrow 2H + O$

2. Ion-ion Recombinations:

$O^+ + O^-$	$\rightarrow 2O$
$O^+ + O_2^-$	$\rightarrow O + O_2$
$O_2^+ + O^-$	$\rightarrow O_2 + O$
$O_4^+ + O_2^-$	$\rightarrow 2O_2 + 2O$
$H_2O^+ + O^-$	$\rightarrow H_2O + O$

3. Detachment and ion conversions

$O^- + O$	$\rightarrow O_2 + e$
$O_2^- + O$	$\rightarrow O_3 + e$
$N^+ + O$	$\rightarrow O^+ + N$
$N^+ + O_2$	$\rightarrow NO^+ + O$
$N_2^+ + O$	$\rightarrow NO^+ + N$
$N_2^+ + O$	$\rightarrow O^+ + N_2$
$O^+ + N_2$	$\rightarrow N_2^+ + O$
$O^+ + O_2$	$\rightarrow O_2^+ + O$
$OH^+ + OH$	$\rightarrow H_2O^+ + O$
$H_2O^+ + O$	$\rightarrow O_2^+ + H_2$

4. Reactions involving excited species:

$O_2(a^1\Delta_g) + N$	$\rightarrow NO + O$
$O(^1D) + H_2O$	$\rightarrow 2OH$
$O(^1D) + H_2O$	$\rightarrow H_2 + O_2$
$O(^1D) + N_2$	$\rightarrow O + N_2$
$N_2(A^3\Sigma_u^+) + O_2$	$\rightarrow N_2 + O + O$
$N_2(A^3\Sigma_u^+) + O_2$	$\rightarrow N_2O + O$
$N_2(a'^1\Sigma_u^-) + O_2$	$\rightarrow N_2 + O + O$
$N_2(a'^1\Sigma_u^-) + NO$	$\rightarrow N_2 + N + O$
$N_2(A^3\Sigma_u^+) + N_2(a'^1\Sigma_u^-)$	$\rightarrow N_2^+ + e$
$N_2(a'^1\Sigma_u^-) + N_2(a'^1\Sigma_u^-)$	$\rightarrow N_2^+ + e$
$O_2(a^1\Delta_g) + O_3$	$\rightarrow 2O_2 + O$
$O_2(a^1\Delta_g) + H$	$\rightarrow OH + O$
$O_2(a^1\Delta_g) + HO_2$	$\rightarrow OH + O + O_2$

5. Reactions involving radicals with background gas:

$N + O_2$	$\rightarrow NO + O$
$O + O + N_2$	$\rightarrow O_2 + N_2$
$O + O + O_2$	$\rightarrow O_2 + O_2$
$O + O_2 + N_2$	$\rightarrow O_3 + N_2$
$O + O_2 + O_2$	$\rightarrow O_3 + O_2$
$O + O_3$	$\rightarrow O_2 + O_2$
$O + HO_2$	$\rightarrow OH + O_2$
$O + N_2$	$\rightarrow NO + N$
$O + H_2O$	$\rightarrow 2OH$
$OH + O$	$\rightarrow O_2 + H$
$OH + OH$	$\rightarrow H_2O + O$

Table 1. Simplified set of reactions leading to production and loss of atomic oxygen in non equilibrium discharge in humid air

4.3 Electron basic data and energy distribution function

The input data needed to feed models are interaction potentials or collision cross sections, transport and reaction coefficients for electrons, ions and neutrals (i.e. radicals and excited species) interacting with the background gas. During the discharge development and propagation, the primary interactions are due to electrons which are the most energetic species. Thus electron-molecule collisions lead to the formation of the primary active species (dissociated, excited and ionized molecules). In order to accurately know the formation rate of the primary active species, electron energy distribution function (EEDF) have to be accurately known because it contains the complete information on the primary processes generating the studied non thermal plasmas. EEDF is obviously solution of Boltzmann equation of weakly ionized gas. The method recommended here to solve Boltzmann equation for the calculation of EEDF and then for electron transport and reaction coefficients has been described elsewhere (Yousfi 1996). It is based on the multi-term development of the distribution function (see in Fig. 9, the significant deviation between a Maxwell distribution, a two-term EEDF and a multi-term EEDF). The dominant interaction processes considered for electron Boltzmann equation are those between electrons and molecules in their ground state. However, the interactions between electrons and excited molecules have also to be considered as for instance superelastic collisions (molecular de-excitation) or stepwise ionization (ionization of a metastable state).

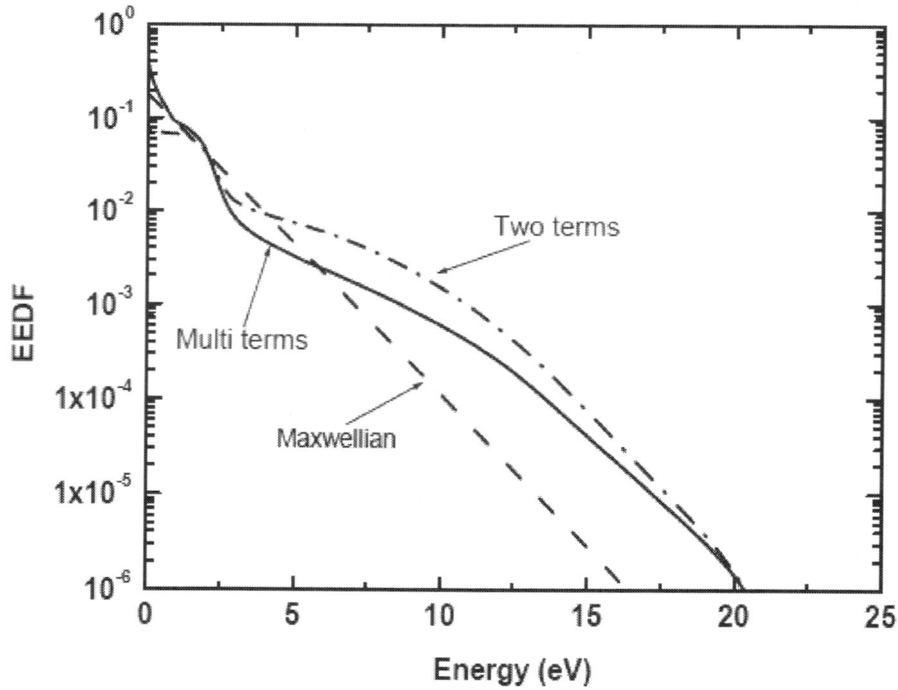

Fig. 9. EEDF as a function of electron energy in a humid gas mixture (76% N_2 12% CO_2 6% O_2 6% H_2O) for an electric magnitude corresponding to the secondary streamer head or the primary streamer channel (E/N=120 Td)

Elastic collisions (using the Davidov operator for energy exchange and thermal agitation of molecules) and inelastic collisions (rotational, vibrational and electronic excitations, together with ionization and attachment) have also to be taken into account. Under these conditions, Boltzmann equation solution allows the calculation of the different electron transport and reaction coefficients measured in classical drift tube experiments. Then from EEDF of the different orders, we can obtain all the needed electron basic data such as excitation, ionization and attachment rate coefficients, and also electron drift velocity, transversal and longitudinal diffusion coefficients.

4.5 Necessity to use validated set of collision cross sections for distribution function computation

4.5.1 Electron-molecule collision cross sections

The use of an accurate EEDF is not sufficient, it is also necessary to use validated set of collision cross sections for the interactions of electrons with every molecules involved in the studied gas mixture (for example e-N_2, e-O_2, and e- H_2O in the case of discharge in humid air at atmospheric pressure). The procedure of validation of every set of the electron-molecule collision cross sections (Yousfi et al 1996) is based on the known swarm unfolding technique summarized in the flowchart of fig 10. Figure 11 shows the adjustment done in the specific case of electron-H_2O set on the ionization cross section to better fit the recent measurements of the effective ionization coefficients based on time resolved Townsend experiment (de Urquijo et al 2007).

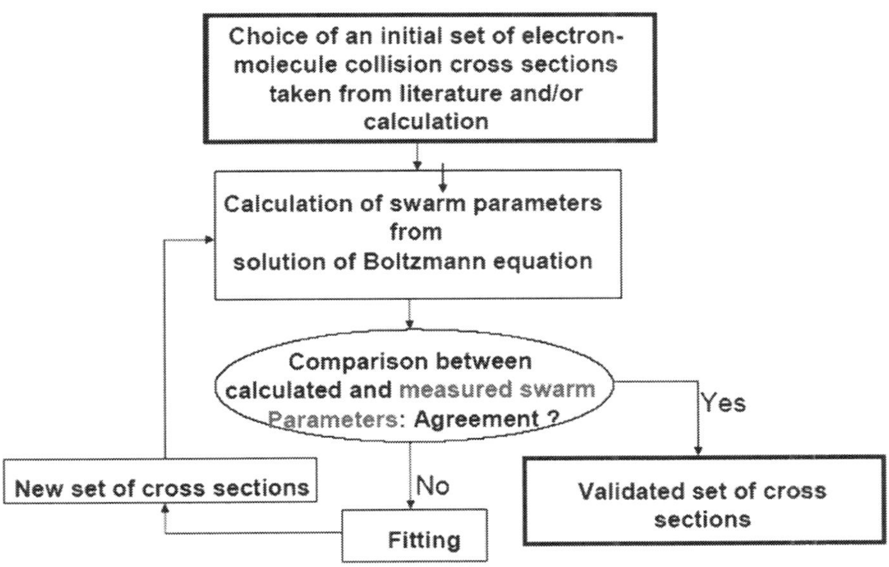

Fig. 10. Simplified flow chart of the fitting method of collision cross sections from Boltzmann equation solution (Yousfi 1996)

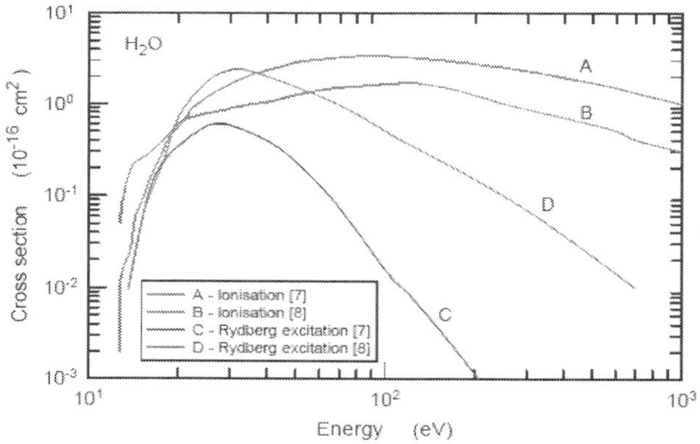

Fig. 11. a. Ionization and Rydberg excitation cross sections, taken from Yousfi 1996 (A and C [7]), and fitted by Yousfi et al 2010b (B and D [8]), from comparisons with recent Pulsed Towsend measurements of the effective ionization coefficients in H_2O and H_2O-N_2 mixtures (Ruiz et al 2010)

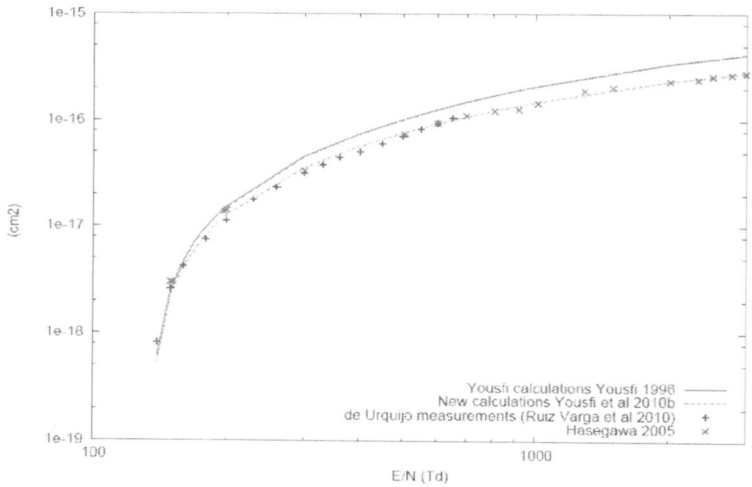

Fig. 11. b. Effective ionisation coefficient of electron in H_2O: comparison between calculation, measurements and literature data from Pulsed Townsend de Urquijo et al 2007 and Hasegawa et al 2005. The results, taken from Yousfi et al 2010b and Yousfi 1996, show that green curve is the best fit

4.5.2 Ion-molecule collision cross sections

It is also necessary to use validated sets of ion-gas collision cross sections because the discharge dynamics is also dependent on ion-gas collisions during the secondary streamer evolution and even in certain cases during the primary streamer evolution (Bekstein et al

2010). The involved ions in the discharge dynamics and in the ion chemistry in the case of humid air molecules are obviously the parent ions (N_2^+ or O_2^+ or H_2O^+) with the dissociated ions (N^+ or O^+ or O^-) and also some polyatomic ions (N_4^+or O_4^+ or etc.) which can be created at atmospheric pressure following a three body reaction ($N_2^+ + 2N_2 \rightarrow N_4^+ + N_2$ or $O_2^+ + 2O_2 \rightarrow O_4^+ + O_2$) or two body reactions (interactions between two nitrogen or oxygen metastables) during the discharge dynamics and therefore can affect its development (Bekstein et al 2010). The transport and reaction coefficients of such ions, in the case of for instance a discharge in air, can be calculated from validated sets of collision cross sections for N_4^+ and O_4^+ ion in N_2 and in O_2 by using a JWKB method to calculate elastic momentum collision cross sections (Bekstein et al 2010) from a 12-6-4 or 8-6-4 core interaction potential *V(r)* well adapted for diatomic and polyatomic ions.

$$V(r) = \frac{n\varepsilon_m}{n\,(3+\gamma) - 12\,(1+\gamma)}\left[\frac{12}{n}(1+\gamma)\left(\frac{r_m - a}{r-a}\right)^n - 4\gamma\left(\frac{r_m - a}{r-a}\right)^6 - 3\,(1-\gamma)\left(\frac{r_m - a}{r-a}\right)^4\right]$$

r is the intermolecular distance, ε_m the minimum energy of the potential, r_m the position of the minimum, n is the power of the repulsive part of the potential, γ is a strength factor and a is the shift between the mass center and the charge center (see Bekstein et al 2010 for details on the calculation and fitting on ion-molecule collision cross sections from *V(r)*). Fig. 12b shows an example of the obtained set of elastic and inelastic ion-molecule collision cross sections for systems O_4^+/N_2 and O_4^+/O_2 systems. Fig 12b shows the reduced mobility O_4^+ polyatomic ion in N_2, pure O_2 and in air calculated from Monte Carlo method using the ion-molecule cross sections shown in Fig. 12a.

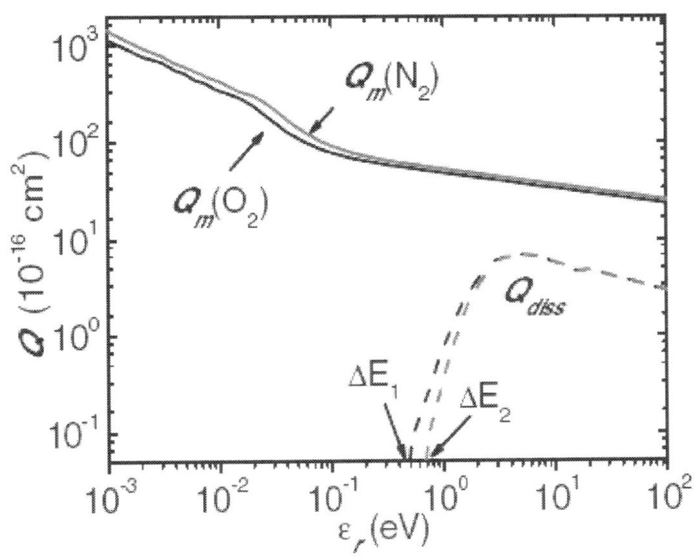

Fig. 12. a. O_4^+/O_2 (black) and O_4^+/N_2 (red lines) collision cross sections (taken from Bekstein et al 2010)

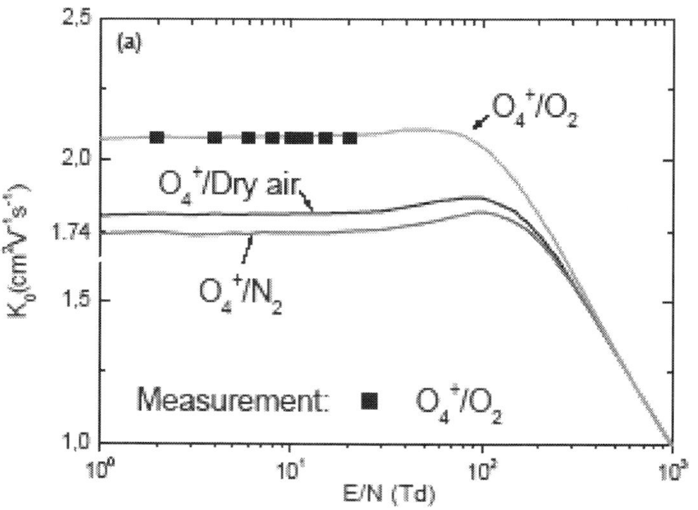

Fig. 12. b. Reduced mobility for O_4^+ ion in O_2, , N_2 and dry air(80%N_2+20%O_2) calculated from Monte Carlo simulation (lines) and compared to available experimental data from Ellis et al 1976 (symbol) for O_4^+/O_2 system (taken from Bekstein et al 2010)

4.6 Example of the effect of the choice of ion basic data on streamer dynamics and active species production

The consideration of the previous basic data more particularly those of polyatomic ions (as for instance O_4^+) on the streamer dynamics modelling has obviously a significant effect on for instance the determination of the active species (as e.g. atomic radicals O and N) formation inside the ionized channel of the streamer during primary and secondary development. The effect of consideration of O_4^+ ion on streamer characteristics such as velocity, electric field propagation and charged particle densities is already discussed in Bekstein et al, 2010. In the following a focus is given specifically on the evolution of radicals like O and N atoms. Fig. 13 shows in the case of positive corona discharge between point-to-plane electrodes, the time evolution of the mean density (integrated over the whole gap distance from 0 up to 4mm) of radicals O and N produced during the propagation of primary streamer (from initial time up to 60 ns), the development of secondary streamer (up to about 75ns) and during the discharge relaxation (up to 200 ns). Radicals O and N can be (from such discharge modelling) quantified and localized during the discharge propagation and relaxation. We observe that these atomic active species which are very useful to identify and quantify for environmental and biomedical plasma applications, are mainly produced in the secondary streamer and discharge relaxation stages (due to the dissociative excitation and attachment of oxygen and nitrogen molecule). Such results are coherent with Ono & Oda 2004 measurements using UV Laser absorption spectroscopy. Furthermore we also observe, due to the better efficiency of O_2 dissociation, that O density is higher than N density despite the higher proportion of N_2 in dry air. Last, it is worth noting that the non consideration of the polyatomic ion overestimates, as expected, the densities of O and N radicals; this emphasizes the importance of the polyatomic ion transport and reaction kinetics.

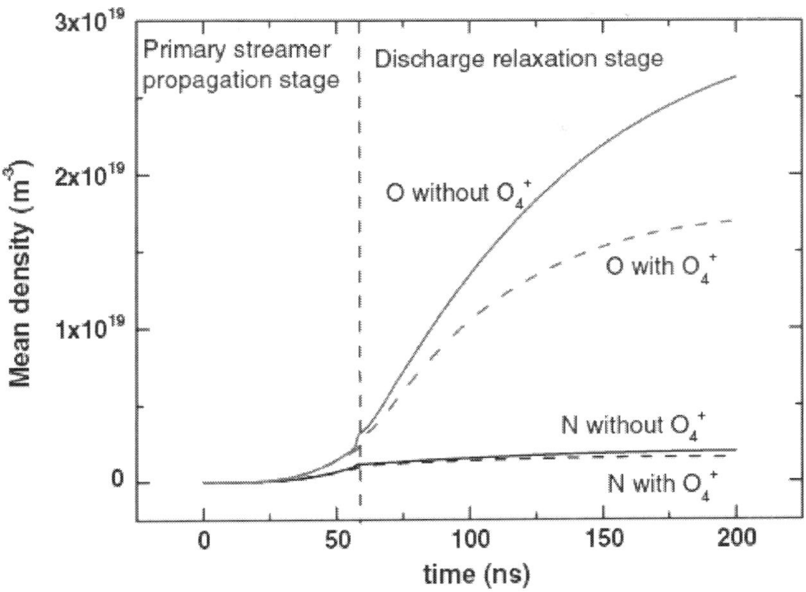

Fig. 13. Space integrated O and N radicals densities (integration over the whole space from 0 up to 4 mm) as a function of time in the case of a DC point-to-plane corona discharge in dry air at atmospheric pressure and a DC voltage of 5.3 kV (taken from Bekstein et al 2010)

5. Illustrative results

Two examples have been given in this section to illustrate the use of low temperature and non thermal plasma sources generating active species at both reduced and atmospheric pressures in the case of bacteria decontamination and bio material treatment.

5.1 Bacteria decontamination using sources of active species at reduced and atmospheric pressure

In the flowing afterglow discharge in pure N_2 at reduced pressure, the active species already identified (Villeger et al 2008) as the main decontamination vector are N atoms. The increase of the injected microwave power P_{MW} from 100 to 300 watts induces a 70% increase of the N concentration in the late afterglow reactor (Boudam et al 2007). Fig. 15 shows that such P_{MW} increase allows to obtain a 6 log decrease of the initial bacteria population after 30 min of exposure at room temperature. The microbiological protocole is described by Sarrette et al 2010. Fig. 15 also shows that in the case of the plasma jet in ambient air (CR-AP), a similar trend was obtained with a diminution of the distance d between the discharge and the exposed bacterial film.

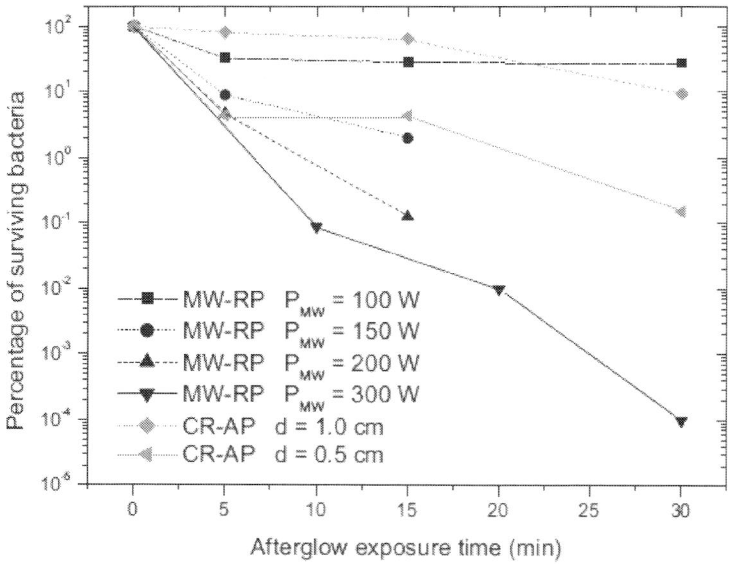

Fig. 14. Effect of increase of the concentration of the afterglow active species on the E. coli inactivation kinetics and effect of distance variation from the plasma jet. P_{MW} is the microwave power injected in reduced pressure discharge working in pure nitrogen (1 slm) at a 5 Torr (MR-RP) and d is the distance between the plasma jet in ambient air (CR-AP) and the exposed bacterial film (taken from Sarrette et al 2010).

This first example clearly emphasizes that the inactivation of E. coli bacteria can occur by using either a selective active species (atomic nitrogen) in the case of flowing afterglow discharge where the gas composition is well controlled or a mixture of active species (not clearly identified and quantified) in the case of the plasma jet in ambient air. This means that when the identification of the species really active in the biomedical processes, it is interesting to control totally the gas composition as in the case of flowing afterglow discharge at reduced pressure.

5.2 Collagen treatment using low temperature plasma jet in ambient air

Biomaterials based on collagen can be used as substitutes of the extracellular matrix for the realization of for instance skin substitutes. In order to develop new biophysical treatments to increase the durability and the stability of such biomaterials, plasma jet in ambient air has been tested (Delaunay et al 2010a and b) for the treatment of type I collagen which is the most abundant type in mammalian cells. Fig. 15 shows the Differential Scanning Calorimetry (DSC) graph of the control collagen sample (without plasma treatment) compared to the DSC graphs of collagen samples exposed to the ambient air plasma jet. Several exposure times are considered (5, 10 and 60 mn). A large endothermic phenomenon is observed for the different collagen samples between 50°C and 150°C. This can be attributed to the evaporation and vaporization of residual bound water in collagen (Samouillan et al 1999). A second endothermic event is observed above 200°C for all the samples with a specific shape for each sample. This can be attributed to the denaturation of collagen. The later, distinct of degradation, implies that the rupture of peptide bonds, leads to the formation of an amorphous polymer. This more particularly means that the plasma treatment stabilizes the collagen structure because firstly there is a shift towards higher temperature range of the collagen denaturation and secondly there is a stiffening of the chains by a cross-linking action when compared to the control sample (collagen without plasma treatment). The thermal denaturation of collagen shows interesting information on the effects of plasma jet treatment on the triple helical structure and on the collagen stability. Further analyses are obviously needed to better quantify the plasma treatment on collagen by using the expertise of our colleagues of polymer physics (Samouillan et al 1999) and also biochemists in order to analyze the biomaterial functionalization.

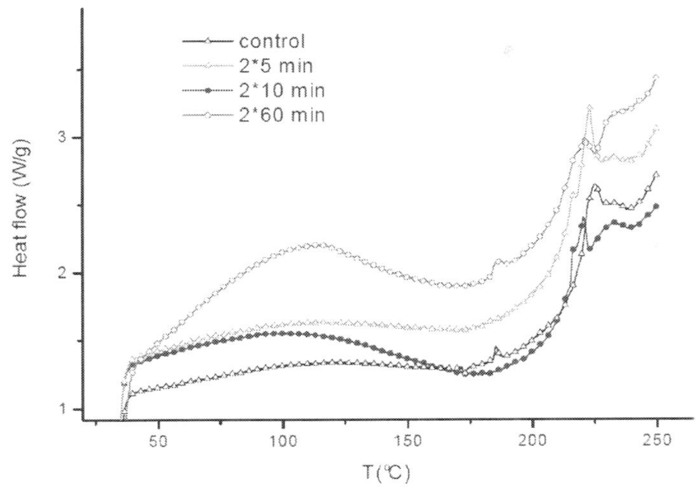

Fig. 15. Differential Scanning Calorimetry graphs of freeze dried collagen samples: comparison between control sample and treated (recto/verso) sample at different time exposures.

6. Conclusion

The optimizations of low temperature and non thermal plasmas have to be done in close collaboration between the plasma and biomedical researchers. For a given application concerning for instance decontamination or biomaterial functionalization or plasma medicine (as blood coagulation, wound healing, etc.) the role of the biomedical researcher is to finely analyze the effect of the different plasmas while the role of the plasma researcher is to provide a "tailored plasma" for the application. In fact, iterations are needed between plasma and biomedical researchers in order to identify and to select the plasma species (for instance a specific radical or a specific photon wavelength or a specific charged particle energy, etc.) really active in a given biomedical application.

In order to reach their goal, the plasma researchers need to use the experimental diagnostics and also modelling tools to better known and characterize the low temperature and non thermal plasma as a function of the different operating parameters such as gas composition and pressure, shape and magnitude of power supply, geometry and design of the plasma reactor. To better understand and control the generation of active species more particularly in the case of streamer discharges at atmospheric pressure, further works are needed in both the experimental diagnostics and modeling of low temperature and non thermal plasmas. These works can concerns:

- the quantification of the spatio-temporal concentrations of radical and excited species (metastable and vibration) by using of advanced experiments such as LIF or TALIF and CRDS techniques adapted to the short transient regimes and filamentary discharge structure.
- the study of streamer branching phenomena by using fast imagery and 3D discharge dynamics modelling
- the physical understanding of photo-ionisation, photo-emission and secondary electrode processes (role of gas and surface on streamer development) that more particularly needs VUV and UV measurements of the short live excited species
- the model validation: further works are required on basic data for transport, chemistry and kinetics processes particularly in the case of polyatomic ions, excited species and radical interactions with gas and surface, etc.

Once developed and mastered the tools and the techniques of the characterization of the low temperature plasmas for their identification and quantification, the ultimate goal is to develop sources of active species fulfilling the following features:

1. production of selective active species well identified and well quantified,
2. very good efficiency of the production of the selected active species (i.e. high ratio between produced species and dissipated energy) and
3. last and not least the sources of active species have to be easily transportable, easily usable and without danger for the user.

7. References

Abahazem A., N. Merbahi, O. Ducasse, O. Eichwald, and M. Yousfi, 2008, IEEE Transactions on Plasma Science 36, 924,

Abahazem A., A. Mraihi, N. Merbahi, M. Yousfi, and O. Eichwald, 2011, IEEE Transactions on Plasma Science,

Allen N. L. and D. C. Faircloth, 2003, IEEE Transactions on Dielectrics and Electrical Insulation Vol. 10, 295

Bekstein A., M. Yousfi, M. Benhenni, O. Ducasse, and O. Eichwald, 2010, "Drift and reactions of positive tetratomic ions in dry, atmospheric air: Their effects on the dynamics of primary and secondary streamers", J. Appl. Phys. 107, 103308

Bhoj A. N. and M. J. Kushner, 2008, Plasma Sources Sci. Technol. 17 035024

Boudam M.K., B. Saoudi, M. Moisan, A. Ricard, 2007, J. Phys. D: Appl. Phys. 40, 1694

Briels Tanja M. P., Eddie M. van Veldhuizen, and Ute Ebert, 2005, Branching of Positive Discharge Streamers in Air at Varying Pressures IEEE Transactions On Plasma Science, Vol. 33,

Casanovas, A. M.· Casanovas, J. Lagarde F.· Belarbi A., 1992, J. Appl Phys, 72, pp. 3344-3354

Creyghton, Y., 1994, "Positive pulsed corona" Ph.D. thesis, Eindhoven University of Technology, The Netherlands d'Agostino R., Pietro Favia, 2008, *"Nano-Structured Cell-Adhesive and Cell-Repulsive Plasma-Deposited Coatings: Chemical and Topographical Effects on Keratinocyte Adhesion"* Plasma Process. Polym. 5, 540–551

Delaunay F., V. Samouillan, J.P. Gardou, N. Merbahi, J. Dandurand, C. Lacabanne, M. Yousfi, 2010, Development and characterization of plasma and laser treated collagen for biomedical applications XVIIIth Annual Meeting of the French Society of the Extracellular Matrix Biology, March 8 - 10, Paris

Delaunay F., N. Merbahi, V. Samouillan, J.P. Gardou, J. Dandurand, M. Yousfi, C. Lacabanne, , 2010, "Non thermal atmospheric pressure plasma treatment and characterization of collagen for biomedical applications, Int Conf on Plasma medicine ICPM3 - Greifswald, 19th - 24th september

Desmet T, Rino Morent, Nathalie De Geyter, Christophe Leys, Etienne Schacht, and Peter Dubruel, 2009, "Non thermal Plasma Technology as a Versatile Strategy for Polymeric Biomaterials Surface Modification: A Review", *Biomacromolecules, Vol. 10, No. 9,2351-2378*

de Urquijo J, A. M. Juarez, J. C. Rodríguez-Luna, and J. S. Ramos-Salas, 2007, IEEE Trans. Plasma Science, Vol. 35, No. 5, 1204-1209

Dorai R. and M. J. Kushner, 2003, J. Phys. D 36, 1075

Duan Y., C. Huang, Q. Yu, 2005, IEEE Trans. Plasma Sci. 33,328

Ebeling D., Westphall M. S., Scalf M, Smith L M, 2000, Analytical chemistry vol. 72, n°21, pp. 5158-5161

Eichwald O., M. Yousfi, A. Hennad, M. Benabdessadok, 1997, J. Appl. Phys. 82, 4781

Eichwald O., M. Yousfi, P. Bayle, M. Jugroot , 1998,J. Appl. Phys. 84, 4704

Eichwald O., N A Guntoro, M Yousfi and M Benhenni., 2002 J. Phys. D: Appl. Phys. 35 439-450

Eichwald O., O. Ducasse, D. Dubois, A. Abahazem, N. Merbahi, M. Benhenni, M. Yousfi , 2008, J . Phys D:Appl Phys 41, 234002

Eliasson B and Kogelschatz U, 1988, *Appl. Phys.* B 46 229–303

Ellis H.W., R.Y. Pai, E.W. McDaniel, E.A. Mason, L.A. Viehland, 1976, Atom. Data Nucl. Table 17 177

Fang Z, Y Qiu and E Kuffel, 2004, J. Phys. D: Appl. Phys. 37 2261

Fridman G, G Friedman, A Gutsol, A B. Shekhter, V N. Vasilets, A. Fridman, 2008, Plasma Process. Polym. 5

Gardou J.P., N. Merbahi, M. Yousfi, 2009, ICPIG, July 12-17, Cancún, México

Gorry Peter A. ; Whitehead J. Christopher ; Jinhui Wu, 2007, Plasma processes and polymers 4, 556-562

Gui-Bing Zhao, Morris D. Argyle, and Maciej Radosz, 2007, J. Appl. Phys. **101**, 033303

Hasegawa H, H Date, M. Shimozuma, , 2007, J. Phys D: Appl. Phys, 40, 2495

Hayashi M., 1989, Nonequilibrium Processes in Partially Ionized Gases, edited by M. Capitelli Plenum, New York,

Held B. and R. Peyrous, 1999, Czechoslovak Journal of Physics, 49, pp 301-320

Herron J T, 1999, Evaluated Chemical Kinetics Data for Reactions of $N(^2D)$, $N(^2P)$, and N_2 $(A^3\Sigma_u^+)$ in the Gas Phase, J. Phys. Chem. Ref. Data, Vol. 28, 1453 No. 5

Kanzari Z., M. Yousfi and A. Hamani, 1998, "Modeling and basic data for streamer dynamics in N_2 and O_2 discharges", J. Appl. Phys., 84 (8), 4161-4169

Kelly-Wintenberg K., T. C. Montie, C. Brickman, 1998, J. R. Roth, A. K. Carr, K. Sorge, L. C. Wadsworth, and P. P.-Y. Tsai, J. Industr. Microbiology and Biotechnology, vol. 20, pp. 69–74

Kempkens H., Uhlenbusch, 2000, J. Plasma sources science & technology 9, pp. 441-540

Kieft I. E., D. Darios, A. J. M. Roks, E. Stoffels, 2005, IEEE Trans. Plasma Sci. 33, 771.

Kim Hyun-Ha, 2004, Plasma Process. Polym. 1, 91

Kim GonJun, S. R. Park, G. C. Kim, Jae Koo (J.K.) Lee, , 2010, *"Targeted Cancer Treatment Using Anti-EGFR and -TFR Antibody-Conjugated Gold Nanoparticles Stimulated by Nonthermal Air Plasma"*, Plasma Medecine, Vol 1 Issue 1, pp45-5

Kozlov K. V., R. Brandenburg, H.E. Wagner, A.M. Morozov and P. Michel, , 2005, "Investigation of the filamentary and diffuse mode of barrier discharges in N2/O2 mixtures at atmospheric pressure by cross correlation spectroscopy", J. Phys. D: Appl. Phys., Vol. 38, pp. 518–529

Kunhardt E. E., 2000, IEEE Trans. Plasma Science 28, 189

Laroussi M., 2002, IEEE Transactions on Plasma Science 30, 1409

Laroussi M., X. Lu, V. Kolobov and R. Arslanbenkov, 2004, "Power consideration in the pulsed dielectric barrier discharge at atmospheric pressure", J. Appl. Phys.,Vol. 96, pp. 328-330

M. Laroussi, X. Lu, 2005, Appl. Phys. Lett. 87, 113902.

Laroussi M., T. Akan, 2007, *"Arc-Free Atmospheric Pressure Cold Plasma Jets: A Review"* Plasma Process. Polym. 4, 777–788

Lee HW, G Y Park, Y S Seo, Y H Im, S B Shim and H J Lee, 2011, "Modelling of atmospheric pressure plasmas for biomedical applications J. Phys. D: Appl. Phys. 44, 053001 (27pp)

Liu S. and M. Neiger ,"Excitation of dielectric barrier discharges by unipolar submicrosecond square pulses", J. Phys. D: Appl. Phys, Vol. 34, pp. 1632-1638, 2001

Lloyd G, G Friedman, S Jafri, G Schultz, A Fridman, K Harding, 2010, *"Gas plasma:Medical uses and development in wound care"*, Plasma Process. Polym. 7, 194-211

Marchal F., N Sewraj, G Jabbour, P Rodriguez Akerreta and G Ledru, 2010, Temperature dependence of xenon excimer formations using two photon absorption laser induced fluorescence, J Phys B: At. Mol. Opt. Phys

Merbahi N, A Abahazem, O Eichwald, M Yousfi and D. Dubois, 2008, The European Physical Journal: Appl Phys, 42,55- 62,

Merbahi N, Gardou J P , M Yousfi, 2011, J Appl. Phys

Merbahi N, M. Yousfi, O. Eichwald, 2011, *Device for emitting a plasma jet from the atmospheric pressure air at ambient temperature and pressure, and use of said device"*, N° of the international Publication of the patent: WO 2011/00170 A1, date of publication 6/01/2011, Holder : UPS et CNRS

Moreau E, 2007, J. Phys. D: Appl. Phys. 40, 605–636

Morfill GE, M G Kong, 2009, JL Zimmerman, *"Focus on Plasma Medicine,"*, New J. of Phys., 11

Nair S. A., T Nozaki, and K Okazaki, 2007, Applied Chemistry, Ind. Eng. Chem. Res. 46, 3486-3496

Panousis E, N Merbahi, F Clément, A Ricard, M Yousfi, L Papageorghiou, J- F Loiseau, O Eichwald, B Held and

Penetrante M. and S. E. Schultheis, 1993, *Non- thermal Plasma Techniques for Pollution Control*, Parts A&B, edited by Springer-Verlag, Berlin- Heidelberg

Ochkin V. N.; Savinov S. Y. ; Tskhai S. N. ; Czarnetzki U.; Schulz-Von Der Gathen V. ; Döbele H. F., 1998, IEEE Trans on Plasma Science 26, pp. 1502-1513

Oda T., Y. Yamashita, K. Takezawa, R. Ono, 2006, Thin Solid Films 506– 507, 669 - 673

Ohyama R., K Inoue, J S Chang, 2007, J. Phys. D: Appl. Phys. 40 573-578

Ono R and Oda T, 2004, *J. Phys. D: Appl. Phys.* 37 730

Ono R., Y. Yamashita, K. Takezawa and T. Oda, 2005, J. Phys. D: Appl. Phys. 38, 2812–2816

Pointu A.M., A. Ricard, B. Dodet, E. Odic, J. Larbre, M. Ganciu, 2005,J. Phys. D 38, 1905

Ricard A. Optical spectroscopy on processing plasmas : cathode magnetron sputtering and flowing post-discharges for elastomer activation and medical sterilization, 2005 ,Thin Solid Films, 475, p. 1

Ricard A., J.Henriques , S.Cousty , S.Villeger and J.Amorim, 2007 , *Determination of N , H and O – atom densities in N_2-H_2 and in N_2-O_2 gasmixtures by optical actinometry in flowing microwave discharges and by NO titration in post-discharges*, Plasma Processes and Polymers 4 , S965

G. Ruíz-Vargas, M. Yousfi, J. de Urquijo, 2010, 'Electron transport coefficients in the mixtures of H_20 with N_2, O_2, CO_2 and dry air for the optimization of non-thermal atmospheric pressure plasmas' J. Phys D: Appl. Phys 43 455201

Samouillan V, Dandurand-Lods J, Lamure A, Maurel E, Lacabanne C, Gerosa G, Venturini A, Casarotto A, Gherardini L, Spina, 1999, M. Thermal analysis characterization of aortic tissues for cardiac valve bioprostheses. J Biomed Mat Res 46, 531-538

Sardella E., Loredana Detomaso, Roberto Gristina, Giorgio S. Senesi, Hossein Agheli, Duncan S. Sutherland,

Stancu G D., M Janda, F Kaddouri, D A. Lacoste and C O. Laux , , 2009, *J. Phys. Chem. A*

Srivastava, N.; Wang, C.; Dibble, T. S., 2009, The European Physical Journal D - Atomic, Molecular and Optical Physics, 54, pp. 77-86

Sarrette JP, S Cousty, N Merbahi, A Nègre-Salvayre and F Clément, 2010, "Observation of antibacterial effects obtained at atmospheric and reduced pressures in afterglow conditions", Eur. Phys. J. Appl. Phys. 49 1, 13108

Spyrou N, 2009, IEEE Trans Plasma Science, 37, 1004-1015

Stoffels E, Anton J. M. Roks, Leo E. Deelman, 2008, *Delayed Effects of Cold Atmospheric Plasma on Vascular Cells*, Plasma Process. Polym. 5, 599–605

Timatkov V.V., G.J. Pietsch, A.B. Saveliev, M.V. Sokolova and A.G Temnikov, 2005, J. Phys.D : Applied Physics 38 877-886

Villeger S. , J.P Sarrette , A.Ricard, 2005, "Synergy between N and O atom action and substrate temperature in a stérilization process using a flowing N2-O2 microwave post-discharge". Plasma Processes and Polymers , 2 , 709

Villeger S., J.P. Sarrette, B. Rouffet, S. Cousty and A. Ricard, 2008, "Treatment of flat and hollow substrates by a pure nitrogen flowing post discharge. Application to bacterial decontamination in low diameter tubes", Eur. Phys. J. Appl. Phys., 42, 25-32

Wetman KD, K Dieter, E Kindel, T von Woedtke, M Hähnel, M Stieber, R Brandenburg, 2010, "*Atmospheric pressure plasma sources: prospectives tools for plasma Medicine*", Pure and Appl. Chem. , 82(6), 1223-1237

Winands G. J. J.' Liu Z., Pemen A. J. M. ; Van Heesch E. J. M. ; Yan K. ; Van Veldhuizen E. M, 2006, J Phys. D, Appl Phys, 39, 3010-3017

Yousfi M. and M.D. Benabdessadok, 1996, J. Appl. Phys., 80 (12), 6619-6631

Yousfi M, A Bekstein , N Merbahi , O Eichwald , O Ducasse , M Benhenni and J P Gardou, 2010, « Basic data for atmospheric pressure non-thermal plasma investigations in environmental and biomedical applications", Plasma Sources Sci. Technol. 19 034004

M. Yousfi, J. de Urquijo, A. Bekstein, E. Basurto, O. Eichwald, J. L. HernÁndez-Ávila, M. Benhenni, A. M. Juarez Reyes, N. Merbahi, 2010, "Measured and calculated electron transport coefficients for H_2O and N_2-H_2O", XVIII International Conference on Gas Discharges and their Applications, Greifswald (Germany) 5-10 September

6

Thermal Responsive Shape Memory Polymers for Biomedical Applications

Jianwen Xu and Jie Song
Department of Orthopedics & Physical Rehabilitation, Department of Cell Biology, University of Massachusetts Medical School, Worcester, USA

1. Introduction

Shape memory polymers (SMPs) are a type of polymeric materials that can be programmed to memorize a less-constrained shape/configuration, subsequently assume a strained temporary shape/configuration, and then revert to the memorized shape/configuration upon triggering by an external stimulus(Lendlein & Kelch, 2002). Such responsiveness to stimuli is reminiscent of the adaptive responses universally observed in living organisms. Based on the nature of the external stimulus, SMPs can be categorized into light-responsive SMPs, chemical-responsive SMPs, magnetic field-responsive SMPs, and thermal-responsive SMPs, etc. Thermal-responsive SMPs are one of the most studied systems and will be the focus of this chapter.

Shape memory effect is not a universal property of polymeric materials. Polymer networks comprising of both net-points and reversible switching components, which are responsible for maintaining the dimensional stability and determining reversible thermal response of the polymer, respectively, have the potential to be programmed to exhibit shape memory effect. Processing histories and programming conditions also impact the shape memory effect of an SMP. The intrinsic mechanism for shape memory behavior in thermal responsive SMPs is the reversible freezing and activation of polymeric chain motion in the switching segments below and above the transition temperature (T_{trans}), respectively. Shape memory properties have been reported in a wide range of polymers including, but not limited to, polyurethanes, epoxies, polyolefins and polyesters (Behl & Lendlein, 2007a; Behl, 2010; Lendlein & Kelch, 2002; Liu, 2007; Mather, 2009).

The earliest report of shape memory effect dated back to the 1940s (Liu, 2007). Industrial applications of the shape memory effect took place in the 1950s when chemist Paul Cook, founder of Raychem Corporation, invented heat shrink tubings using radiation-crosslinked polyethylenes (Dole, 1981). The term "shape memory polymer" became better known as shape memory poly(norborene), developed by the French company CDF-Chimie, was commercialized in Japan by Nippon Zeon Company in the 1980s under the brand name Norsorex. Poly(trans-isoprene) and poly(styrene-butadiene) with shape memory effect were subsequently developed by two other Japanese companies (Leng, 2010). These events ushered in the first golden age of SMP research, which had primarily focused on polyene-based systems until segmental polyurethane-based SMPs were introduced by Mitsubishi

Heavy Industry (MHI) in the early 1990s (Hayashi, 1995; Ito, 1996; Takahashi, 1996; Tobushi, 1996; Tobushi, 1997; Tobushi, 2001). The flexibility of urethane chemistries enabled the development of shape memory polyurethanes with a wide range of mechanical properties and glass transition temperatures (T_g's) for individual applications. The publication of a series of landmark papers by Lendlein et al. since 2002 (Lendlein, 2001; Lendlein & Kelch, 2002; Lendlein & Langer, 2002), exploring the potential application of SMPs in modern medicine ushered in a second surge in SMP research, with >100 SMP-related patents and research articles published annually (Liu, 2007).

Shape memory polymers as "smart" materials have been extensively reviewed in recent literature (Behl & Lendlein, 2007a; b; Behl, 2010; Lendlein & Kelch, 2002; Liu, 2007; Madbouly & Lendlein, 2010; Mather, 2009; Rousseau, 2008; Sokolowski, 2007; Wagermaier, 2010). This chapter briefly reviews the fundamental principles of thermal responsive SMPs and discusses the challenges of SMPs for biomedical applications. Instead of providing an exhaustive citation of recent literatures, we choose to highlight some key concepts and a few examples revealing the structure-property relationship of SMPs that have inspired our on-going work in this area.

2. Fundamental principles of SMPs and common characterization techniques

The driving force for shape recovery of an SMP is the recoiling of polymeric chains from a strained configuration (temporary state) to a less-ordered configuration ("memorized" state), namely, entropy elasticity. The "memorized" state could be the most relaxed, equilibrated configuration as the material was prepared. Upon deformation at a higher temperature ($T > T_{trans}$), the original orientations of the chain segments are altered and the net-points are dislocated, resulting in new sets of local chain-chain interactions. The temporarily deformed shape can be fixed as the material cools ($T < T_{trans}$), provided that the newly formed chain-chain interactions are strong enough to overcome the tendency of the chain segments for elastic recoiling. Upon triggering by a higher temperature ($T > T_{trans}$), the increased entropy of chain segments overcomes the constraining local chain-chain interactions, permitting the recoiling of chain segments to a more disordered state.

The net-points of an SMP network, which maintain its dimensional stability, could be either covalent or physically crosslinked. The switching components that reversibly respond to temperature changes could be either amorphous or semicrystalline. Thus, SMPs could be classified into four main categories (Lendlein & Kelch, 2002; Liu, 2007; Rousseau, 2008) based on the nature of net-points and switching components: (1) chemically crosslinked net-points with amorphous switching compnents; (2) chemically crosslinked net-points with semicrystalline switching components; (3) physically crosslinked net-points with amorphous switching components; (4) physically crosslinked net-points with semicrystalline switching componetns. According to the polymer classification convention, the first two categories belong to thermosets and the last two belong to thermoplastics, respectively (Gedde, 1995). All four types of SMPs have been realized (Alteheld, 2005; Jeon, 2000; Lendlein, 2001; Ping, 2005).

In thermoplastic SMPs, the chain entanglements or local crystalline domains formed by strong chain-chain interactions can serve as the physical crosslinking sites. The advantages of thermoplastic SMPs include their moldability with different permanent shapes/ configurations, high shape deformation range, and the ease for blending with other polymers and additives. On the other hand, the molecular weight of the polymer chains in thermoplastic SMPs need to be sufficiently high in order to enable effective entanglement or distinctive phase separation. Due to the dynamic nature and temperature-dependency of these physical crosslinks, the original network points could be destroyed during the deformation with a loss of stored elastic energy, resulting in incomplete shape recovery.

By contrast, thermoset SMPs rarely show creeps (Gedde, 1995). Chemically crosslinked SMPs generally exhibit better strain fixing ratios and strain recovery ratios, faster strain recovery rates and larger shape recovery stress, but lower strain-to-failure values. Such a combination of properties of thermoset SMPs may arise from their higher crosslinking densities and the ability of the chemical crosslinks to better withstand tensile deformations. The main disadvantages of thermoset SMPs are the need for tailored polymer processing and their inability to be reprocessed into a new shape/configuration after being chemically crosslinked, which may not be a concern when the SMP is designed for one time applications, for instance, as *in vivo* tissue engineering scaffolds.

An ideal SMP system may lie at the interface of thermoplastics and thermosets. Optimization through rational molecular and network designs, combined with the choice of appropriate processing programs, is the key for successful, application-driven design of SMPs.

In essence, the shape memory property is a combination of thermal and mechanical properties. To facilitate subsequent discussions on SMP performances, key terms and techniques used to describe and characterize the shape memory properties of SMPs are defined and summarized below.

Transition temperature (T_{trans}) is the temperature around which a material changes from one state to another. T_{trans} could be either melting temperature (T_m) or glass transition temperature (T_g). T_{tran} is usually determined by differential scanning calorimetry (DSC), thermomechanical analysis (TMA) or dynamic mechanical thermal analysis (DMA). DSC measures the change in heat capacity, TMA measures the change in coefficient of thermal expansion, while DMA measures the change in elastic modulus during the thermal transition. Due to intrinsic polydispersity in molecular weights and imperfect spatial distribution of network chains, the unique thermal characteristics of a polymer should be defined as a temperature range rather than at one specific temperature. For the ease of comparison, however, a single T_{trans} (T_m or T_g) value taken from the peak or midpoint of a broader transition is often reported in literature.

Melting temperature (T_m) is the temperature at which a material changes from solid to liquid state. In polymers, T_m is the peak temperature at which a semicrystalline phase melts into an amorphous state. Such a melting process usually takes place within a relative narrow range (<20 °C), thus it is acceptable to report T_m as a single value.

Glass transition temperature (T_g) is the temperature beyond which a polymer turns from a hard, glass-like state to a rubber-like state. For the ease of comparison of conventional polymers, a single T_g value taken from the midpoint of a broader transition is often used in literature. However, since the width of glass transition have a profound impact on the shape memory performance of SMPs, it will be more appropriate to report the width of the transition along with the mid-point T_g value, or to report the onset glass transition temperature (T_g^{onset}) and the ending glass transition temperature (T_g^{end}) along with the mid-point T_g value.

Stress (σ) is defined as the force exerted on the material per area. The ultimate tensile stress that leads to the tensile failure of an SMP, or the ultimate tensile strength, as well as the lowest stress that produces a permanent deformation in an SMP, or the yield strength, are both utilized in the characterization of SMPs.

Strain (ε) is defined as the deformation per unit length due to stress. The strain-to-failure value indicates the maximum strain that a SMP could reach under external stress.

Modulus (E) is also referred as Young's modulus or elastic modulus. It is the slope of the linear elastic region of a stress-strain curve. E changes significantly with temperature in thermal-responsive SMPs. The glassy state modulus of an SMP at a lower temperature can be several orders of magnitude higher than its rubbery state modulus at a higher temperature. The rubbery state modulus of an SMP, indicative of the density of crosslinks, has only minimal influence on the free-strain recovery behavior (e.g. shape recovery rate and shape recover percentage) except when the crosslinking density is extremely low. However, the rubbery state modulus of an SMP dictates the recovery stress during the fixed-strain recovery. The recovery stress is proportional to the energy stored as a deformed SMP is being cooled to fix its temporary shape/configuration. Since the deformation of an SMP usually takes place at its rubbery state, the energy stored could be approximated as the product of its rubbery state modulus and the imposed strain.

Shape fixing components are defined as the domain or net-point, either covalently crosslinked or physically formed (e.g. via physical entanglement or H-bonding), in an SMP network that maintains the dimensional stability during the deformation and subsequent recovery.

Shape switching components are the polymeric chains in an SMP network that can switch from one state to another in response to the temperature change, which are responsible for the temperature-dependent deformation and recovery.

Shape deforming temperature (T_d) is the working temperature at which SMP is strained to a temporary shape. The relationship of T_d relative to T_{trans} (below, at or above) has significant impact on the shape memory performance of an SMP.

Temporary shape fixing temperature (T_f) is the working temperature at which the temporary shape of a deformed SMP is fixed. T_f is usually lower than the T_{trans}.

Shape recovery temperature (T_r) is the working temperature at which an SMP is triggered to recover from its fixed temporary shape. T_r is usually higher than T_{trans} and is often chosen to be the same as the T_d.

Cyclic thermo-mechanical test is a widely used quantitative analysis of shape memory performance using a mechanical testing instrument equipped with a temperature control unit (Knight, 2008; Lendlein & Kelch, 2002; Wagermaier, 2010). The test can be carried out in either stress-controlled or strain-controlled mode. In a stress-controlled cyclic thermo-mechanical test, a predefined stress and temperature ramping are applied to the SMP and the strain is recorded over time. In a strain-controlled cyclic thermo-mechanical test, a predefined strain and temperature ramping are applied to the SMP and the stress is recorded over time. A typical stress-controlled cyclic thermo-mechanical test in the Nth cycle constitutes 4 distinctive steps (Fig. 1):

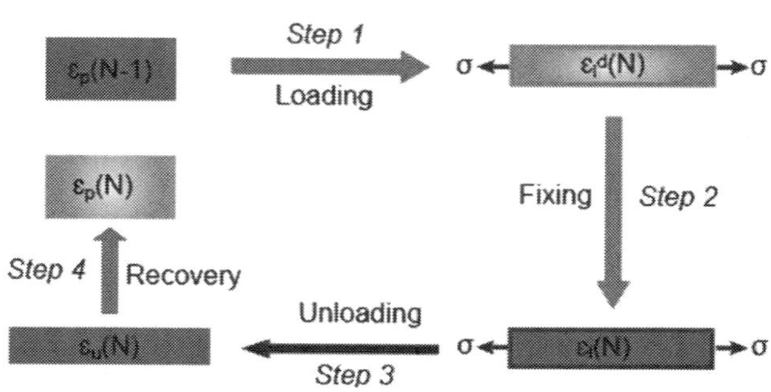

Fig. 1. Programming steps in a stress-controlled cyclic thermo-mechanical test of an SMP. Denotations: p = permanent, l = with loading, d = deformation temperature T_d, u = unloading

Step 1. Equilibrating an SMP with a recorded permanent strain $\varepsilon_p(N\text{-}1)$ at deformation temperature T_d, followed by subjecting the SMP to predefined deformation stress σ at T_d. The deformed sample length at T_d is recorded as ε_l^d (N).

Step 2. Fixing the temporary length ε_l^d (N) by cooling the SMP to a lower fixing temperature (T_f) under constant loading σ. The recorded fixed strain at T_f under loading is ε_l (N).

Step 3. Unloading the stress to zero or a specific lower constrain stress (σ_c). The resulting strain after unloading is recorded as $\varepsilon_u(N)$.

Step 4. Recovering the shape under either zero stress or a specific constrain stress σ_c at T_r. The final recovered strain is recorded as $\varepsilon_p(N)$. In a **free-strain recovery** mode, the SMP recovers without external constrains either as a function of temperature during a transient heating or as a function of time during an isothermal hold. In the alternative **fixed-strain recovery** mode, stress is generated within the SMP under full deformation constraint either as a function of temperature during a transient heating or as a function of time during an isothermal hold. **Shape recovery stress (E_r)**, defined as the stress that a SMP exhibits during recovery, could be recorded during this mode.

Shape fixing ratio (R_f) is used to evaluate how stably can an SMP be held in a strained temporary shape. It is defined as the ratio of the deformation after unloading versus the deformation at T_f under the loading σ, as calculated per Equation (1):

$$R_f = \frac{\varepsilon_u(N) - \varepsilon_p(N-1)}{\varepsilon_l(N) - \varepsilon_p(N-1)} \tag{1}$$

Shape recovery ratio (R_r) is used to evaluate how completely an SMP recovers to its memorized state (permanent shape). It is defined as the ratio of the recovered deformation at T_r versus the fixed deformation under stress at T_d, as calculated per Equation (2):

$$R_r = \frac{\varepsilon_u(N) - \varepsilon_p(N)}{\varepsilon_u(N) - \varepsilon_p(N-1)} \tag{2}$$

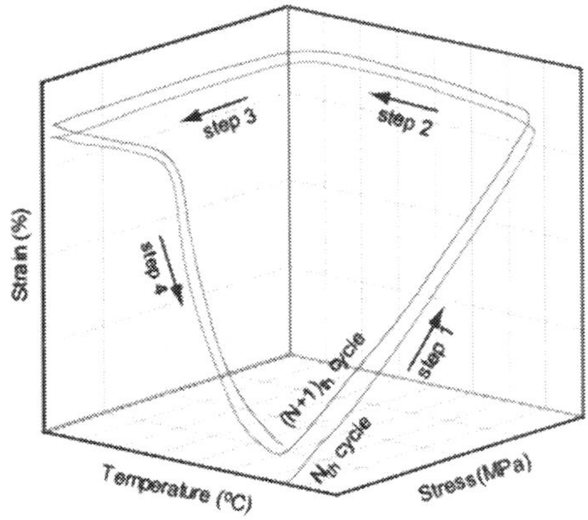

Fig. 2. A representative 3-D plot for presenting cyclic thermo-mechanical testing results.

Shape recovery time (t) is the time that it takes for an SMP to reach its recoverable strain at T_r. It characterizes how fast an SMP responds to the stimulus. This parameter is mostly reported by studies that video-record real-time shape changes

Cyclic thermo-mechanical testing data are most commonly presented in a three-dimensional (3-D) plot with temperature, stress and strain as X, Y, and Z axis (Figure 2), respectively.(Knight, 2008; Lee, 2008; Wagermaier, 2010) Alternatively, the data can be presented in a two-dimension (2-D) graph with multiple Y axes representing stress, strain and temperature plotting against time on the X axis (Fig.3).(Lendlein, 2001; Xie, 2010).

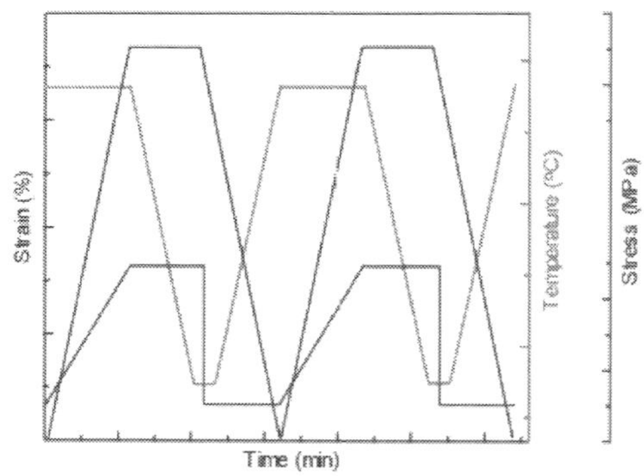

Fig. 3. A representative 2-D plot for presenting cyclic thermo-mechanical testing results. The lines represent a hypothetically ideal SMP with 100% fixing ratio and and 100% recovery ratio.

3. Biomedical SMPs: Applications and challenges

The unique properties of SMPs present enormous opportunities for the design of next-generation less invasive, resorbable smart medical implants, tissue scaffolds and medical devices. Traditional commercial SMPs, including polyurethane-based, polystyrene-based, cyanate ester-based, and epoxy-based SMPs, were not originally designed for biomedical applications. However, as recently reviewed by Sokolowski, Mather, Lendlein and their colleagues (Lendlein, 2010; Mather, 2009; Sokolowski, 2007), a wide range of potential biomedical applications based on SMPs have already emerged or are currently being pursued.

The first SMP-based biomedical application was demonstrated by Hayashi and colleagues who developed SMP-based catheters, which would soften at body temperature, potentially reducing the risks for soft tissue / organ injuries during their surgical delivery (Utsumi, 1995). Maitland et al. designed a thermoset polyurethane SMP-based microactuator for treating strokes (Maitland, 2002; Small, 2007). The microactuator was coupled to an optical fiber and was set in a straight configuration for easy surgical insertion. Upon reaching the targeted blood clot, laser heating was applied to activate the SMP to form a pre-cast corkscrew shape to facilitate the capturing of the thrombus. In order to reach the necessary temperature (65-85 °C) required for actuating the devices, however, significant engineering challenges of the SMP in terms of its optical properties and device geometries had to be met.

In addition, SMP-based biodegradable self-expanding and drug eluting stents (Wache, 2003; Xue, 2010; Yakacki, 2007), biodegradable self-deployable intragastric implants for treating obesity (Klausner, 2003; Pagano & Serezin, 2009), self-fitting vascular and coronary grafts (Sokolowski, 2007), patient-specific customized orthopedic devices (Sokolowski, 2007), tissue engineering scaffolds (Cui, 2011; Filion, 2011; Neuss, 2009; Xu & Song, 2010), and dynamic cell culture substrates (Davis, 2011) have also been explored.

One of the most studied biomedical SMPs is cold hibernated elastic memory (CHEM)-processed polyurethane foams for endovascular treatment of aneurysm in animals (Metcalfe, 2003). The pre-compressed CHEM foams were used to occlude aneurysms in dogs as they resumed an expanded, porous configuration, activated by the body heat, to produce near-complete obliteration of aneurysms, resulting in improved angiographic scores in 3 weeks.

Comparing to shape memory alloys (SMAs) that have been broadly used in stents, the SMP counterparts offer the advantages of being lightweight, ease of processing, higher recovery strain, and programmable degradability (El Feninat, 2002). The relatively low recovery stress, slow recovery rate, and the one-way shape memory of most existing SMPs, however, present important yet exciting challenges for the molecular/network design of biocompatible and biodegradable SMPs as high-performance, expandable and resorbable stents.

4. Recent progress on the network design and shape memory programming of SMPs

To realize the enormous potential and address the multifaceted challenges of SMPs for biomedical applications, innovative macromolecular designs and network engineering, nanotechnology, and creative shape memory programming techniques have been pursued to improve the shape memory performance within a physiologically relevant temperature range. In this section, we review a few examples that help illustrate how specific properties underlying the fundamental shape memory performance can be improved, followed by an example illustrating how multiple functional requirements may be integrated for biomedical applications.

4.1 SMP with high recovery stress

The recovery stress of an SMP positively correlates with the energy stored during its deformation. Most SMPs are deformed in the rubbery state where their typical elastic moduli are in the order of several megapascals (MPa), thus limiting the amount of energy that could be stored and resulting in relatively low shape recovery stress, especially when compared with SMA. A low shape recovery stress could result in incomplete expansive shape recovery within a spatially constraint environment such as a collapsed vertebral disc or a narrowed blood vessel.

To improve the rubbery state elastic modulus, either the crosslinking density of a thermoset SMP or the degree of physical crosslinking in a thermoplastic SMP could be increased. Alternatively, one may improve the rubbery state elastic modulus by incorporating fillers within the SMP network. For instance, SMPs reinforced with SiC particles, carbon powders, carbon nanotubes (CNT), glass fibers or Kevlar fibers showed improved elastic modulus and shape recovery stress but decreased shape recovery percentage (Gall, 2000; Gall, 2002;

Liu, 2009; Liu, 2004; Madbouly & Lendlein, 2010). Carbon-based nanoparticles, nanotubes, and nanofiber fillers also introduce electrical conductive properties to the SMPs, enabling potential electrical field-driven triggering. More recently, Miaudet et al. strengthened polyvinyl alcohol (PVA) SMP fibers with a large fraction of CNT (Miaudet, 2007). Significant broadening of the glass transition (T_g: 50 to 200 °C) was observed for the CNT-PVA fiber versus the neat PVA fiber (T_g: ~80 °C), with much improved storage modulus both at the glassy state and at the rubbery state. When deformed at 70 or 90 °C, the CNT-PVA fiber exhibited a maximal stress of ~150 MPa, one to two orders of magnitude greater than the stress generated by conventional SMPs. However, the reinforced CNT-PVA fiber suffered from incomplete shape fixation (R_f < 60%) and no data on the shape recovery time was reported. Another special phenomenon observed in this system was the so-called temperature memory effect, in which the temperature correlating with the peak shape recovery stress during heating was identical to the deformation temperature.

4.2 Fully recoverable high-strain SMPs

One of the most important advantages of SMPs over SMAs is their significantly larger deformation strains. Although deformation strains over several hundred percentages have been reported for SMPs, most of these strains could not be fully recovered. The development of SMPs with fully recoverable high-strains will be of significant value to applications requiring dramatic yet complete shape changes.

Thermoplastic SMPs usually exhibit high strain-to-failure but not all of the strains is recoverable. Due to plastic deformation/irreversible damage of physically crosslinked net-points, R_r's of thermoplastic SMPs are usually far less than 100%. By contrast, thermoset SMPs usually have high R_r's yet their strain-to-failure tend not to be high. Gall's group proposed that an ideal high-strain SMP may exist at the boundary of a thermoset and a thermoplastic, and should have evenly distributed long chains tethered by light enough crosslinking (Voit, 2010). They systematically studied an acrylate crosslinking system to maximize its fully recoverable strain capacity by adjusting the composition of the co-monomers and crosslinkers. The acrylate network were prepared by crosslinking methyl acrylate (MA), methyl methacrylate (MMA), and isobornyl acrylate (IBoA) with crosslinkers such as poly(ethylene glycol) dimethacrylate (PEGDMA), bisphenol A ethoxylate di(meth)acrylate (BPAEDMA) or a bifunctional crosslinker with both crosslinking and photoinitiating functionalities. SMPs with varied glass transitions and high recoverable strains were obtained. During the optimization of a base polymer composition (19:1/MA:IBoA, wt%; 0.02 mol% initiator) using varied crosslinker BPAEDMA contents, they found that the SMPs with low loading of the crosslinker BPAEDMA (≤0.100wt%) were thermoplastic in nature and displayed inconsistent recoverability from high-strain deformations. With the content of BPAEDMA increasing to 0.014 and 0.027 mol%, the materials could be strained repeatedly to >800%, although some residual strains of 8 and 5% could not be fully recovered, respectively. At the BPAEDMA content of 0.054 mol%, the material still exhibited a fully recoverable high strain-to-failure of 800%. Further increase of BPAEDMA content resulted in the decrease of strain-to-failure. Photoinitiator content and crosslinker length also exerted significant effect on the recovery strain. These data suggested that designing a fully crosslinked network with crosslink spacing that is large and evenly distributed is the key in achieving fully recoverable strain capacity.

4.3 SMPs with sharp transition temperatures

Biomedical SMPs that are designed to thermally deploy (e.g. via catheter heating) *in vivo* should ideally possess a sharp thermal transition slightly above body temperature. Such a thermal property is important to prevent premature shape recovery as the SMP is being delivered in a minimally invasive configuration to its targeted location at body temperature and to minimize potential cellular and tissue damage when it is subsequently triggered to deploy.

For both chemically and physically crosslinked SMPs, the shape switching segments could be either crystalline or amorphous. The width of thermal transition of an SMP is dependent on the distribution of relaxation time associated with the molecular mobility of polymer chains, which in turn is dictated by the chemical composition and network structure of the SMP. Crystalline segments usually exhibit a sharp transition with a relatively narrow temperature range while amorphous segments tend to display a glass transition range tens of degrees wide. The maximum shape recovery rate seems to increase with the narrowing of glass transitions.

A broad transition temperature range has dual effects on the shape memory properties. One may take advantage of the broad transition range to program multi-stage shape memory effects or temperature memory effects, or to enable higher shape recovery stress on one end. For instance, it was shown that when deformation was carried out at a temperature lower than the T_g in an epoxy thermoset, it resulted in a lower shape recovery temperature and higher shape recovery stress (Gall, 2005; Liu, 2004).

On the other hand, a broad transition temperature could also have negative impact on the shape memory performance, for instance, resulting in less stable/incomplete shape fixing, premature shape recovery, and/or slower shape recovery. For SMPs with narrow T_{trans} windows, fixing a temporary shape at a temperature 20 °C below the T_{trans} and triggering the shape recovery at a temperature 20 °C above the T_{trans} are usually adequate in achieving good shape fixing and recovery. For SMPs with broad transition windows, however, some percentages of the switching segments would still remain mobile at 20 °C below the T_{trans}, and some switching components may start to recover prematurely at a temperature far below its T_{trans}. For example, 20% of the shape recovery of a poly(MMA-co-PEGDA)-based SMP took place at a temperature at as low as >40 °C below its T_g of 92 °C (Yakacki, 2008). These disadvantages could cause problems for biomedical applications where an SMP implant needs to be delivered in a stably held minimally invasive configuration and remain so until a safe temperature triggers its rapid deployment. Premature deployment at an unintended *in vivo* location could have grave consequences to the patient.

Predictable shape recovery is conventionally considered more obtainable by SMPs with crystalline switching segments. However, recent work shows that it is possible to design SMP networks with amorphous switching segments to display glass transitions as narrow as 10 °C. The key is to keep the chain segments between netpoints as identical as possible, which can be accomplished by crosslinking well-defined star-branched macromers. For instance, Nagahama et al. prepared biodegradable polyurethane SMPs by crosslinking 8-arm star-branched poly(ε -caprolactone) (PCL) macromers, containing 10 or 20 PCL repeating units per arm, with hexamethylene diisocyanate (Nagahama, 2009). The resulting SMPs both showed outstanding strain fixing ratio (R_f > 97%) and strain recovery ratio (Rr ≈ 100%). The SMP crosslinked from macromers containing longer PCL arms displayed complete shape recovery within a 6 °C range (47-53 °C) that correlated well with its T_m of 49 °C. Interestingly, the SMP crosslinked from macromers containing shorted PCL arms exhibited a more temperature-sensitive recovery, accomplishing 90% strain recovery within a 2 °C heating window (37-39 °C) that was below its T_m of 43 °C and 100% recovery in 10 s at the T_m.

Nair et al. recently reported homogenous SMP networks prepared by thiol-ene photo-polymerization that exhibited glass transitions as narrow as 12 °C (Nair, 2010). By tuning the network compositions, two thiol-ene SMPs with T_g's around 30-40 °C were obtained. These materials exhibited excellent shape fixing at room temperature, distinct shape memory actuation response, and a rapid shape recovery rate (5%/min versus the 1.8-4.2%/min commonly observed with other SMPs).

4.4 SMPs with multi-shape memory effect

It's generally accepted that the number of shapes an SMP can memorize correlates with the number of discrete reversible phase transitions within its network. Conventional SMPs are designed to memorize only one permanent shape that corresponds to the most relaxed state of the switching segments, exhibiting the so-called dual-shape memory effect. The first example of triple-shape memory effect was reported by Bellin et al. where two types of polymeric chains with discrete transition temperatures were incorporated within a crosslinked network (Bellin, 2006). One of the polymer networks containing poly(ε-caprolactone) (PCL) segments and poly(cyclohexyl methacrylate) (PCHMA) segments, named MACL, exhibited a T_m around 50 °C and a T_g around 140 °C. The second network containing PCL segments and poly(oligomer polyethylene glycol monomethyl ether methacrylate) (PPEGMA), named CLEG, exhibited two T_m's above 50 °C and around 17-39 °C depending on the content of PPEGMA. For shape memory programming, a sample adopting a shape C was deformed to shape B at a temperature (T_{high}) above the higher one of the two T_{trans}'s, and then shape B was fixed by cooling the sample to a temperature (T_{mid}) between the two T_{trans}'s before it was further deformed into shape A at T_{mid} and fixed by cooling below the lower temperature of the two T_{trans}'s. During the shape recovery, the sample was heated above T_{high} where shape B and Shape C were recovered sequentially. Both MACL and CLEG engineered with appropriate compositions were able to display such a triple-shape memory effect. It's noteworthy that the deformed shapes B and A were not necessarily unidirectional, which opens the opportunity for applications where complex and multi-directional shape recovery is required. Tuning the triple-shape memory effect in these systems, however, required fine adjustments of the ratio of the two discrete phases. For example, the triple-shape memory effect was only observed for the MACL networks at PCL content of 40-60 wt% and for the CLEG networks at PCL content of 30-60 wt%. It was also found that R_f increased with increasing content of the component forming the domain responsible for the transition. In addition, low R_f's were observed during the programming. In the case of the MACL network, the shape fixing ratio of B following deformation from C was relatively poor (R_f = 48% to 87%), likely due to the fact that polymeric chains exhibiting the higher T_{trans} and those exhibiting the lower T_{trans} could both be affected during this delicate programming step.

Using a different approach, Xie et al. realized triple shape memory effect in a crosslinked macroscopic polymer bilayers with two well separated phase transitions (Xie, 2009). The bilayer SMPs were fabricated by curing an epoxy polymer layer L exhibiting a lower

T_g (38 °C) on top of another pre-formed epoxy polymer layer H exhibiting a higher T_g (78 °C). A similar programming process as described above was used to program the triple-shape memory effect. Similarly, poor R_f's were observed after the first deformation-fixing cycle. Strong interfacial bonding between the two macroscopic layers was found to be critical for accomplishing the triple shape memory effect using this approach. Because of the generalizability of this method, it may be extended for the fabrication of multiple-shape memory effect in an SMP consisting of more than two macroscopic layers.

More recently, Xie designed a unique SMP system with multiple-shape memory effect using a single neat polymer, perfluorosulphonic acid ionomer (PFSA) (Xie, 2010). PFSA is a commercial thermoplastic with a polytetrafluoroethylene backbone and perfluoroether sulfonic acid side chains (Fig. 4a). It has a broad glass transition over 55-130 °C (Fig. 4b) corresponding to the short-range segmental motions within the electrostatic network. PFSA exhibits dual shape memory effect with excellent R_f and R_r (~100%) regardless whether the employed T_d and T_r are at the onset, the mid-point, or the ending of the glass transition window. However, it was found that the deformation strain introduced at a higher T_d could not be recovered fully with a lower T_r, and a well-defined multi-stage recovery was observed when the sample was heated in a staged manner (Fig. 5). Deformation temperature memory effect was also observed in PFSA. Such a phenomenon was also observed in a strengthened PVA SMP (Voit, 2010), although no multiple-shape memory effect was reported. A broad glass transition such as the one in PFSA could be viewed as a collection of an infinite numbers of sharp transitions. At a given T_d or T_f, only a portion of the collective transitions was activated or frozen, resulting in the multi-stage shape memory behaviors. Such a phenomenon is also expected in other amorphous or semicrystalline SMPs with broad reversible thermal transitions, which could serve as a more feasible approach to engineer SMPs with multi-shape memory effects.

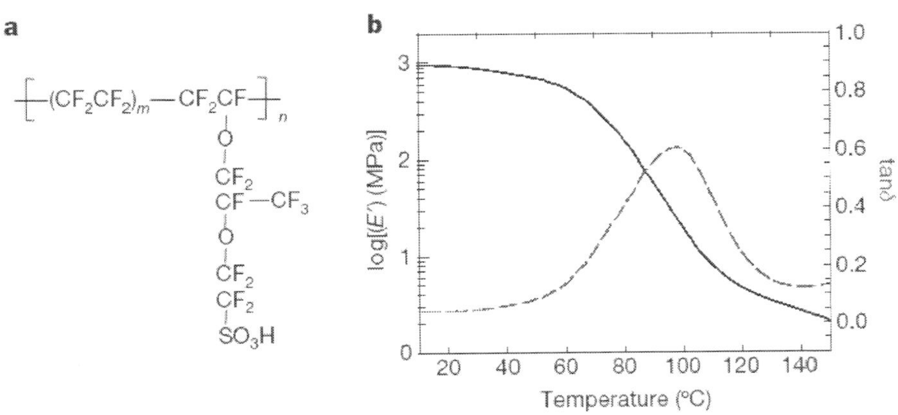

Fig. 4. Structure and dynamic mechanical properties of PFSA. a, Structure of PFSA, b, Dynamic mechanical analysis curve of PFSA.
(Adapted with permission from (Xie, 2010). 2010. Nature Publishing Group Inc.)

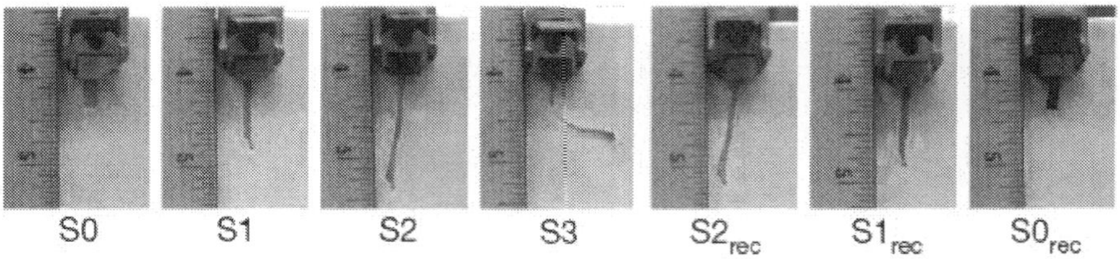

Fig. 5. Quadruple-shape memory properties of PFSA. S0: permanent shape; S1: first temporary shape (T_d^1: 140 °C); S2: second temporary shape (T_d^2: 107 °C); S3: third temporary shape (T_d^3: 68°C); $S2_{rec}$: recovered second temporary shape (T_r^1: 68°C); $S1_{rec}$: recovered first temporary shape (T_r2: 107 °C); $S0_{rec}$: recovered permanent shape (T_r^3: 140 °C). (Adapted with permission from (Xie, 2010). 2010. Nature Publishing Group Inc.)

4.5 SMPs with multiple functional properties

As discussed in Section 2, *in vivo* applications of SMPs often require that multiple factors governing the efficiency and safety of their clinical use be considered. Combining adequate mechanical properties, efficient shape memory effects, suitable degradability and biofunctionality in one material design is challenging yet necessary for biomedical SMPs. For example, we envision that a "smart" SMP bone substitute may be fabricated with a permanent configuration that precisely matches with a patient's defect configuration (e.g. guided by X-rays or MRI scans). Such a SMP scaffold can be deformed into a minimally invasive shape to facilitate its surgical insertion. Once reaching its targeted location, the scaffold can then be thermally triggered to conform to the defect to provide the necessary supportive functions, structurally and/or mechanically. The scaffold should also be ideally resorbable as it induces new bone ingrowth. For such an application, the SMP network needs to exhibit adequate mechanical strength at body temperature, both before and after the thermal deployment, and should have the ability to rapidly and completely recover at a physiological safe triggering temperature. Finally, such an SMP should also have tunable degradation rates potentially matching with new bone ingrowth rate.

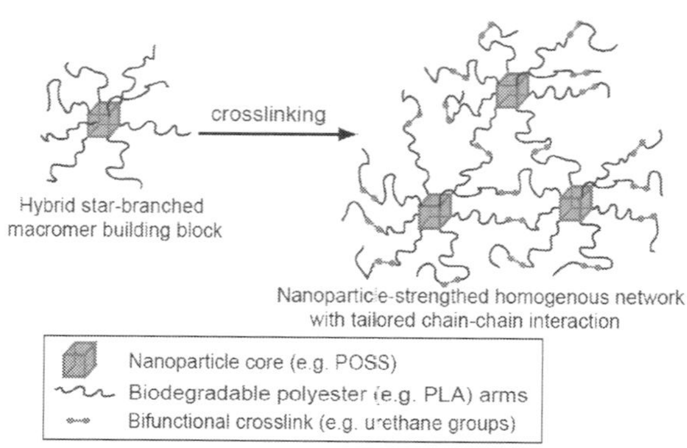

Fig. 6. Depiction of a multi-functional SMP network. (Adapted with permission from (Xu & Song, 2010). 2010, the National Academy of Sciences, USA.)

To achieve complete freezing of chain segment motion below T_{trans} (temporary shape fixation) and full activation of all chain segments above T_{trans} (shape recovery), a homogenous SMP network consisting of identical chains with tunable chain-chain interactions would be ideal. We recently demonstrated that a network crosslinked from well-defined star-branched macromer containing bulky rigid core could meet such requirements (Fig. 6) (Xu & Song, 2010). The bulky, rigid, symmetric core was designed to define the spatial distribution of polyester arms and decrease excessive chain-chain interactions upon crosslinking. The multiple reactive ends of the macromer were designed to achieve adequate mechanical strength via high-density crosslinking and desired bioactivity via selective end-group functionalization. By using the strategy of crosslinking of pre-formed macromers, a wide range of chemistries could be applied for preparing well-defined macromer with tunable chemical compositions and thus degradation profiles.

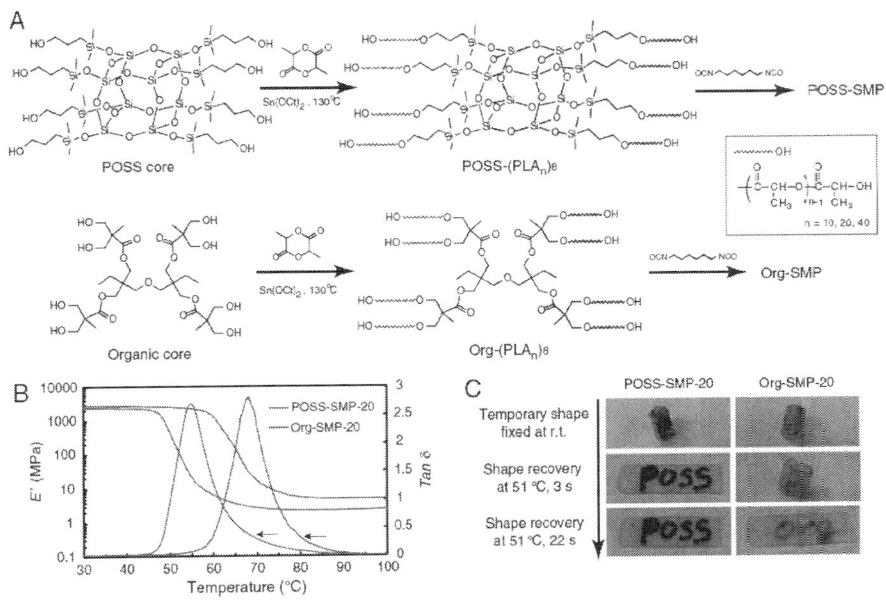

Fig. 7. Preparation and thermal mechanical properties of SMPs containing POSS (POSS-SMP) vs. organic (Org-SMP) anchors: (A) synthesis and crosslinking of macromers; (B) Storage modulus (E')-temperature and loss angle (Tan δ)-temperature (denoted by black arrows) curves of POSS-SMP-20 vs. Org-SMP-20; (C) Recovery rates of POSS-SMP-20 (red arrows) vs. Org-SMP-20 (blue arrows) from an identical rolled-up temporary shape (left panel) to fully extended rectangle (30.0 mm × 6.0 mm × 0.5 mm) in water at 51 °C. (Adapted with permission from (Xu & Song, 2010). 2010, the National Academy of Sciences, USA.)

Specifically, we designed a nanoparticle-mediated homogeneous SMP network that exhibited an extraordinary combination of stable temporary shape fixation and rapid and full shape recovery around physiological temperature with excellent mechanical properties (Xu & Song, 2010). Cubic polyhedral oligomeric silsesquioxane (POSS) was chosen as the core nanoparticle and POSS-centered, 8-arm polyester macromer, (POSS-$(PLA_n)_8$ (n = 10, 20, 40), were pre-synthesized by ring-opening polymerization of D,L-lactide (Fig. 7A). Upon crosslinking by diisocyanates, a POSS-modulated SMP network (POSS-SMP) was formed. A control network (Org-SMP) crosslinked from a less bulky and more flexible all-organic macromer, (Org-$(PLA_n)_8$ (n = 10, 20, 40), were also prepared to facilitate a comparative study of the role of the core structure on the thermal mechanical properties of the SMP network.

The unique capability of the bulky and symmetric POSS core in modulating spatial distribution and interaction of chains enabled the formation of a highly crosslinked POSS-SMP network with homogenous and less entangled microstructure. Although POSS-SMP and Org-SMP possessed the same crosslinking density and equally narrow glass transitions, POSS-SMP had significantly lower T_g than its Org-SMP counterpart (Fig. 7B). The effect of POSS core on the interaction of polymeric arms within the nanostructured molecular network also translated, on a macroscopic scale, into more rapid shape recovery at a lower triggering temperature. For example, shape memory performance testing demonstrated that both POSS-SMP-20 and Org-SMP-20 could be stably fixed at a temporary shape within seconds upon cooling to room temperature, indicating complete freezing of chain segment motions below the T_g in both networks. At 51 °C, the rate of shape recovery of POSS-SMP-20 (<3 s) was much faster than that of Org-SMP-20 (>20 s) (Fig. 7C), although they both recovered at a similar rate (<1 s) at 73 °C.

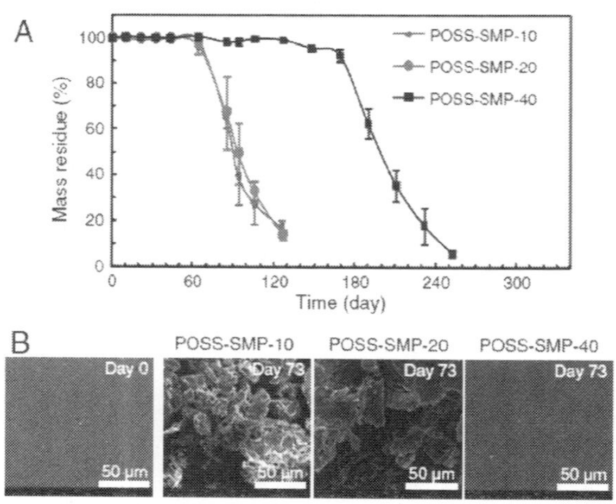

Fig. 8. *In vitro* hydrolytic degradation of POSS-SMPs: (A) %Mass residue of POSS-SMPs in PBS (pH 7.4) as a function of time and PLA arm length. A sample size of 3 was applied. (B) SEM micrographs of POSS-SMPs before and after 73-day incubation in PBS at 37 °C. (Adapted with permission from (Xu & Song, 2010). 2010, the National Academy of Sciences, USA.)

The effect of the POSS core on the thermal mechanical properties of the SMP network was further exemplified by the glass transition change as a function of PLA chain length. In contrast to Org-SMPs where the T_g's decreased with the increase of chain length as a result

of lower crosslinking density, the T_g's in POSS-SMPs increased from 42.8 °C at n= 10 to 48.4 °C at n=40. The storage modulus of POSS-SMPs and Org-SMPs at the rubbery state both decreased with the increase of PLA chain length n, consistent with the expected lower crosslinking densities at longer inter-netpoint chain lengths.
All POSS-SMPs (n=10, 20, and 40) exhibited a T_g slightly above body temperature (~ 50 °C). Equally important, they all exhibited an extremely narrow glass transition range, with peak widths at the half peak height (WHPH) less than 10 °C, accompanied by sharp storage modulus changes of up to 3 orders of magnitude around the glass transitions. By contrast, most conventional SMP networks exhibit wide glass transitions (WHPH > 20 °C) with no more than 2 orders of magnitude modulus change around the T_{trans}. Such a narrow glass transition endowed POSS-SMPs with excellent shape fixing at body temperature, which was slightly below their T_g's, and instant recovery at a safe triggering temperature slightly above their T_g's. Indeed, we showed that all POSS-SMPs exhibited stable temporary shape fixing at room temperature for >1 year, instant and complete recovery around 50 °C, and over 2-GPa storage modulus at body temperature. These properties combined make the POSS-SMPs uniquely suited for weight-bearing *in vivo* applications, for instance, as self-fitting bone tissue engineering scaffolds that can be delivered in a minimally invasive fashion to an area of defect and subsequently deployed to conform to the defect.
Moreover, we demonstrated that the degradability of POSS-SMPs could be tuned by the lengths of the PLA arms of the presynthesized macromers (Figure 8). The POSS-SMPs with shorter PLA arms degraded much faster than those with longer PLA arms. The tunable degradation profiles make it possible to make customized scaffold according to the tissue healing rate. Moreover, the multiple -OH end-groups on the macromer provide extra anchors for further attachment of bioactive molecules, as demonstrated by the covalent coupling of fluorescently tagged RGD peptide using "click" chemistry. Finally, using a rat subcutaneous implantation model, we showed that POSS-SMPs were minimally immunogenic and did not elicit pathologic abnormities in any vital/scavenger organs one year after implantation (Filion, 2011).

5. Conclusion

In summary, despite significant progress on the macromolecular engineering, network formation strategies, shape memory programming / processing techniques in SMPs, the development of SMPs suitable for biomedical applications remains to be a challenging topic. Each SMP system we discussed above has its unique advantages and disadvantages, and provides valuable hints to an integrated solution to the design of biomedical SMPs.

6. Acknowledgements

This work was supported by the National Institutes of Health grants R01AR055615 and R01GM088678.

7. References

Alteheld A, Feng YK, Kelch S & Lendlein A. (2005).Biodegradable, amorphous copolyester-urethane networks having shape-memory properties. *Angewandte Chemie-International Edition*; Vol.44, No.8, pp. 1188-1192, ISSN 1433-7851

Behl M & Lendlein A. (2007a).Shape-memory polymers. *Materials Today*; Vol.10, No.4, pp. 20-28, ISSN 1369-7021

Behl M & Lendlein A. (2007b).Actively moving polymers. *Soft Matter*; Vol.3, No.1, pp. 58-67, ISSN 1744-683X

Behl M, Razzaq MY & Lendlein A. (2010).Multifunctional Shape-Memory Polymers. *Advanced Materials*; Vol.22, No.31, pp. 3388-3410, ISSN 0935-9648

Bellin I, Kelch S, Langer R & Lendlein A. (2006).Polymeric triple-shape materials. *Proceedings of the National Academy of Sciences of the United States of America*; Vol.103, No.48, pp. 18043-18047, ISSN 0027-8424

Cui J, Kratz K, Heuchel M, Hiebl B & Lendlein A. (2011).Mechanically active scaffolds from radio-opaque shape-memory polymer-based composites. *Polymers for Advanced Technologies*; Vol.22, No.1, pp. 180-189, ISSN 1042-7147

Davis KA, Burke KA, Mather PT & Henderson JH. (2011).Dynamic cell behavior on shape memory polymer substrates. *Biomaterials*; Vol.32, No.9, pp. 2285-2293, ISSN 0142-9612

Dole M. (1981).History of the Irradiation Cross-Linking of Polyethylene. *Journal of Macromolecular Science-Chemistry*; Vol.A 15, No.7, pp. 1403-1409, ISSN 0022-233X

El Feninat F, Laroche G, Fiset M & Mantovani D. (2002).Shape memory materials for biomedical applications. *Advanced Engineering Materials*; Vol.4, No.3, pp. 91-104, ISSN 1438-1656

Filion TM, Xu JW, Prasad ML & Song J. (2011).In vivo tissue responses to thermal-responsive shape memory polymer nanocomposites. *Biomaterials*; Vol.32, No.4, pp. 985-991, ISSN 0142-9612

Gall K, Mikulas M, Munshi NA, Beavers F & Tupper M. (2000).Carbon fiber reinforced shape memory polymer composites. *Journal of Intelligent Material Systems and Structures*; Vol.11, No.11, pp. 877-886, ISSN 1045-389X

Gall K, Dunn ML, Liu YP, Finch D, Lake M & Munshi NA. (2002).Shape memory polymer nanocomposites. *Acta Materialia*; Vol.50, No.20, pp. 5115-5126, ISSN 1359-6454

Gall K, Yakacki CM, Liu YP, Shandas R, Willett N & Anseth KS. (2005).Thermomechanics of the shape memory effect in polymers for biomedical applications. *Journal of Biomedical Materials Research Part A*; Vol.73A, No.3, pp. 339-348, ISSN 1549-3296

Gedde UW. (1995). *Polymer Physics*, Kluwer Academic Publishers, ISBN 0412626403,

Hayashi S, Kondo S, Kapadia P & Ushioda E. (1995).Room-Temperature-Functional Shape-Memory Polymers. *Plastics Engineering*; Vol.51, No.2, pp. 29-31, ISSN 0091-9578

Ito K, Abe K, Li HL, Ujihira Y, Ishikawa N & Hayashi S. (1996).Variation of free volume size and content of shape memory polymer polyurethane upon temperature studied by positron annihilation lifetime techniques and infrared spectroscopy. *Journal of Radioanalytical and Nuclear Chemistry-Articles*; Vol.211, No.1, pp. 53-60, ISSN 0236-5731

Jeon HG, Mather PT & Haddad TS. (2000).Shape memory and nanostructure in poly(norbornyl-POSS) copolymers. *Polymer International*; Vol.49, No.5, pp. 453-457, ISSN 0959-8103

Klausner EA, Lavy E, Friedman M & Hoffman A. (2003).Expandable gastroretentive dosage forms. *Journal of Controlled Release*; Vol.90, No.2, pp. 143-162, ISSN 0168-3659

Knight PT, Lee KM, Qin H & Mather PT. (2008).Biodegradable thermoplastic polyurethanes incorporating polyhedral oligosilsesquioxane. *Biomacromolecules*; Vol.9, No.9, pp. 2458-2467, ISSN 1525-7797

Lee KM, Knight PT, Chung T & Mather PT. (2008).Polycaprolactone-POSS chemical/physical double networks. *Macromolecules*; Vol.41, No.13, pp. 4730-4738, ISSN 0024-9297

Lendlein A, Schmidt AM & Langer R. (2001).AB-polymer networks based on oligo(epsilon-caprolactone) segments showing shape-memory properties. *Proceedings of the National Academy of Sciences of the United States of America*; Vol.98, No.3, pp. 842-847, ISSN 0027-8424

Lendlein A & Kelch S. (2002).Shape-memory polymers. *Angewandte Chemie-International Edition*; Vol.41, No.12, pp. 2034-2057, ISSN 1433-7851

Lendlein A & Langer R. (2002).Biodegradable, elastic shape-memory polymers for potential biomedical applications. *Science*; Vol.296, No.5573, pp. 1673-1676, ISSN 0036-8075

Lendlein A, Behl M, Hiebl B & Wischke C. (2010).Shape-memory polymers as a technology platform for biomedical applications. *Expert Review of Medical Devices*; Vol.7, No.3, pp. 357-379, ISSN 1743-4440

Leng J, (Ed). (2010). *Shape-Memory Polymers and Multifunctional Composites*, CRC Press, ISBN 9781420090192

Liu C, Qin H & Mather PT. (2007).Review of progress in shape-memory polymers. *Journal of Materials Chemistry*; Vol.17, No.16, pp. 1543-1558, ISSN 0959-9428

Liu YJ, Lv HB, Lan X, Leng JS & Du SY. (2009).Review of electro-active shape-memory polymer composite. *Composites Science and Technology*; Vol.69, No.13, pp. 2064-2068, ISSN 0266-3538

Liu YP, Gall K, Dunn ML & McCluskey P. (2004).Thermomechanics of shape memory polymer nanocomposites. *Mechanics of Materials*; Vol.36, No.10, pp. 929-940, ISSN 0167-6636

Madbouly SA & Lendlein A. (2010).Shape-Memory Polymer Composites. *Shape-Memory Polymers*; Vol.226, pp. 41-95, ISSN 0065-3195

Maitland DJ, Metzger MF, Schumann D, Lee A & Wilson TS. (2002).Photothermal properties of shape memory polymer micro-actuators for treating stroke. *Lasers in Surgery and Medicine*; Vol.30, No.1, pp. 1-11, ISSN 0196-8092

Mather PT, Luo XF & Rousseau IA. (2009).Shape Memory Polymer Research. *Annual Review of Materials Research*; Vol.39, pp. 445-471, ISSN 1531-7331

Metcalfe A, Desfaits AC, Salazkin I, Yahia L, Sokolowski WM & Raymond J. (2003).Cold hibernated elastic memory foams for endovascular interventions. *Biomaterials*; Vol.24, No.3, pp. 491-497, ISSN 0142-9612

Miaudet P, Derre A, Maugey M, Zakri C, Piccione PM, Inoubli R & Poulin P. (2007).Shape and temperature memory of nanocomposites with broadened glass transition. *Science*; Vol.318, No.5854, pp. 1294-1296, ISSN 0036-8075

Nagahama K, Ueda Y, Ouchi T & Ohya Y. (2009).Biodegradable Shape-Memory Polymers Exhibiting Sharp Thermal Transitions and Controlled Drug Release. *Biomacromolecules*; Vol.10, No.7, pp. 1789-1794, ISSN 1525-7797

Nair DP, Cramer NB, Scott TF, Bowman CN & Shandas R. (2010).Photopolymerized thiol-ene systems as shape memory polymers. *Polymer*; Vol.51, No.19, pp. 4383-4389, ISSN 0032-3861

Neuss S, Blomenkamp I, Stainforth R, Boltersdorf D, Jansen M, Butz N, Perez-Bouza A & Knuchel R. (2009).The use of a shape-memory poly(is an element of-caprolactone)dimethacrylate network as a tissue engineering scaffold. *Biomaterials*; Vol.30, No.9, pp. 1697-1705, ISSN 0142-9612

Pagano P & Serezin DR, inventors; Compagnie Europeenne d'Elude et de Dispositifs pour L'lmplantation par Laparoscopie (Vienne, FR) assignee. Shape memory intragastric balloon. France patent 2009/0093838. 2009 2009.

Ping P, Wang WS, Chen XS & Jing XB. (2005).Poly(epsilon-caprolactone) polyurethane and its shape-memory property. *Biomacromolecules*; Vol.6, No.2, pp. 587-592, ISSN 1525-7797

Rousseau IA. (2008).Challenges of Shape Memory Polymers: A Review of the Progress Toward Overcoming SMP's Limitations. *Polymer Engineering and Science*; Vol.48, No.11, pp. 2075-2089, ISSN 0032-3888

Small W, Wilson TS, Buckley PR, Benett WJ, Loge JA, Hartman J & Maitland DJ. (2007).Prototype fabrication and preliminary in vitro testing of a shape memory endovascular thrombectomy device. *Ieee Transactions on Biomedical Engineering*; Vol.54, No.9, pp. 1657-1666, ISSN 0018-9294

Sokolowski W, Metcalfe A, Hayashi S, Yahia L & Raymond J. (2007).Medical applications of shape memory polymers. *Biomedical Materials*; Vol.2, No.1, pp. S23-S27, ISSN 1748-6041

Takahashi T, Hayashi N & Hayashi S. (1996).Structure and properties of shape-memory polyurethane block copolymers. *Journal of Applied Polymer Science*; Vol.60, No.7, pp. 1061-1069, ISSN 0021-8995

Tobushi H, Hara H, Yamada E & Hayashi S. (1996).Thermomechanical properties in a thin film of shape memory polymer of polyurethane series. *Smart Materials & Structures*; Vol.5, No.4, pp. 483-491, ISSN 0964-1726

Tobushi H, Hashimoto T, Hayashi S & Yamada E. (1997).Thermomechanical constitutive modeling in shape memory polymer of polyurethane series. *Journal of Intelligent Material Systems and Structures*; Vol.8, No.8, pp. 711-718, ISSN 1045-389X

Tobushi H, Okumura K, Endo M & Hayashi S. (2001).Thermomechanical properties of polyurethane shape-memory polymer foam. *Shape Memory Materials and Its Applications*; Vol.394-3, pp. 577-580, ISSN 0255-5476

Utsumi A, Morita Y, Kaide T, Onishi K & Hayashi S, inventors; Mitsubishi Cable Indudtries, Ltd., Amagasaki

Mitsubishi Jukogyo Kabushiki Kaisha, Tokyo, assignee. Catheter with body temperature glass transtion region. Japan patent 5441489. 1995 Aug. 15, 1995.

Voit W, Ware T, Dasari RR, Smith P, Danz L, Simon D, Barlow S, Marder SR & Gall K. (2010).High-Strain Shape-Memory Polymers. *Advanced Functional Materials*; Vol.20, No.1, pp. 162-171, ISSN 1616-301X

Wache HM, Tartakowska DJ, Hentrich A & Wagner MH. (2003).Development of a polymer stent with shape memory effect as a drug delivery system. *Journal of Materials Science-Materials in Medicine*; Vol.14, No.2, pp. 109-112, ISSN 0957-4530

Wagermaier W, Kratz K, Heuchel M & Lendlein A. (2010).Characterization Methods for Shape-Memory Polymers. *Shape-Memory Polymers*; Vol.226, pp. 97-145, ISSN 0065-3195

Xie T, Xiao XC & Cheng YT. (2009).Revealing Triple-Shape Memory Effect by Polymer Bilayers. *Macromolecular Rapid Communications*; Vol.30, No.21, pp. 1823-1827, ISSN 1022-1336

Xie T. (2010).Tunable polymer multi-shape memory effect. *Nature*; Vol.464, No.7286, pp. 267-270, ISSN 0028-0836

Xu JW & Song J. (2010).High performance shape memory polymer networks based on rigid nanoparticle cores. *Proceedings of the National Academy of Sciences of the United States of America*; Vol.107, No.17, pp. 7652-7657, ISSN 0027-8424

Xue LA, Dai SY & Li Z. (2010).Biodegradable shape-memory block co-polymers for fast self-expandable stents. *Biomaterials*; Vol.31, No.32, pp. 8132-8140, ISSN 0142-9612

Yakacki CM, Shandas R, Lanning C, Rech B, Eckstein A & Gall K. (2007).Unconstrained recovery characterization of shape-memory polymer networks for cardiovascular applications. *Biomaterials*; Vol.28, No.14, pp. 2255-2263, ISSN 0142-9612

Yakacki CM, Shandas R, Safranski D, Ortega AM, Sassaman K & Gall K. (2008).Strong, tailored, biocompatible shape-memory polymer networks. *Advanced Functional Materials*; Vol.18, No.16, pp. 2428-2435, ISSN 1616-301X

7

Biocompatible Phosphorus Containing Photopolymers

Claudia Dworak
Institute of Applied Synthetic Chemistry, Vienna University of Technology, Vienna Austria

1. Introduction

Radical photopolymerization is the key technique to prepare films and coatings in an environmentally friendly way within the fraction of a second. During the last decade this technique has found access to many other categories, as for example rapid prototyping, manufacturing of printed circuits boards, dental filling materials and other biomedical applications. Photopolymers display several advantages compared to classical thermally cured materials like polylactic acid (PLA). Their most important features are: easy processability and implantation; it is possible to perform the photopolymerization in vivo and ex vivo, which allows for minimal invasive surgery; preparation of complex shaped polymeric scaffolds; spatial and temporal control of the polymerization process; versatility of the formulations and good storage stability of the formulations under the most appropriate conditions until use.

Considering these many advantages, photopolymerized networks have found a broad application spectrum in drug delivery (Liat & Seliktar 2010; Censi et. al. 2009; Clapper et. al. 2007)) tissue engineering (Schuster et. al. 2009; Ma et. al. 2010) cell encapsulation (Nuttelman et. al. 2008; Declerq et. al. 2008), biomimetic coatings (Naik et. al. 2003), contact lenses (Xu et. al. 2010), and dental restorative materials (Anseth et. al. 1996). In current biomedical research, great efforts are undertaken to obtain superior materials for tissue restoration, because the loss of tissue by an accident or disease as well as bone defects are crucial topics for our aging society. The human body as a complex and sensitive biological system provides a great challenge for the development of appropriate materials in the field of tissue engineering. Therefore, the requirements for such biocompatible materials are high: they must display proper mechanical strength, they should be degradable after cells initiate the re-growth of tissue and last but not least these materials, respectively their degradation products, must be safe concerning human health. This chapter will provide a general review on the photopolymerization technology, discuss some biomedical application fields, emphasize still open potentials or challenges and report some of the work that has been carried out so far to further develop this technology, for example the use of monomers based on phosphorus containing vinyl esters.

2. Radical photopolymerization

A simple photopolymerizable system consists of a monomer, a photoinitiator and a light source. To fulfil the targeted application, such a formulation can be amended with other additives, e.g. other type of monomer, crosslinkers, bioactive molecules, drugs etc. Upon irradiation with UV or visible light, light-sensitive compounds, so-called photoinitiators, are able to decompose into free radical species, that can initiate polymerization in a monomer formulation to deliver crosslinked networks.

2.1 Photoinitiators

The key component of a photopolymerizable formulation is the photoinitiator. It should show a high absorption at a specific wavelength of light, thus generating the radical initiating species. For biomedical applications also the biocompatibility, the water solubility, stability and cytotoxictity of a photoinitiator should be considered (Fouassier 1995). There are three major classes of photoinitiators depending on the cleavage mechanism: radical formation can occur by photocleavage, hydrogen abstraction and cationic polymerization. Cationic photoinitiators are generally not applicable for tissue engineering due to the formation of protonic acids. A complete list of photoinitiators would be beyond the scope of this review, but it is worth mentioning at least a few of them: e.g. eosin Y (Desai et. al. 2010) 2,2-dimethoxy-2-phenyl acetophenone, (Nijst et. al. 2007; Niu & Bhatia 2002), Irgacure 2959 (Leach & Schmidt 2002), Irgacure 651 (Peng et. al. 2007), camphorquinone/amine, where the amine is triethylamine, triethanolamine or ethyl 4-*N,N*-dimethylamino benzoate. They have been used as photoinitiators for tissue engineering, drug delivery and cell encapsulation.

2.2 Photopolymerizable materials

While photopolymerization with UV/Vis light works well for many applications, there are some difficulties for the use in tissue engineering. The main problem is, that most of the monomers are cytotoxic and one cannot rule out, that some residual (meth)acrylate groups remain unreacted in the cured polymer. To circumvent this problem, macro-monomers, or macromers are in use (Figure 1a and 1b). Monomers, that have been investigated extensively are (di)methacrlyic or (di)acrylic derivatives of poly(ethylene glycol), PEG (Liu et. al. 2008; Polizzotti et. al. 2008; Lavanant et. al. 2010) poly(vinyl alcohol) and its derivatives (Martens et. al. 2003; Mawad et. al. 2006), ethylene glycol-lactic acid copolymers (Shah et. al. 2006), poly(anhydrides) (Shi et. al. 2010; Burkoth), urethanes (Werkmeister et. al. 2010), polysaccharides (Matsuda & Magoshi, 2002), like dextran (Liu & Chan-Park, 2010), collagen (Gonen-Wadmany et. al. 2007), hyaluronic acid (Baier et. al. 2003; Burdick, 2005), diethyl fumarate (Hou et. al 2009; Sharifi et. al. 2009) and many others. PEG has been used for long as biomaterial due to its high hydrophilicity, thus reducing the adsorption of proteins and allowing to alter the interaction of materials with tissues and cells. For the synthesis of methacrylate end-capped oligo esters like ethylene glycol lactic acid a PEG chain is used as initiator for the ring opening polymerization of D,L lactide, glycolide or ε-caproplactone (Sawhney et. al. 1993; Davis et. al. 2003). Anhydrides such as carboxyphenoxy propane with methacrylic groups have been described as injectable materials for bone regeneration (Burkoth et. al. 2000)

Furthermore, photopolymerizable monomers are able to deliver partially degradable or non-degradable polymer networks. However, polyacrylates and polymethacrylates are unable to undergo full degradation due to the formation of a non-degradable hydrocarbon backbone. To control the degradation process, it is possible to add easily hydrolyzable chemical bonds to the monomer (e.g. esters, anhydrides, amides), or to decrease the molecular weight of the monomer, or to change the hydrophilic/hydrophobic nature of the monomer. The molecular weight (MW) determines whether the network is loosely (high MW) or dense (low MW). In a dense network, degradation is slowed down as the cleavage of the bonds is hindered.

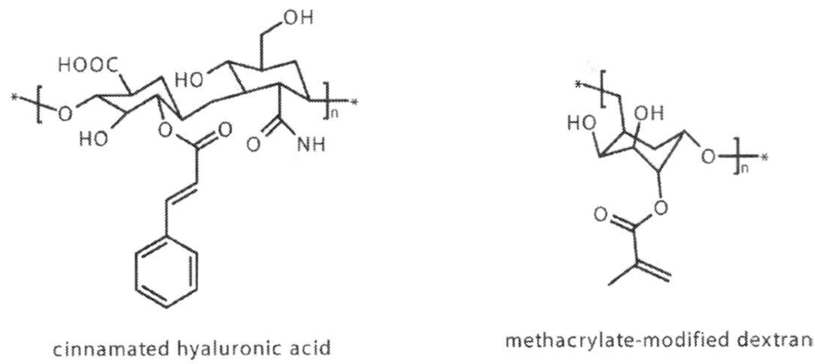

Fig. 1. a. Chemical structures of photopolymerizable glycomonomers for tissue engineering

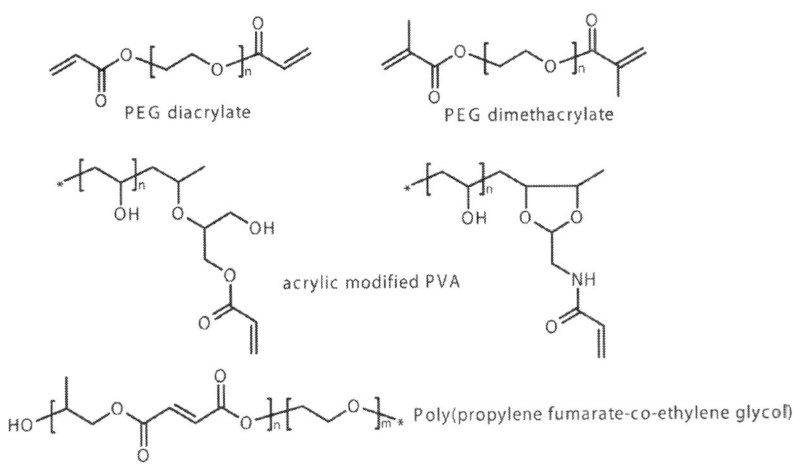

Fig. 1. b. Chemical structures of photopolymerizable monomers for tissue engineering

For example, Sawhney et. al. prepared photopolymerizable, bioerodible hydrogels based on PEG-co-poly(α-hydroxy acid) diacrylate macromers (Sawhney et. al. 1993). A more detailed overview is given by Ifkovits & Burdick (2007). Such materials are suitable as injectable biomaterials, although certain challenges must be met. As already stated before, unreacted monomer can significantly influence the mechanical properties as well as the biocompatibility and should therefore be avoided. However, full double bond conversion is almost never achieved due to limited mobility of the polymerizing molecules. Another restricting condition is the exothermic reaction of the radical polymerization, resulting in an elevated temperature in vivo. Nevertheless, of some materials reports of successful curing in vivo without severe damage on the surrounding tissue have been obtained (Hill-West, 1994). Another major issue of tissue engineering apart from curing in vivo is the delivery of living cells to the injured tissue. Therefore, water-soluble macromers, which give highly hydrated polymers upon curing, are used for the photoencapsulation of living cells (Burkoth et. al. 2000).

In comparison to thermoplastics, photocured polymers display several outstanding advantages, especially easy processing and tailor made mechanical properties due to the formation of crosslinked networks. However, there are also some disadvantages to be accepted. For example, the toxicity and skin irritancy of (meth)acrylate based monomers limit their application in biomedicine. The reason for such drawbacks can be found within the high reactivity of the acrylate double bond towards Michael Addition reaction with amino or thiol groups of biologic molecules like proteins or DNA. Monomers based on diethyl fumarate (Figure 1b) display less toxicity, but also less photoreactivity. Another approach is the use of thiol-ene chemistry (Rydholm 2008), which offers the possibility to tune the mechanical properties of photopolymerizable formulations, in order to control the cell-material interactions. To obtain lower molecular weight fragments also radical ring opening polymerization can be applied, which leads to the formation of ester groups in the polymer backbone (Hiraguri et. al. 2006).

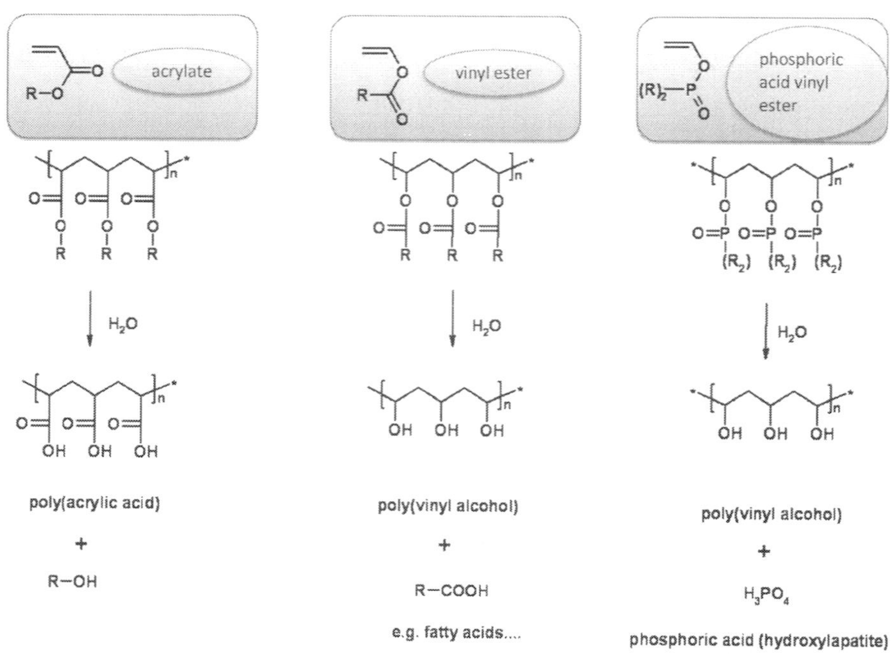

Scheme 1. Degradation of polymers

In summary, there exists only a limited number of reactive groups, that are applicable as biocompatible photopolymers. Therefore, the focus of photopolymers for biomedical research switches to alternative polymerizable groups. It is well known, that vinyl acetate delivers an easily cured polymer with low cytotoxicity, that finds wide-spread use in food industry. However, there are only few vinyl ester monomers commercially available and most of them are monovinyl esters. Recently, Heller et al (2009) synthesized a large number of vinyl esters to study their hence unknown photoreactivity, mechanical properties and their behaviour towards biological systems. In a further step it seemed of interest to prepare a series of monomers based on phosphorus containing vinyl esters (Dworak et. al; 2010), as many of the most important biochemicals, including DNA and RNA, are organophosphates. Another major drawback of crosslinked acrylates is their main degradation product: polyacrylic acid. It is stable towards biodegradation and its transport within the human body is quite difficult. The local decrease of the pH by the presence of the polyacid might also provoke adverse effects on cells. As a remedy poly(vinyl esters) can form non-toxic poly(vinyl alcohol) as degradation product, which is widely applied in drug, food and cosmetic industry (Scheme 1).

3. Biocompatible phosphorus containing photopolymers

Basically, vinyl esters of phosphoric acid, which resemble the monomer type II (Figure 1) own a broad application spectrum as insecticides (Zhang & Casida, 2000) and pharmaceutical industry (Kumpulainen et. al., 2005), but they are also able to undergo radical photopolymerization. Acrylate and methacrylate based phosphoesters are mainly in use as flame-retardant materials. Unfortunately, scaffolds made of poly(meth)acrylates might result in polyacid degradation products, which are rather stable towards biodegradation and furthermore cannot be transported easily within the human body as already discussed in the previous chapter. In contrast to that, monovinyl and divinyl esters of phosphoric acid provide linear, respectively crosslinked polymers, that can undergo hydrolyzation (Hayashi, 1978). Thus, from such polymer types it can be expected, that they form non-toxic polyvinyl alcohol based degradation products and phosphates.

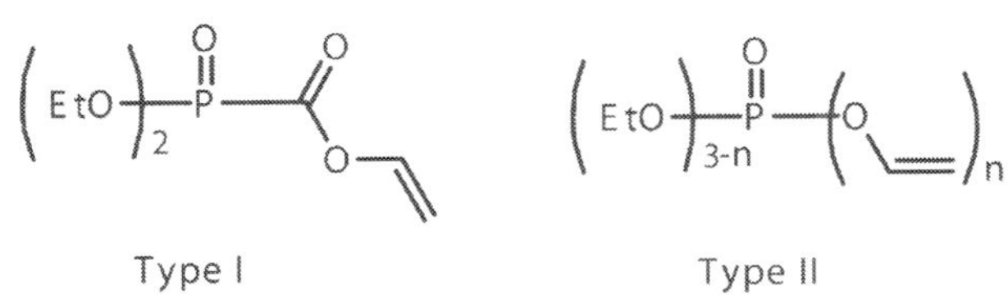

Fig. 2. Monomers based on phosphorus containing vinyl esters

Synthesis of such phosphorus-based vinyl esters is simple and straight forward. For type I a Michaelis-Arbuzov reaction can be applied, starting form triethyl phosphate and chlorovinyl formate. The second type of vinyl esters of phosphoric acid is prepared in a two-step synthesis. First the lithium enolate of vinyl alcohol is prepared by the cycloreversion reaction of THF with n-butyl lithium at room temperature (Bates et. al., 1972). The enolate is then converted with a mono-, di- or trichloride of phosphoric acid to the corresponding vinyl ester of phosphoric acid.

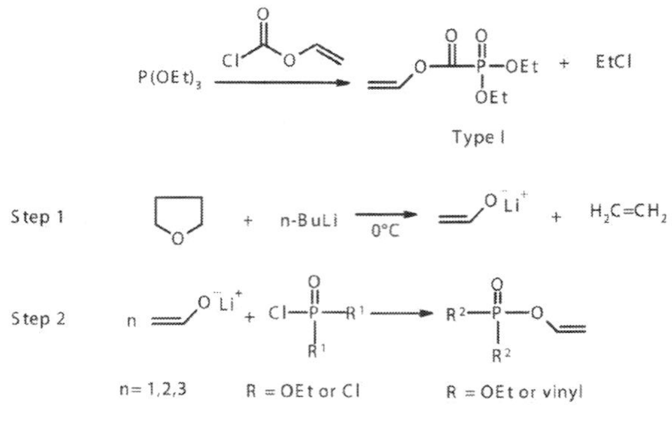

Scheme 2. Synthesis of vinyl esters Type I and Type II

Suitable reference compounds are classical acrylates and methacrylates; poly (ε-caprolactone), PCL, and PLA as representatives for biocompatible thermoplastics.

3.1 Photoreactivity

One of the most important requirement for such new monomers is their photoreactivity. By photo-differential scanning calorimetry (DSC) experiments it is possible to determine the performance of a formulation. The reactivity can be derived from the time, which is needed to reach the maximum polymerization heat (t_{max}, s). The double bond conversion (DBC) and the maximum rate of polymerization (R_{Pmax}, mol L^{-1} s^{-1}) give additional information on the performance of a photo-curable system. R_{Pmax} is calculated from the height of the maximum (h, mW mg^{-1}), and the density of the monomers (ρ, g L^{-1}) using equation 1.

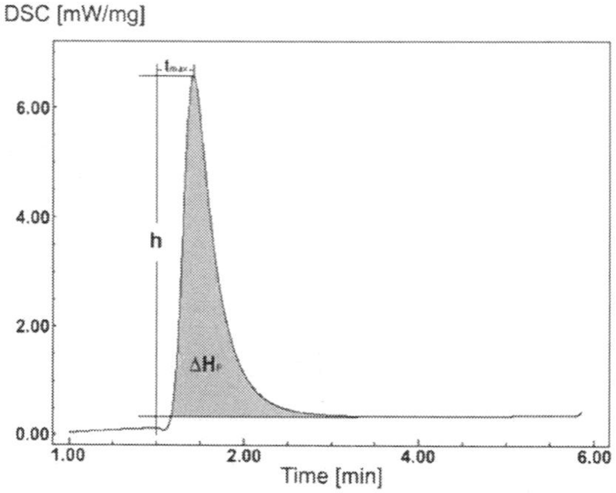

Fig. 3. Example for a photo-DSC plot and the parameters, that can be obtained

$$R_{P\max} = \frac{h \times \rho}{\Delta H_{0,P}} \qquad (1)$$

To obtain knowledge on the photoreactivity of a monomer it is also essential to know the theoretical polymerisation heat ($\Delta H_{0,p}$, J mol^{-1}). A well established method (Hoyle et. al., 1999) to determine this value is to cure monomer formulations by photo-DSC. Thus the actual heat of polymerization (H_P, J g^{-1}) evolved under this conditions is determined. In combination with the DBC obtained from ATR-IR analysis of the sample after curing by photo-DSC it is possible to calculate the theoretical polymerization heat using equation 2, where M_M (g mol^{-1}) is the molecular weight of the monomer.

$$\Delta H_{0,P} = \frac{H_P \times M_M}{DBC} \qquad (2)$$

For evaluation of the monomer reactivity and in terms of calculating their $\Delta H_{0,P}$ peak fitting can be used (PeakFit V4.12, SSI) to determine the DBC of the polymers. This method has already been established by Lemon et. al. (2007) for the investigation of hydrogen bonding in methacrylate-based monomers and polymers. In case of vinyl esters the decrease of the C=C stretching vibration at 1640 cm-1 in the monomer and the polymer spectrum, for (meth)acrylates the vibration at 1660 cm^{-1} is applicable. The P=O vibration at 1265 cm^{-1} served as reference for the phosphorus-based compounds, whereas for acrylates, methacrylates and common vinyl esters the C=O bond at 1740 cm^{-1} is suitable for this purpose.

The DBC of the phosphorus-containingvinyl monomers, obtained by peak fit analysis of the ATR-IR spectra, is rather high (~90%) - as expected. Also t_{max}, the time to reach the maximum polymerization rate, was in the range of the reference methacrylates. Generally, vinyl esters showed higher values for the $\Delta H_{0,P}$ than the reference acrylates and methacrylates, which is also in good accordance with experiments already stated in literature (Roper et. al. 2006).

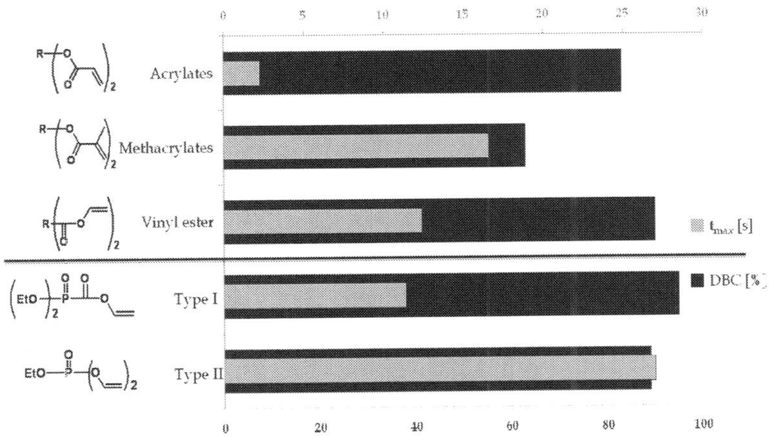

Fig. 4. Photo-Differential Scanning Calorimetry data for the phosphormonomers, Type I and II, as well as for reference acrylates and methacrylates

3.2 Cytotoxicity

Generally, photopolymers are well known to release several components into the environment after curing. These compounds might be residual monomer, molecules derived from the photoinitiator or similar products of degradation processes. With respect to their application in medicine and tissue regeneration, it is absolutely necessary to evaluate the influence of such compounds on cell proliferation and differentiation. Cell viability and multiplication as well as alkaline phosphatase (ALP) activity of osteoblasts are sensitive indicators of any substance for their compatibility with the biological tasks of the cells. Especially the ALP-activity is an important indicator whether osteoblasts proceed in their cell differentiation process or are blocked by a reagent. To compare the toxicity of the monomers, MC3T3-E1 cells were incubated with increasing amounts of the monomers. Then the concentration was approximated at which half of the cells survived. This concentration was denominated as LC_{50}. Although, some differences between cell viability and cell number were found, both parameters were comparable for all investigated monomers (Table 1). In this match vinyl esters with/without phosphorus moieties had the least influence on cell multiplication. Compared to methacrylates, which are already in use as biomaterials (e.g. poly(methyl methacrylate) as component in dental filling formulations), ALP activity was significantly better for the vinyl ester-based monomers. It could be demonstrated, that some of the vinyl ester compounds even stimulated the cell differentiation process, visible by an increase of ALP activity over 100% compared to the control group. Short chain fatty acids differentially regulate proliferation and differentiation of cultured cells. Most studies are based on butyrate and the tumor drug valproate (Oki & Issa, 2006). Both regulate proliferation and differentiation by inhibiting histone deacetylase activity, which is an important regulator of gene expression and cell differentiation. It might be speculated, that the increase of ALP activity of the vinyl esters is the result of a similar mechanism.

	phospho vinyl esters	**vinyl esters**	**methacrylates**
Viability [LC_{50}]	3-12 mM	3-10 mM	1-3 mM
Cell number [LC_{50}]	5-16 mM	2-10 mM	0.8-2 mM
ALP-activity [% of control group]	60-123	40-135	6

Table 1. Influence of the monomers on cell multiplication, viability and ALP activity of osteoblast-like cells

3.3 Mechanical testing

Mechanical properties of a material can be easily screened by the nanoindentation method. It allows a very fast and material-saving comparison of some basic mechanical properties of the investigated polymers. From the recorded load versus displacement data the indentation modulus (YM_{IT}) and indentation hardness (H_{IT}) can be extracted (Schiffmann, 2007; Oliver & Pharr, 2007). H_{IT} is calculated starting from the maximum force F_{max} by applying equations 3 and 4:

$$H_{IT} = \frac{F_{max}}{24.5 \times h_c^2} \tag{3}$$

$$h_c = h_{max} - \varepsilon\left(h_{max} - h_r\right) \quad (4)$$

where F_{max} is the maximum force, h_{max} is the penetration depth at maximum force, h_r is the intersection of the tangent of the unloading curve at maximum load with the x-axis, and ε is the indenter constant.
YM_{IT} is calculated starting from the slope of the unloading curve´s tangent at the maximum load as shown in equations 5 and 6.

$$YM_{IT} = \frac{1-(\nu_s)^2}{\frac{1}{YM_r} - \frac{1-(\nu_s)^2}{YM_i}} \quad (5)$$

$$YM_r = \frac{\sqrt{\pi} \times s}{2 \times \sqrt{A_p}} \quad (6)$$

With ν_s being the Poisson´s ratio of the indenter tip, YM_r the reduced modulus of the indentation contact in [MPa], YM_i the modulus of the indenter tip in [MPa], S the contact strength in [N/m] (defined as the resistance of two particles against their mutual displacement) and A_P the projected area in [m²].
As shown in Figure 5, the mechanical properties of all investigated photopolymers materials superseded the reference material PCL which is used as biodegradable polymer for various biomedical applications, e.g. bone replacement or tissue engineering. Astonishingly, the highly crosslinked Type II polymer with n=3 exhibited even better mechanical properties than the semicrystalline reference PLA which finds also wide-spread use as biodegradable material. Moreover, the IM of this polymer already approached that of human bone (Lewis & Nyman, 2008) and also an extraordinary high hardness was found for this compound.

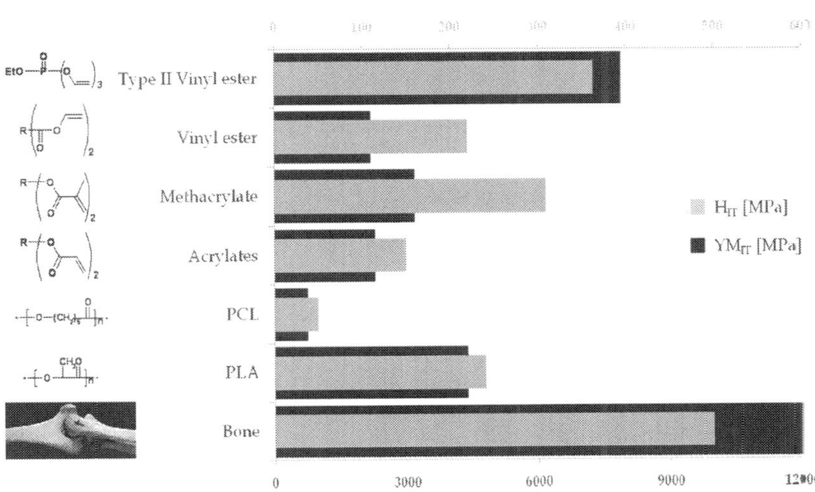

Fig. 5. Mechanical Properties of the phosphorus containing polymers determined by nanoindentaion experiments

3.4 Degradation behaviour

Hydrolytic degradation of polymers is a desired feature especially for bone replacement materials. In the ideal case, the polymeric material will start degradation after the cultivation with bone cells and the initiation of bone re-growth. An important point is also the nature of the degradation products, which should of course be non-toxic towards the human body. From the degradation of polyphosphoesters it is known, that the breakdown of such polymers by hydrolytic or enzymatic cleavage delivers finally phosphates and alcohol derivatives (Wang et. al. 2001; Wachiralarpphaithoon et. al. 2007). Several other phosphorus based degradation products could be expected as it was shown in another study dealing with the hydrolytic degradation mechanisms of polyphosphoesters (Baran & Penczek 1995). However, it can be assumed in the case of the vinyl ester based phosphopolymers that during the surface erosion and/or degradation process non-toxic polyvinyl alcohol is released from such materials.
Recent studies (Heller et. al. 2011) have proven that degradation rates of cross-linked vinyl esters are significantly higher than for PLA, PCL or their acrylate counterparts under acidic conditions (Figure 6). This was confirmed in model experiments with low molecular polymer-analogous compounds. An explanation could be given by the less sterically hindered C=O group of polyvinyl esters compared to polyacrylates. Surprisingly, the polymers of Type II phosphoric acid vinyl esters showed almost similar degradation times under acidic and alkaline conditions, exceeding the other investigated materials at low pH values. This rather fast degradation under acidic hydrolysis might be favourable for its use as bone replacement material, as the bone-destroying cells, the osteoclasts also form an acidic milieu during the bone-resorption process.

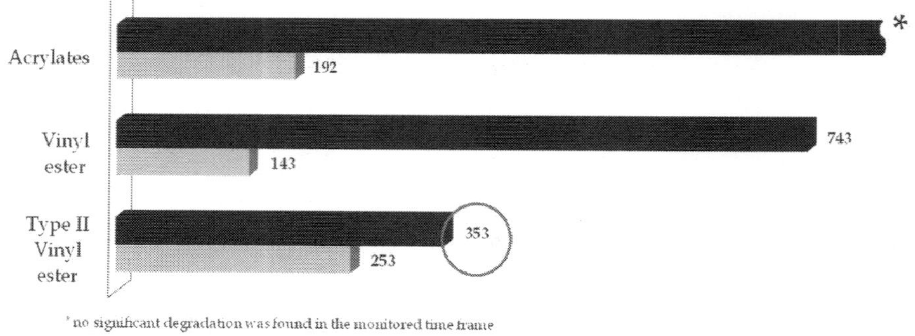

Fig. 6. Data for erosion behaviour of the phosphorus-containing photopolymers compared to PLA

4. Conclusion

Biocompatible photopolymerizable polymers with a polyvinyl alcohol backbone are promising alternatives to common thermoplastic materials like PLA, as photopolymerization offers a wide range of processing technologies. Besides, vinyl esters show great advantages compared to acrylates and methacrylates, which are standard materials for soft tissue replacement. In contrast to non-toxic vinyl esters, scaffolds based on classical polyacrylates proved to be harmful because of their residual functional groups, that provoke adverse effects on the cells already adhered to the scaffolds surface by Michael addition to amino or thiol containing groups in proteins or DNA. To further improve biocompatibility of the monomers, polymers and degradation products, aiming at future applications in bone replacement surgery, a phosphorus moiety can be introduced onto these vinyl esters. The advantage of such polymers is clear: the products of hydrolytic degradation are phosphoric acid or phosphates and non-toxic polyvinyl alcohol, which finds widespread use as glue on stamps, as component of chewing gums and also as additive in medical drugs. By Photo-DSC experiments good photoreactivity was found for the phosphorus-containing monomers, comparable to common vinyl esters. With respect to their use as medical implants, the cytotoxicity, hydrolytic degradation and mechanical properties of the obtained polymers were tested. Cell viability and measurements on the development of alkaline phosphatase-activity revealed a low cytotoxicity. Surprisingly, some phosphorus containing vinyl esters exhibited even a stimulatory effect on the osteoblast cells´ differentiation process. By nanoindentation measurements the hardness and elastic modulus of the polymers was determined. These showed mechanical stability almost in the range of human bone, actually without the addition of any filling material.

5. Acknowledgment

Financial support by the Austrian Science Fund FWF for this project, P19769-N14, is gratefully acknowledged.

6. References

Anseth, KS; Goodner, MD; Reil, MA; Kannurpatti, AR; Newman, SM; Bowman, CN. (1996) The influence of comonomer composition on dimethacrylate resin properties for dental composites. *Journal of Dental Research*, 75 (8),1607-1612.

Baier LJ; Bivens KA; Patrick CW; Schmidt CE. (2003) Photocrosslinked hyaluronic acid hydrogels: natural, biodegradable tissue engineering scaffolds. *Biotechnology and bioengineering*, 82 (5), 578-89.

Baran, J; Penczek, S. (1995) Hydrolysis of Polyesters of Phosphoric Acid. 1. Kinetics and the pH Profile. *Macromolecules,* 28 (15), 5167-5176.

Bates RB, Kroposki LM, Potter DE. (1972) Cycloreversion of anions from tetrahydrofurans. A convenient synthesis of lithium enolates of aldehydes. *J Org Chem*, 37, 560-562.

Burdick, JA; Chung, C; Jia, X; Randolph, MA.; Langer, R. (2005) Controlled Degradation and Mechanical Behavior of Photopolymerized Hyaluronic Acid Networks. *Biomacromolecules*, 6 (1), 386-391.

Burkoth, AK.; Burdick, J; Anseth, KS. (2000) Surface and bulk modifications to photocrosslinked polyanhydrides to control degradation behavior. *Journal of Biomedical Materials Research,* 51 (3), 352-359.

Censi, R; Vermonden T; van Steenbergen MJ; Deschout, H; Braeckmans K; De Smedt SC; van Nostrum CF, di Martino P, Hennink WE. (2009) Photopolymerized thermosensitive hydrogels for tailorable diffusion-controlled protein delivery. *Journal of Controlled Release*, 140 (3), 230-236.

Clapper JD; Skeie JM; Mullins RF; Guymon CA. (2007). Development and characterization of photopolymerizable biodegradable materials from PEG-PLA-PEG block macromonomers. *Polymer*, 48 (22), 6554-6564.

Davis KA; Burdick, JA; Anseth, KS. (2003) Photoinitiated crosslinked degradable copolymer networks for tissue engineering applications. *Biomaterials*, 24, 2485-2495.

Declercq, HA; Gorski, TL; Tielens, SP; Schacht, EH; Cornelissen, MJ. (2005) Encapsulation of osteoblast seeded microcarriers into injectable, photopolymerizable three-dimensional scaffolds based on D,L-lactide and ε -caprolactone. *Biomacromolecules*, 6 (3), 1608-1614.

Desai, PN; Yuan, Q; Yang, H. (2010) Synthesis and Characterization of Photocurable Polyamidoamine Dendrimer Hydrogels as a Versatile Platform for Tissue Engineering and Drug Delivery. *Biomacromolecules*, 11 (3), 666-673.

Dworak, C; Koch, T; Varga, F; Liska, R. (2010) Photopolymerization of Biocompatible Phosphorus-containing Vinyl esters and Vinyl carbamates. *Journal of Polymer Science Part A: Polymer Chemistry*, 48, 2916-2924.

Fouassier, JP. (1995) Photoinitiators and Photosensitizers. In *Photoinitiation, photopolymerization and photocuring*; 11-15, Hanser New York

Gonen-Wadmany, M; Oss-Ronen, L; Seliktar, D. (2007) Protein-polymer conjugates for forming photopolymerizable biomimetic hydrogels for tissue engineering. *Biomaterials*, 28 (26), 3876-3886.

Hayashi K. (1978) Radical polymerization and co-polymerization of some vinylphosphates. Die Makromolekulare Chemie, 179 (7), 1753-1763.

Heller, C; Schwentenwein, M; Russmüller, G; Koch, T; Moser, D; Schopper, C; Varga, F; Stampfl, J; Liska, R. (2011) Vinylcarbonates and Vinylcarbamates: Biocompatible Monomers for Radical Photopolymerization. *Journal of Polymer Science, Part A: Polymer Chemistry*, 49, 650-661.

Heller, C; Schwentenwein, M; Russmueller, G; Varga, F; Stampfl, J; Liska, R. (2009) Vinyl esters: Low cytotoxicity monomers for the fabrication of biocompatible 3D scaffolds by lithography based additive manufacturing. *Journal of Polymer Science, Part A: Polymer Chemistry*, 47 (24), 6941-6954.

Hill-West JL; Chowdhury SM; Sawhney AS; Pathak CP; Dunn RC; Hubbell JA. (1994) Prevention of postoperative adhesions in the rat by in situ photopolymerization of bioresorbable hydrogel barriers. *Obstetrics and gynecology*, 83(1), 59-64.

Hiraguri J; Katase K; Tokiwa, Y. (2006) Synthesis of Biodegradable Hydrogel by Radical Ring-Opening Polymerization of 2-Methylene-1,3,6-Trioxocane. *Journal of Macromolecular Science, Part A: Pure and Applied Chemistry*, 43 (7), 1021-1027.

Hou Q; Grijpma DW; Feijen J. (2009) Creep-resistant elastomeric networks prepared by photocrosslinking fumaric acid monoethyl ester-functionalized poly(trimethylene carbonate) oligomers. *Acta biomaterialia*, 5 (5), 1543-51.

Hoyle, CE; Miller, CW; Jonsson, ES. (1999) Photochemistry and photopolymerization of maleimides. *Trends in Photochemistry & Photobiology*, 5, 149-167.

Ifkovits, JL; Burdick, JA. (2007) Review: Photopolymerizable and Degradable Biomaterials for Tissue Engineering Applications. *Tissue engineering*, 10, 2369-2385.

Kumpulainen H; Järvinen T; Saari R; Lehtonen M; Vepsäläinen J. (2005) An efficient strategy for the synthesis of 1-chloroethyl phosphates and phosphoroamidates. *Journal of Organic Chemistry*, 70 (22), 9056-9058.

Lavanant, L; Pullin, B; Hubbell, JA; Klok, H-A. (2010) A Facile Strategy for the Modification of Polyethylene Substrates with Non-Fouling, Bioactive Poly (poly (ethylene glycol) methacrylate) Brushes. *Macromolecular Bioscience*, 10 (1), 101-108.

Leach, JB; Schmidt, CE. (2004) Characterization of protein release from photocrosslinkable hyaluronic acid-polyethylene glycol hydrogel tissue engineering scaffolds. *Biomaterials*, 26 (2), 125-135.

Lemon, MT; Jones, MS; Stansbury, JW. (2007) hydrogen bonding interactions in methacrylate monomers and polymers. *Journal of Biomedical Materials Research Part A*, 33, 734-746.

Lewis, G; Nyman, JS. (2008) The use of nanoindentation for characterizing the properties of mineralized hard tissues: state-of-the art review. *Journal of Biomedical Materials Research, Part B: Applied Biomaterials*, 87 B(1), 286-301.

Liat O-R, Seliktar D. (2010). Photopolymerizable hydrogels made from polymer-conjugated albumin for affinity-based drug delivery. *Advanced Biomaterials*, 1, B45-B52.

Liu, VA; Bhatia, SN. (2002) Three-dimensional photopatterning of hydrogels containing living cells. *Biomedical Microdevices*, 4 (4), 257-266.

Liu, Y; Chan-Park, MB. (2010) A biomimetic hydrogel based on methacrylated dextran -graft-lysine and gelatin for 3D smooth muscle cell culture. *Biomaterials*, 31 (6), 1158-1170.

Liu B; Lewis AK; Shen W. (2008). Physical Hydrogels Photo-Cross-Linked from Self-Assembled Macromers for Potential Use in Tissue Engineering. *Biomacromolecules*, 10 (12), 3182-3187.

Ma, G; Yang D; Li, Q; Wang K; Chen B; Kennedy J; Nie J. (2010). Injectable hydrogels based on chitosan derivative/polyethylene glycol dimethacrylate/N,N-dimethylacrylamide as bone tissue engineering matrix. *Carbohydrate Polymers*, 79 (3), 620-627.

Martens, PJ; Bryant, SJ; Anseth, KS. (2003) Tailoring the Degradation of Hydrogels Formed from Multivinyl Poly (ethylene glycol) and Poly (vinyl alcohol) Macromers for Cartilage Tissue Engineering. *Biomacromolecules*, 4 (2), 283-292.

Matsuda, T; Magoshi, T. (2002) Preparation of Vinylated Polysaccharides and Photofabrication of Tubular Scaffolds as Potential Use in Tissue Engineering. *Biomacromolecules*, 3 (5), 942-950.

Mawad, D; Martens, PJ; Odell, RA.; Poole-Warren, LA. (2006) The effect of redox polymerization on degradation and cell responses to poly (vinyl alcohol) hydrogels. *Biomaterials*, 28 (6), 947-955.

Naik, RR; Brott, LL; Rodriguez, F; Agarwal, G; Kirkpatrick, SM.; Stone, MO. (2003) Bio-inspired approaches and biologically derived materials for coatings. *Progress in Organic Coatings* 47 (3-4), 249-255.

Nijst, CLE; Bruggeman, JP.; Karp, JM.; Ferreira, L; Zumbuehl, A; Bettinger, CJ.; Langer, R. (2007) Synthesis and Characterization of Photocurable Elastomers from Poly(glycerol-co-sebacate). *Biomacromolecules*, 8 (10), 3067-3073.

Nuttelman CR, Rice MA, Rydholm AE, Salinas CN, Shah, DN, Anseth KS. (2008). Macromolecular monomers for the synthesis of hydrogel niches and their application in cell encapsulation and tissue engineering. *Progress in Polymer Science*, 33 (2), 167-179.

Oki, Y; Issa, J-P. (2006) Review: recent clinical trials in epigenetic therapy. *Reviews on Recent Clinical Trials*, 1 (2), 169-182.

Oliver, WC; Pharr, GM. (2004) Measurement of hardness and elastic modulus by instrumented indentation: advances in understanding and refinements to methodology. *Journal of Materials Research*, 19 (1), 3-20.

Peng, HT; Martineau L; Shek PN. (2007) Hydrogel-elastomer composite biomaterials: 1. Preparation of interpenetrating polymer networks and in vitro characterization of swelling stability and mechanical properties. *J Mater Sci: Mater Med*, 18, 975–986.

Polizzotti, BD; Fairbanks, BD; Anseth, KS. (2008) Three-Dimensional Biochemical Patterning of Click-Based Composite Hydrogels via Thiolene Photopolymerization. *Biomacromolecules*, 9 (4), 1084-1087.

Roper, TM; Hoyle, CE; Magers, DH. (2006). Reaction enthalpies of monomers involved in photopolymerization. In *Photochemistry and UV-curing. New Trends*. J.P. Fouassier Ed.; 253-264. Research Signpost, India.

Rydholm, AE; Held, NL; Danielle SW; Bowman, CN; Anseth, KS. (2008) Modifying network chemistry in thiol-acrylate photopolymers through postpolymerization functionalization to control cell-material interactions. *Journal of Biomedical Materials Research, Part A*, 86 A(1), 23-30

Sawhney, AS, Pathak, CP; Hubbell, GA. (1993) Bioerodible hydrogels based on photopolymerized poly(ethylene glycol)-co-poly(α-hydroxy acid) diacrylate emacromers. *Macromolecules*, 26, 581-587.

Schiffmann, KI. (2007) Area function calibration in nanoindentation using the hardness instead of Young's modulus of fused silica as a reference value. *International Journal of Materials Research*, 98 (5), 424-429

Schuster M; Turecek C; Weigel G; Saf R; Stampfl J; Varga F; Liska R. (2009). Gelatin-based photopolymers for bone replacement materials. *Journal of Polymer Science, Part A: Polymer Chemistry*, 47 (24), 7078-7089.

Shah, NM; Pool, MD; Metters, AT. (2006) Influence of Network Structure on the Degradation of Photo-Cross-Linked PLA-b-PEG-b-PLA Hydrogels. *Biomacromolecules*, 7 (11), 3171-3177.

Sharifi S; Imani M; Mirzadeh H; Atai M.; Ziaee F.; Bakhshi R. (2009) Synthesis, characterization, and biocompatibility of novel injectable, biodegradable, and in situ crosslinkable polycarbonate-based macromers. *Journal of biomedical materials research. Part A*, 90 (3), 830-43.

Shi, Q; Zhong, S; Chen, Y; Whitaker, A. (2010) Photo-crosslinking copolymers based polyanhydride and 1G polyamidoamine-methacrylamide as bone tissue engineering: Synthesis, characterization, and in vitro degradation. *Polymer Degradation and Stability*, 95 (10), 1961-1968.

Wachiralarpphaithoon C; Iwasaki Y; Akiyoshi K. (2007) Enzyme-degradable phosphorylcholine porous hydrogels cross-linked with polyphosphoesters for cell matrices. *Biomaterials*, 28 (6), 984-993.

Wang, J; Mao, H-Q; Leong, KW. (2001) A Novel Biodegradable Gene Carrier Based on Polyphosphoester. *Journal of the American Chemical Society*, 123 (38), 9480-9481.

Werkmeister, JA; Adhikari, R; White, JF; Tebb, TA; Le, TPT; Taing, HC; Mayadunne, R; Gunatillake, PA; Danon, SJ; Ramshaw, JAM. (2010) Biodegradable and injectable cure-on-demand polyurethane scaffolds for regeneration of articular cartilage. *Acta Biomaterialia*, 6 (9), 3471-3481.

Xu, J; Li, X; Sun, F. (2010) Cyclodextrin-containing hydrogels for contact lenses as a platform for drug incorporation and release. *Acta Biomaterialia*, 6 (2), 486-493.

Zhang, N; Casida, JE. (2000) Convenient syntheses of biologically relevant vinyl and divinyl phosphates by selective dealkylation of the corresponding phosphites. *Synthesis*, 10, 1454-1458

8

Coating Nanomagnetic Particles for Biomedical Applications

Ângela Andrade[1], Roberta Ferreira[2], José Fabris[3] and Rosana Domingues[2]
[1]*Department of Chemistry, ICEB, Federal University of Ouro Preto*
[2]*Department of Chemistry, ICEx, Federal University of Minas Gerais*
[3]*Federal University of Jequitinhonha and Mucuri Valleys, Diamantina, Minas Gerais*
Brazil

1. Introduction

Magnetic particles with dimensions ranging from the nanometer to the micrometer scales are being used in an increasing number of medical applications, since the mid-1970s. The most important properties of magnetic particles for clinical diagnostics and medical therapies are clearly nontoxicity, biocompatiblilty, injectability, and high-level accumulation in the target tissue or specific organ, being strictly and spatially confined to the planned region of the internal body (Ito et al., 2005). The unique feature of NMPs to be guided by an external magnetic field has been used in magnetic resonance imaging (MRI), tissue repair, hyperthermia, drug delivery, and in cell separation (Duguet et al., 2006; Gupta & Gupta, 2005; Gupta et al., 2007; Mccarthy et al., 2007). For these biomedical applications, magnetic particles exhibiting superparamagnetic behavior at room temperature are preferred because they do not retain any magnetism after removal of the magnetic field. For NMPs, this behavior can be explained by their extraordinarily reduced sizes (Mørup et al., 1976; Pfannes, 1997). The magnetization relaxation depends on KV/kT (Gupta & Gupta, 2005; Gupta et al., 2007) in which K is the particle anisotropy constant, V is particle volume, k is Boltzmann's constant and T is temperature. At a certain reduced size (volume), KV becomes comparable to the thermal energy kT. As a result, the magnetization of the particle fluctuates rapidly from one direction to another due to the thermal agitation, leaving no net magnetic moment. At this magnetic stage, the particle is said to be superparamagnetic (Xu & Sun, 2007). Fig. 1 shows a magnetization curve obtained by Andrade *et al* for a NMPs with particle size of 7 nm (Andrade et al., 2009). This shows that a particle can be magnetized under an external magnetic field (H), reaching a maximum moment (M) when the field is strong enough. However, there is no remnant magnetic moment, i.e. without an external magnetic field, the net moment of the particle is randomized to zero. Therefore, these superparamagnetic nanoparticles are very useful for biomedical applications as they are not subject to strong magnetic interactions in the dispersion and are readily stabilized in physiological conditions (Gupta & Gupta, 2005; Neuberger et al., 2005; Sonvico et al., 2005).

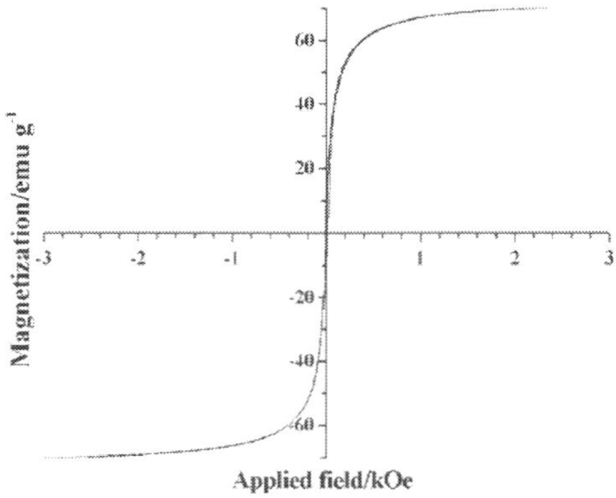

Fig. 1. Magnetization curve for NMPs with the applied magnetic field. This hysteresis loop indicates nearly zero value for coercivity and magnetic remanence.

Among superparamagnetic nanoparticles, iron oxide nanoparticles such as magnetite (Fe_3O_4) or its oxidized form maghemite (γ-Fe_2O_3) are by far the most commonly employed in biomedical applications, as their biocompatibility has already been proven (Schwertmann & Cornell, 2000; Souza et al., 2008). Highly magnetic materials such as cobalt and nickel are toxic, susceptible to oxidation and hence are of little interest. Nanoparticles of magnetic iron oxides, are usually modified through the formation the formation of few atomic layers of polymer/surfactant or inorganic metallic (such as gold) or oxide surfaces (such as silica or alumina), which prevents agglomeration and also allows further functionalization by attaching various biomolecules (Berry & Curtis, 2003; Ferreira et al., 2009).
NMPs with suitable surface characteristics have potential applications both *in vitro* and *in vivo*. Information about the way the magnetic particle system is prepared and its surface is modified must be accompanied by its full characterization, by determining particles size distribution and morphology, their surface chemistry and, obviously, magnetic properties. All these features are critically important, if the material is planned and destined for application in medical practices (Andrade et al., 2009). This review covers most of these essential topics with illustrative examples of applications of monodisperse NMPs in clinical diagnostics, magnetic separation and human medical therapy.

2. Application of magnetic nanoparticles

Uses of NMPs in biotechnology and biomedicine have dramatically increased over the last few of years. They can be grouped into two broader categories, depending on the methodology: *in vitro* and *in vivo* procedures. For *in vitro* applications, the main use is in diagnostic and separation/labeling of biomolecules, such as protein, cell, DNA/RNA, microorganism, for *in vivo*, applications can be further split into (i) diagnoses (magnetic resonance imaging (MRI)) and (ii) therapies (drug delivery and hyperthermia).
The applications of superparamagnetic nanoparticles in biomedicine can be rationalized as follows: firstly, the superparamagnetic nanoparticles are a class of intrinsically ordered magnetic materials. As their magnetic signal is generated by application of external strong magnetic field it far exceeds that signal from any of the known biomolecules. This makes

them readily identified by a magnet or magnetic sensor from an ocean of biomolecules. Secondly, at diameters less than 20 nm, these particles are smaller than or comparable to a cell (10–100 µm), a virus (20–450 nm), a protein (5–50 nm) or a gene (2 nm wide and 10–100 nm long). These, plus their capability of being manipulated under an external magnetic field, provide controllable means of magnetically tagging biomolecules, leading to potentially highly efficient bioseparation, highly sensitive biosensing and magnetic resonance imaging (MRI) contrast enhancement, as well as site-specific drug delivery (Dobson, 2006; Gupta & Gupta, 2005; Neuberger et al., 2005; Sunderland et al., 2006). Such particles also respond resonantly to an alternating magnetic field, allowing the transfer of magnetic energy to the particles as a form of heat. This has been proposed to be one of the key approaches to successful cancer therapy in the future (Hilger et al., 2005; Ito et al., 2005).

These potential biomedical applications of NMPs require that the nanoparticles be monodisperse, meaning that each individual nanoparticle has identical physical and chemical properties allowing controlled biodistribution, bioelimination and contrast effects (Andrade *et al.*, 2011).

In the absence of any surface coating, NMPs have hydrophobic surfaces with a large surface area to volume ratio. Due to hydrophobic interactions between the particles, they tend to agglomerate forming large clusters. Coating favors the effective stabilization and dispersion ability of NMPs. Besides this, coatings making them better water- or oil-soluble thus providing better conditions for functionalization to form conjugate biomolecules. A variety of experimental approaches have been proposed and used to coat NMPs, including *in situ* and post-synthesis coating (Laconte et al., 2005). In the *in situ* approach, the NMPs are coated with some stabilizer such as surfactants or polymers during the synthesis process. Various surfactants, e.g., oleic acid, sodium oleate, dodecylamine, sodium dodecylbenzene sulphonate have been used in the synthesis of NMPs. These surfactants always form a double layer on the surfaces of magnetic particles turning them more stable (Shen et al., 1999; Shen et al., 2001; Wooding et al., 1991). Surfactants such as polymers, cyclodextrins and large capping ligands stabilize nanoparticles trough steric repulsion of interparticle interaction. However, small-molecules like carboxylates and phosphates engage the electrostatic mechanism in aqueous medium. Magnetic nanoparticles stabilized by electrostatic layer and steric layer are showed in Fig. 2.

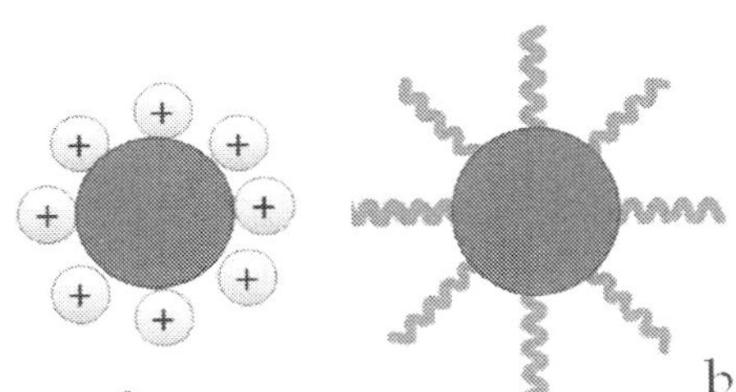

Fig. 2. Nanoparticles stabilized by: a) electrostatic layer and b) steric layer.

Polymeric coating materials may be either synthetic or natural. Examples of synthetic polymers are: poly (ethyleneglycol) (PEG) (Suzuki et al., 1995), poly (vinyl alcohol) (PVA) (Lee et al., 1996), poly (lactic acid) (PLA) (Gomez-Lopera et al., 2001), polyethylene

(Chatterjee et al., 2002) and block copolymer (Harris et al., 2003). Natural polymers include dextran (Paul et al., 2004), chitosan (Hassan et al., 1992) and starch (Veiga et al., 2000).
The post-synthesis coating methods for NMPs make use of a variety of materials, including monolayer ligands, polymers, combinations of polymers and biomolecules such as phospholipids and carbohydrates, and inorganic materials, such as silica (Kobayashi et al., 2003) and gold (Kinoshita et al., 2003). These coatings not only provide stability to nanoparticles in solution but also help in binding the several biological ligands on the nanoparticle surface, as needed for medical applications. The aim of surface functionalization of magnetic composite particles, such as polymer-coated NMPs and silica coated NMPs, is to introduce some functional groups on the surface intending to immobile biomolecules and biological ligands, such as antibodies, proteins, transferring (Berry et al., 2004), folic acid (Zhang et al., 2002). These can be attached onto the polymer surfaces coating the magnetic nanoparticles, by chemical coupling, to make the particles target-specific.
Surface functional groups are usually introduced into magnetic particles-polymer systems by two main methods: copolymerization and chemical modification of the preformed polymer. In copolymerization, a large amount of functional groups are usually buried in the polymer and only a low surface density of functional groups is obtained. Chemical modification has been reported to be an efficient way to obtain abundant functional groups on the surface of magnetic particles (Liu et al., 2005; 2004a, 2004b; Ma et al., 2005a, 2005b). However, in some reactions, due to high acid or strong oxidation effect, the magnetic iron oxide inside the composite particles gets deteriorated, thus resulting in the loss of magnetic properties.
For silica coated magnetic particles, the functional groups are usually introduced by silanation using silane coupling agents (Levy et al., 2002; Liu et al., 2004c, 2004d). A typical silane coupling agent has the structure of $Y\text{–}(CH_2)n\text{–}Si\text{–}X_3$, where X represents the alkoxy or halide groups and Y, the organic functional groups, including amine, thiol, carboxylic, phosphate, vinyl, cyanide, and methacrylate. The $Si\text{-}X_3$ group hydrolyzes readily in the presence of water and catalyst to form silanol groups which couple with surface silanol groups, forming Si-O-M bonds upon dehydration. As a result, the organic functional groups (Y) remain reactive on the surface. This unique feature of silane coupling agents has made silanation a widely used method in modifying surface properties and introducing functional groups on particles. A large volume of literature is available for the surface functionalization of magnetic silica particles by silanation (Berry & Curtis, 2003; Dong et al., 2008; Koneracka et al., 1999; Sulek et al.).

2.1 Magnetic separation

The processes of isolation and separation of specific molecules are used in almost all areas of biosciences and biotechnology, and are the most documented and currently the most useful application of NMPs (Lucena et al., 2011 ; Smith et al., 2006).
The basic principle of magnetic separation is relatively simple. NMPs with an immobilized affinity or hydrophobic ligand or ion-exchange groups are mixed with a sample containing the target compound. Following an incubation period, when the target compound binds to the NMPs, the magnetic complex is easily and rapidly separated from the sample using an appropriate magnetic separator Fig 3. The system can be reused several times. After washing out contaminants, the eluted magnetic material will be ready for new usage.

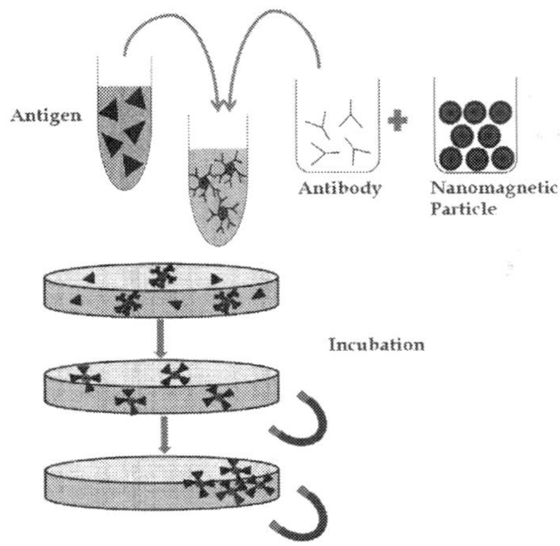

Fig. 3. Magnetic separation of antigens with antibody-functionalized NMPs

Compared to other standard separation procedures, such as chromatography and centrifuges, magnetic separation has several advantages: it is usually very simple and can be performed directly in crude samples containing suspended solid materials. In fact, magnetic separation is the only feasible method for recovery of small magnetic particles in the presence of biological debris and other fouling materials of similar size (Safarik & Safarikova, 2004). Magnetic separation has wide application in biotechnology and biomedicine. The protein separation with organosilane, such as carboxyl, aldehyde, amine, and thiol groups, and also assembled silica coated NMPs was achieved for model proteins such as bovine serum albumin (BSA) and lysozyme (LSZ) at different pH conditions. A work on using these amino functionalized silica coated NMPs for protein purification indicates that they have many advantages such as easy preparation, low cost, easy handling and rapid purification. These particles have extensive potential for serving as a very useful tool for facilitating biotechnology applications (Chang et al., 2008). Ma et al. had developed magnetic poly (methacrylate-divinylbenzene) (mPMA-DVB) microspheres with copper ions capable of binding proteins that display metal affinity. It was showed a high adsorption capacity of the microspheres with rather low non-specific adsorption when the model protein, bovine hemoglobin (BHb), was adopted to investigate (Ma et al., 2005a). A simple and efficient method for protein separation using hydrophobic pocket-modified Si-NMPs was demonstrated by Chang et al. Silica-coated NMPs (Si-NMPs) with alkyl as the hydrophobic pockets of target proteins such as BSA was prepared. It was demonstrated the efficient adsorption or desorption depends on the hydrophobic pockets size adsorption. The study showed an appropriate surface modification technique to prepare system can be used in clinical diagnoses and protein/enzyme recognition processes (Chang et al., 2010).

Array-based bioassay is a promising approach for DNA, protein, and microbe analyses (Macbeath & Schreiber, 2000; Mark Schena, 1995; Wilson & Nock, 2003). Currently, fluorescence and chemiluminescence technologies are used as a standard for the detection on microarrays owing to their high sensitivity, dynamic range, and multiplexing capabilities. However, this approach has the disadvantage in that the signal from the labels is often reduced in intensity because of photo-degradation. To improve the performance of the array-based assay, the development of molecular labels for bioassay is an important issue for improving detection sensitivity. As one of the attractive materials for the assay system, nanoparticles conjugated with biological molecules have been proposed for use as a label (Amemiya et al., 2005; Baselt et al., 1998; Goldman et al., 2004; Park et al., 2002; Reichert et al., 2000). NMPs are detectable by measuring their magnetism. They are unaffected by the measurement process, and the samples may be stored indefinitely (Richardson et al., 2001). Detection techniques based on magnetic labels are simple to perform and inexpensive in terms of instrumentation compared with the fluorescence detection method, and therefore they are suitable for miniaturization of the detection system (Edelstein et al., 2000; Richardson et al., 2001). NMPs are also much less costly than fluorescent dyes including quantum dots.

NMPs also have been coated with amorphous silica shells for enhanced surface reactivity and RNA and DNA purification (Park & Chang, 2007)**Error! Reference source not found.**. DNA is a polyanionic molecule due to the presence of phosphate groups on the nucleic acid backbone and is conveniently captured on a polymeric resin or other metal/inorganic supports with positively charged functional groups. However, current DNA purification methods suffer from several drawbacks that make them unsuitable for the manufacture of pharmaceutical grade. They often involve the use of solvents, toxic chemicals such as cesium chloride, ethidium bromide, phenol, and chloroform, or animal-derived enzymes such as ribonuclease A and lysozyme that are either not approved or not recommended by regulatory agencies. Finally, many techniques were designed to produce small quantities of DNA for laboratory use and are not suitable for the production of therapeutic materials at larger scale (Park & Chang, 2007). Surface modifications of NMPs with suitable intermediates are commonly used to extract the desired target. The driving forces for adsorption processes are hydrophobic, electrostatic, and ligand binding interactions (Donselaar et al., 1997; Massart & Cabuil, 1987). Desorptions of the biomolecules from the magnetic particles could be achieved by using high concentration salts, changing pH, and temperature, for undergoing conformational changes. An example is a sensitive and selective method for DNA detection related to HIV gene using nanoparticle-based Raman tags and magnetic nanoparticles as immobilization and separation tool have developed by Liang et al (Liang et al., 2007). The method based on DNA hybridization uses biocompatible Ag/SiO_2 nanoparticle-based Raman tags functionalized with oligonucleotides applied as detection tool and the amino group functionalized silica-coated magnetic nanoparticles with captures trands as immobilization and separation tool. In addition to facilitate separation, the magnetic nanoparticles led to enhances the Raman signal. However, despite the potential benefits of this technology, it still remains limited to analytical or laboratory scales rather than preparative scale, largely due to low binding capacity of magnetic particles. In magnetic separation, classical proteinaceous ligands, such as streptavidin, antibodies, protein A, protein G, tripsin, inhibitors and cofactors are used most often throughout protein separation. In recent years, some other pseudo affinity ligands, such as triazine dyes (Ma et al., 2006b; Odabaš & Denizli, 2004), metal ions (Akgöl et al., 2004; Ma et al., 2006a; O'brien et al., 1996) have gained much interest. Classical proteinaceous ligands suffer from the disadvantage of high cost, low binding capacity on immobilization, and liability to sanitizing agents used to regenerate the supports. In comparison, pseudo affinity ligands (e.g., metal ions) offer the advantage of low cost, high stability, and easy coupling to the supports with high density, resulting in high-capacity supports. Thus, pseudo affinity ligands are more suitable for large-scale protein separation (O'brien et al., 1996, 1997;

Odabaš et al., 2004). NMPs have been used in separation of target cells from a heterogeneous cell mixture. A novel MHC/peptide complex-conjugated bacterial magnetic particle was developed for separation of melanoma-specific cytotoxic T lymphocytes (CTLs). CTLs are essential in anticancer and antivirus immunity and purification of CTLs from heterogeneous immune cells is desired for an efficient immunotherapy and fundamental research. In the work proposed by Takahashi et al. CTLs were successfully separated from stimulated peripheral blood mononuclear cells derived from a vaccinated melanoma patient (Takahashi et al., 2009).

2.2 Magnetic target drug delivery and magnetic guided gene transfection

The major disadvantage of most drugs for tumour chemotherapy is their relative non-specificity. The drugs are administered intravenously for general system distribution, resulting in deleterious side effects as they attack normal, healthy cells in addition to the target tumour cells. Preferably, the drugs should be localized to the tumourous site. In the late 1970s researchers proposed the use of magnetic carriers to target drugs to specific sites within the body (Widder et al., 1978; Senyei et al., 2009). The attachment of drugs to magnetic particles can be used to reduce drug doses and potential side effects on healthy tissues and the costs associated with drug treatment. The size, charge and surface chemistry of the magnetic particles are particularly important in affecting both blood circulation time as well as bioavailability of the particles within the body (Berry & Curtis, 2003). In addition, magnetic properties and internalization of particles depend strongly on the size of the NMPs and the surrounding magnetic field strength. Also, some hydrodynamic parameters, such as blood flow rate, particle concentration, infusion route play significant roles. Since the 1970s, a variety of NMPs and microparticle carriers have been developed to deliver drugs to specific target sites *in vivo*. The optimization of these carriers has continued to this day. Generally, the magnetic particle core is coated with biocompatible polymers to be used for the intravenous applications. Recently, inorganic coatings such as silica and gold have been developed. The coating acts to shield the magnetic particle from the surrounding environment and can also be functionalized by attaching functional groups, e.g., biotin, avidin and other molecules.

A treatment of hepatocellular carcinoma (HCC) via trans-arterial chemoembolization in the hepatic-artery applying therapeutic magnetic microcarriers (TMMC) was proposed by Pouponneau et al. TMMC is constituted of biodegradable poly (D,L-lactic-co-glycolic acid) microparticles loaded with doxorubicin as antitumour drug and iron-cobalt nanoparticles. *In vitro* and *in vivo* studies showed that the magnetic resonance navigation was successfully carried out using endovascular steering of the TMMC. This work had showed the capability of MRN to enhance drug targeting in deep tissue (Pouponneau et al., 2009).

Several researchers have studied NMPs as drug carriers for paclitaxel. In one interesting study, poly-D,L-lactide-co-glycolide nanospheres loaded with biocompatible magnetic fluid and anticancer drug taxol were prepared with efficiency encapsulation and sufficient magnetization to be used as magnetic carrier (Koneracká et al., 2008). A new group of candidates as anticancer drugs were proposed by Hwu et al. Paclitaxel-conjugated nanoparticles were synthesized by using Fe_3O_4 and Au as nanoparticles and functioned as drug carriers of paclitaxel which was liberated in the presence of phosphodiesterase. Hydrophilic and hydrophobic paclitaxel conjugates were produced by synthesizing Au-NPs through different methods (Hwu et al., 2008).

Magnetically guided gene transfection (magnetofection) is another way to enhance the performance of nucleic acid and gene delivery for both, *in vivo* or *in vitro* essays (Schillinger et al., 2005). The fundamental principle of magnetofection is simple and comprises the steps of: a) formulating a magnetic vector composed of a therapeutic gene and surface modified NMPs; b) adding it to the medium covering cultured cells; c) injecting it systemically via the blood stream or applying it locally to a target tissue, and d) applying a magnetic field in order to direct the vector towards the target cells or retain it in the target tissue. It has been proved that magnetofection can greatly improve the efficacy of nucleic acid delivery and it is a powerful tool in cancer therapy.

Until now, only a small number of clinical trials with magnetic drug targeting has been performing. The first clinical trial using magnetically targeted drug was conducted Lubbe et al. in 1996 (Lübbe et al., 1996). This phase I clinical trial was performed using nanomagnetic particles loaded epirubicin in patients with advanced cancers or sarcomas. They demonstrated that the infusion of ferrofluids was well tolerated in most of the 14 patients studied and successfully directed to the tumour site in 6 patients. In 2002, Koda et al. applied doxorubicin coupled to a magnetic particle (MTC-DOX) carrier in patients with hepatocellular carcinoma. In this study, 22 patients were studied and the tumours were targeted successfully in 20 of them (Koda et al., 2002). Another clinical trial was performed by Wilson et al. in 2004 using MTC-DOX. The particles were directed to the tumour sites by magnets and monitored by MRI image. The results showed the drug had treated between 64 and 91% of tumour volume (Wilson et al., 2004).

2.3 Magnetic resonance imaging and cancer diagnosis

Magnetic resonance imaging (MRI) is a very common noninvasive method for diagnosing soft tissue and early cartilage pathologies. The method principle is based on the fact that the relaxation times of hydrogen atoms are influenced by the medium and, in particular, the disease medium. The disease processes alters molecular shapes and/or cell behavior which can be identified from molecular imaging. This insight allows the early detection of disease, so the prognoses, the effective treatment, and, personalized drugs and treatment times can be prescribed. Hence, molecular imaging is one promising tool to promote laboratory and clinical progress (Gamarra et al., 2010). The demand for innovative contrast agents encouraged the studies in the synthesis and coating of NMPs. NMPs probes for biomedical applications are comprised of nanoscale superparamagnetic iron oxide cores of magnetite and/or maghemite which are encapsulated in natural or synthetic polymers, silica and Au coatings. Cobalt ferrite (Morais et al., 2004) and gallium chelates were also used (Flacke et al., 2001; Louie et al., 2000).

The performance of the magnetic iron oxide contrast agents can be evaluated by their clearance, cell response, and toxicity. Particles sizes over 200 nm undergo mechanical filtration by the spleen and liver. Particles below 10 nm are rapidly removed during extravasations and renal clearance (Gupta & Wells, 2004). Amphiphilic coatings increase the circulation time of NMPs from minutes to hours which enhances the targeting potential of the contrast agent. One important problem related to the NMPs is finding the dose necessary to MRI detection. Some techniques which involves intracellular trapping (Kelly et al., 2005) have being of particular worth. In this approach, receptor-mediated uptake of NMPs is exploited to accrue elevated levels of the contrast agent within the desired cells.

2.4 Magnetic nanoparticle induced hyperthermia

Hyperthermia is a cancer therapy which consists in heating selectively tumour zones. Those zones have less blood vessels and are less oxygenated than health ones. Consequently, they are more sensible and died when the local temperature increases above 43 °C. Among the methods used for this therapy are induction heating, capacitive heating and hot water. The great advantage of this therapy is the fact that, in principle, all kinds of tumour cells can be treated. However, it is needed to control the temperature rising to prevent the death of health cells. Magnetic hyperthermia is another method to induce hyperthermia using NMPs. In this approach, NMPs are firstly introduced into the desired tissues and then guided by an external magnetic field. An externally applied oscillating magnetic field induces the hyperthermia as illustrated in Fig 4. (Ferreira et al., 2011; Jordan et al., 2009; Mitsumori et al., 1994; Wada et al., 2001).

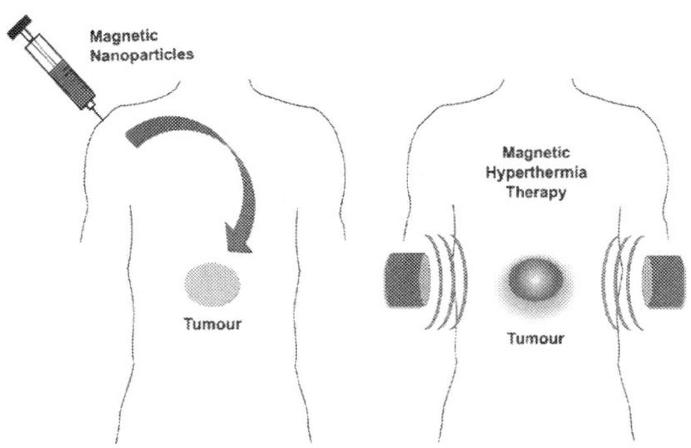

Fig. 4. Sketch showing the general procedure for the endovenous injection of the NMPs suspension into the human body: (a) the particles are first injected in a tumour and, then, (b) an externally applied alternating magnetic field induces the hyperthermia.

In 1979, Gordon *et al.* first proposed the concept of inducing intracellular hyperthermia it means, the magnetic field heating effects in a scale smaller than that of biological cell diameters (Gordon et al., 1979). They believed that intracellular hyperthermia should be more efficacy than the extracellular one since the cell membranes are not good thermal conductors and could act as thermal barriers. In this process, the cells can be selectively killed by the heat generated by nanomediators located inside the cell. Gordon *et al.* also showed that NMPs colloidal suspension injected intravenously can be phagocytized by cancer cells and after application of alternating magnetic field the cancer cells were selectively destroyed. In a more recent study, Wilhelm et al. showed that maghemite anionic nanoparticles are efficiently captured by human prostatic tumour cells (PC3) and concentrate within intracellular vesicles (Wilhelm et al., 2007). After these works, some researchers have proposed modifications on superparamagnetic particle surfaces to obtain magnetic colloidal ferrofluids to provide hyperthermia treatments. Magnetite nanoparticles(Fe_3O_4) coated with sodium oleate and poly(ethylene glycol) partially inhibited the growth of cancerous B16 cell sat the highest tested dose (2.1 mg/ml of Fe_3O_4 in MFPEG (Zavisova et al., 2011). In the presence of external alternating magnetic field bimagnetic Fe/Fe_3O_4 core/shell nanoparticles encapsulated by dopamine-oligoethylene glycol ligands showed considerable anti-tumour effect on murine B16-F10 melanoma.

Decrease in tumour size was observed 24hrs after intravenous administration of the NMPs followed by three days of alternating magnetic field. This study showed attenuation of the tumour without the undesirable side effects associated with traditional cancer therapy (Balivada et al., 2010).
Kim et al. developed promising materials to be applied in magnetic targeted hyperthermia based on chitosan-coated nanomagnetic particles. The hyperthermic thermoseed generated a temperature rise of 23°C under an alternating magnetic field and the capturing rate of the nanomagnetic particles was 96% under an external magnetic field of 0.4 T. The study showed that chitosan-coated nanomagnetic particles were biocompatible and exhibited higher affinity of KB carcinoma cells than L929 normal cells magnetic (Kim et al., 2009).
The potential hyperthermia application of magnetic fluids based on magnetite coated by biocompatible starch layer was studied by Linh et al. (Linh et al., 2009). The investigation of the heating ability was performed on magnetic fluid samples with particles concentration varying from 3 to 15 mg/ml under an alternating magnetic field with frequency of 184 kHz and field strength of 12 kA/m. The results obtained for sample with minimal iron oxide concentration are particularly of interest for applications in the heating therapy because this sample combined the high specific loss power value (129 W/g) with the saturation temperature of 45°C, which is appropriate for cancer treatment application.
Several works have studied magnetoliposomes in hyperthermia cancer treatment. An example is the study using magnetite cationic liposomes (MCLs) as a mediator of local hyperthermia to treatment of rat mammary cancer under alternating magnetic field with frequency 360 kHz. MCLs were infused into the rat tumour by using an infusion pump to obtain approximately 2 mg MCL per mL tumour volume. The rats were exposed to 3 series of hyperthermia treatments for 30 min each. The treated tumours were well controlled over a 30-day observation period showing an induction of immunological antitumour activity mediated by the MCLs (Motoyama et al., 2008).
The use of anti-HER2 immunoliposomes containing nanomagnetic particles (HMLs) for anti-HER2 antibody therapy and tumour-specific hyperthermia has been exploited for many researche groups. The first time that the combination of anti-HER2 antibody therapy and tumour-specific hyperthermia displaying a strong cytotoxic effect was in the study published by Ito et al. (Ito et al., 2004b). In this study, anti-HER2 immunoliposomes magnetite nanoparticles were synthesized. Analysis of combined effect of anti-HER2 antibody and hyperthermic treatment was performed on SKBr3 breast cancer cells *in vitro* showing strong cytotoxic effects after the cells heated at 42.5°C and incorporation of more than 60% of magnetite nanoparticles into SKBr3. Kikumory et al. investigated the retention ability of HML and the hyperthermic effects of HMLs on the subcutaneous tumours of breast cancer in nude mice. HMLs were injected into subcutaneous cancer nodules of BT474 (high HER2 expression) or SKOV3 (low HER2 expression) cells in nude mice and exposed to an alternating magnetic field, but HMLs accumulation was observed only in BT474 tumours. After hyperthermic treatment, tumour temperature increased to 45 °C, while the body temperature stayed around 38 °C. Tumour regression was observed and sustained for 10 weeks after hyperthermia (Kikumori et al., 2009).
The ability to conduct magnetic hyperthermia upon exposure to low-frequency alternating magnetic field and the biocompatibility were evaluated in maghemite nanoparticles embedded in a ordered mesoupourous silica-matrix MMS. Cell culture experiments showed that MMS particles were efficiently internalized by human A549, Saos-2 and HepG2 cells and presented good biocompatibility. Magnetic hyperthermia tests performed under

alternating magnetic field at a frequency of 100 kHz and a magnetic field intensity of 200 Oe. It was observed that in low concentration of MMS (48mg.mL^{-1}) the temperature in the culture medium increased to 44 °C in 30 min and the cell viability index dropped to about 0.5. When the tests were performed in high concentration (80 mg.mL^{-1}) cells increased the temperature of culture medium to 50 °C in 25 min and the cell viability index decreased to 0.8 (Martín-Saavedra et al., 2010).
The influence of the oleic acid surface coating on Fe_3O_4 and $NiFe_2O_4$ nanoparticles on their magnetic and calorimetric characterization was investigated. Fe_3O_4 (particle sizes of 15–20 and 20–30 nm) and $NiFe_2O_4$ (particle sizes of 20 30 nm) were dispersed in oleic acid. The temperature rising in the oleic-acid-coated nanoparticles was greater than that of the uncoated ones. The viscosity dependence on the self-heating temperature of Fe_3O_4 under an alternating magnetic field was measured. The temperature rise for both Fe_3O_4 particle sizes exhibited a strong dependence on viscosity and magnetic field frequency. Moreover, *in vitro* cytotoxicity test of Fe_3O_4 and $NiFe_2O_4$ was performed using human cervical carcinoma cells (HeLa), and the cytotoxicity of $NiFe_2O_4$ was compared to that of Fe_3O_4.

2.5 Tissue engineering using nanomagnetic particles

The application of nanomagnetic particles in tissue engineering has increased in the last years. These materials can allow develop new tissues in vitro with function and anatomical structure similar to original. The method consists in develop degradable tissue scaffolds to grow new tissues (Langer, 1993). It is possible to culture the principal cell (the keratinocyte) of the epidermis and use these cells to reconstitute human tissue (Bell et al., 1981; Yannas et al., 1982). Ito el al. proposed the use of magnetite cationic lipossomes (MCLs) in a novel methodology (Mag-TE) to construct multilayered keratinocyte sheets and collect the sheets without enzymatic treatment in presence of magnetic field. It was possible obtain keratinocytes further stratified and, subsequently, 10-layered epidermal sheets (Ito et al., 2004a). The technique Mag-TE was applied to construct heterotypic layered coculture system of rat hepatocytes and human aortic endothelial cells (HAECs). In this study, HAECs accumulated onto hepatocyte monolayers at sites where a magnet was positioned, and then adhered to form heterotypic, layered construct with tight and close contact. Albumin secretion was enhanced in the homotypic hepatocyte culture in presence of a magnetic force compared with the culture without magnets (Ito et al., 2004c).

3. Conclusion

Recent progress in nanomaterials syntheses has proved that solution-phase syntheses are capable of producing monodisperse NMPs with controlled chemical and magnetic properties. Surface modification and functionalization allows the NMPs to attach to various biomolecules, making them promising magnetic labels for bioseparation, biodetection and contrast enhancement of magnetic resonance imaging. Moreover, they can act as contrast agent and drug delivery system simultaneously which enhances the probability of success of many therapy diseases. Once the issues in toxicity, biodistribution and bioeleimination of these nanoparticles in a biological system are solved, the functionalized monodisperse nanoparticles will serve as powerful magnetic labels or delivery vehicles for highly sensitive/efficient biosensing, drug delivery and magnetic fluid hyperthermia applications.

4. Acknowledgment

We acknowledge the Brazilian agencies Fundação de Amparo à Pesquisa do Estado de Minas Gerais (FAPEMIG), Conselho Nacional de Desenvolvimento Científico e Tecnológico (CNPq), and Coordenação de Aperfeiçoamento de Pessoal de Nível Superior (CAPES) for the financial support. CAPES also grants the Visiting Professor PVNS fellowship to JDF at Federal University of Jequitinhonha and Mucuri Valleys.

5. References

Akgol, S., Turkmen, D., & Denizli, A. (2004). Cu (II) incorporated, histidine containing, magnetic metal complexing beads as specific sorbents for the metal chelate affinity of albumin. *Journal of Applied Polymer Science*, Vol. 93, No.6, (September 2004), pp. 2669-2677, ISSN 1097-4628

Amemiya, Y., Tanaka, T., Yoza, B., & Matsunaga, T. (2005). Novel detection system for biomolecules using nano-sized bacterial magnetic particles and magnetic force microscopy. *Journal of Biotechnology*, Vol. 120, No. 3, (November 2005), pp. 308-314, ISSN 0168-1656

Andrade, A.L., Souza, D.M., Pereira, M.C., Fabris, J.D., & Domingues, R.Z. (2009). Magnetic properties of nanoparticles obtained by different chemical routes. *Journal of Nanoscience and Nanotechnology*, Vol. 9, No. 3, (March 2003), pp. 2081-2087, ISSN 1533-4880

Andrade, A.L., Souza, D.M., Pereira, M.C., Fabris, J.D., & Domingues, R.Z. (2010). pH effect on the synthesis of magnetite nanoparticles by the chemical reduction-precipitation method. *Química Nova*, Vol. 33, No. 3, (February 2010), pp. 524-527, ISSN 0100-4042

Andrade, A.L., Domingues, R. Z., Fabris, J.D., & Goes, A. M. (2011). How safe are magnetic iron oxides to coat nanoparticles used in technical procedures of clinical diagnostics and therapy?, In: *Toxic Effects of Nanomaterials*, Haseeb Khan, Danvers MA, Bentham eBooks, Retrieved from
<http://www.benthamscience.com/ebooks/forthcomingtitles.htm#T>

Balivada, S., Rachakatla, R.S., Wang, H.W., Samarakoon, T.N., Dani, R.K., Pyle, M., Kroh, F.O., Walker, B., Leaym, X., & Koper, O.B. (2010). A/C magnetic hyperthermia of melanoma mediated by iron (0)/iron oxide core/shell magnetic nanoparticles: a mouse study. *BMC Cancer*, Vol. 10, No. 119, (March 2010), pp. 1-9, ISSN 1471-2407

Baselt, D.R., Lee, G.U., Natesan, M., Metzger, S.W., Sheehan, P.E., & Colton, R.J. (1998). A biosensor based on magnetoresistance technology. *Biosensors and Bioelectronics*, Vol. 13, No. 7-8, (October 1998), pp. 731-739, ISSN 0956-5663

Bell, E., Ehrlich, H.P., Buttle, D.J., & Nakatsuji, T. (1981). Living tissue formed *in vitro* and accepted as skin-equivalent tissue of full thickness. *Science (New York, NY)*, Vol. 211, No. 4486, (March 1981), pp. 1052, ISSN 0036-8075

Berry, C.C., & Curtis, A.S.G. (2003). Functionalisation of magnetic nanoparticles for applications in biomedicine. *Journal of Physics D: Applied Physics*, Vol. 36, No. 13, (June 2003), pp. R198-R206, ISSN 0022-3727

Berry, C.C., Charles, S., Wells, S., Dalby, M.J., & Curtis, A.S.G. (2004). The influence of transferrin stabilised magnetic nanoparticles on human dermal fibroblasts in culture. *International Journal of Pharmaceutics*, Vol. 269, No. 1, (January 2004), pp. 211-225, ISSN 0378-5173

Chang, J.H., Kang, K.H., Choi, J., & Jeong, Y.K. (2008). High efficiency protein separation with organosilane assembled silica coated magnetic nanoparticles. *Superlattices and Microstructures*, Vol. 44, No. 4-5, (October 2008), pp. 442-448, ISSN 0749-6036

Chang, J.H., Lee, J., Jeong, Y., Lee J.H.; Kim, I.J., & Park, S.E. (2010). Hydrophobic partitioning approach to efficient protein separation with magnetic nanoparticles. *Analytical Biochemistry*, Vol. 405, No.1, (October 2010), pp. 135-137, ISSN 0003-2697

Chatterjee, J., Haik, Y., & Chen, C.J. (2002). Polyethylene magnetic nanoparticle: a new magnetic material for biomedical applications. *Journal of Magnetism and Magnetic Materials*, Vol. 246, No. 3, (May 2002), pp. 382-391, ISSN 0304-8853

Dobson, J. (2006). Magnetic nanoparticles for drug delivery. *Drug Development Research*, Vol. 67, No. 1, (May 2006), pp. 55-60, ISSN 0272-4391

Dong, J., Xu, Z.H. & Wang, F. (2008). Engineering and characterization of mesoporous silica-coated magnetic particles for mercury removal from industrial effluents. *Applied Surface Science*, Vol. 254, No. 11, (March 2008), pp. 3522-3530, ISSN 0169-4332

Donselaar, L.N., Philipse, A.P., & Suurmond J. (1997). Concentration-dependent sedimentation of dilute magnetic fluids and magnetic silica dispersions. *Langmuir*, Vol. 13, No. 23, (November 1997), pp. 6018-6025, ISSN 0743-7463

Duguet, E., Vasseur, S., Mornet, S., & Devoisselle J.M. (2006). Magnetic nanoparticles and their applications in medicine. *Nanomedicine*, Vol. 1, No. 2, (August 2006), pp. 157-168, ISSN 1743-5889

Edelstein, R.L., Tamanaha, C.R., Sheehan, P.E., Miller, M.M., Baselt, D.R., Whitman, L.J., & Colton, R.J. (2000). The BARC biosensor applied to the detection of biological warfare agents. *Biosensors and Bioelectronics*, Vol. 14, No. 10-11, (January 2000), pp. 805-813, ISSN 0956-5663

Ferreira, R.V., Fabris, J.D., & Domingues, R.Z. (2011). Magnetite: Structure, properties and applications of chapter, In: *Magnetite: Structure, properties and applications*, Dawn M. Angrove, Nova Science Publishers, ISBN 978-1-61761-839-0

Ferreira, R.V.; Pereira, I.L.S.; Cavalcante, L.C.D.; Gamarra, L.F.; Carneiro, S.M.; Amaro, E.; Fabris, J.D.; Domingues, R.Z. & Andrade A.L. (2009). Synthesis and characterization of silica-coated nanoparticles of magnetite. *Hyperfine Interactions*, Vol.195, (September 2009), pp. 265-274

Flacke, S., Fischer, S., Scott, M.J., Fuhrhop, R.J., Allen, J.S., McLean, M., Winter, P., Sicard, G.A., Gaffney, P.J., Wickline, S.A. & Lanza, G.M. (2001). Novel MRI contrast agent for molecular imaging of fibrin: implications for detecting vulnerable plaques. *Circulation*, Vol. 104, No. 11, pp. 1280-1285, 0009-7322

Gamarra, L.F., Mamani, J.B., Carneiro, S.M., Fabris, J.D., Ferreira, R.V., Domingues, R.Z., Cornejo, D.R., Pontuschka, W.M., & Amaro, E. (2010). Characterization of superparamagnetic iron oxide coated with silicone used as contrast agent for magnetic resonance image for the gastrointestinal tract. *Journal of Nanoscience and Nanotechnology*, Vol. 10, No. 2, (February 2010), pp. 1153-1158, ISSN 1533-4880

Goldman, E.R., Clapp, A.R., Anderson, G.P., Uyeda, H.T., Mauro, J.M., Medintz, I.L., & Mattoussi, H. (2004). Multiplexed toxin analysis using four colors of quantum dot fluororeagents. *Analytical Chemistry*, Vol. 76, No. 3, (February 2004) pp. 684-688, ISSN 0003-2700

Gomez-Lopera, S.A., Plaza, R.C., & Delgado, A.V. (2001). Synthesis and characterization of spherical magnetite/biodegradable polymer composite particles. *Journal of Colloid and Interface Science*, Vol. 240, No. 1, (August 2001), pp. 40-47, ISSN 0021-9797

Gordon, R.T., Hines, J.R., & Gordon, D. (1979). Intracellular hyperthermia a biophysical approach to cancer treatment via intracellular temperature and biophysical alterations. *Medical Hypotheses*, Vol. 5, No. 1, (January 1979), pp. 83-102, ISSN 0306-9877

Gupta, A.K., & Wells, S. (2004). Surface-modified superparamagnetic nanoparticles for drug delivery: preparation, characterization, and cytotoxicity studies. *IEEE Transactions on Nanobioscience*, Vol. 3, No. 1, (March 2004), pp. 66-73, ISSN 1536-1241

Gupta, A.K., & Gupta, M. (2005). Synthesis and surface engineering of iron oxide nanoparticles for biomedical applications. *Biomaterials*, Vol. 26, No. 18, (June 2005), pp. 3995-4021, ISSN 0142-9612

Gupta, A.K., Naregalkar, R.R., Vaidya, V.D., & Gupta, M. (2007). Recent advances on surface engineering of magnetic iron oxide nanoparticles and their biomedical applications. *Nanomedicine*, Vol. 2, No. 1, (February 2007), pp. 23-39, ISSN 1743-5889

Harris, L.A., Goff, J.D., Carmichael, A.Y., Riffle, J.S., Harburn, J.J., Pierre, T.G.S., & Saunders, M. (2003). Magnetite nanoparticle dispersions stabilized with triblock copolymers. *Chemistry of Materials*, Vol. 15, No. 6, (March 2003), pp. 1367-1377, ISSN 0897-4756

Hassan, E.E., Parish, R.C., & Gallo, J.M. (1992). Optimized formulation of magnetic chitosan microspheres containing the anticancer agent, oxantrazole. *Pharmaceutical research*, Vol. 9, No. 3, (March 1992), pp. 390-397, ISSN 0724-8741

Hilger, I., Hergt, R., & Kaiser, W.A. (2005). Use of magnetic nanoparticle heating in the treatment of breast cancer. *IEE Proceedings-Nanobiotechnology*, Vol. 152, No. 1, (February 2005), pp. 33-39, ISSN 1740-9748

Hwu, J.R., Lin, Y.S., Josephraja, T., Hsu, M.H., Cheng, F.Y., Yeh, C.S., Su, W.C., & Shieh, D.B. (2009). Targeted Paclitaxel by conjugation to iron oxide and gold nanoparticles. *Journal of the American Chemical Society*, Vol. 131, No. 1, (January 2009), pp. 66-68, ISSN 0002-7863

Ito, A., Hayashida, M., Honda, H., Hata, K.I., Kagami, H., Ueda, M., & Kobayashi, T. (2004a). Construction and harvest of multilayered keratinocyte sheets using magnetite nanoparticles and magnetic force. *Tissue Engineering*, Vol. 10, No. 5-6, (May 2004), pp. 873-880, ISSN 1076-3279

Ito, A., Kuga, Y., Honda, H., Kikkawa, H., Horiuchi, A., Watanabe, Y., & Kobayashi, T. (2004b). Magnetite nanoparticle-loaded anti-HER2 immunoliposomes for combination of antibody therapy with hyperthermia. *Cancer Letters*, Vol. 212, No. 2, (August 2004), pp. 167-175, ISSN 0304-3835

Ito, A., Takizawa, Y., Honda, H., Hata, K.I., Kagami, H., Ueda, M., & Kobayashi, T. (2004c). Tissue engineering using magnetite nanoparticles and magnetic force: heterotypic layers of cocultured hepatocytes and endothelial cells. *Tissue Engineering*, Vol. 10, No. 5-6, (May 2004), pp. 833-840, ISSN 1076-3279

Ito, A., Shinkai, M., Honda, H., & Kobayashi, T. (2005). Medical application of functionalized magnetic nanoparticles. *Journal of Bioscience and Bioengineering*, Vol. 100, No. 1, (July 2005), pp. 1-11, ISSN 1389-1723

Jordan, A., Wust, P., Fahling, H., John, W., Hinz, A., & Felix, R. (2009). Inductive heating of ferrimagnetic particles and magnetic fluids: physical evaluation of their potential for hyperthermia. *International Journal of Hyperthermia*, Vol. 25, No. 7, (January 2009), pp. 499-511, ISSN 0265-6736

Kelly, K.A., Allport, J.R., Tsourkas, A., Shinde-Patil, V.R., Josephson, L., & Weissleder, R. (2005). Detection of vascular adhesion molecule-1 expression using a novel multimodal nanoparticle. *Circulation Research*, Vol. 96, No. 3, (February 2005), pp. 327-336, ISSN 0009-7330

Kikumori, T., Kobayashi, T., Sawaki, M., & Imai, T. (2009). Anti-cancer effect of hyperthermia on breast cancer by magnetite nanoparticle-loaded anti-HER2 immunoliposomes. *Breast Cancer Research and Treatment*, Vol. 113, No. 3, (February 2009), pp. 435-441, ISSN 0167-6806

Kim, D.H., Kim, K.N., Kim, K.M., & Lee, Y.K. (2009). Targeting to carcinoma cells with chitosan and starch coated magnetic nanoparticles for magnetic hyperthermia. *Journal of Biomedical Materials Research Part A*, Vol. 88, No. 1, (January 2009), pp. 1-11, ISSN 1549-3296

Kinoshita, T., Seino, S., Okitsu, K., Nakayama, T., Nakagawa, T., & Yamamoto, T.A. (2003). Magnetic evaluation of nanostructure of gold-iron composite particles synthesized by a reverse micelle method. *Journal of Alloys and Compounds*, Vol. 359, No. 1-2, (September 2003), pp. 46-50, ISSN 0925-8388

Kobayashi, Y., Horie, M., Konno, M., Rodriguez-Gonzalez, B., & Liz-Marzan, L.M. (2003). Preparation and properties of silica-coated cobalt nanoparticles. *Journal of Physical Chenistry B*, Vol. 107, No. 30, (July 2003), pp. 7420-7425, ISSN 1520-6106

Koda, J., Venook, A., Walser, E., & Goodwin, S. (2002). A multicenter, phase I/II trial of hepatic intra-arterial delivery of doxorubicin hydrochloride adsorbed to magnetic targeted carriers in patients with hepatocellular carcinoma. *European Journal of Cancer*, Vol. 38, Suppl 7, (Nov. 2002), pp. S18-S18, ISSN 0959-8049

Koneracka, M., Kopcansk, P., Antalik, M., Timko, M., Ramchand, C.N., Lobo, D., Mehta, R.V., & Upadhyay, R.V. (1999). Immobilization of proteins and enzymes to fine magnetic particles. *Journal of Magnetism and Magnetic Materials*, Vol. 201, No. 1-3, (July 1999), pp. 427-430, ISSN 0304-8853

Koneracka, M., Muckova, M., Zavisova, V., Tomasovicova, N., Kopcansky, P., Timko, M., Jurikova, A., Csach, K., Kavecansky, V., & Lancz, G. (2008). Encapsulation of anticancer drug and magnetic particles in biodegradable polymer nanospheres. *Journal of Physics: Condensed Matter*, Vol. 20, No. 20, (May 2008) pp. 204151, ISSN 0953-8984

LaConte, L., Nitin, N., & Bao, G. (2005). Magnetic nanoparticle probes. *Materials Today*, Vol .8, No. 5, (May 2005), pp. 32-38, ISSN 1369-7021

Langer, R., & Vacanti, J.P. (1993). Tissue engineering. *Science*, Vol. 260, No. 510, (May 1993), pp. 920–926, ISSN 0036-8075

Lee, J., Isobe, T., & Senna, M. (1996). Preparation of ultrafine Fe_3O_4 particles by precipitation in the presence of PVA at high pH. *Journal of Colloid and Interface Science*, Vol 177, No. 2, (February 1996), pp. 490-494, ISSN 0021-9797

Levy, L., Sahoo, Y., Kim, K.S., Bergey, E.J., & Prasad, P.N. (2002). Nanochemistry: Synthesis and characterization of multifunctional nanoclinics for biological applications. *Chemical Materials*, Vol. 14, No. 9, (September 2002), pp. 3715-3721, ISSN 0897-4756

Liang, Y., Gong, J.L., Huang, Y., Zheng, Y., Jiang, J.H., Shen, G.L., & Yu, R.Q. (2007). Biocompatible core-shell nanoparticle-based surface-enhanced Raman scattering probes for detection of DNA related to HIV gene using silica-coated magnetic nanoparticles as separation tools. *Talanta*, Vol. 72, No. 2, (April 2007), pp. 443-449, ISSN 0039-9140

Linh, P.H., Thach, P.V., Tuan, N.A., Thuan, N.C., Manh, D.H., Phuc, N.X., & Hong, L.V. (2009). Magnetic fluid based on Fe_3O_4 nanoparticles: Preparation and hyperthermia application. *Journal of Physics: Conference Series*, Vol. 187, No. 1, (September 2009), pp. 012069

Liu, X.Q., Guan, Y.P., Ma, Z.Y., & Liu H.Z. (2004a). Surface modification and characterization of magnetic polymer nanospheres prepared by miniemulsion polymerization. *Langmuir*, Vol. 20, No. 23, (November 2004), pp. 10278-10282, ISSN 0743-7463

Liu, X.Q., Guan, Y.P., Yang, Y., Ma, Z.Y., Wu, X.B., & Liu, H.Z. (2004b). Preparation of superparamagnetic immunomicrospheres and application for antibody purification. *Journal of Applied Polymer Science*, Vol. 94, No. 5, (December 2004), pp. 2205-2211, ISSN 0021-8995

Liu, X.Q., Ma, Z.Y., Xing, J.M., & Liu H.Z. (2004c). Preparation and characterization of amino-silane modified superparamagnetic silica nanospheres. *Journal of Magnetism and Magnetic Materials*, Vol. 270, No. 1-2, (March 2004), pp. 1-6, ISSN 0304-8853

Liu, X.Q., Xing, J.M., Guan, Y.P., Shan, G.B, & Liu, H.Z. (2004d). Synthesis of amino-silane modified superparamagnetic silica supports and their use for protein immobilization. *Colloids and Surfaces A: Physicochemical and Engineering Aspects*, Vol. 238, No. 1-3, (May 2004), pp. 127-131, ISSN 0927-7757

Liu, X.Q., Guan, Y.P. Liu, H.Z., Ma, Z.Y., Yang, Y. & Wu, X.B. (2005). Preparation and characterization of magnetic polymer nanospheres with high protein binding capacity. *Journal of Magnetism and Magnetic Materials*, Vol. 293, No. 1, (May 2005) pp. 111-118, ISSN 0304-8853

Louie, A.Y., Huber, M.M., Ahrens, E.T., Rothbacher, U., Moats, R., Jacobs, R.E., Fraser, S.E., & Meade, T.J. (2000). *In vivo* visualization of gene expression using magnetic resonance imaging. *Nature Biotechnology*, Vol. 18, No. 3, (March 2000), pp. 321-325, ISSN 1087-0156

Lubbe, A.S., Bergemann, C., Huhnt, W., Fricke, T., Riess, H., Brock, J.W., & Huhn, D. (1996). Preclinical experiences with magnetic drug targeting: tolerance and efficacy. *Cancer Research*, Vol. 56, No. 20, (October 1996), pp. 4694-4701, ISSN 0008-5472

Lucena, R., Simonet, B.M., Cardenas, S., & Valcarcel, M. (2011). Potential of nanoparticles in sample preparation. *Journal of Chromatography A*, Vol. 1218, No. 4, (January 2011), pp. 620-637, ISSN 0021-9673

Ma, Z.Y., Guan, Y.P., Liu, X.Q., & Liu, H.Z. (2005a). Preparation and characterization of micron-sized non-porous magnetic polymer microspheres with immobilized metal affinity ligands by modified suspension polymerization. *Journal of Applied Polymer Science*, Vol. 96, No. 6, (June 2005), pp. 2174-2180, ISSN 0021-8995

Ma, Z.Y., Guan, Y.P., Liu, X.Q., & Liu H.Z. (2005b). Synthesis of magnetic chelator for high-capacity immobilized metal affinity adsorption of protein by cerium initiated graft polymerization. *Langmuir*, Vol. 21, No. 15, (July 2005), pp. 6987-6994, ISSN 0743-7463

Ma, Z.Y, Guan, Y.P, & Liu, H.Z. (2006a). Superparamagnetic silica nanoparticles with immobilized metal affinity ligands for protein adsorption. *Journal of Magnetism and Magnetic Materials*, Vol. 301, No. 2, (June 2006), pp. 469-477, ISSN 0304-8853

Ma, Z.Y., Guan, Y.P., & Liu, H.Z. (2006b). Affinity adsorption of albumin on Cibacron Blue F3GA-coupled non-porous micrometer-sized magnetic polymer microspheres. *Reactive and Functional Polymers*, Vol. 66, No. 6, (June 2006), pp. 618-624, ISSN 1381-5148

MacBeath, G., & Schreiber, S.L. (2000). Printing proteins as microarrays for high-throughput function determination. *Science*, Vol. 289, No. 5485, (September 2000), pp. 1760-1763, ISSN 0036-8075

Martin-Saavedra F.M., Ruiz-Hernandez E., Bore A., Arcos D., Vallet-Regi M., Vilaboa N. (2010) Magnetic mesoporous silica spheres for hyperthermia therapy. *Acta Biomaterialia*, Vol. 6, No. 12, (December 2010), pp. 4522-4531, ISSN 1742-7061

Massart, R., & Cabuil, V. (1987). Effect of some parameters on the formation of colloidal magnetite in alkaline medium: yield and particle size control. *Journal de Chimie Physique et de Physico-Chimie Biologique*, Vol. 84, No. 7-8, pp. 967–973, ISSN 0021-7689

McCarthy, J.R., Kelly, K.A., Sun, E.Y., & Weissleder, R. (2007). Targeted delivery of multifunctional magnetic nanoparticles. *Nanomedicine*, Vol. 2, No. 2, (April 2007), pp. 153-167, ISSN 1743-5889

Mitsumori, M., Hiraoka, M., Shibata, T., Okuno, Y., Masunaga, S., Koishi, M., Okajima, K., Nagata, Y., Nishimura, Y., Abe, M., Ohura, K., Hasegawa, M., Nagae, H., & Ebisawa, Y. (1994). Development of intraarterial hyperthermia using a dextran-magnetite complex. *International Journal of Hyperthermia*, Vol. 10, No. 6, (November-December 1994), pp. 785-793, ISSN 0265-6736

Morais, P.C., Gravina, P.P., Bakuzis, A.F., Neto, K.S., & Lima, E.C.D. (2004), Magneto-optical properties of ionic magnetic fluids: The effect of the nanoparticle surface passivation. *Physica Status Solidi (c)*, Vol. 1, No. 12, (December 2004), pp. 3575-3578, ISSN 1610-1642

Morup, S., Topsoe, H., & Lipka, J. (1976). Modified theory for Mössbauer spectra of superparamagnetic particles: Application to Fe_3O_4. *Le Journal de Physique Colloques*, Vol. 37, No. 6, (December 1976), pp. C6 287- C6 290, 0449-1947

Motoyama, J., Yamashita, N., Morino, T., Tanaka, M., Kobayashi, T., & Honda, H. (2008). Hyperthermic treatment of DMBA-induced rat mammary cancer using magnetic nanoparticles. *Biomagnetic Research and Technology*, Vol. 6, No. 2, (February 2008), pp. 1-6, ISSN 1477-044X

Neuberger, T., Schopf, B., Hofmann, H., Hofmann, M., & Rechenberg, B. (2005). Superparamagnetic nanoparticles for biomedical applications: Possibilities and limitations of a new drug delivery system. *Journal of Magnetism and Magnetic Materials*, Vol. 293, No. 1, (May 2005) pp. 483-496, ISSN 0304-8853

OBrien, S.M., Sloane, R.P., Thomas, O.R.T., & Dunnill, P. (1997). Characterisation of non-porous magnetic chelator supports and their use to recover polyhistidine-tailed T4 lysozyme from a crude *E. coli* extract. *Journal of Biotechnology*, Vol. 54, No. 1, (April 1997), pp. 53-67, ISSN 0168-1656

OBrien, S.M., Thomas, O.R.T., & Dunnill, P. (1996). Non-porous magnetic chelator supports for protein recovery by immobilised metal affinity adsorption. *Journal of Biotechnology*, Vol. 50, No. 1, (September 1996), pp. 13-25, ISSN 0168-1656

Odabasi, M., & Denizli, A. (2004a). Cibacron Blue F3GA attached magnetic poly (2 hydroxyethyl methacrylate) beads for human serum albumin adsorption. *Polymer International*, Vol. 53, No. 3, (March 2004), pp. 332-338, ISSN 0959-8103

Odabasi, M., Uzun, L., & Denizli, A. (2004b). Porous magnetic chelator support for albumin adsorption by immobilized metal affinity separation. *Journal of Applied Polymer Science*, Vol. 93, No. 5, (September 2004), pp. 2501-2510, ISSN 0021-8995

Park, M.E., & Chang, J.H. (2007). High throughput human DNA purification with aminosilanes tailored silica-coated magnetic nanoparticles. *Materials Science and Engineering: C - Biomimetic and Supramolecular Systems*, Vol. 27, No. 5-8, (September 2007), pp. 1232-1235, ISSN 0928-4931

Park, S.J., Taton, T.A., & Mirkin, C.A. (2002). Array-based electrical detection of DNA with nanoparticle probes. *Science*, Vol. 295, No. 5559, (February 2002), pp. 1503-1506, ISSN 0036-8075

Paul, K.G,; Frigo, T.B., Groman J.Y., & Groman, E.V. (2004). Synthesis of ultrasmall superparamagnetic iron oxides using reduced polysaccharides. *Bioconjugate Chemistry*, Vol. 15, No. 2, (March-April 2004), pp. 394-401, ISSN 1043-1802

Pfannes, H.D. (1997). Simple theory of superparamagnetism and spin-tunneling in Mössbauer spectroscopy. *Hyperfine Interactions*, Vol. 110, No. 1-2, (September 1997), pp. 127-134, ISSN 0304-3843

Pouponneau, P., Leroux, J.C., Soulez, G., Gaboury, L., & Martel S. (2011). Co-encapsulation of magnetic nanoparticles and doxorubicin into biodegradable microcarriers for deep tissue targeting by vascular MRI navigation. *Biomaterials*, Vol. 32, No. 13, (May 2011), pp. 3481-3486, ISSN 0142-9612

Reichert, J., Csaki, A., Kohler, J.M., & Fritzsche, W. (2000). Chip-based optical detection of DNA hybridization by means of nanobead labeling. *Analitical Chemistry*, Vol. 72, No. 24, (December 2000), pp. 6025-6029, ISSN 0003-2700

Richardson, J., Hill, A., Luxton, R., & Hawkins, P. (2001). A novel measuring system for the determination of paramagnetic particle labels for use in magneto-immunoassays. *Biosensors and Bioelectronics*, Vol. 16, No. 9-12, (December 2001), pp. 1127-1132, ISSN 0956-5663

Safarik, I., & Safarikova, M. (2004). Magnetic techniques for the isolation and purification of proteins and peptides. *BioMagnetic Research and Technology*, Vol. 2, No. 1, (November 2004), pp. 1-17, ISSN 1477-044X

Schena, M., Shalon, D., Davis, R.W., & Brown, P.O. (1995). Quantitative monitoring of gene expression patterns with a complementary DNA microarray. *Science*, Vol. 270, No. 5235, (October 1995), pp. 467-470, ISSN 0036-8075

Schillinger, U., Brill, T., Rudolph, C., Huth, S., Gersting, S., Krotz, F., Hirschberger, J., Berġemann, C., & Plank, C. (2005). Advances in magnetofection--magnetically guided nucleic acid delivery. *Journal of Magnetism and Magnetic Materials*, Vol. 293, No. 1, (May 2005), pp. 501-508, ISSN 0304-8853

Schwertmann, U., & Cornell, R.M. (2000). *Iron oxides in the laboratory*, Wiley Online Library, available from http://onlinelibrary.wiley.com/doi/10.1002/9783527613229.fmatter/summary

Senyei, A., Widder, K., & Czerlinski, G. (1978). Magnetic guidance of drug carrying microspheres. *Journal of Applied Physics*, Vol. 49, No. 6, (January 1978), pp. 3578-3583, ISSN 0021-8979

Shen, L.F., Laibinis, P.E., & Hatton, T.A. (1999). Bilayer surfactant stabilized magnetic fluids: Synthesis and interactions at interfaces. *Langmuir*, Vol. 15, No. 2, (January 1999), pp. 447-453, ISSN 0743-7463

Shen, L.F., Stachowiak, A., Fateen, S.E.K., Laibinis, P.E., & Hatton, T.A. (2001). Structure of alkanoic acid stabilized magnetic fluids. A small-angle neutron and light scattering analysis. *Langmuir*, Vol. 17, No. 2, (January 2001), pp. 288-299, ISSN 0743-7463

Smith, J.E., Wang, L., & Tan, W.T. (2006). Bioconjugated silica-coated nanoparticles for bioseparation and bioanalysis. *Trac Trends in Analytical Chemistry*, Vol. 25, No. 9, (October 2006), pp. 848-855, ISSN 0165-9936

Sonvico, F., Dubernet, C., Colombo, P., & Couvreur, P. (2005). Metallic colloid nanotechnology, applications in diagnosis and therapeutics. *Current Pharmaceutical Design*, Vol. 11, No. 16, (June 2005), pp. 2091-2105, ISSN 1381-6128

Souza, D.M., Andrade, A.L., Fabris, J.D., Valério, P., Goes, A.M., Leite, M.F., & Domingues R.Z. (2008). Synthesis and *in vitro* evaluation of toxicity of silica-coated magnetite nanoparticles. *Journal of Non-Crystalline Solids*, Vol. 354, No. 42-44, (November 2008), pp. 4894-4897, ISSN 0022-3093

Sulek, F., Drofenik, M., Habulin, M., & Knez, Z. (2010). Surface functionalization of silica-coated magnetic nanoparticles for covalent attachment of cholesterol oxidase. *Journal of Magnetism and Magnetic Materials*, Vol. 322, No. 2, (January 2010), pp. 179-185, ISSN 0304-8853

Sunderland, C.J., Steiert, M., Talmadge, J.E., Derfus, A.M., & Barry S.E. (2006). Targeted nanoparticles for detecting and treating cancer. *Drug Development Research*, Vol. 67, No. 1, (January 2006), pp. 70-93, ISSN 0272-4391

Suzuki, M., Shinkai, M., Kamihira, M., & Kobayashi, T. (1995). Preparation and characteristics of magnetite-labeled antibody with the use of poly (ethylene glycol) derivatives. *Biotechnology and Applied Biochemistry*, Vol. 21, No. 3, (June 1995), pp. 335-345, ISSN 0885-4513

Takahashi, M., Akiyama, Y., Ikezumi, J., Nagata, T., Yoshino, T., Lizuka, A., Yamaguchi, K., & Matsunaga, T. (2009). Magnetic separation of melanoma-specific cytotoxic T lymphocytes from a vaccinated melanoma patient's blood using MHC/peptide complex-conjugated bacterial magnetic particles. *Bioconjugate Chemistry*, Vol. 20, No. 2, (February 2009), pp. 304-309, ISSN 1043-1802

Veiga, V., Ryan, D.H., Sourty, E., Llanes, F., & Marchessault, R.H. (2000). Formation and characterization of superparamagnetic cross-linked high amylose starch. *Carbohydrate Polymers*, Vol. 42, No. 4, (August 2000), pp. 353-357, ISSN 0144-8617

Wada, S., Yue, L., Tazawa, K., Furuta, I., Nagae, H., Takemori, S., & Minamimura T. (2001). New local hyperthermia using dextran magnetite complex (DM) for oral cavity: Experimental study in normal hamster tongue. *Oral Diseases*, Vol. 7, No. 3, (May 2001), pp. 192-195, ISSN 1354-523X

Widder, K.J., Senyel, A.E., & Scarpelli, G.D. (1978). Magnetic microspheres: a model system of site specific drug delivery *in vivo, Proceedings of the Society for Experimental Biology and Medicine*, Vol. 158, No. 2, (June 1978), pp. 141-146, ISSN 1525-1373

Wilhelm, C., Fortin, J.P., & Gazeau, F. (2007). Tumour cell toxicity of intracellular hyperthermia mediated by magnetic nanoparticles. *Journal of Nanoscience and Nanotechnology*, Vol. 7, No. 8, (August 2007), pp. 2933-2937, ISSN 1533-4880

Wilson, D.S., & Nock, S. (2003). Recent developments in protein microarray technology. *Angewandte Chemie International Edition*, Vol. 42, No. 5, (January 2003), pp. 494-500, ISSN 1433-7851

Wilson, M.W., Kerlan, R.K., Fidelman, N.A., Venook, A.P., LaBerge, J.M., Koda, J., & Gordon, R.L. (2004). Hepatocellular carcinoma: Regional therapy with a magnetic targeted carrier bound to doxorubicin in a dual MR imaging/conventional angiography suite—initial experience with four patients. *Radiology*, Vol. 230, No. 1, (January 2004), pp. 287-293, ISSN 0033-8419

Wooding, A., Kilner, M., & Lambrick, D.B. (1991). Studies of the double surfactant layer stabilization of water-based magnetic fluids. *Journal of Colloid and Interface Science*, Vol. 144, No. 1, (June 1991), pp. 236-242, ISSN 0021-9797

Xu, C.J., & Sun, S.H. (2007). Monodisperse magnetic nanoparticles for biomedical applications. *Polymer International*, Vol. 56, No. 7, (July 2007), pp. 821-826, ISSN 0959-8103

Yannas, I.V., Burke, J.F., Orgill, D.P., & Skrabut E.M. (1982). Wound tissue can utilize a polymeric template to synthesize a functional extension of skin. *Science*, Vol. 215, No. 4529, (January 1982), pp. 174-176, ISSN 0036-8075

Zavisova, V., Koneracka, M., Muckova, M., Lazova, J., Jurikova, A., Lancz, G., Tomasovicova, N., Timko, M., Kovac, J., Vavra, I., Fabian, M., Feoktystov, A.V., Garamus, V.M., Avdeev, M.V., & Kopcansky, P. (2011). Magnetic fluid with poly (ethylene glycol) with moderate anticancer activity. *Journal of Magnetism and Magnetic Materials*, Vol. 323, No. 10, (May 2010), pp. 1408-1412, ISSN 0304-8853

Zhang, Y., Kohler, N., & Zhang, M. (2002). Surface modification of superparamagnetic magnetite nanoparticles and their intracellular uptake. *Biomaterials*, Vol. 23, No. 7, (April 2002), pp. 1553-1561, ISSN 0142-9612

9

Effect of Texture on Success Rates of Implants

Abdelilah Benmarouane
UFR Sciences Exactes et Naturelles, LACMDTI, Reims Cedex 2, France

1. Introduction

The aim of the present study was to study the interface implant-bone by synchrotron radiation and neutron diffraction, the implant has two faces the first one coated with hydroxyapatite and the second uncoated. In orthopaedic surgery, Titanium alloy (Ti-Al-4V) implants are currently coated with hydroxyapatite (HAp), Ca_{10} $(PO_4)_6$ $(OH)_2$, in order to obtain a stable and functional direct connection between the bone and the implant. At the implant-bone interface, the new bone reconstituted after two months of implantation must have the same properties like the natural bone in order to have good mechanical properties at the interface with the implant. Therefore, we studied the texture of the reconstituted bone crystals at the interface applying two non-destructive diffraction methods, as well as the influence of the coating on crystallinity index. The required high spatial resolution was achieved utilizing high-energy synchrotron radiation on ID15 at ESRF in Grenoble, France, and the second method was done by neutron diffraction, the high-intensity with two-axis diffractometer was used, equipped with variable resolution: D20, at Institut Max von Laue-Paul Langevin (ILL) in Grenoble, France.
In orthopaedic surgery, it is necessary to use biocompatible implants in order to have good mechanical and fracture resistance. Bone is a composite material whose components are primarily collagen and HAp. The c-axes of the apatite crystallites and the collagen fibres are preferentially oriented, e.g., in the long bones in the directions of the stresses that the bones need to withstand. HAp crystallizes in the hexagonal system and its unit cell parameters are a=9,4 Å and c=6,8 Å its space group is P63/m. Bone occurs in two principal structural forms: cortical, or compact bone, which forms a dense matrix, and spongy bone. We use cortical bone in this work.
The long-term success of biomedical implants largely depends on the stable fixation of the implant to bones. Composite materials, in which metals have coated with ceramics, have been extensively reported as an alternative to plain materials in favour of a long-term fixation. The development of bioactive ceramic-alloy structures for implants has focused by the idea of combining the bioactivity of ceramics with the mechanical properties of selected metallic alloys. Ti-6Al-4V presents good mechanical proprieties and is biocompatible. HAp has low mechanical strength, but has a very good osteointegration and biocompatibility. The idea is to combine these two materials in order to have mechanical strength and good osteointegration proprieties at the interface. Plasma spraying is the most popular method for coating implant parts with HAp. In order to improve these coatings, it is necessary to investigate the texture and crystallinity evolutions of the bone's crystal structure, as a function of the distance from the implant-interface.

2. Materials and method

The success of the biomaterial used in implantology necessarily depends on the interface between implant and bone. Among many biological parameters on the mechanical level, the lifetime of the implant depends on the distribution of the regenerated HAp crystals at the interface with implant. The reconstructed orientation of these crystals should respect the preferred orientation of crystals of the bone of origin. The advantage of this protocol is to test the effect of implant coating with a layer of HAp crystals on the properties of the reconstructed bone. We will use an implant Ti-6Al-4V parallelepiped with one face was coated with a deposit of HAp hoping to observe a different behavior of the distribution of HAp crystals in the bone between the coated surface and the face unpaved.

2.1 Plasma thermal spraying "PTS"

The plasma thermal spraying "PTS" has been applied to deposit the HAp onto a titanium substrate. It is a powerful tool for the high rate deposition of thin coatings with low cost precursors. It is necessary to choose the thickness of HAp between 60 and 120 μm in order to satisfy the clinic application. PTS process consists in introducing solid particles in a high-temperature and relatively high-velocity gas jet, where the particles are eventually melted and projected onto the substrate to form the deposed coating, layer by layer. The plasma jet accelerates and heats the particles in a highly complex manner, strongly depending not only on plasma thermal spraying setup, but also on individual particle trajectories, actually determining the thermal history of the latter.

2.2 Bones sample

In this study, we use the implant constituted by Ti-6Al-4V (20x5x2mm) with two faces: the first face coated with HAp (80μm) and the second face uncoated. The implant was been inserted in the tibia bone of a sheep respecting the clinical protocols. The sheep has been pre-medicated and anesthetized. Two separate longitudinal incisions, 5 cm long, have been made on tibia bone. Corresponding to each skin incision, the cortex of the head of the tibia has been exposed, and a 5 mm wide and 20 mm long strip of peri-osteal tissue has been

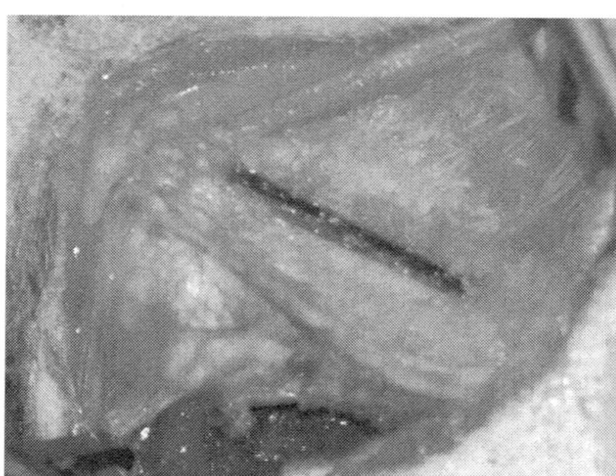

Fig. 1. Implant inserted in sheep tibia

removed. Using an oscillating saw, two longitudinal slots have been made at about 120° from each other on the circumference of the bone. The implant has been introduced in one of these slots, the other remains as a control. After 60 days of implantation, the sample constituted by implant and bone has been extracted and preserved in the ethanol in order to keep them under the best conditions before measurements. The specimen has been prepared in the Pius Branzeu Centre of Laparoscopic Surgery and Microsurgery (Romania).
The sample will be characterize by synchrotron diffraction at ESRF and after by neutron diffraction at ILL in order to compare the results of this two techniques by studying the texture and crystallinity of the new bone reconstituted at the interface with implant.

2.3 Texture

The preferred orientation or texture is defined by a non-random distribution of crystals in the polycrystalline material. The study of preferred orientation is an important technique for understanding the structures of polycrystalline materials. One of the main problems in materials science is to link the physical properties of anisotropic polycrystalline material to the preferential alignment of the components in the preferred directions. For many years the development of textured metal or textured polymer is area research subject in improving the behaviour and life of components. Several areas of research are relevant today as electronics: the development of thin films, the texture not only controls the electrical properties but also the mechanical stability of films. In our study, the texture is present in biomaterials, yet the relationship between the mechanical properties of bone and alignment of hydroxyapatite crystals in bone has never been studied in spatial resolution, who laid the groundwork for the analysis of texture in biomaterials. In many cases, the characterization of texture has an important influence in the resolution and refinement of powder diffraction patterns. In an effort to characterize texture at all scales, from micrometer to the centimeter, researchers have used an increasing range of techniques to characterize quantitatively the texture. In this context, the use of large facilities such as synchrotrons and neutron sources, is particularly important and finds a new application in biomaterials.

2.4 Neutron diffraction study

With the neutrons diffraction, it's very necessary to remove the organic part from the bone in order to reduce the intense incoherent scattering of neutrons by hydrogen and that is done by heat treatment. The heat treatment does not affect the preferred orientation of the mineral bone crystallites and crystallinity. With synchrotron we can do the measurement without remove the organic part.
By neutron diffraction, we used the high-intensity two-axis diffractometer with variable resolution: D20, at Institut Max von Laue-Paul Langevin (ILL) in Grenoble, France. D20 provides a high flux of up to 108 cm−2 s−1 at the sample position and medium to high resolution. It is equipped with a large linear curved position sensitive detector (PSD) permitting numerous short-time measurements. The PSD has an aperture of 153.6° with 10 cells per degree (2θ). It operates in a wide range of wavelengths. It is used either for fast data-acquisition, e.g. time-resolved powder diffraction or texture measurements, or for diffraction experiments that require accurate intensity measurements, e.g. investigations of disordered systems or physisorbed layers. D20 is particularly suited for real-time measurements and offers different sample environments, among others a vacuum vessel and an Eulerian cradle for texture measurements.

The sample has been mounted in the Euler cradle. The scan was made with step sizes of 10° for $\Delta\varphi$ and $\Delta\chi$, with φ from 0 to 360° and χ from 0° to 90°, and ω constant at 90°. The data acquisition was done during the motor motion of φ. Every 1° of rotation, the motor stopped for a fixed amount of time, and after rotation of 10°, the accumulated acquisition during these ten steps of motor motion is attributed to the average angle of φ. This method enabled us to gain one hour of dead time normally spent on motor motion, without losing information on the orientations of crystallites. The size of beam was 9 mm × 0.5 mm and λ = 2.4 Å. It takes 6 hours for each slice of 0.5 mm of the tibia.

2.5 Synchrotron diffraction study

For the study by synchrotron diffraction, we used the high spatial resolution utilizing high-energy synchrotron radiation with a monochromatic beam of 88.9 keV on ID15 at the European Synchrotron Radiation Facilities ESRF in Grenoble. A Mar345 image plate detector was set at 1m from the sample to allow a complete collection of the Debye-Scherrer rings. In order to obtain a complete pole figure, it is enough to rotate the sample in the axial direction. The synchrotron radiation scan was carried out from 0° to 180° in 10° steps at a step time of 120s, beam size : 300µm and λ=0,14Å.

2.6 Material Analyzed Using Diffraction techniques "MAUD" program

In the texture analysis field, we need the sophisticated tools in order to get the maximum information from the analyzed material using diffraction techniques. Currently, very powerful tools can gather in a short time a large quantity of data. It is difficult to process all this data in a traditional way of consuming even with very powerful workstations. The processing time by computer from the latest generation was now significantly reduced. However, the amount of data collected also increases with measurement time granted to the user, time is always the same and limited. Several informations of data collected by the instruments were lost or never used. The solution is to develop new analytical tools that we can process more data and optimize the measurement time allowed for each user who wants to use large instruments. Material Analyzed Using Diffraction Techniques "MAUD" program meets this need.
L. Luttorotti has developed particularly powerful software based on the Rietveld method for quantitative analysis with two modes of refinement. MAUD program is written in Java and allows to adopt all the current machines at ILL and ESRF.

2.7 Results and discussion

The data were analyzed in order to define the structure of the HAp in tibia bone and texture. The Fig.2 shows all diffractions patterns of HAp in the bone at 6 mm from the interface with implant.
In the first, we refine all parameters of HAp structures, and after we refine the texture of HAp using the MAUD program. For presenting the orientations of tibia bone, we trace the pole figures of HAp in bone at 6mm from the implant. This distance is very far from the interface in order to show how the HAp crystallites are oriented in unperturbated parts of the bone, the pole figures tracing in this distance indicating the reference of orientations for this work. The reconstructed pole figures from Rietveld texture analysis with MAUD program of a tibia bone showing the little preferred orientation of HAp crystallites when comparing the reflection (002) and the (111) reflections. We choose the reflection (002) for the study the texture and (111) a measure of the crystallinity of the HAp at the interface with implant.

2.8 Result of synchrotron radiation

ID15B has a 2D detector, the image consist by the Debye-Scherrer rings at the interface with the implant (Fig. 2).

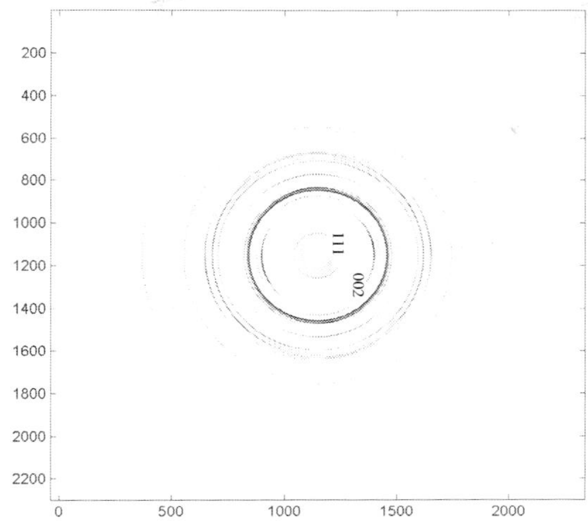

Fig. 2. Diffraction image of tibia bone at the interface with the implant.

In order to get the data for Rietveld analysis, the one-dimensional diffraction patterns were obtained by integration of the diffraction rings along each ring in 10° steps, we get 684 diffraction patterns (Fig. 8). It is necessary to refine the crystal's structure and texture in order to trace the pole figures at the interface with implant.

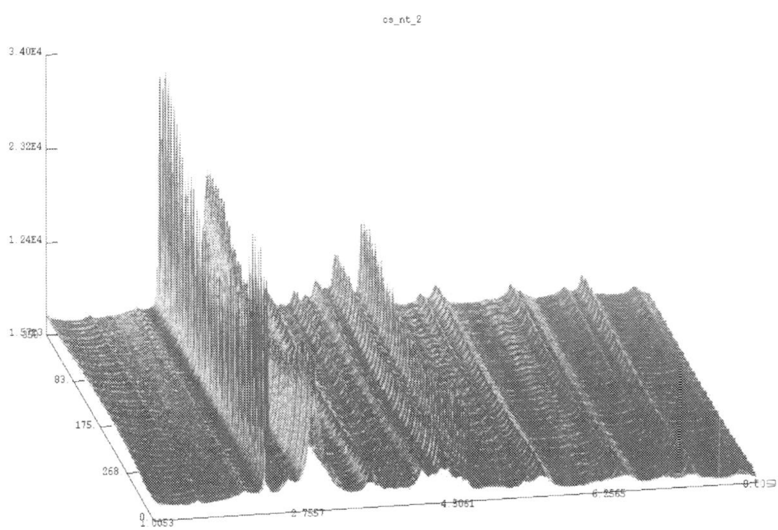

Fig. 3. 684 diffractions patterns of HAp

In the first, we refine the sum of all data in order to calculate the parameters structures of HAp Fig. 4.

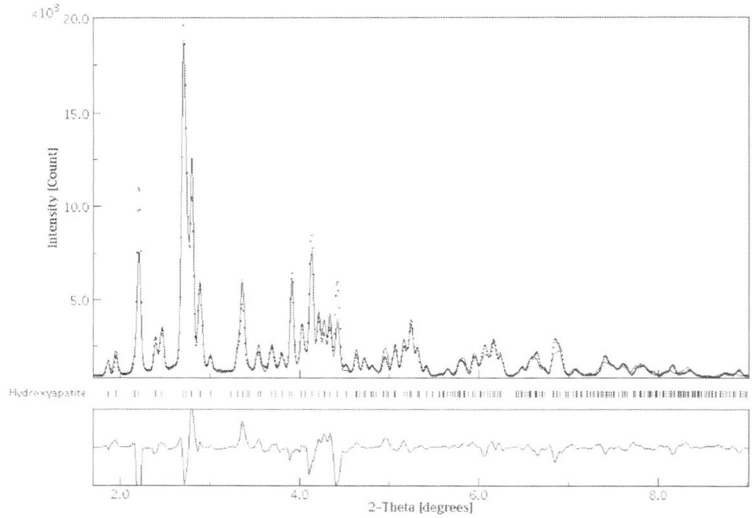

Fig. 4. Reitveld refinement of sum of all data

The second step is the refinement the texture and to trace the pole figures. The all structure parameters have been and the texture of 684 diffraction patterns has been refined simultaneously by introducing the texture parameters on MAUD program.

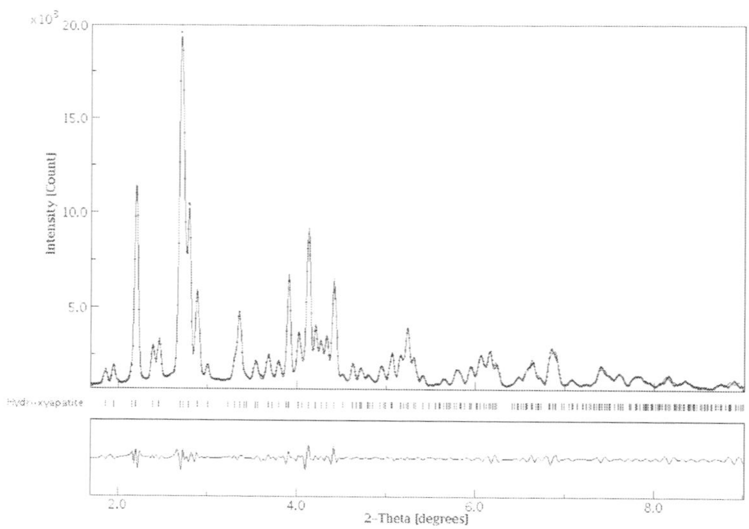

Fig. 5. Reitveld refinement of sum of all data with texture parameters

The figure 6 represents the pole figures obtained from a layer (0,3 × 0,3 mm^2) of bone, very far from the implant in order to have the reference and to show how the HAp crystallites are oriented in the unperturbed part of bone.

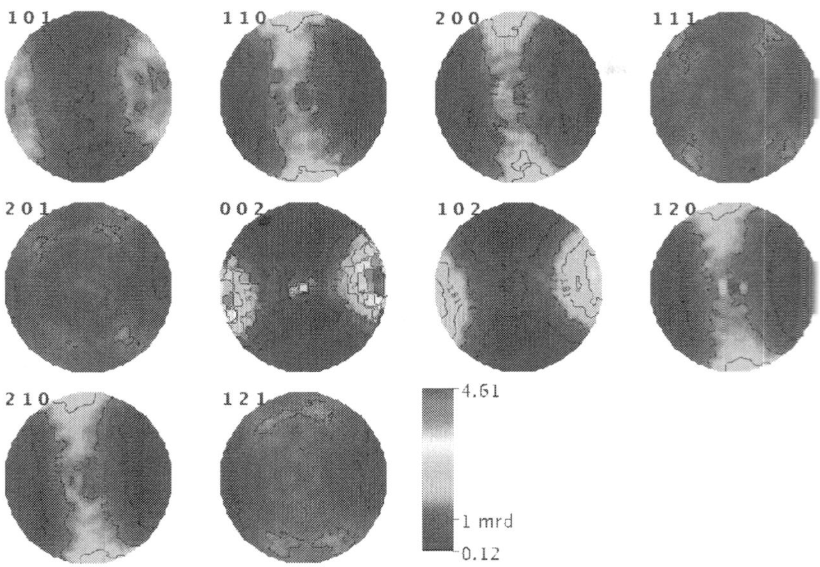

Fig. 6. Pole figures of tibia bone at 6mm from the interface bone-implant

The reflection (002) was choose for the study the texture and (111) for characterizing the HAp crystallinity evolution at the interface with implant.
The pole figures at the interface with face coated and uncoated were traced in figures 7 and 8.

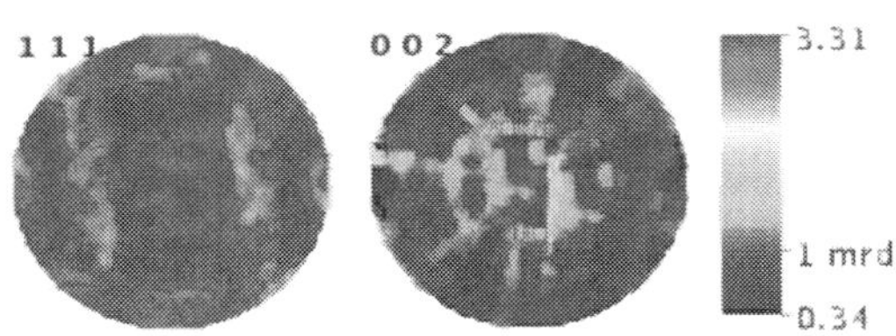

Fig. 7. Pole figures of tibia bone's at the interface with the face coated with HAp

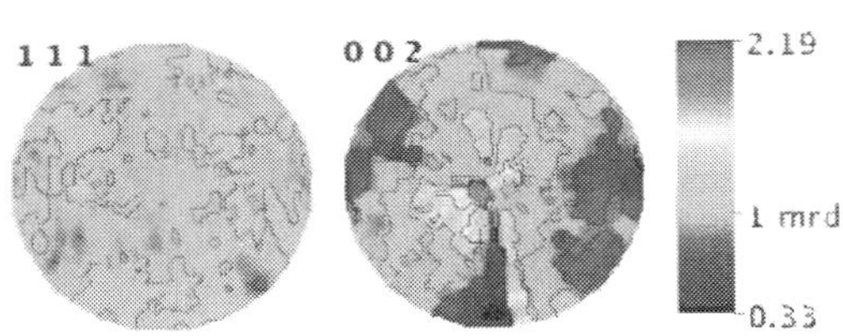

Fig. 8. Pole figures of tibia bone's at the interface with the face uncoated

At the interface with the face uncoated (Fig. 8), the pole figure (002) shows several orientations of the HAp crystallite's.
We get the preferred orientation like the unperturbated parts of the bone (Fig. 9), after 2,4 mm from the uncoated interface.

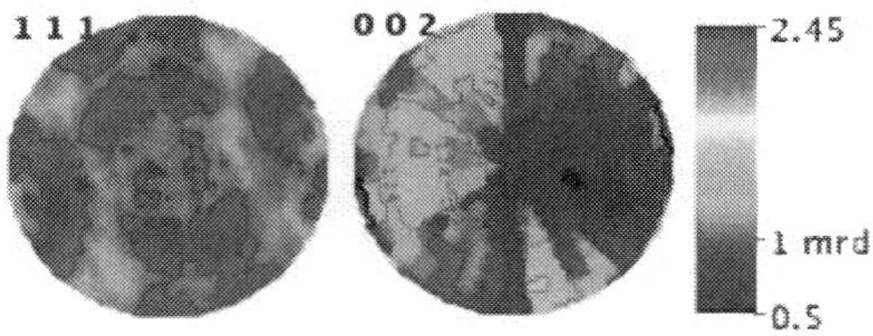

Fig. 9. Pole figures at 2,4 mm from the interface with the face uncoated

2.8.1 Results of neutron diffraction

With neutron diffraction, we got 360 diffraction patterns; like the synchrotron diffraction data, the all structure parameters have been refined and after the 360 diffraction patterns have been refined simultaneously by introducing the texture parameters on MAUD program. The figure 10 represents the pole figures obtained from a layer (0.5×9 mm^2) of unperturbed bones very far from the interface.

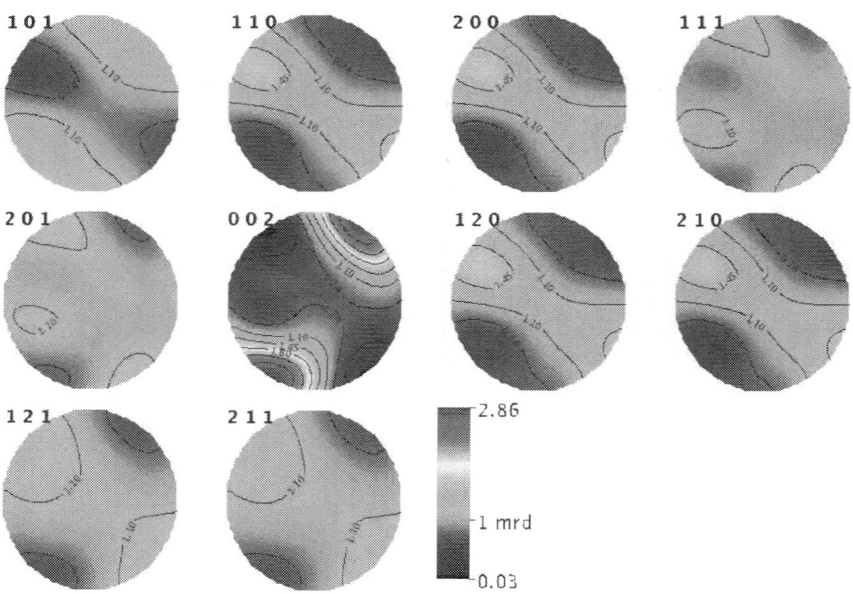

Fig. 10. Pole figures of tibia sheep bone by Neutron diffraction

The figure 10 reveals that the reconstructed pole figures from Rietveld texture analysis with MAUD of a tibia bone showing the little preferred orientation of HAp crystallites when comparing the reflection (002) and the (111) reflections, like the pole figures measured by synchrotron radiation. The pole figures at the interface with face coated and uncoated were traced in figures 11 and 12.

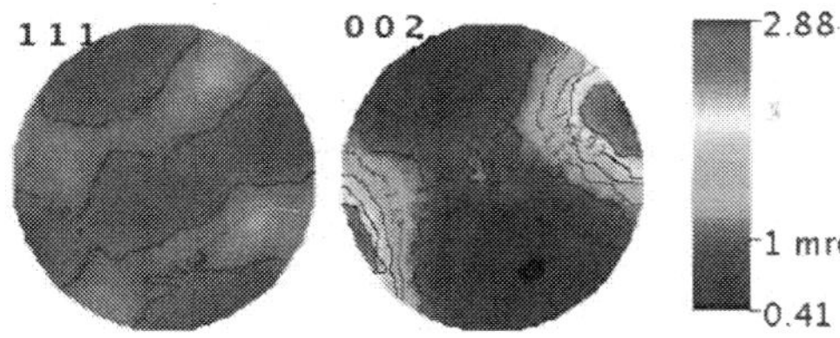

Fig. 11. Pole figures at the interface with face coated with Hap

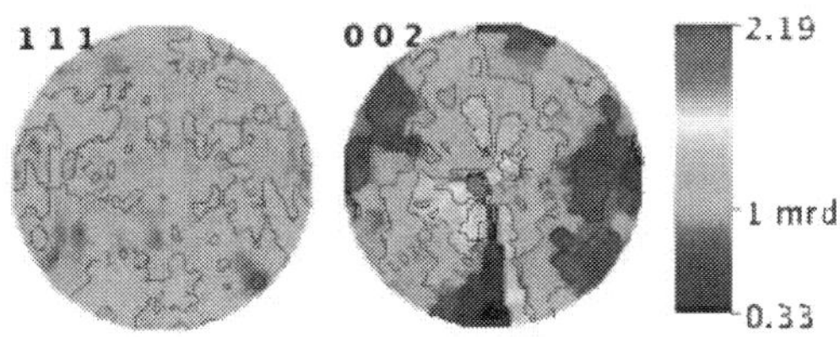

Fig. 12. Pole figures at the interface with face uncoated

AT the interface with the implant, the reconstituted bone at the interface with the face coated with HAp show the preferred orientation like the tibia bone. However, at the interface with the face uncoated (Fig. 6), the pole figure (002) show several orientations of the HAp crystallite's. At the interface with the face coated with HAp the new bone reconstituted conserves the preferred orientation of natural bone.

2.9 Crystallinity study by neutron diffraction and synchrotron radiation

The crystallinity index evolution has been measured from the interface with the implant. Therefore, we measured the intensity of the peak (1 1 1), because it is not affected by texture. The sheep tibia was measured with beam size of 0,5 mm by neutron diffraction and 0,3 mm by synchrotron radiation. The refinement was be done by MAUD.

The evolution of the crystallinity index has been traced from the interface with the implant coated with HAp and uncoated.

The crystallinity index of (111) peaks revealed that at the interface, the measurement by synchrotron diffraction is more intense than the measurement by neutron diffraction (Fig. 13) at the interface with the face coated with HAp and uncoated. At the interface with the fac coated with HAp the crystallinity is very high, the coating favoured the crystallinity by 20% compared with the face uncoated.

The results of the new bone crystals at the interface obtained by the synchrotron radiation and neutron diffraction study are particularly interesting and reveal a great advantage of the HAp coated implant interface on the crystallinity anf texture. At the interface with implant coated with HAp, the crystallinity is more intense and the new bone has the same orientation of the tibia's bone.

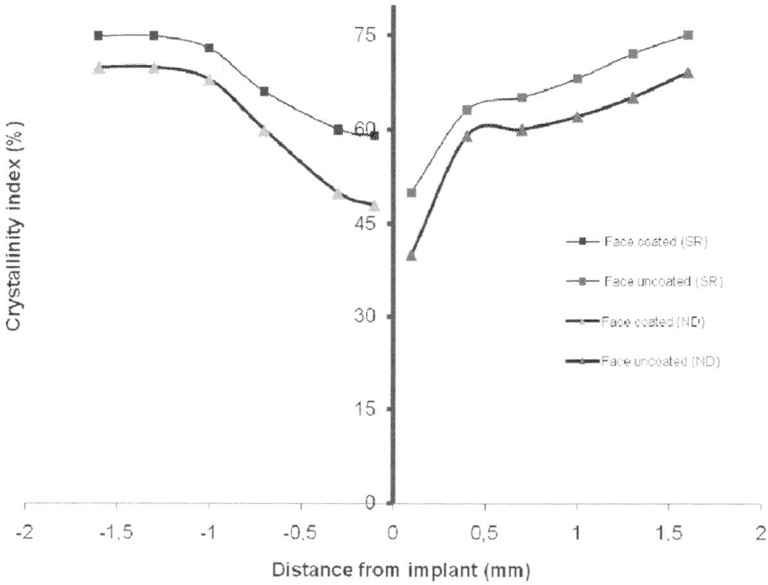

Fig. 13. Crystallinity index of the HAp at the interface with implant, ND: Neutron diffraction and SR: Synchrotron Radiation

3. Conclusion

The method of characterizing the texture and crystallinity, which uses the technique of neutron diffraction and synchrotron radiation at high spatial resolution, finds an application in implantology. In mechanical terms, the success of bone regeneration around implants depends directly on the orientation distribution and crystallinity index of HAp crystals in reconstituted bone after implantation. The non-destructive methods study allows also to compare the results from the faces coated with HAp and uncoated. The texture of HAp crystallites in new bone around the implant and crystallinity are the preferable conditions for successful implantation. If the implant was coated with HAp, the new HAp crystallites preserve the preferred orientation of HAp inside the bone. If the implant is uncoated, the orientation of HAp crystallites were changed, in this case we have several orientations, this situation generates the perturbations and the mechanical properties at the interface will be very low, therefore the crakes will appear and the implant can be rejected. At the coated interface, the bone has a high crystallinity index and has the same orientation like the natural bone; therefore, the bond constituted presents good mechanical properties. This study reveals that it is necessary to cover implants with HAp in order to have good mechanical properties at the interface with implant and increase the lifetime of the implant. by the two methods at the interface, we have the same orientation of the HAp crystallites like the originally orientation of the tibia bone. The characterization with synchrotron radiation reveal that the texture and the crystallinity of the HAp crystallites at the interface are more intense than the measurement by neutron diffraction, and show after 60 days of regeneration that the crystallinity index of HAp at 1 mm from the interface with the implant is similar to crystallinity index of the original tibia bone (at 2 mm from the interface). The bond reconstructed at the interface with the face caoted with HAp is very strength and it is one of the most important factors indicative of the reliability of fixing the implant to the bone tissue. Ti-6Al-4V coated with HAp by PTS, offers the potential of combining the superior mechanical performance of the metal component with the excellent biological responses possible of HAp. The two techniques confirm that it is necessary to use the implant coated with HAp in order to improve the lifetime of implants.

The success of the biomaterial used in implantology necessarily depends on the interface between implant and bone, so bone restored after several months of implantation.

Therefore, in this study the high resolution of the synchrotron radiation and neutron diffraction allow to characterize the interface and show the texture effects of the new bone crystallites at the interface bone-implant on the success rate of the implant.

4. Acknowledgment

The authors would like to thank the Pius Branzeu Center of laparoscopic Surgery and Microsurgery (Romania) for the samples preparation.

5. References

J.M.S. Skakle and R.M. Aspden: J. App. Cryst., Vol. 35 (2002), p. 506

R.C. Barroso, L.F. Oliveira, C.R. Castrob, J.C. Limab, D. Brazb, R. T. Lopesb, R. Droppac, G. Trombad, L. Mancinid, F. Zaninid, L. Rigone, and D. Dreossie: Nuclear Instruments and Methods in Physics Research A Vol. 579 (2007), p. 318

G. E. Bacon, P. J. Bacon and R. K. Griffiths: J. Appl. Cryst. Vol. 12 (1979), p. 99

H. Sitepu: J. Appl. Cryst. Vol. 35 (2002), p. 274

A. Benmarouane, T. Hansen and A. Lodini: Physica B Vol. 350 (2004), p. E611

A. Benmarouane, T. Hansen P. Millet and A. Lodini, Solid State Phenomena Vol. 105 (2005), p.427.

H.-R. Wenk., Y. Xie, L. Lutterotti, L. Ratschbacher, J. Richardson: J. Appl. Cryst. Vol. 34, (2001), p. 442

S. Matthies, H.-R. Wenk and G. W. Vinel: J. Appl. Cryst. Vol. 21 (1988), p. 285

A. Benmarouane, T. Hansen P. Millet and A. Lodini: Materials Science Forum, 2006, 524, 951-956

A. Benmarouane, T. Hansen and A. Lodini, Physica B, Vol. 350 (2004), p. E611

J.M.S. Skaklea and R.M. Aspdenb, J. App. Cryst., Vol. 35 (2002), p. 506

A. Benmarouane, T. Hansen P. Millet and A. Lodini Materials Science Forum, Vol. 524 (2006), p. 951

H. Sitepu, Assessment of preferred orientation with neutron powder diffraction data, J. Appl. Cryst. (2002), 25274-277

H.-R. Wenk and S. Grigull, Synchrotron texture analysis with area detectors, J. Appl Cryst. (2003). 36, 1040-1049

H-R Wenk and P Van Houtte, Texture and anisotropy. Rep. Prog. Phys. (2004). 67, 1367-1428.

H.-R. Wenk, L. Cont, Y. Xie, L. Lutterotti, L. Ratschbacher and J. Richardson, Rietveld texture analysis of Dabie Shan eclogite from TOF neutron diffraction spactra. J. Appl. Cryst. (2001). 34, 442-453

G. E. Bacon and A. E. Goodship, the orientation of the mineral crystals in the radius and tibia of the sheep, and its variation with age, J. Anat. (1991). 179, 15-22

H.J. Bunge, Texture-the key to physics in polycrystalline matter. Materials Science Forum (1998). 273, 3-14

K. El Ghazouli, Nouvelle méthode d'analyse, par la diffraction des rayons X, des variations de texture dans les couches minces. Thèse de l'Institut supérieur de génie mécanique et productique, Metz (1998)

Caglioti G., Paoletti A., Ricci F P., Choice of collimators for a crystal spectrometer for neutron diffraction. Nuclear Instruments, (1958) 3, 223

H. M. Rietveld, A profil refinement method for nuclear and magnetic structures, J. Appl. Cryst. (1969) 2, 65.

H. J. Bunge and C. Esling, The harmonic Method. Dans " Preferred Orientation in Deformed Metals ansd Rocks:An Introduction to modern Texture Analysis" pages: 109-119, Edited by H. R. Wenk

S. Matthies, G. W. Vinel, Physica Status Solidi B (1982). 112, K111-K114

Matthies S., Wenk H. -R (1985). In "Preferred orientation in deformed metals and rocks: an introduction to modern texture analysis",H. -R. Wenk editor, Academic Press inc. pp 139-147

K. Pawlik, Materials Science Frum, (1993). 133-136, 151-156

H. Schaeben (1991). In "Advances and applications of quantitative texture analysis", H.-J. Bunge, C. Esling, Eds. DGM. Oberusel, Germany, pp 109-118.

L. Cont, D. Chateigner, L. Lutterotti, J. Ricote, M.L. Colzada, J. Mendiola, Ferroelectrics, (2002). 267, 323-328.

M. Morales, D. Chateigner, L. Lutterotti, J. Ricote, Materials Sciences Forum, (2002). 408-412, 1055-1060.

H. Sitepu, W.W. Schmahl, R.b. Von Dreele, Use of the generalized spherical harmonic model for describing crystallographic texture in polycrystalline NiTi shape-memory alloy with time-of-flight neutron powder diffraction data, Appl. Phys. A, (2002). 74, S1677.

R. Adell, B. Erikkson, U. Lekholm, P. Branemark, T. Jemt, International Journal of Oral and Maxillofacial Implants, 5, (1990), 347-359.

P. Fogarassy, D. Gerday and A. Lodini, Agglomerated nanostructured particles disintegration during the plasma thermal spraying process, Mechanics Research Communications 32 (2005) 221–239

10

Magnetic Particle Induction and Its Importance in Biofilm Research

Amy M. Anderson[1], Bryan M. Spears[1], Helen V. Lubarsky[2], Irvine Davidson[2], Sabine U. Gerbersdorf[3] and David M. Paterson[2]
[1]Centre for Ecology and Hydrology - Edinburgh, Penicuik, Midlothian,
[2]Sediment Ecology Research Group, Scottish Oceans Institute,
University of St Andrews, Fife,
[3]Institute of Hydraulic Engineering, University Stuttgart, Stuttgart,
[1,2]Scotland
[3]Germany

1. Introduction

Since the mid-twentieth century scientists have been aware that aquatic bacteria are more abundant as biofilms on solid surfaces than as suspended free cells (ZoBell, 1943). The last few decades have seen significant advancement in our understanding of the development of biofilms and the processes occurring within these colonies of adhered microorganisms (Coenye & Nelis, 2010; Hall-Stoodley et al., 2004). Two features in particular distinguish microorganisms in biofilms from their free-living counterparts. The first is their ability to produce a coherent extracellular polymeric matrix (containing polysaccharides, proteins and DNA) which results in firmer attachment to the surface (Costerton et al., 1987; Donlan & Costerton, 2002). The other is the coordinated behaviour of the cells embedded in this matrix due to communication by a process known as quorum sensing. Quorum sensing is the secretion and detection of inducer molecules that accumulate as a function of cell density. At a threshold population density the accumulated autoinducers bind to cellular receptors activating transcription of certain genes (Costerton & Lapin-Scott, 1995; Hall-Stoodley et al., 2004; Nadell et al., 2008; Sauer, 2003).

While the existence of a biofilm is beneficial in many settings, for example in waste water treatment plants where they play an essential role in flocculation and nutrient removal (Nicolella et al., 2000; Wagner & Loy, 2002), their presence can also be extremely harmful or costly. Biofilms are implicated in numerous diseases, including cystic fibrosis and tuberculosis (Lam et al., 1980; Singh et al., 2000); they also contaminate food, its packaging and the water distribution network thereby posing a serious threat to human health (Flemming, 2002; Kumar & Anand, 1998; LeChavalier et al., 1987). Microorganism colonization and extracellular polymeric substance (EPS) secretion on man-made structures such as heat exchangers and the hulls of ships can result in decreased performance and increased operating costs (Meesters et al., 2003; Schultz et al., 2011). As such, biofilms have become a priority subject in many research areas in recent years. Publications in the fields of biomedicine (Guo et al., 2008; Morton et al., 1998), waste water treatment (Liu & Fang, 2003; Pollard, 2010), ecology (Lubarsky et al., 2010; Yallop et al., 2000), food science (Carpentier &

Cerf, 1993) and biotechnology (Flemming & Wingender, 2001; Houghton & Quarmby, 1999) serve to highlight the wide ranging importance of biofilms and their secretions of EPS.
Technological developments originating in different fields will have translational value. We report here on the MagPI (**Mag**netic **P**article **I**nduction) System, one such development in the field of environmental science. The MagPI System uses magnetic induction of ferrous particles to quantify the adhesive capacity of a test surface. As the "stickiness" of surfaces can often be attributed to the presence of a biofilm the MagPI System can be used to evaluate biofilm formation and state of development. Previously, measurements of this process have been conducted using large laboratory scale systems that can be both expensive and labour intensive. A variety of relevant procedures and devices are presented (Table 1).
In this paper we will review the key phases in the development of the MagPI System, outline the procedures for use, review its current applications and highlight uses for this device that will be of relevance to biomedical sciences.

2. Technical aspects and development of the MagPI System

The MagPI System has been developed by a multidisciplinary team led by the University of St Andrews. Initially the goal of development was to produce a device that could sensitively measure the adhesive capacity of sediment surfaces. The adhesive capacity or retentive ability of the sediment surface is a proxy for bed stability. Several devices based on different approaches already exist to measure sediment stability, e.g. water flow [Sedflume (McNeil et al., 1996); SETEG (Haag et al., 2001)], water jets [CSM (Paterson, 1989)] and propellers [EROMES (Schuenemann & Kuehl, 1991)]. To measure sediment stability these devices require that bed failure occurs. The MagPI System is capable of repeatedly measuring changes in surface properties below the point of bed failure (incipient erosion) that are undetectable by these other devices. For example, changes in adhesion during early stages of biofilm formation. As such, its use will fill a gap in our knowledge of properties and behaviour of surfaces and sediments (Larson et al., 2009).

2.1 The electromagnet

In the early stages of construction commercially available magnets were tested for their suitability. However, common problems included too large a surface area to be useful in observing particle reaction to the increasing magnetic force or inadequate strength to uplift the test particles. As a result, electromagnets were specially constructed by coiling insulated copper wire around a ferrous alloy core (Figure 1). The wire gauge, core dimensions and the number of turns in the coil can be varied between models to create electromagnets with different ranges.

2.2 Ferrous test particles

The test particles (Figure 1) are composed of a mixture of ferrous materials mixed with fluorescent pigment to increase their visibility (Partrac Ltd., Glasgow, UK). After their production a spectrum of particle sizes exist (80-400 μm). Particles are homogenized by sieving them into different size classes. The targets for MagPI need not be confined to particles. Almost any target design can be envisaged as long as the target is attracted by a magnetic field. So far small metal discs (<1cm diameter) and larger metal spheres (c.f 1-3mm) have also been tested. The choice of target depends on the purpose of the study.

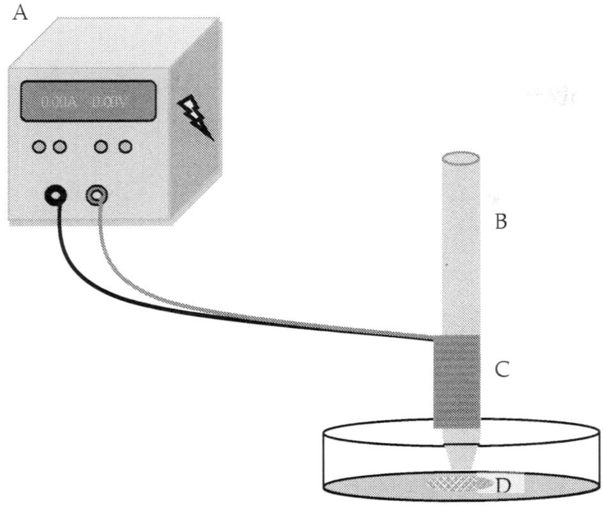

Fig. 1. Schematic diagram of the MagPI system. A) Voltage and current variable power supply. B) Aluminium rod. Acts as a heat sink and can be attached to a micromanipulator or clamp when MagPI system is in use to hold it at a set height above test surface. C) Ferrous alloy core around which copper wire is coiled. The core is waterproofed by coating it in a plastic film. D) Fluorescent ferrous test particles.

3. Standard operating procedure

The laboratory-based MagPI System consists of a variable electromagnet controlled by a power supply capable of producing fine scale increments of current and voltage and the specially designed magnetic particles (Figure 1). To ensure repeatable measurements are taken, magnetic particles of a known size and density must be consistently applied to the test surface in a relatively even single layer. The procedure followed when using the MagPI system in the laboratory is detailed below:

1. Magnetic particles of a known size and density are suspended in water.
2. The particle-water mixture is then drawn into a pipette or syringe. The suspended particles are allowed to settle to the tip of the pipette or syringe.
3. A couple of drops of the mixture are sufficient to distribute a single layer of particles to an area of c. 1 cm^2. This is ejected about 1 cm above the test surface into the overlying medium.
4. The time interval between particle application and retraction depends on the objective of the investigation. If the adhesive capacity of the test surface is in question then the measurement of magnetic force required to uplift the particles from the test surface should be taken immediately. This is the most reliable way to ensure repeatable measurements. Particles left on the surface a period of time before the uplift process begins will become incorporated into the biofilm to some extent. Thus, the strength required to retract the particles is also influenced by the ability of the developing biofilm to entrap particles. The MagPI probe (electromagnet) is lowered into position above the particles (Generally 5 - 10mm from the surface) using a micromanipulator.

Method	Basic procedure	Advantages	Limitations	References
Microscopy (e.g. epifluorescence, laser-scanning confocal, transmission electron, scanning electron)	Varies between different microscopic techniques. For some microscopic methods biofilms are treated with a fixing agent (e.g. formaldehyde, glutaraldehyde) and stained (e.g. with acridine orange, ruthenium red, safranin) prior to imaging.	Non-destructive High resolution images provide information of biofilm morphology, phylogeny and matrix structure and architecture	Labour intensive Require specialist training Costly Pre-treatment can alter specimen morphology Potential for underestimation of biofilm levels if thickness not measured Not quantitative	Lawrence et al., 2003; Morató et al., 2004; Perkins et al., 2006; Priester et al., 2007
Crystal Violet Method	Biofilm cells stained with crystal violet. The dye incorporated into sessile microorganisms is then solubilised and the absorbance of the solution measured.	Affordable Doesn't require specialist training	Time consuming High variations for a same result Efficiency of biofilm removal from surface unknown	Musk et al., 2005; Vesterlund et al., 2005
Flow Cytometry	Adhered microorganisms are removed from their surface (e.g. by sonication). Cells are suspended in a rapidly flowing stream of water that passes by an electronic detection apparatus.	Rapidly obtains and processes data Reveals heterogeneity of cells: numbers, size distribution, physiological and biochemical characteristics	Expensive Requires specialist training Efficiency of biofilm removal from surface unknown	Vives-Rego et al., 2000; Williams et al., 1999
BioFilm Ring Test®	A magnetic bead solution is added to bacterial cultures on a microtitre plate. After a period of incubation a magnet is used to assemble the non-immobilized beads to the bottom of the well. The resulting spot is quantified through specialized image algorithms.	Easy to operate Automated Sensitive to early stages of biofilm formation Results obtained quickly Repeatable	Cannot be used to quantify biofilm formation in nature No information on phylogeny or morphology obtained as with microscopy	Chavant et al., 2007
MagPI System	Magnetic beads are applied to the biofilm and exposed to an incrementally increasing magnetic force. The force at which the beads are recaptured from the surface can be taken as an indication of the extent of biofilm formation.	Easy to operate Inexpensive Can be used to measure biofilm formation on any surface Sensitive to early stages of biofilm formation Non-destructive Results obtained rapidly Repeatable	Not automated No information on phylogeny or morphology obtained as with microscopy	Larson et al., 2009

Table 1. Methods and procedures used for studying biofilms

5. The current to the probe is gradually increased (~ 0.2A increments). As the current increases so too does the magnetic force acting on the particles.

6. Four levels of particle response to the increasing magnetic field have been identified. The fourth level is the least subjective and should therefore be taken as the end point of the experiment (Figure 2).
7. Prior to repeat measurements being taken on the same test surface it is made certain that no particles from a previous measurement remain in the area to be tested.
8. It is advisable to calibrate at the start, during and at end of an experiment to account for changes in the coil resistance that would result in a loss of magnetic field strength.

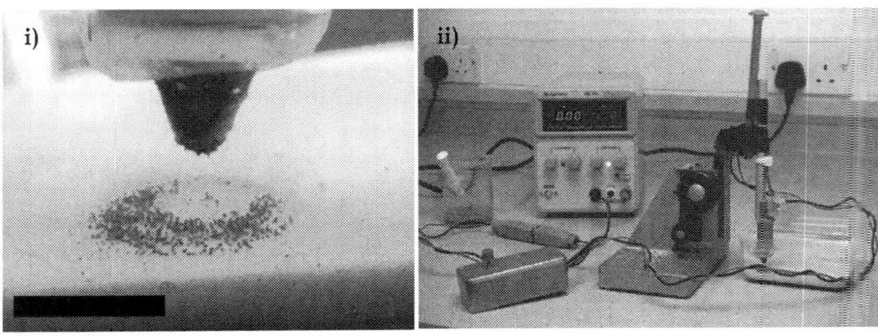

Fig. 2. **i)** Stage 4 of particle response to a magnetic field- complete removal of particles from the test surface below the electromagnet tip, particles can be seen adhering to the electromagnet. (Scale-bar: 1cm) **ii)** MagPI System set-up

4. Calibrations and magnetic force equation

Calibrations enable comparison of results obtained using different MagPI probes or in different laboratories or experiments. To calibrate the device the probe is placed at a set distance above a sensor connected to a Gauss meter. The voltage and current are increased incrementally (0.2V/ ~0.1A per increment) while all other factors remain constant. The magnetic flux density (MFD) for each voltage increase is measured by the Gauss meter in mTesla and recorded. Calibrations have been carried out with the probe submerged in both distilled water and seawater at distances of 5, 7 and 10mm between the probe and the Gauss meter sensor. Each calibration was carried out in triplicate.

No significant difference was found between the freshwater and distilled water calibrations (α=0.05). There was a strong linear relationship between voltage and MFD at all distances (r^2: 5mm = 0.99; 7mm = 0.99; 10mm = 0.99). When measuring the adhesive capacity of a test surface the voltage at which particles are uplifted from the surface (stage 4) is recorded and the MFD can later be calculated from the straight line equation obtained in calibrations (Figure 3).

The attractive magnet force acting on the particles at the point of uplift can be calculated according to the following equation:

Equation 1. $$F= B^2A/ 2\mu_0$$

Where B is the MFD, A is the area of the magnetic pole facing the test surface and μ_0 is the permeability of free space (constant during measurements in the same medium).

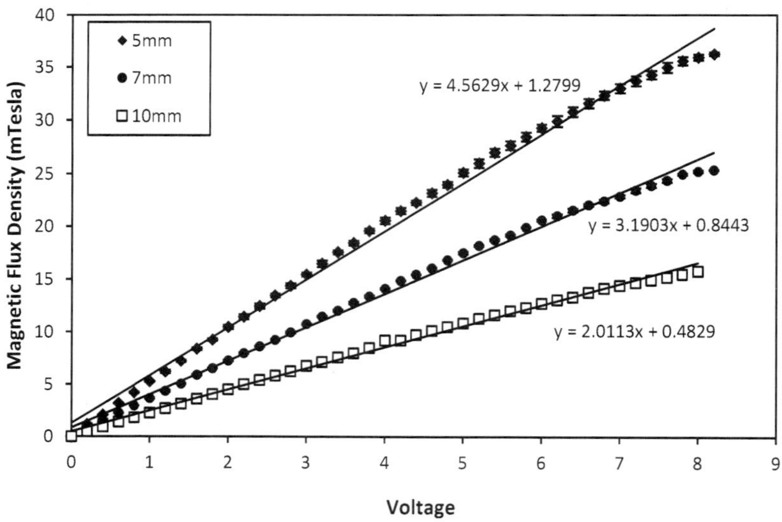

Fig. 3. Seawater calibration curve (n = 3, +/- standard error). Distances reported are MagPI probe from a sensor connected to a Gauss meter.

5. Biofilms in aquatic systems

Biofilms are ubiquitous in benthic aquatic environments (Battin et al., 2003; Larson et al., 2009; Lubarsky et al., 2010) where they regulate a number of important ecosystem services such as nutrient cycling (Battin et al., 2003; Cyr & Morton, 2006), pollutant accumulation (Schlekat et al., 1998; Wolfaardt et al., 1998) and biodegradation (Battin et al., 2003). More recently the influence of benthic microbial assemblages on sediment stability has been proven (Decho, 2000; Gerbersdorf et al., 2008; Spears et al., 2007). Traditionally physico-chemical and biochemical processes were considered to be the most important drivers of sediment stability (Calles, 1983; McNeil & Lick, 2004). Microbial assemblages can enhance the stability of sediment in two ways, either directly, via the presence of physical mats (Dodds, 2003) or indirectly. Benthic microbes indirectly increase stability by secreting EPS which enhances adhesion and cohesion between the EPS molecules and sediment particles (Decho, 1994). Annular flume experiments have shown that the presence of a biofilm at the sediment surface significantly increases the energy required to erode the sediment compared to those sediments without biostabilisation (Droppo et al., 2001). These findings are transferable to the natural environment. Strong correlations between sediment stability, benthic algal biomass and EPS concentration have been observed in marine systems (Sutherland et al., 1998; Yallop et al., 2000). Although biostabilisation has also been observed in freshwater systems (Droppo et al., 2007; Gerbersdorf et al., 2007 & Spears et al, 2007) correlations between the aforementioned parameters are weaker. It is evident that under high electrolyte concentrations the effect of EPS on sediment stability is enhanced (Spears et al., 2008). This emphasizes the need for a device, such as the MagPI System, that is sensitive enough to discern subtle changes in sediment stability across freshwater environments where low ionic concentrations generally place sediment stability below the range measurable by other devices (See section 2). Understanding the processes that control the erodibility and transport of sediments and their associated pollutants is vital for safeguarding the economic and ecological health of aquatic systems (Förstner at al., 2004; Westrich & Förstner, 2005; Wood & Armitage, 1999).

5.1 First applications of the MagPI System

The MagPI System was first introduced by Larson et al. (2009). Calibration data for an earlier prototype was presented and the ability of the MagPI System to precisely detect small differences in adhesion was demonstrated by measurements taken on a variety of abiotic and biotic test surfaces. Since then the MagPI System has contributed significantly to advancement in our understanding of biostabilisation. Until recently research into the biostabilisation of sediments focussed largely on the stabilising effect of benthic microalgae and their carbohydrate-rich EPS (Underwood & Paterson, 2003; Spears et al., 2008; Stal, 2003). The contribution of benthic bacteria was for the most part overlooked despite their omnipresence at sediment surfaces and their ability to produce copious amounts of EPS as recognized from medical (Costerton et al., 1999), biotechnology (Wang et al., 2006) and industrial investigations (Kumar & Anand, 1998). Studies in which the MagPI System has been used to measure sediment stability appear to show that the role of heterotrophic bacteria in biostabilisation far exceeds what was previously thought and may even surpass that of microalgae.

Gerbersdorf et al. (2009) investigated the biostabilisation potential of natural microbial assemblages on a non-cohesive substratum under conditions of nutrient limitation and repletion. Measurements of adhesion / stability obtained by the MagPI System and the Cohesive Strength Meter (CSM) were related to EPS (protein and carbohydrate), bacterial cell numbers, bacterial community composition, diatom biomass and diatom assemblage composition. The sensitivity of the MagPI System was highlighted by the inability of the CSM to determine differences in substratum stability between the control (no microorganisms and no nutrient addition) and early stages of the experimental treatments while the MagPI System indicated a significant increase in adhesive capacity as compared to the control even at this early stage in biofilm development. Nutrient addition appeared to profit the microalgae whereas bacteria dominated in nutrient-deplete cultures. The taxonomic shift between treatments resulted in differences in EPS composition which in turn moderated the biostabilisation capacity: microalgal dominated cultures were found to be less stable than those cultures where bacteria were prolific. Lubarsky et al. (2010) utilised the MagPI System in a comparison of pure bacterial cultures, axenic microalgal cultures and mixed assemblages grown on a non-cohesive substratum in an attempt to elucidate the individual stabilising capacity of the main biofilm components. Pure bacterial cultures had a significantly higher stabilisation potential compared to the microalgae. These results back-up the assertions of Gerbersdorf et al. (2008) that bacteria do play an important role in biostabilisation and can be regarded as "ecosystem engineers". Mixed assemblages were more stable than either pure bacterial cultures or microalgae. However, the hypothesis of a synergistic relationship between the microalgae and bacteria in terms of stability was discounted and it was deemed more likely that in mixed microbial culture the combination of EPS components with different mechanical properties and characteristics accounted for the increase in stability.

6. Biofilms in medicine

In recent years there has been an alarming rise in the occurrence of multi-drug resistant microorganism infections (Fridkin & Gaynes, 1999; Gaynes & Edwards, 2005; Lessa et al., 2009; Livermore, 2000). Two bacterial strains are of particular concern: meticillin-resistant *Staphylococcus aureus* (MRSA) and *Pseudomonas aeruginosa* (Smith & Hunter, 2008). The persistence of these infectious microorganisms, despite measures to control them, is attributed to their existence as biofilms rather than as free-floating cells (Donlan & Costerton, 2002). Microorganisms incorporated into a biofilm have 10 to 1000 times more resistance to antimicrobial agents than planktonic microorganisms (Mah & O'Toole, 2001). An estimated 65 - 80% of infections in the developed world are biofilm related (Coenye & Nelis, 2010). It has been speculated that the emergence of biofilm diseases results from the success of vaccines and antibiotics against diseases originating from planktonic bacteria (Costerton, 2001).

Several mechanisms are considered to be responsible for sessile microorganisms' resistance to antibiotics. They include: i) the delayed or incomplete penetration of antimicrobial agents through the extracellular polymeric matrix in which cells are enclosed (Stewart, 1997; Suci et al., 1994), ii) slower growth rates and metabolism of sessile microorganisms compared to planktonic ones and hence slower uptake of antibiotics (Anwar et al., 1992; Evans et al., 1990) and iii) quorum sensing induction of a biofilm specific phenotype (Mah & O'Toole, 2001; Dagostino et al., 1991; Whiteley et al., 2000). For example, it has been suggested that in *Escherichia coli* biofilms the induction of the rpoS gene instigates a physiological response which in turn leads to antibiotic resistance (Adams & McLean, 1999). The disruption of quorum sensing systems is being investigated as a novel means of preventing or limiting biofilm pathogens (Dong & Zhang, 2005; Stickler et al., 1998). Of the numerous products seen to inhibit quorum sensing in *in vitro* systems a few (halogenated furanones, fungal compounds and garlic extract) have been tested with great success in animal models (Hentzer et al., 2003; Manefield et al., 2002; Rasmussen et al., 2005; Wu et al., 2000, 2004). However, the potential toxicity of furanones and patulins prevents their clinical use and garlic extract would have to be administered to humans in huge quantities to be comparable to the dosage used in mouse experiments (Rasmussen & Givskov, 2006).

6.1 Biofilms and infectious diseases

The chronic pneumonia that affects Cystic Fibrosis (CF) sufferers is one infection for which there is definitive proof of *P.aeruginosa* biofilm involvement. The well established morphological evidence is supplied by the recovery of cells from the airways of CF patients which are embedded in a thick matrix of extracellular material (Costerton et al., 1983; Lam et al., 1980). The hypothesis that the pathogen grows as a biofilm has more recently been reinforced by chemical data. Singh et al. (2000) present *in vitro* data showing that biofilm populations of *P.aeruginosa* produce more butyryl (C4) acyl homoseine lactone (AHL) than the oxyodecanoyl (C12) quorum signal whereas planktonic cells favour production of the C12 signal. Sputum examined directly from CF patients revealed that the ratio of the C4 to C12 signal was comparable to that found in the *in vitro* grown biofilms. Prior to these findings, infections could be classed as biofilm-related based solely on morphological evidence. The addition of this chemical data has established CF pneumonia as the definitive biofilm infection (Costerton, 2001).

CF itself is an autosomal recessive hereditary disease in which a net deficiency of water renders the respiratory mucous more viscous and as a result impairs the mucociliary clearance of inhaled particles from the airways leaving the patient vulnerable to bacterial infection (Donlan & Costerton, 2002). *S.aureus* and *Haemophilus influenzae* infections usually predispose airway colonisation by *P.aeruginosa* (Koch & Hoiby, 1993). Infections due to these strains can generally be controlled by antimicrobial agents. However, antipseudomonal therapy is less effective. By adolescence most Cystic Fibrosis patients will have become chronically infected with *P.aeruginosa* which can be severely debilitating and often fatal (Koch & Hoiby, 1993; Lykzak et al., 2002). The exact mechanisms by which the CF lung becomes colonised with *P.aeruginosa* biofilms are unknown. One hypothesis is that the thick respiratory mucus provides a matrix scaffold and creates a hypoxic environment in which *P.aeruginosa* are believed to thrive (Worlitzsch et al., 2002; Yoon et al., 2002). The second hypothesis is that airway inflammation enhances pseudomonal receptors on the respiratory epithelia to which *P.aeruginosa* can attach (Hall-Stoodley et al., 2004).

CF is just one example of a biofilm related infection. Other diseases in which infectious biofilms are implicated include native valve endocarditis where bacteria or fungi in the blood stream adhere to vascular endothelium and potentially lead to structural damage of the valve tissues (Donlan & Costerton, 2002); Otitis media, a common childhood ear infection (Hall-Stoodley et al., 2006) and Peritontitis, a disease affecting the supporting tissue of teeth (Schaudinn et al., 2009).

6.2 Biofilms on indwelling medical devices

Infectious biofilm formation in the human body is not restricted to biotic surfaces. Indwelling medical devices (e.g. prosthetic heart valves, contact lenses, intrauterine devices and urethral catheters) are susceptible to bacterial adhesion and the subsequent formation of a biofilm. Bacteria may originate from the skin of the patient, health care workers, tap water or other fluid to which the device is exposed (Donlan, 2001). The adhesion of microorganisms to urinary catheters is particularly problematic. Catheter associated urinary tract infections (CAUTI) are the most common hospital acquired infection (Desai et al., 2010). Urinary catheters are tubular, latex or silicon devices inserted into the bladder via the urethra for a variety of purposes including collection of urine during surgery, measuring urine output, prevention of urine retention and control of urinary incontinence (Schumm & Lam, 2008). Urinary catheters are used in enormous numbers in modern medicine. An investigation carried out across eight European countries showed that 11% of hospitalised patients were undergoing catheterisation (Jepsen et al., 1987).

The occurrence of urinary tract infection is related to the length of time a patient is subject to catheterisation. Of those patients undergoing short term catheterisation (up to 7 days) 10 to 50% acquire an infection (Haley et al. 1981; Mulhall et al. 1988) and virtually all patients undergoing long-term catheterisation (longer than 28 days) develop infections (Warren, 1991). While the acquired infections are generally asymptomatic, patients are at risk from a variety of complications that render them more vulnerable than non-catheterized patients. Platt et al. (1982) revealed in a study of hospitalised patients that the development of a urinary tract infection during catheterisation was associated with an almost threefold increase in mortality. Kidney and bladder stones, bladder cancer, bacteraemia and pyelonephritis are among the complications that can potentially afflict catheterised patients (Stickler & Zimakoff, 1994).

The scale of this problem puts the development of catheter surfaces that prevent biofilm formation at the forefront of medical research. The most common antimicrobial compounds in urinary catheters are silver and nitrofurazone. However, their effectiveness is variable between different studies. One review (Schumm & Lam, 2008) concluded that silver alloy catheters did decrease the occurrence of asymptomatic bacteriuria in patients undergoing both short term and long term catheterisation, although this decrease was less pronounced in those patients catheterised for over a week. Desai *et al.* (2010) found that nitrofurazone-impregnated catheters had only a minimal preventative effect in the earlier stages of *E.coli* and *E.faecalis* biofilm development (< 5 days) and that silver impregnation had a negligible effect. The incorporation of a silver releasing device between the drainage tube and catheter was found to provide an antibacterial barrier that could protect against bacterial colonisation for periods of at least 10 days in the bag and 8 days for the tubes and catheters (Stickler et al., 1994). The principle of this device is that as urine flows through it bactericidal silver ions will be released by dissolution.

6.3 The MagPI System in medical research

It is clear that health care providers and medical microbiologists still have some way to go in identifying strategies that will prevent biofilm related infections. The MagPI System could prove to be a very useful tool in these investigations due to its ability to detect early stage biofilm formation. It could, for example, be utilized in the laboratory based development of anti-biofilm coatings and materials for indwelling medical devices or to assess the effectiveness of quorum sensing disruptors and antibiotics on biofilm formation. It could also be used in more frontline actions against biofilm infection such as in hospital disinfection to identify bacterial colonization on equipment. In the case study below (Section 7.0) we have used the MagPI System to investigate the effect of antibiotics on biofilm development in aquatic systems. Although this study was not carried out on bacterial biofilms in a setting relevant to medical science it does demonstrate the straight forward approach of the MagPI system to measuring early-stage biofilm formation and highlights its transitional value between different scientific disciplines. Besides the uses for the MagPI System in sediment ecology research and medical and pharmaceutical research, we have identified numerous fields in which the MagPI System could be utilised (Table 2).

Biofilm Occurrence	Problem/ Effect	Mitigation Efforts	MagPI Potential Use	References
Teeth	Plaque formation and dental caries	Incorporation of antimicrobial agents (e.g. bisbiguandines, metal ions, phenols, quaternary ammonium compounds) into toothpaste and mouth rinses.	Development of anti-plaque products and research into the bacteriology of plaque biofilms.	Marsh, 2011; Rosan & Lamont, 2000
Water distribution network	Clogging of pipes, decrease in water velocity and carrying capacity, Increased corrosion and energy utilisation. Potential contamination by pathogens.	Chemical water treatment e.g. chlorination.	Monitoring biofilm formation. Developing new technologies and treatments.	LeChevalier et al.,1987; Lund & Ormerod, 1995; Momba et al. 2000
Ships' Hulls	Increased surface roughness increases frictional resistance and thus fuel consumption. Decreased top speed and range.	Anti-biofouling coatings which incorporate biocides e.g. Tributyl tin (use is regulated due to their toxicity to non-target marine species) or copper.	Development of non-toxic anti-fouling coatings.	Champ, 2003; Schultz et al., 2010

Biofilm Occurrence	Problem/ Effect	Mitigation Efforts	MagPI Potential Use	References
Food stuff and food packaging	Economic loss due to food spoilage. Serious hygiene problem- adherence of pathogenic microorganism poses threat to human health.	Coatings and paints with antimicrobial agents for factory floors, walls etc. Removal of surface roughness of machinery. Disinfection of factories. Inhibition of biofilm development on food contact surfaces by bioactive compounds (e.g. Nisin).	Monitoring biofilm development in industrial plants. Development of antimicrobial agents for food packaging.	Kumar & Anand, 1998
Fluid flow systems (Industrial system cooling processes)	Decreased efficiency of heat exchangers, corrosion and health risk to workers if there's pathogen contamination.	Chemical water treatment with biocides e.g. hypochlorite, chlorine dioxide, bromine, ozone. Biofiltration.	Development of non-toxic chemical treatments and new technologies. Monitoring biofilm development.	Flemming, 2002; Meester et al., 2003

Table 2. Examples of biofilm occurrence, their effect and ways in which the MagPI could be used to help overcome these problems

7. Case study: The effect of antibiotics on bacterial biostabilisation potential

7.1 Introduction

In recent years awareness of antibiotics as common contaminants of aquatic systems has increased significantly (Kümmerer, 2001, 2009; Santos et al., 2010; Segura et al., 2009). Antibiotics reportedly occur in wastewater treatment plant (WWTP) effluent and surface waters at concentrations ranging from ng l^{-1} to several µg l^{-1} (Costanzo et al., 2005; Hirsch et al., 1999). There are a number of routes via which antibiotics can reach aquatic systems (Figure 4). As an important group of pharmaceuticals antibiotics are used extensively to treat infectious diseases in humans. Following consumption antibiotics are subject to metabolic reactions, such as hydroxylation, cleavage or glucuronation. However, between 30 and 90% of the administered dosage of antibiotics is excreted from the body still in a biologically active form (Jjemba, 2006; Rang et al., 1999). Some of these compounds will later be released into aquatic systems in effluent from WWTPs. Several investigations have shown that residual pharmaceuticals are incompletely removed by waste water treatment procedures (Heberer, 2002; Ternes, 2002; Xu et al., 2007). Antibiotics are also used in huge quantities in animal husbandry and increasingly in aquaculture to protect the health of animals, enhance growth and promote nutritional efficiency (Sarmah et al., 2006). As a result antibiotics also enter surface and ground water after leaching from animal feed and excrement (Christian et al., 2003). Another major contributor of antibiotics to aquatic systems is pharmaceutical manufacturers. Holm et al. (1995) found that groundwater down gradient from landfill used by a pharmaceutical company contained a large variety of sulphonamides at concentrations up to 5mg l^{-1}. Another investigation revealed that antibiotics were occurring in the mg l^{-1} range in effluent from drug manufacturing in India (Larsson et al., 2007).

Antibiotics released into aquatic environments are a concern for several reasons, including: i) contamination of water used for irrigation, drinking or recreation, ii) promotion of bacterial resistance to antibiotics (Kümmerer, 2009), iii) disruption of sewage treatment facilities in which microorganisms perform waste water treatment functions (Gomez et al.,

1996; Campos et al., 2001) and iv) their potential to negatively impact important ecosystem services regulated by microorganisms e.g. denitrification, nitrogen-fixation and organic matter degradation (Costanzo et al., 2005; Hirsch et al., 1999).

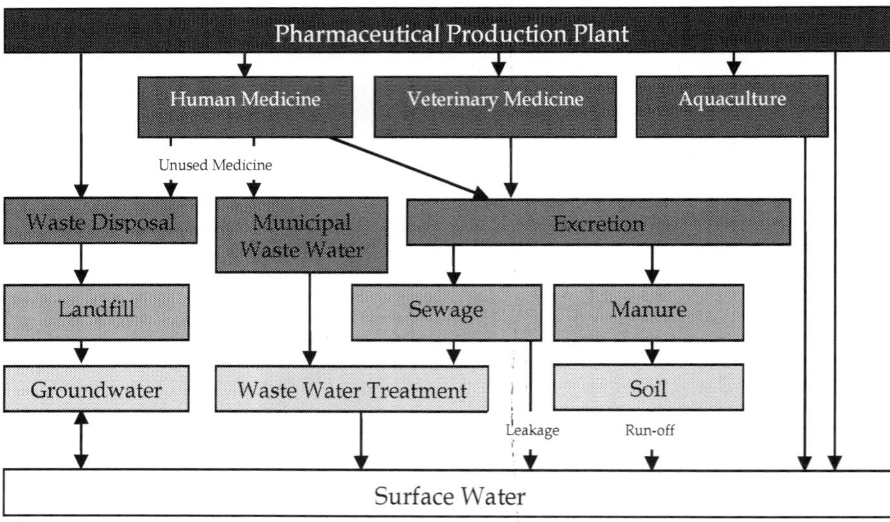

Fig. 4. Schematic diagram showing possible pathways of antibiotics into aquatic systems.

As previously discussed microbial consortia in aquatic systems drive a number of important processes in aquatic ecosystems (Section 5.0). One of these functions is biostabilisation whereby microorganisms living in biofilms at the sediment surface mediate the response of the sediment to erosive forces. Bacteria in biofilms are known to play an important role in sediment stabilisation (Gerbersdorf et al., 2009; Lubarsky et al., 2010). The objective of the present study was to investigate the biostabilisation potential of natural bacterial biofilms when exposed to environmentally relevant concentrations of antibiotics. Understanding the biostabilisation capacity of biofilms and its impairment by pollutants is important for successful sediment management in waterways and coastal zones.

Chloramphenicol, a bacteriostatic antibiotic, was selected for use in this investigation. It inhibits the growth and reproduction of certain bacteria by preventing peptide bond formation and thus disrupts the growth of peptide chains (Brosche & Backhaus, 2010). The use of chloramphenicol in human medicine is restricted due to its toxic properties (Forth at al., 1992) and its use has been completely banned in veterinary medicine since 1995 (BGW, 1996). However, chloramphenicol is still used extensively in aquaculture (Fierro & Olivia, 2009). Chloramphenicol occurs in surface water at relatively low concentrations compared to some other antibiotics, a maximum concentration of $0.06\mu g\ l^{-1}$ has been recorded (Hirsch et al., 1999). The concentrations used in this experiment (5, 10 and $50\mu g\ l^{-1}$) are not environmentally relevant concentrations of chloramphenicol itself. They were chosen to represent concentrations of total antibiotics in surface waters. Hirsch et al. (1999) found that the concentrations of certain antibiotics in surface waters reached $1.7\mu g\ l^{-1}$. The mean concentration of antibiotics in WWTP effluent in the Thames catchment area has been estimated at 62μg l^{-1}. By convention the concentration of antibiotics in surface waters where no measurements exist is taken as 10% of the concentration in WWTP effluent (Hirsch et al., 1999; Singer et al., 2011). Thus, it would not be unrealistic that background total antibiotic concentrations of 5μgl^{-1}, as used in this investigation, exist in some waterways.

Over the course of the experiment the MagPI System was used to measure the adhesive capacity of the substratum, a proxy for sediment stability. It was hypothesised that the MagPI System would detect a negative effect on substratum stability as a result of antibiotic exposure and that this effect would become increasingly pronounced as antibiotic concentration increased.

7.2 Materials and methods

7.2.1 Bacterial cultures

Surface sediment (20mm depth) from the intertidal mud flats of the Eden Estuary (Scotland, 56°22'N, 2°51'W) was mixed with the same volume of 1 μm filtered seawater and sonicated (Ultrasonic bath XB2 50 - 60 Hz) for 10 min to enhance detachment of the bacteria from the sediment, followed by two 10 min periods of centrifugation at 1500 rpm (Mistral E, Sanyo rotor 43122-105). The pellet (sediment fraction) was separated from the supernatant (containing bacterial fraction). The supernatant was centrifuged again, this time at 17000 rpm (Sorval, RC5B/C) for 10 min to obtain a microbial pellet. The resultant supernatant was discarded and the pellet with its associated bacteria was resuspended and passed through a 1.6 μm filter. The filter size was chosen to exclude the smallest expected microalgae from the estuarine sediment. Autoclaved standard nutrient broth (Fluka, peptone 15g l^{-1}, yeast extract 3g l^{-1}, sodium chloride 6g l^{-1}, D (+) glucose 1g l^{-1}) was added to the filtered supernatant (5:1). The bacterial stock cultures were left to establish under constant aeration and temperature (15°C) in the dark for one week prior to the experiment beginning.

7.2.2 Experimental set-up

Glass incubation chambers (L: 105mm, W: 105mm, H: 55mm) were filled to c. 1cm depth with 270 μm glass beads to provide a substratum for biofilm formation. The chambers were filled with 300ml autoclaved seawater (control) that had been spiked with defined concentrations of the antibiotic chloramphenicol (treatments). For the treatments a stock solution of chloramphenicol was prepared followed by dilution with autoclaved seawater (35psu) to the desired concentrations of 5 (T1), 10 (T2) and 50 (T3) μg l^{-1}. The glass chambers, including those for the control, were inoculated with 10ml of the bacterial stock solution to initiate biofilm growth. Four replicates were established for each of the treatments and the control. All incubation chambers were gently aerated and kept at a constant temperature (15°C) in a dark room over the experimental period of 6 days.

7.2.3 Sampling strategy

Sampling was carried out on days 0, 2, and 6. Samples for EPS protein analysis and low-temperature scanning electron microscopy (LTSEM, Figure 7) were obtained using a mini corer (cut-off 2ml syringe) and frozen immediately in liquid nitrogen and stored at -80°C until required for analysis.

7.2.4 Substratum stability

The adhesive capacity, a proxy for bed stability, of the biofilms growing on the glass beads was measured on sampling days by magnetic particle induction (MagPI System). Fluorescent particles of size range 150 - 250μm were applied to the test surface as outlined in Section 3. This particle size range was chosen to best represent the grain size of the substratum. The MagPI probe was set 7mm above the surface of the glass beads. The following equation was used to calculate the magnetic flux density (MFD) at total particle clearance.

Equation 2. $$y = 3.1903x + 0.8443$$

Obtained from the 7mm seawater calibration (Figure 3), where y is the MFD and x is the voltage at particle uplift from the test surface.

7.2.5 EPS extraction and colloidal protein analysis

Cores were placed in safety-lock Eppendorf caps with 2ml of distilled water and rotated for 1.5 hours by a horizontal mixer (Denley Spiramix 5) at room temperature. After centrifugation at 5000rpm (Mistral 3000E Sanyo, rotor 43122-105) for 15 minutes the supernatant was analysed for protein following the modified Lowry procedure (Raunkjaer et al., 1994). Protein concentration was measured by spectrophotometer at 750nm wavelength (BUCK Scientific, CECIL CE3021, UK) and protein concentrations were calculated according to BSA standard (Albumin from bovine serum: Sigma, cat no A 4503-10g) with results reported in μg ml^{-1}.

7.2.6 Statistical analysis

All statistical analysis was conducted using Minitab version 16 (Minitab, Coventry, UK). Substratum stability (mTesla) variation over time and between treatments was assessed using two-way analysis of variance (ANOVA: significance level $P < 0.05$). The unbalanced data set of colloidal protein concentration was tested for variation over time and between treatments by general linear modelling (significance level $P < 0.05$). One-way ANOVA (significance level $P < 0.05$) was applied followed by Tukey's post hoc test to determine which treatments showed a significant difference in adhesive capacity and protein concentration and also to determine for which treatments there was a time effect on the adhesive capacity and protein concentration.

7.3 Results

7.3.1 Substratum stability

A two-way ANOVA indicated significant variation in the response of sediment stability to both time ($P< 0.001$) and treatment ($P< 0.001$). For measurements of adhesive capacity taken directly after experimental set-up (day 0), there was no significant difference ($P= 0.484$) between treatments. On experiment days 2 and 6 there was a strong treatment effect (day 2 $P< 0.001$; day 6 $P= 0.001$). For both days, the mean adhesive capacity of the control was found to be significantly higher than any of the treatments. Statistical testing each day did not reveal a significant difference between the three treatments (Figure 5). One-way ANOVA determined a time effect only for the control ($P= 0.001$) and treatment 2 ($P= 0.012$). For the control measurements of adhesive capacity differed significantly between day 0 and day 2 as well as day 0 and day 6 but no significant difference was found between days 2 and 6. For treatment 2, the adhesive capacity measurements on day 6 differed significantly from day 2 and day 0 but days 0 and 2 of the experiment were not significantly different to each other.

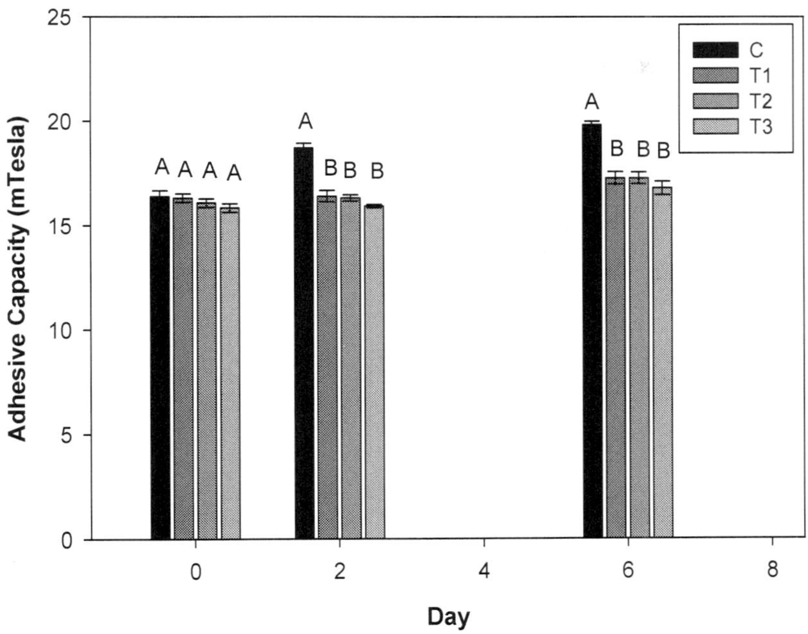

Fig. 5. Mean response (n=4, +/- standard error) of substratum adhesive capacity (proxy for sediment stability) to antibiotic exposure over the experimental period. C= control, T1= low antibiotic concentration (5 µg l^{-1}), T2= medium antibiotic concentration (10 µg l^{-1}), T3= high antibiotic concentration (50 µg l^{-1}). Where treatments do not share a letter denotes a significant difference on that day.

7.3.2 Colloidal protein concentration

There was a significant response to time (P< 0.001) but not treatment (P= 0.087) in colloidal protein concentration. On days 0 and 2 of the experiment no significant difference was found between treatments (Day 0 P= 0.319; Day 2 P= 0.401). One-way ANOVA of protein concentration on day 6 revealed a significant variation between treatments (P= 0.03). T1 (low antibiotic concentration) was significantly higher than the control (C). Neither T1 nor C was significantly different from T2 and T3 on day 6 of the experiment (Figure 6). Statistical testing revealed a time effect only for T1 (P= 0.001) and T2 (P= 0.012). For T1, the protein concentration differed significantly between day 0 and day 6 and no significant difference was found between days 2 and day 6 or day 2 and day 0. For treatment 2, the protein concentration on day 6 differed significantly from days 0 and 2 but protein concentration on days 0 and 2 were not significantly different.

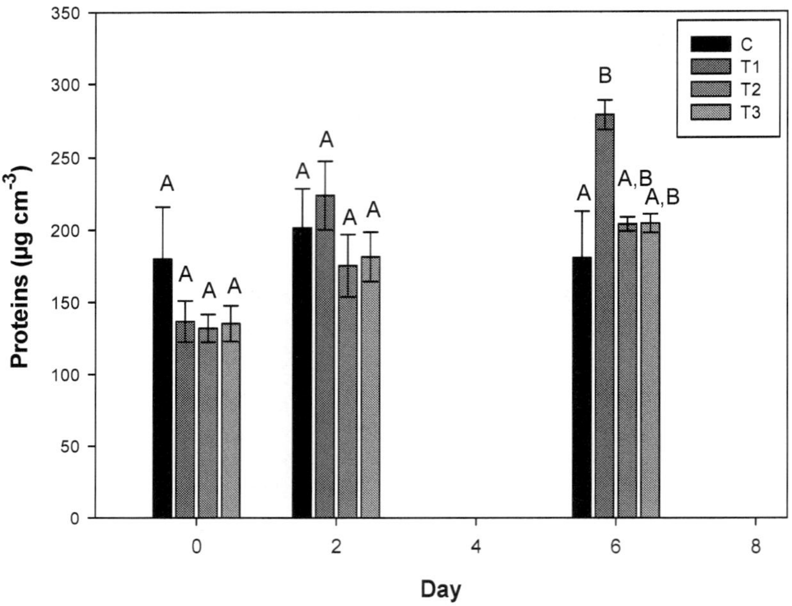

Fig. 6. Mean response (n=4, +/- standard error) of colloidal protein concentration to antibiotic exposure over the experimental period. C= control, T1= low antibiotic concentration (5 µg l^{-1}), T2= medium antibiotic concentration (10 µg l^{-1}), T3= high antibiotic concentration (50 µg l^{-1}). Where treatments do not share a letter denotes a significant difference on that day.

7.4 Discussion

If the results for the adhesive capacity measured by magnetic particle induction are taken as a proxy for biofilm formation then it would appear that biofilm development was significantly higher on the substratum surface of the control when compared to all treatments. No significant time effect on the adhesive capacity was found for treatments 1 and 3. As the substratum was composed wholly of non-cohesive glass beads the binding force observed in the control and in treatment 2 (on day 6 only) must have been due to bacterial adhesion and EPS secretion. The control had a significantly higher adhesive capacity than each of the treatments on days 2 and 6 of the experiment. This suggests that the biostabilisation potential of bacteria is affected by antibiotics at concentrations likely to be found in natural surface waters. In the event of an influenza pandemic the amount of antibiotics reaching surface waters is predicted to increase. Singer et al. (2011) project a mean total antibiotic concentration of 15µg l^{-1} and a maximum concentration of 80µg l^{-1} in the Thames catchment area in the event of a severe pandemic. Our results for the adhesive capacity of treatment 3 (50 µg l^{-1}) suggest that the biostabilisation potential of bacteria in aquatic systems would be significantly affected in the event of a severe influenza pandemic.

To-date the majority of studies addressing the effects of pharmaceuticals on aquatic microorganisms have been conducted using concentrations greater than those observed in the environment (Halling-Sorensen, 2001; Kümmerer et al., 2000; Pomati et al., 2004). Of the investigations conducted using environmentally relevant concentrations of antibiotics there has been a strong indication that antibiotics in aquatic ecosystems have the potential to influence biotic processes (Costanzo et al., 2005). Schreiber and Szewzyk (2008) conducted an experiment using environmentally relevant concentrations (0.5 - 50μg l^{-1}) of antibiotics. They found that antibiotic exposure enhanced, inhibited or had no influence on the initial adhesion of bacteria to a surface. The effect was dependent on the selected pharmaceutical, the bacterial strain and the adhesion surface as well as antibiotic concentration. In aquatic systems there are a myriad of antibiotics present all of which function differently. In addition biofilms are not composed solely of bacteria, other microorganisms, microalgae for example, may also be present in surface sediment biofilms. Our results highlight the need for investigations into the effect of pharmaceuticals at concentrations occurring in surface waters on biostabilisation as well as other important ecosystem services conducted by microorganisms in aquatic ecosystems.

As previously discussed (Section 5.0) EPS production by microorganisms adhered to the sediment surface is thought to significantly increase its stability (Underwood & Paterson, 2003). Traditionally, microalgae and their polysaccharide-rich EPS were considered to be the principal binding force (Underwood & Paterson, 2003). However, recent work suggests that biofilm bacteria and bacterial EPS which is estimated to contain up to 60% protein (Flemming & Wingender, 2001) are more important for biostabilisation than previously considered and that a synergistic effect between EPS protein and EPS carbohydrate might strengthen their binding forces (Gerbersdorf et al., 2008; Lubarsky et al., 2010). In spite of this, no correlation was found ($\alpha = 0.05$) between substratum adhesiveness and colloidal protein. Adhesive capacity results imply that there is no biofilm formation for treatment 1 and 3 but that biofilm formation was not inhibited in treatment 2 or in the control. However, if we take protein concentration rather than the MagPI System measurements as an indication of biofilm formation then it would appear that there was no biofilm formation in the control as there is no significant time effect on protein concentration. Both adhesive capacity results and protein concentration suggest the development of biofilms in treatment 2. A time effect on the protein concentration of treatment 1 was also observed and the protein concentration was found to be significantly higher for treatment 1 than for the control on the final day of the experiment. The higher colloidal protein concentration observed in treatment 1 on the final day of the experiment may be the product of a stress response by the bacteria to antibiotic exposure. Studies have shown that at subinhibitory levels some antibiotics stimulate EPS production by certain bacteria (Rachid et al., 2000). The lack of correlation between protein concentration and adhesive capacity in this experiment may indicate that proteins do not actually play a very important role in biostabilisation in this experimental system. Alternatively, exposure of the bacterial cultures to chloramphenicol may not necessarily affect the quantity of the EPS as much as the quality. It is possible that the higher molecular weight fraction of EPS protein is responsible for the binding characteristics that have been observed in natural bacterial assemblages (Lubarsky et al., 2010). Inhibition of peptide bond formation by chloramphenicol may result in the excretion of only small molecular weight protein molecules which have no influence on sediment stability.

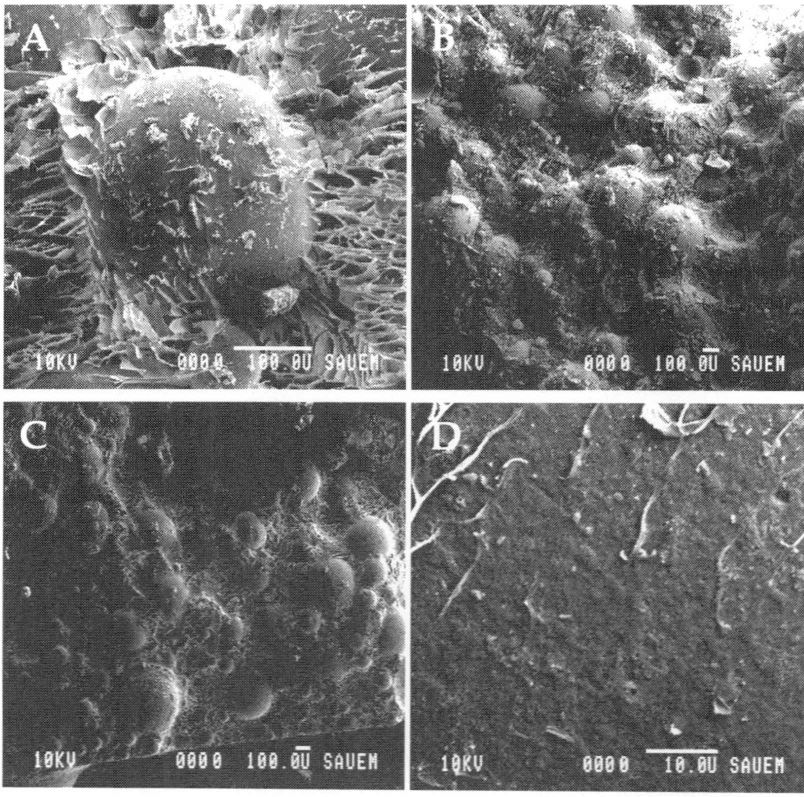

Fig. 7. Low- temperature scanning electronmicroscopy (LTSEM) images of biofilms on glass beads. **A**: Day 0, control. Low organic matter cover, honeycomb structure around bead is water; **B:** Day 6, T3; **C:** Day 6, T2; **D:** Close-up of biofilm on glass bead surface, Day 6, T1.

7.5 Conclusion

The adhesive capacity results for this experiment successfully demonstrate the ability of the MagPI System to determine subtle changes in surface adhesion as a result of biofilm formation. The stability of the non-cohesive glass bead substratum was significantly increased during the experimental period for the control. Although there was a detrimental effect on biostabilisation as a result of the bacteria being exposed to antibiotics in the treatments the effect was not as hypothesised; the adhesive capacity was not found to decrease with increasing chloramphenicol concentration. It must be considered that this experiment targeted only one group of biofilm microorganisms and used a single compound. As such these findings cannot be taken as conclusive proof that the levels of antibiotics found in our waterways are having a damaging effect on the sediment stabilisation potential of biofilms. They do however highlight the need for further investigations using a mixture of antibiotics at environmentally relevant concentrations and varied microbial assemblages. Future work should also calibrate MagPI System measurements of adhesive capacity against biological variables other than EPS protein concentration, for example bacterial cell numbers or EPS carbohydrate concentration.

8. Summary

Biofilms have become an important research topic across numerous scientific disciplines in recent years. While their presence can be desirable or beneficial in some situations, it can be incredibly harmful or costly in others. Bacterial biofilms can be particularly harmful to human health and pose a serious challenge in modern medicine. The last decade has seen a significant increase in the occurrence of multi-drug resistant microorganism infections. The persistence of these infectious microorganisms is attributed to their existence as biofilms rather than as free-floating cells. It is thought that microorganisms in biofilms have 10 to 100 times more resistance to antibiotics than their planktonic counterparts. Biofilm research in medical science, as well as in many other fields, has previously been conducted using time-consuming procedures or large laboratory scale systems that can be both expensive and labour intensive. The MagPI System presented in this paper is an alternative method for biofilm detection. It uses magnetic induction of ferrous particles to quantify the adhesive capacity of a test surface. As the "stickiness" of surfaces can often be attributed to the presence and growth phase of a biofilm the MagPI System can be used to evaluate biofilm formation and state of development. This system has already been used with much success in the field of sediment ecology and we propose its use across a number of other fields where research questions require a measure of adhesion or extent of biofilm formation. The MagPI System may be especially useful in medical science. It could, for example, be used in the development of anti-microbial indwelling medical devices, to evaluate the effect of antibiotics on biofilm formation or in the disinfection of healthcare facilities. In summary, the MagPI System combines a highly variable system, of logistic ease and relatively low cost providing a means of repeatedly and non-destructively quantifying the adhesive capacity of a test surface as a result of biofilm formation.

9. Acknowledgements

We thank R. Aspden and R.W. Hussin for their laboratory assistance. This research was funded by the Natural Environment Research Council (UK) through an "Innovations A" grant. We also thank A. Singer for his helpful advice on antibiotics in aquatic ecosystems.

10. References

Anwar, H., J. L. Strap, K. Chen & J. W. Costerton. (1992). Dynamic interactions of biofilms of mucoid *Pseudomonas aeruginosa* with tobramycin and piperacillin. *Antimicrob. Agents Chemother.* Vol. 36, pp. 1208–1214.

Adams, J. L. & R. J. C., McLean. (1999). Impact of rpoS deletion on Escherichia coli biofilms. *Appl. Environ. Microbiol.* Vol. 65, pp. 4285–4287

Battin, T.J., L.A., Kaplan, J.D., Newbold & C.M.E., Hansen. (2003). Contributions of microbial biofilms to ecosystem processes in stream mesocosms. *Nature.* Vol. 426, pp. 439-442

Brosche, S. & T., Backhaus. (2010). Toxicity of five protein synthesis inhibiting antibiotics and their mixture to limnic bacterial communities. *Aquatic Toxicology*. Vol. 99, pp. 457–465

Calles, B. (1983). Settling processes in a saline environment. *Geografiska Annaler. SeriesA. Physical Geography*. Vol. 65, pp. 159–166

Campos, J.L., J.M., Garrido, R., Mendez & J.M., Lema. (2001). Effect of two broad-spectrum antibiotics on activity and stability of continuous nitrifying system. *Applied Biochemistry and Biotechnology*. Vol. 95, pp. 1–10

Carpentier, B. & O., Cerf. (1993). Biofilms and their consequences, with particular reference to hygiene in the food industry. *Journal of Applied Microbiology*. Vol. 75, pp. 499-511

Champ, M.A. (2003). Economic and environmental impacts on ports and harbors from the convention to ban harmful marine anti-fouling systems. *Marine Pollution Bulletin*. Vol. 46, pp. 935–940

Chavant, P., B., Gaillard-Martinie, R., Talon, M., Hébraud & T., Bernardi. (2007). A new device for rapid evaluation of biofilms formation potential by bacteria. *Journal of Microbial Methods*. Vol. 68, pp. 605-612

Christian, T., R.J., Schneider, H.A., Färber, D., Skutlarek, M.T., Meyer & H.E., Goldbach. (2003). Determination of Antibiotic Residues in Manure, Soil, and Surface Waters. *Acta hydrochim. hydrobiol.* Vol. 31, pp. 36–44

Coenye, T. & H.J., Nelis. (2010). In vitro and in vivo model systems to study microbial biofilm formation. *Journal of Microbiological Methods*. Vol. 83, pp. 89-105

Costanzo, S.D., J., Murby & J., Bates. (2005). Ecosystem response to antibiotics entering the aquatic environment. *Marine Pollution Bulletin*. Vol. 51, pp. 218–223

Costerton, J. W., J., Lam, K., Lam & R., Chan. (1983). The role of the microcolony mode of growth in the pathogenesis of Pseudomonas aeruginosa infections. *Rev. Infect. Dis.* Vol. 5, pp. 867–873

Costerton, J. W., K.-J., Cheng, G. G. Geesey, T. I. Ladd, J. C. Nickel, M. Dasgupta, & T. J. Marrie. (1987). Bacterial biofilms in nature and disease. *Annu. Rev. Microbiol.* Vol. 41, pp. 435–464

Costerton, J. W. & H. M., Lappin-Scott. (1995). Introduction to microbial biofilms. In: *Microbial Biofilms*. H. M. Lappin-Scott & J. W. Costerton (ed.), pp. 1-11, Cambridge University Press, Cambridge, United Kingdom.

Costerton, J. W., P. S., Stewart, & E. P., Greenberg. 1999. Bacterial biofilms: a common cause of persistent infections. *Science*. Vol. 284, pp. 1318–1322

Costerton, J.W. (2001). Cystic fibrosis pathogenesis and the role of biofilms in persistent infection. *Trends in Microbiology*. Vol.9, pp. 50-52

Cyr, H., & K.E., Morton. (2006). Distribution of biofilm exopolymeric substances in littoral sediments of Canadian Shield lakes: effects of light and substrate. *Canadian Journal of Fisheries and Aquatic Sciences*. Vol. 63, pp. 1763–1776

Dagostino, L., A. E. Goodman & K. C. Marshall. (1991). Physiological responses induced in bacteria adhering to surfaces. *Biofouling*. Vol. 4, pp. 113–119

Decho, A. W. (1994). Molecular scale events influencing the macroscale cohesiveness of exopolymers. In: *Biostabilisation of Sediment*, W. E. Krumbein, D. M. Paterson and L. J. Stal (eds.), pp. 135–148, BIS Verlag, Oldenburg

Decho, A.W., (2000). Microbial biofilms in intertidal systems: an overview. *Continental Shelf Research*. Vol. 20, pp. 1257–1273

Desai, D.G., K.S., Liao, M.E., Cevallos & B.W., Trautner. (2010). Silver of nitrofurazone impregnation of urinary catheters has a minimal effect on uropathogen adherence. *The Journal of Urology*. Vol. 184, pp. 2565-2571

Dodds, W. K. (2003). The role of periphyton in phosphorus retention in shallow freshwater aquatic systems. *Journal of Phycology*. Vol. 39, pp. 840–849

Dong, Y-H. & L-H., Zhang. (2005). Quorum sensing and quorum- quenching enzymes. *The Journal of Microbiology*. Vol. 43, pp. 101-109

Donlan, R.M. (2001). Biofilms and device-associated infections. *Emerging Infectious Diseases*. Vol. 7, pp. 277-281

Donlan, R.M. & J.W., Costerton. (2002). Biofilms: Survival mechanisms of clinically relevant microorganisms. *Clin. Microbiol. Rev*. Vol. 15, pp. 167-193

Droppo, I.G., Y.L., Lau & C., Mitchell. (2001). The effect of depositional history on contaminated bed sediment stability. The Science of the Total Environment Vol. 266, pp. 7-13

Evans, D. J., D. G. Allison, M. R. W. Brown & P. Gilbert. (1990). Effect of growth-rate on resistance of gram-negative biofilms to cetrimide. *J. Antimicrob. Chemother*. Vol. 26, pp. 473–478.

Fierro, J. & D., Oliva. (2009). Effect of antibiotic treatment on the growth and survival of juvenile northern Chilean scallop, Argopecten purpuratus Lamarck (1819), and associated microflora in experimental cultures. *Aquaculture Research*. Vol. 40, pp. 1358–1362

Flemming, H.C., (2002). Biofouling in water systems - cases, causes and counter measures. *Applied Microbiology and Biotechnology*. Vol. 59, pp. 629-640

Flemming, H.C. & J., Wingender. (2001). Relevance of microbial extracellular polymeric substances (EPSs)-Part I:Structural and ecological aspects. Water Science And Technology. Vol. 43, pp. 1-8

Förstner, U., S., Heise, R., Schwartz, B., Westrich & W., Ahlf. (2004). Historical contaminated sediments and soils at river basin scale. *J. Soils Sediments*. Vol. 4, pp. 247-260

Fridkin, S.K. & R.P., Gaynes (1999). Antimicrobial resistance in intensive care units. *Clinics in Chest Medicine*. Vol. 20, pp. 303-316

Gabriel, M.M., M.S., Mayo, L.L., May et al. (1996). In vitro evaluation of the efficacy of a silver-coated catheter. *Current Microbiology*. Vol. 33

Gaynes, R., J.R., Edwards & The National Nosocomial Infections Surveillance System. (2005). Overview of nosocomial infectionscaused by gram-negative bacilli. *Healthcare Epidemiology*. Vol. 41, pp. 848-854

Gerbersdorf, S.U., W., Manz & D.M., Paterson. (2008). The engineering potential of natural benthic bacterial assemblages in terms of the erosion resistance of sediments. *Fems Microbiology Ecology*. Vol. 66, pp. 282-294

Gerbersdorf, S.U., R., Bittner, H., Lubarsky, W., Manz & D.M., Paterson. (2009). Microbial assemblages as ecosystem engineers of sediment stability. *Journal of Soils and Sediments*. Vol. 9, pp. 640-652

Gomez, J., R., Mendez & J.M., Lema. (1996). The effect of antibiotics on nitrification processes—batch assays. *Applied Biochemistry and Biotechnology*. Vol. 57, pp. 869–876

Guo, L.H., H.L., Wang, X.D., Liu & J., Duan. (2008). Identification of protein differences between two clinical isolates of Streptococcus mutans by proteomic analysis. *Oral Microbiology Immunology*. Vol. 23, pp. 105-111

Haag, I., U., Kern & B., Westrich. (2001). Erosion investigation and sediment quality measurements for a comprehensive risk assessment of contaminated aquatic sediments. *The Science of the Total Environment*. Vol. 266, pp. 249-257

Haley, R.W., D.H., Culver, J.W., White, W.M., Morgan & T.G., Emori. (1985). The national nosocomial infection rate. *Am. J. Epidemiol*. Vol. 121, pp. 159-167

Halling-Sorensen, B. (2001). Inhibition of aerobic growth and nitrification of bacteria in sewage sludge by antibacterial agents. *Arch. Environ. Contam. Toxicol*. Vol. 40, pp. 451–460

Hall-Stoodley, L., J.W., Costerton & P., Stoodley. (2004). Bacterial biofilms: from the natural environment to infectious diseases. *Nat Rev Microbiol*. Vol. 2, pp. 95–108

Hall-Stoodley, L., F.Z., Hu, A., Gieseke, L., Nistico, D., Nguyen, J., Hayes, *et al*. (2006) Direct detection of bacterial biofilms on the middle-ear mucosa of children with chronic otitis media. *JAMA*. Vol. 296, pp. 202–211

Hentzer, M., H., Wu, J.B., Andersen, K., Riedel, T.B., Rasmussen, N., Bagge, N., Kumar, M.A., Schembri, Z., Song, P., Kristoffersen, M., Manefield, J.W., Costerton, S., Molin, L., Eberl, P., Steinberg, S., Kjelleberg, N., Hoiby & M., Givskov. (2003). Attenuation of Pseudomonas aeruginosa virulence by quorum sensing inhibitors. *EMBO J*. Vol. 22, pp. 3803–3815

Herberer, T. (2002). Occurrence, fate, and removal of pharmaceutical residues in the aquatic environment: a review of recent research data. *Toxicology Letters*. Vol. 131, pp. 5–17

Hirsch, R., T., Ternes, K., Haberer & K-L., Kratz. (1999). Occurrence of antibiotics in the aquatic environment. *Science of the Total Environment*. Vol. 225, pp. 109-118

Holm JV, K., Ruegge, P.L., Bjerg & T.H., Christensen. (1999) Occurrence and distribution of pharmaceutical organic compounds in the groundwater down gradient of a landfill - Grindsted, Denmark. Environ Sci Technol. Vol. 5, pp.1415-1420

Houghton, J.I. & J. Quarmby. (1999). Biopolymers in wastewater treatment. *Current Opinion in Biotechnology*. Vol. 10, pp. 259-262

Jepsen, O.B., S.O., Larsen, J., Dankert et al. (1982). Urinary tract infection and bacteraemia in hospitalized patients- a European multiculture prevalence survey on nosocomial infection. *Journal of Hospital Infection*. Vol. 3, pp. 241-252

Jjemba P.K. (2006). Excretion and ecotoxicity of pharmaceutical and personal care products in the environment. *Ecotixicol. Environ. Saf.* Vol. 63, pp. 113-130

Johnson, J.R., P., Delavar & M., Azar (1999). Activities of a nitrofurazone- containing urinary catheter and a silver hydrogel catheter against multidrug- resistant bacteria characteristic of catheter- associated urinary tract infections. *Antimicrob. Agents Chemother*. Vol. 43

Koch, C., & N., Hoiby. (1993). Pathogenesis of cystic fibrosis. *Lancet*. Vol. 341, pp. 1065–1069

Kumar, C.G. & S.K., Anand. (1998). Significance of microbial biofilms in food industry: a review. *International Journal of Food Microbiology*. Vol. 42, pp. 9-27

Kümmerer, K., A., Al-Ahmad & V., Mersch-Sundermann.(2000). Biodegradability of some antibiotics, elimination of the genotoxicity and affection of wastewater bacteria in a simple test. *Chemosphere*. Vol. 40, pp. 701–710

Kümmerer, K. (2001).Drugs in the environment: emission of drugs, diagnostic aids and disinfectants into wastewater by hospitals in relation to other sources - a review. *Chemosphere*. Vol. 45, pp. 957-96

Kümmerer, K. (2009). Antibiotics in the aquatic environment - A review - Part II. *Chemosphere*. Vol. 75, pp. 435–441

Lam, J., R., Chan, K., Lam & J.W., Costerton. (1980). Production of mucoid microcolonies by Pseudomonas aeruginosa within infected lungs in Cystic Fibrosis. *Infection and Immunity*. Vol. 28, pp. 546-556

Lawrence, J.R., G.D.W., Swerhone, G.G., Leppard, T., Araki, X., Zhang, M.M., West & A.P., Hitchcock. (2003). Scanning transmission X-ray, laser scanning, and transmission Electron microscopy mapping of the exopolymeric matrix of microbial biofilms. *Applied and Environmental Microbiology*. Vol. 69, pp. 5543-5554

LeChevallier, M.W., T.M., Babcock & R.G., Lee. (1987). Examination and characterization of distribution system biofilms. *Appl. Environ. Microbiol.* Vol. 53, pp. 2714-2724

Larson, F., H., Lubarsky, S.U., Gerbersdorf & D.M., Paterson. (2009). Surface adhesionmeasurements in aquatic biofilms using magnetic particle induction: MagPI. *Limnology and Oceanography-Methods*. Vol. 7, pp. 490-497

Larsson, T.A., C., de Pedro & N., Paxeus. (2007). Effluent from drug manufacturers contains extremely high levels of pharmaceuticals. *J. Hazard. Mater.* Vol. 148, pp. 751-755

LeChevalier, M.W., T.M., Bancock & R.G., Lee. (1987). Examination and Characterization of distribution system biofilms. *Appl. Environ. Microbiol.* Vol. 53, pp. 2714-2724

Lessa, F., J.R., Edwards, S.K., Fridkin, F.C., Tenover, T.C., Horan & R.J., Gorwitz. (2009). Trends in Incidence of Late-Onset Methicillin-Resistant Staphylococcus aureus Infection in Neonatal Intensive Care Units: Data From the National Nosocomial Infections Surveillance System, 1995-2004. *Pediatric Infectious Disease Journal* Vol. 28, pp. 577-581

Liu, H. & H.H.P., Fang. (2002). Hydrogen production from wastewater by acidogenic granular sludge. *Water Science and Technology*. Vol. 47, pp. 153–158

Livermore, D.M. (2000). Antibiotic resistance in Staphylococci. *Int. J. Antimicrob. Agents* Vol. 16, pp. 3-10

Lubarsky, H.V., C., Hubas, M., Chocholek, F., Larson, W., Manz, D.M., Paterson & S.U., Gerbersdorf. (2010). The stabilisation potential of individual and mixed assemblages of natural bacteria and microalgae. PLoS ONE 5(11): e13794. doi:10.1371/journal.pone.0013794

Lund, V. & K., Ormerod. (1995). The influence of disinfection processes on biofilm formation in water distribution systems. *Water research*. Vol. 29, pp. 1013-1021

Lyczak, J. B., C.L., Cannon & G..B., Pier. (2002). Lung infections associated with cystic fibrosis. *Clin. Microbiol. Rev.* Vol. 15, pp. 194–222.

Mah, T. F. & G.A., O'Toole. (2001). Mechanisms of biofilm resistance to antimicrobial agents. *Trends Microbiol.* Vol. 9, pp. 34–39

Manefield, M., T.B., Rasmussen, M., Henzter, J.B., Andersen, P., Steinberg, S., Kjelleberg & M., Givskov. (2002). Halogenated furanones inhibit quorum sensing through accelerated LuxR turnover. *Microbiology*. Vol. 148, pp. 1119–1127

Marsh, P.D., A., Moter & D.A., Devine. (2011).Dental plaque biofilms: communities, conflict and control. *Periodontology 2000*. Vol. 55, pp. 16–35

McNeil, J., C., Taylor & W., Lick. (1996). Measurements of erosion of undisturbed bottom sediments with depth. J.Hydraul. Engin. Vol. 122, pp. 316-324.

McNeil, J. & W., Lick. (2004). Erosion Rates and Bulk Properties of Sediments From the Kalamazoo River. *Journal of Great Lakes research*. Vol. 30, pp. 407-418

Meesters, K.P.H., J.W., Van Groenestijn & J., Gerriste. (2003). Biofouling reduction in recirculating cooling systems through biofiltration of process water. *Water Research*. Vol. 37, pp. 525–532

Momba, M.N.B., R., Kfir, S.N., Venter & T.E., Cloete. (2000). An overview of biofilms formation in water distribution systems and its impact on the deterioration of water quality. *Water SA*. Vol. 26, pp. 59-66

Morató, J., F., Codony & J., Mas. (2004). Microscopy techniques applied for monitoring the development of aquatic biofilms. In: Current *Issues on Multidisciplinary Microscopy Research and Education*, pp. 93–10, FORMATEX

Morton, L.H.G., D. L. A., Greenway, C. C., Gaylarde & S. B. Surman. (1998). Consideration of some implications of to biocides the resistance of biofilms. *International Biodeterioration & Biodegradation*. Vol. 41, pp. 247-259

Mulhall, A.B., R.G., Chapman & R.A., Row. (1988). Bacteriuria during indwelling urethral catheterisation. *Journal of Hospital Infections*. Vol. 11, pp. 253-262

Musk, D.J., D.A., Banko & P.J., Hergenrother. (2005). Iron salts perturb biofilms formation and disrupt existing biofilms of Pseudomonas aeruginosa. *Chem. Biol*. Vol. 12, pp. 789–79

Nadell, C.D., J.B., Xavier, S.A., Levin & K.R., Foster. (2008). The evolution of quorum sensing in bacterial. *PLoS Biol*. Vol. 6(1): e14. doi:10.1371/journal.pbio.0060014

Nicolella, C., M.C.M., van Loosdrecht & J.J., Heijnen. (2000). Wastewater treatment with particulate biofilm reactors. *J. Biotechnology*. Vol. 80, pp. 1-33

Paterson, D. M. (1989). Short-term changes in the erodibility of intertidal cohesive sediments related to the migratory behavior of epipelic diatoms. *Limnol. Oceanogr*. Vol. 34, pp. 223-234.

Perkins, R.G., I.R., Davidson, D.M., Paterson, H., Sun, J., Watson & M.A., Player. (2006). Low-temperature SEM imaging of polymer structure in engineered and natural sediments and the implications regarding stability. *Geoderma*. Vol. 134, pp. 48-55

Platt, R., B.F., Polk, B., Murdock & B., Rosner. (1982). Mortality associated with nosocmial urinary-tract infection. *N. Engl. J. Med.* Vol. 307, pp. 637-642

Pollard, P.C., (2010). Bacterial activity in plant (Schoenoplectus validus) biofilmsof constructed wetlands. *Water Research*. Vol. 44, pp. 5939-5948

Pomati, F., A.G., Netting, D.C., Brett & A., Neilan. (2004). Effects of erythromycin, tetracycline and ibuprofen on the growth of Synechocystis sp. and Lemna minor. *Aquatic Toxicology*. Vol. 67, pp. 387–396

Priester, L.H., A.M., Horst, J.L., Saleta, L.A.K., Mertes, & P.A., Holden. (2007). Enhanced visualization of microbial biofilms by staining and environmental scanning electron microscopy. *Journal of Microbiological Methods*. Vol. 68, pp. 577 - 58

Rachid, S., K., Ohlsen, W., Witte, J., Hacker, & W., Ziebuhr. (2000). Effect of subinhibitory antibiotic concentrations on polysaccharide intercellular adhesin expression in biofilm-forming *Staphylococcus epidermidis*. *Antimicrob Agents Chemother*. Vol. 44, pp. 3357–3363

Rang, H.P., M.M., Dale & J.M., Ritter. (1999). Pharmacology. Churchill Livingstone, Edinburgh.

Rasmussen, T.B., M.E., Skindersoe, T., Bjarnsholt, R.K., Phipps, K.B., Christensen, P.O., Jensen, J.B., Andersen, B., Koch, T.O., Larsen, M., Hentzer, L., Eberl, N., Hoiby & M., Givskov. (2005). Identity and effects of quorum-sensing inhibitors produced by Penicillium species. *Microbiology*. Vol. 151, pp. 1325–1340

Rasmussen, T.B, & M., Givskov. (2006). Quorum-sensing inhibitors as anti-pathogenic drugs. International *Journal of Medical Microbiology*. Vol. 296, pp. 149–161

Raunkjaer K, T., Hvitvedjacobsen & P.H., Nielsen. (1994). Measurement of pools of protein, carbohydrate and lipid in domestic waste-water. *Water Research*. Vol. 28, pp. 251-262

Rosan, L. & R.J., Lamont. (2000). Dental plaque formation. *Microbes and Infection*. Vol. 2, pp. 1599−1607

Santos L. H.M.L.M., A.N., Araújo, A., Fachini, A., Pena, C., Delerue-Matos & M.C.B.S.M. Montenegro. (2010). Ecotoxicological aspects related to the presence of pharmaceuticals in the aquatic environment. *Journal of Hazardous Materials*. Vol. 175, pp. 45-95

Sarmah, A.K., M.T., Meyer & A.B.A. Boxall. (2006). A global perspective on the use, sales, exposure pathways, occurrence, fate and effects of veterinary antibiotics (VAs) in the environment. *Chemosphere*. Vol. 65, pp. 725-759

Sauer, K., (2003). The genomics and proteomics of biofilm formation. *Genome Biology*. Vol. 4, Article 219

Schaudinn, C., A., Gorur, D., Keller, P.P., Sedghizadeh & J.W., Costerton. (2009). Periodontitis: An archetypical biofilm disease. *JADA*. Vol. 140, pp. 978-986

Schlekat, C.E., A.W., Decho & G.T., Chandler. (1998). Sorption of cadmium to bacterial extracellular polymeric sediement coatings under estuarine conditions. *Environmental Toxicology and Chemistry*. Vol. 17, pp. 1867–1874

Schreiber, F. & U., Szewzyk. (2008). Environmentally relevant concentrations of pharmaceuticals influence the initial adhesion of bacteria. *Aquatic Toxicology*. Vol. 87, pp. 227–233

Schuenemann, M. & H., Kuehl. (1991). Experimental investigations of the erosional behaviour of naturally formed mud from the Elbe estuary and adjacent Wadden sea, Germany. In: *Nearshore and Estuarine Cohesive Sediment*, A. J. Mehta (ed.), pp. 314-330, American Geophysical Union, Washington, USA

Schultz, M. P., J.A., Bendick, E.R., Holm & W.M., Hertel. (2011). Economic impact of biofouling on a naval surface ship. *Biofouling*. Vol. 27, pp. 87-98

Schumm, K. & T.B., Lam. (2008). Types of urethral catheters for management of short-term voiding problems in hospitalised adults (Review). *The Cochrane Library*. CD004013

Segura, P.A., M., François, C., Gagnon & S., Sauve. (2010). Review of the occurrence of anti-infectives in contaminated wastewaters and natural and drinking waters. *Environmental Health Perspectives*. Vol. 117, pp. 675-684

Singer, A.C., V., Colizza, H., Schmitt, J., Andrews, D., Balcan, W.E., Huang, V.D.J. Keller, A., Vespignani & R.J., Williams. (2011). Assessing the Ecotoxicologic Hazards of a Pandemic Influenza Medical Response. *Environmental Health Perspective*. doi:10.1289/ehp.1002757

Singh, P.K., A.L., Schaefer, M.R., Parsek, T.O., Moninger, M.J., Welsh & E.P., Greenberg. (2000). Quorum-sensing signals indicate that cystic fibrosis lungs are infected with bacterial biofilms. *Nature*. Vol. 407, pp. 762-764

Smith, K. & I.S., Hunter. (2008). Efficacy of common hospital biocides with biofilms of multi-drug resistant clinical isolates. *Journal of Medical Microbiology*. Vol. 57, pp. 966-973

Spears, B. M., J., Funnell, J., Saunders & D.M., Paterson. (2007). On the boundaries: sediment stability measurements across aquatic ecosystems. In: *Sediment Dynamics and Pollutant Mobility in Rivers: An Interdisciplinary Approach*, B. Westrich & U. Föstner (eds.), pp. 68–79, Springer: Berlin, Heidelberg

Spears, B.M., J.E., Saunders, I., Davidson & D.M., Paterson. (2008). Microalgal sediment biostabilisation along a salinity gradient in the Eden Estuary, Scotland: unravelling a paradox. *Marine and Freshwater Research*. Vol. 59, pp. 313–321

Stal, L.J., (2003). Microphytobenthos, their extracellular polymeric substances,and the morphogenesis of intertidal sediments. *Geomicrobiology Journal*. Vol. 20, pp. 463-478

Stewart, P.S. & J.W., Costerton. (2001). Antibiotic resistance of bacteria in biofilms. *The Lancet*. Vol. 358, pp. 135-138

Stickler, D.J. & J., Zimakoff. (1994). Complications of urinary tract infections associated with devices used for long-term bladder management. *Journal of Hospital Infections*. Vol. 28, pp. 177-194.

Stickler, D., N. Morris, M.-C. Moreno & N. Sabbuba. (1998). Studies on the formation of crystalline bacterial biofilms on urethral catheters. *Eur.J. Clin. Microbiol. Infect. Dis.* Vol. 17, pp. 649–652.

Suci, P.A., M.W., Mittelman, F.P., Yu & G.G., Geesey. (1994). Investigation of ciprofloxacin penetration into Pseudomonas aeruginosa biofilms. *Antimicrob Agents Chemother*. Vol. 38, pp. 2125-2133.

Sutherland, T. F., J., Grant & C.L., Amos. (1998).The effect of carbohydrate production by the diatom *Nitzschia curvilineata* on the erodibility of sediment. *Limnology and Oceanography*. Vol. 43, pp. 65–72

Ternes, T.A., M., Meisenheimer,D., McDowell, F., Sacher, H.J., Brauch, B.H., Gulde, G., Preuss, U., Wilme & N.Z., Seibert. (2002). Removal of pharmaceut icals during drinking water treatment. *Environmental Science and Technology*. Vol. 36, pp. 3855-3863

Underwood, G.J.C. & D.M., Paterson. (2003). The importance of extracellular carbohydrate production by marine epipelic diatoms. *Advances in Botanical Research*. Vol. 40, pp. 183-240.

Vesterlund, J., Paltta, M., Karp & A.C., Ouwehand. (2005). Measurement of bacterial adhesion -in vitro evaluation of different methods. *J. MicroBiol. Methods*. Vol. 60, pp. 225–233

Vives-Rego, J., P., Lebaron & G., Nebe-von Caron. (2000). Current and future applications of flow cytometry in aquatic microbiology. *FEMS Microbiology Reviews*. Vol. 24 pp. 429-448

Wagner, W. & A., Loy. (2002) Bacterial community composition and function in sewage treatment systems. *Current Opinion in Biotechnology*. Vol. 13, pp. 218–227

Wang, Z., L., Liu, J., Yeo & W., Cai. (2006). Effects of extracellular polymeric substances on aerobic granulation in sequencing batch reactors. Chemosphere. Vol. 63, pp. 1728-1735

Warren J.W. (1991). The catheter and urinary tract infection. *Medical Clinics of North America*. Vol. 75, pp. 481-493

Westrich, B. & U., Förstner. (2005). Sediment dynamics and pollutant mobility in rivers (SEDYMO). *J. Soils & Sediments*. Vol. 5, pp. 197-200

Whiteley, M., G., Bangera, R.E., Bumgarner, M.R., Parsek, G.M., Teitzel, S., Lory & E. P., Greenberg. (2001). Gene expression in *Pseudomonas aeruginosa* biofilms. *Nature*. Vol. 413, pp. 860-864

Williams, I., F., Paul, D., Lloyd, R., Jepras, I., Critchley, M., Newman, J., Warrack, T., Giokarini, A.J. Hayes , P.F., Randerson & W. A., Venables. (1999). Flow cytometry and other techniques show that Staphylococcus aureus undergoes significant physiological changes in the early stages of surface-attached culture. *Microbiology*. Vol. 145, pp. 1325-1333

Wolfaardt, G.M., J.R., Lawrence, R.D., Robarts & D.E., Caldwell (1988). In situ characterization of biofilm exopolymers involved in the accumulation of chlorinated organics. *Microbial Ecology*. Vol. 35, pp. 213–223.

Worlitzsch, D., R., Tarran, M., Ulrich, U., Schwab, A., Cekici, K.C., Meyer, P., Birrer, G., Bellon, J., Berger, T., Weiss, K., Botzenhart, J.R. Yankaskas, S., Randell, R.C., Boucher & G. Döring. (2002). Effects of reduced mucus oxygen concentration in airway *Pseudomonas* infections of cystic fibrosis patients. *J. Clin. Invest.* Vol. 109, pp. 317–325

Wood, P. & P., Armitage. (1999). Sediment deposition in a small lowland stream-management implications. *Regulated Rivers: Research & Management*. Vol. 15, pp. 199-210

Wu, H., Z., Song, M., Hentzer, J.B., Andersen, A., Heydorn, K., Mathee, C., Moser, L., Eberl, S., Molin, N., Hoiby & M., Givskov. (2000). Detection of N-acylhomoserine lactones in lung tissues of mice infected with Pseudomonas aeruginosa. *Microbiology*. Vol. 146, pp. 2481–2493

Wu, H., Song, M., Hentzer, J.B., Andersen, S., Molin, M., Givskov & N., Hoiby. (2004). Synthetic furanones inhibit quorum-sensing and enhance bacterial clearance in Pseudomonas aeruginosa lung infection in mice. *J. Antimicrob. Chemother.* Vol. 53, pp. 1054–1061

Xu WH, G., Zhang , X.D., Li, S.C., Zou, P., Li, Z.H., Hu & J., Li. (2007). Occurrence and elimination of antibiotics at four sewage treatment plants in the Pearl River Delta (PRD), South China. *Water Research.* Vol. 41, pp. 4526–4534

Yallop, M.L., D.M., Paterson & P., Wellsbury. (2000). Interrelationships between rates of microbial production, exopolymer production, microbial biomass, and sediment stability in biofilms of intertidal sediments. Microbial Ecology 39: 116-127

Yoon S.S., R.F., Hennigan, G.M., Hilliard, U.A., Ochsner, K., Parvatiyar, M.C., Kamani, H.L., Allen, T.R., DeKievit, P.R., Gardner, U., Schwab, J.J., Rowe, B.H., Iglewski, T.R., McDermott, R.P., Mason, D.J., Wozniak, R.E.W., Hancock, M.R., Parsek, T.L., Noah, R.C., Boucher & D.J., Hassett. (2002). Pseudomonas aeruginosa anaerobic respiration in biofilms: relationships to cystic fibrosis pathogenesis. *Developmental Cell.* Vol. 3, pp. 593–603

Zobell, C.E., (1943). The effect of solid surfaces upon bacterial activity. *J. Bacteriol.,* Vol. 46, pp. 39–56

11

Biocompatible Polyamides and Polyurethanes Containing Phospholipid Moiety

Yu Nagase and Kenji Horiguchi
Department of Applied Chemistry
Graduate School of Engineering, Tokai University
Japan

1. Introduction

The non-thrombogenic biomaterial has been received a great interest for the development of medical devices or implants in these few decades. When any medical device contacts with flowing blood or internal organs, the material surface of device should avoid the initiation of the process leading to a thrombosis. Such a biocompatible property of artificial biomaterials is a very important factor to use the materials for long-term implantable devices, extracorporeal circulation and intravenous catheters sensors. Although a lot of medical devices are used clinically, the universal non-thrombogenic material has not yet been developed and these devices have been limited to be used for long-term implantation.

On the other hand, phospholipids are the main components of cell membranes and act as interesting substances in biological and biomedical fields (Chapman, 1968; Gregoriadis & Allison, 1980; Hayward & Chapman, 1984). Several attempts have been made to translate the natural compatibility between blood and phospholipid membranes for the application of medical devices. The phosphorylcholine (PC) group is a polar component of phospholipid molecules, which covers the surface of cell membranes. It has been well known that synthetic polymer materials containing PC group exhibit biocompatibility including blood compatibility (Sugiyama *et al.*, 1995; Ohishi *et al.*, 1997; Gong *et al.*, 2005). Especially, the so-called MPC polymer, which is typically a copolymer of 2-methacryloyloxyethyl phosphorylcholine (MPC) with butyl methacrylate, has been reported as ideal non-thrombogenic and excellent biocompatible materials (Ishihara *et al.*, 1990a, 1990b, 1991; Ueda *et al.*, 1992). This polymer was designed based on the inspiration from the outer surface of the cell membrane, *i.e.* the biomembrane, which is mainly constructed of natural phospholipid molecules. In particular, the adhesion and the activation of platelets were completely suppressed on the surface of the MPC polymer, and the amount of plasma proteins adsorbed on the surface of MPC polymer film was clearly decreased. Since PC group consists of a zwitterion, MPC polymer behaves as an entire neutrality molecule and exhibited no interaction with specific ions in the living organism. Furthermore, the applications to medical devices and other uses have been greatly advanced in these years (Sawada *et al.*, 2006; Patel *et al.*, 2005; Iwasaki *et al.*, 1997; Uchiyama *et al.*, 2002; Ye *et al.*, 2006; Goda & Ishihara, 2006; Snyder *et al.*, 2007). Therefore, MPC polymers are useful polymeric biomaterials not only in the biomedical field but also in the tissue engineering and bioengineering fields.

However, most of MPC polymers do not possess the enough durability to several solvents such as alcohols, the thermal stability and the mechanical strength, which were derived from the polymethacrylate type main chain structure. Then, if these physical properties of MPC polymers improved satisfactorily while maintaining the excellent biocompatibility, novel biocompatible polymer materials could be developed. Recently, we have succeeded in synthesizing a novel diamine monomer containing PC moiety and preparing aromatic polyamides and poly(urethane-urea)s from the monomer (Nagase *et al.*, 2007, 2008; Horiguchi *et al.*, 2008). In addition, PC group was also introduced into ethyl cellulose by polymer reaction using carboxylic compound containing PC group (Tadokoro *et al.*, 2007). It was found that the obtained polymers exhibited the excellent biocompatibility derived from PC unit in addition to the processability, the durability to solvents, the thermal stability and the mechanical strength, which were derived from the main chain components.
In this chapter, the synthetic pathway of novel aromatic diamine monomers containing PC moiety will be described at first. Then, we will describe the preparations of high molecular weight aromatic polyamides and poly(urethane-urea)s containing PC group, which are obtained by polycondensation and polyaddition using these monomers. Furthermore, the physical properties such as solubility, thermal property, biological function as blood compatibility, and surface property of the obtained polyamides will be discussed to reveal the possibility of a durable biocompatible polymer material.

2. Diamine monomer containing phospholipid moiety

At first, our history of development of novel aromatic diamine compound will be described. The synthetic route of the diamine monomer containing PC group, 2-(3,5-diaminophenylcarbonyloxy)ethyl phosphorylcholine (DAPC), is shown in Scheme 1. The starting material, a dinitro compound (**1**), was prepared by the reaction of 3,5-dinitrobenzoyl chloride with excess amount of ethylene glycol in good yield. Then, the reaction of **1** with 2-chloro-2-oxo-1,3,2-dioxaphospholane (COP) yielded a phospholane compound (**2**), which was an intermediate of phosphorylcholine compound. The purification of **2** by a silica-gel column chromatography was difficult because it was easily hydrolyzed. However, the extraction of the crude products with chloroform followed by washing with distilled water gave the pure product of **2**. Next, DAPC was obtained by opening the cyclic phosphoric ester moiety of **2** with trimethylamine, followed by the reduction of the nitro groups of **3** with H_2 catalyzed by Pd. The chemical structure of DAPC was confirmed by IR and ^{1}H-NMR spectra. In the IR spectra of DAPC, a broad adsorption peak in the region of 3400-3150 cm^{-1} was observed as the amino groups, and the PC group was identified by the peak at 1228 and 1076 cm^{-1}. This aromatic diamine compound, DAPC, would be a useful monomer for the syntheses of various aromatic polymers, such as polyamides, polyimides, polyureas and poly(urethane-urea)s that have PC group in the side chain.
Next, the synthesis of copolyamide was carried out by the polycondensation of DAPC with isophthaloyl chloride and another diamine comonomer. As the comonomer, 4,4′-diamino-3,3′-dimethyldiphenylmethane was used to make the polymer soluble in some solvents. Namely, the aromatic copolyamides containing PC group could be successfully prepared from DAPC, whose composition of DAPC unit was 21 mol%. A homopolyamide without PC group was prepared from 4,4′-diamino-3,3′-dimethyldiphenylmethane and isophthaloyl chloride to compare the biocompatible properties with PC-containing copolyamide.

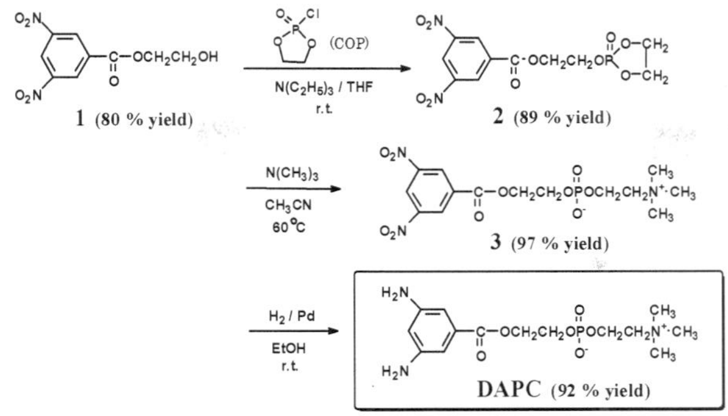

Scheme 1. Synthesis of diamine monomer containing PC moiety (DAPC).

The thin films of these polyamides were prepared by coating of the NMP solutions of the polymers on poly(ethylene terephthalate) (PET) plates, and the blood compatibility of the coating films was evaluated by contacting the coated plates with a human blood. Fig. 1 shows SEM pictures of the two film surfaces of PC-containing copolyamide and homopolyamide without PC unit after contact with human platelet-rich plasma (PRP) for 60 min. The numerous adherent platelets on the homopolyamide surface were observed as large aggregates. In contrast, the platelets were significantly suppressed on the copolyamide film surfaces as shown in Fig. 1(a). These results clearly indicated that PC-containing copolyamide exhibited the excellent blood compatibility and PC unit in the copolyamide was an important element to develop the blood compatibility. Furthermore, the composition of the PC unit was a dominant factor in the reduction of the platelet adhesion (Nagase *et al.*, 2007). These results would be due to the PC unit located at the surface of the polymer film, where the surface is covered with PC unit, and the interaction between the polymer surface and blood ingredients such as cells and platelets is very weak.

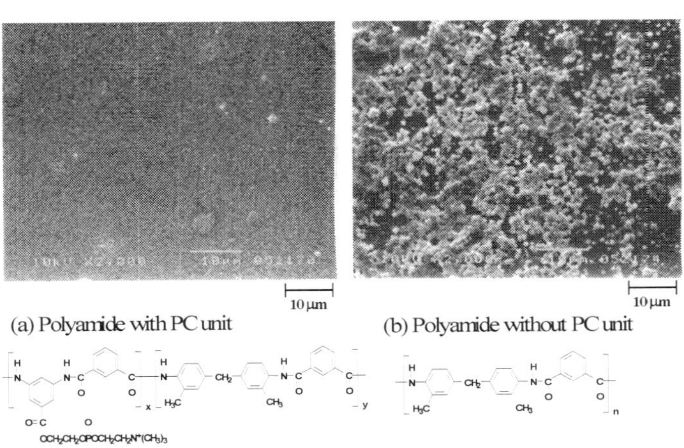

Fig. 1. SEM pictures of polyamide film surfaces with and without PC unit after contact with human PRP for 60 min at 37°C. (x 2,000)

However, the molecular weight and the PC content of copolyamides from DAPC were not enough to produce a self-standing film and to exhibit the higher biocompatibility, respectively, which would be due to the low reactivity and also the highly hygroscopic property of DAPC. Thus, we have projected a new structure of high molecular weight polymer in order to create the practical biomaterials for several applications, which exhibit the excellent biocompatibility in addition to the processability, the durability to solvents, the thermal stability and the mechanical strength. For this purpose, we designed a new diamine monomer containing PC group, 2-[3,5-bis(4-aminophenoxy)phenylcarbonyloxy]ethyl phosphorylcholine (BAPPC in Scheme 2), to solve these problems of DAPC. BAPPC is expected to show the higher reactivity in the polymerization than DAPC, which would be due to the relatively higher reactive amino groups on *p*-position of phenoxy groups.
The synthetic route of the new PC-containing diamine monomer is outlined in Scheme 2. Two kinds of monomers were prepared, which have the different spacer structures between 3,5-bis(4-aminophenoxy)phenyl and PC groups. If the longer and flexible spacer could be introduced into the monomer structure, it is expected that the PC group in the polymer would be easily oriented on the surface because of the mobility of flexible spacer. Then, two compounds, **6a** and **6b**, were prepared as intermediates, which were obtained by the esterification of **5** with ethylene glycol and tri(ethylene glycol), respectively. From **6a** and **6b**, the two diamine monomers, BAPPC-1 and 2, were prepared according to the same pathway as the preparation of DAPC in Scheme 1. Although the several reaction steps are necessary to prepare these monomers, all of the reaction steps proceeded smoothly in high yields. This novel diamine monomers, BAPPC-1 and 2, would be useful for the synthesis of various aromatic polymers which has PC group in the side chain.

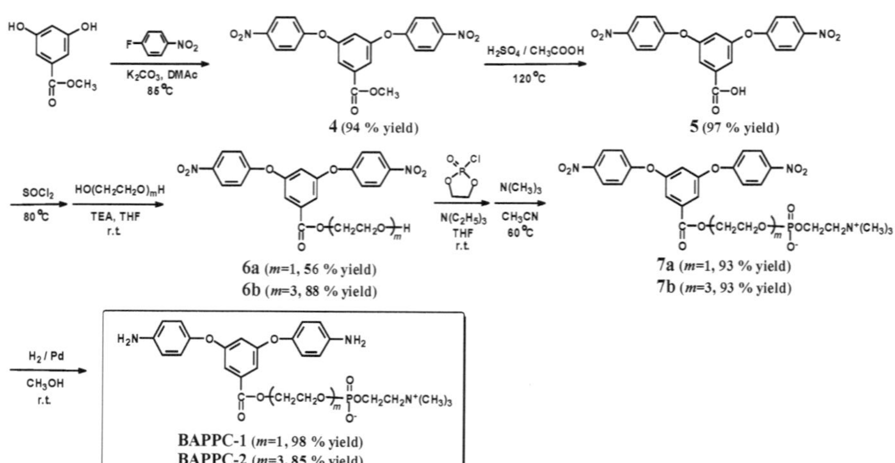

Scheme 2. Synthesis of diamine monomers containing PC moiety (BAPPC).

3. Aromatic polyamides containing phospholipid moiety

In general, the aromatic polyamides are insoluble in many solvents, thermally stable up to 300℃ and mechanically tough materials, which are used in a lot of electric devices and motorcars. Therefore, we attempted to prepare aromatic polyamides containing PC group in the side chain by using the PC-containing diamine monomers, which would lead to new biocompatible polyamides derived from the characteristics of phospholipid moiety.

3.1 Preparation

The preparations of copolyamides were carried out by the polycondensations of BAPPC-1 or 2 with isophthaloyl chloride and another diamine comonomer, as shown in Scheme 3. As the comonomer, 2,2-Bis[4-(amino-phenyloxy)phenyl]propane (BAP) was used to make the polymer soluble in some solvents. On the other hand, a polyamide without PC group (PA) was prepared from BAP and isophthaloyl chloride to compare the physical property with PC-containing copolyamides. Table 1 summarizes the results of polymerizations. Eight kinds of copolyamides with different spacer structures and contents of PC unit were prepared by changing the ratio of monomers in the feed of polymerization. The obtained copolyamides had the number-average molecular weights (*Mn*) more than 10^5., while the *Mn* of polyamides prepared from DAPC in Scheme 1 was in the order of 10^3 - 10^4. Therefore, it is suggested that this novel diamine monomer containing PC group has high reactivity in the polymerization, and would be useful for the preparations of other high molecular weight polymers such as polyimide and polyurea containing PC group.

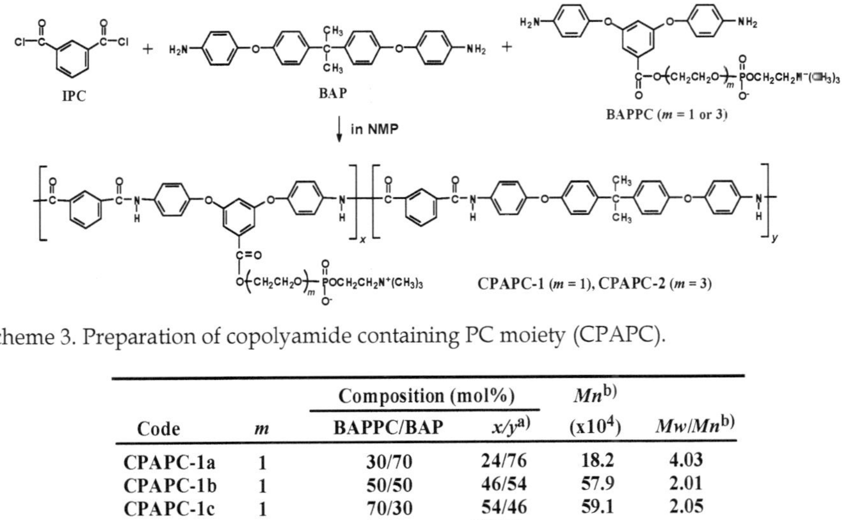

Scheme 3. Preparation of copolyamide containing PC moiety (CPAPC).

Code	*m*	Composition (mol%) BAPPC/BAP	*x/y*[a)]	*Mn*[b)] (x10^4)	*Mw/Mn*[b)]
CPAPC-1a	1	30/70	24/76	18.2	4.03
CPAPC-1b	1	50/50	46/54	57.9	2.01
CPAPC-1c	1	70/30	54/46	59.1	2.05
CPAPC-1d	1	100/ 0	100/ 0	--	--
CPAPC-2a	3	30/70	28/72	11.3	3.21
CPAPC-2b	3	50/50	45/55	22.8	3.14
CPAPC-2c	3	70/30	57/43	24.9	3.31
CPAPC-2d	3	100/ 0	100/ 0	36.0	2.06
PA	--	0/100	0/100	49.0	2.34

a) The copolymer composition, *x/y*, was determined by ^{1}H-NMR.
b) Number-average and weight-average molecular weights (*Mn* and *Mw*) were estimated by gel permeation chromatgraphy using DMF as eluent.

Table 1. Results of polycondensations.

These copolyamides were soluble in aprotic polar solvents, such as dimethylformamide (DMF), dimethylsulfoxide (DMSO) and *N*-methyl-2-pyrrolidinone (NMP), at room temperature, whereas they were insoluble in water, methanol, ethanol, acetone and other ordinary organic solvents. This solubility in specific solvents is advantageous in the processing for medical devices, and the insolubility in other solvents enables the material durable. On the other hand, PC-containing homopolyamides, CPAPC-1d and CPAPC-2d in Table 1, exhibited the less solubility than the copolyamides. For example, CPAPC-1d was insoluble in DMF, therefore, the gel permeation chromatography to determine the molecular weight could not be measured. It is considered that such homopolyamides with high content of PC unit has a strong molecular interaction between polar PC group and amide bond or other PC group to make the polymer insoluble in solvents. Therefore, the copolymerization of BAPPC with other diamine monomer would be effective to obtain soluble and processable polymer material.

3.2 Biocompatibility

The blood compatibility of the copolyamide was evaluated by contacting the copolyamide films with human blood. Circular pieces of PET plates (diameter: 14 mm, thickness: 0.2 mm) were dipped in polymer solutions in NMP for 30 min, and the obtained polymer-coated PET plates were dried. Then, the homogeneous coating films on PET plates were prepared from CPAPC-2 series and other polymers. The polymer-coated PET plates were contacted with phosphate-buffered solution (PBS, pH=7.4) at r.t. for overnight to equilibrate the surface, then human whole blood or PRP was poured onto the plates and incubated for 60 min at 37°C. After the incubation, whole blood and platelet-rich plasma (PRP) were removed with an aspirator, and the plates were rinsed three times with PBS, and then 0.7 ml of 2.5 vol.% glutaraldehyde in PBS was poured onto each plate, and the materials were maintained at room temperature for 2 h in order to fix the blood components on the plates. After the fixation, it had been rinsed five times with distilled water, and then the plate was freeze-dried. The surfaces of the polymer-coated plates were observed with a scanning electron microscope (SEM), and the number of adhered platelets was estimated by the procedure written in our literature (Nagase *et al.*, 2007).

Fig. 2 shows the SEM pictures of PA and CPAPC-2c and 2d film surfaces after contact with PRP. As seen in this figure, it was clarified that the large aggregates of the human platelets occurred on polyamide (PA) film, where a lot of adhered platelets were observed. On the contrary, PC-containing copolyamide films resisted the adhesion of platelets.

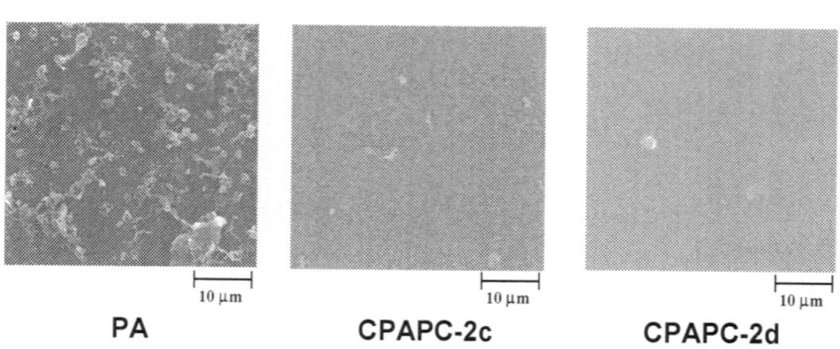

Fig. 2. SEM pictures of polyamide film surfaces with and without PC unit after contact with human PRP. (x 2,000)

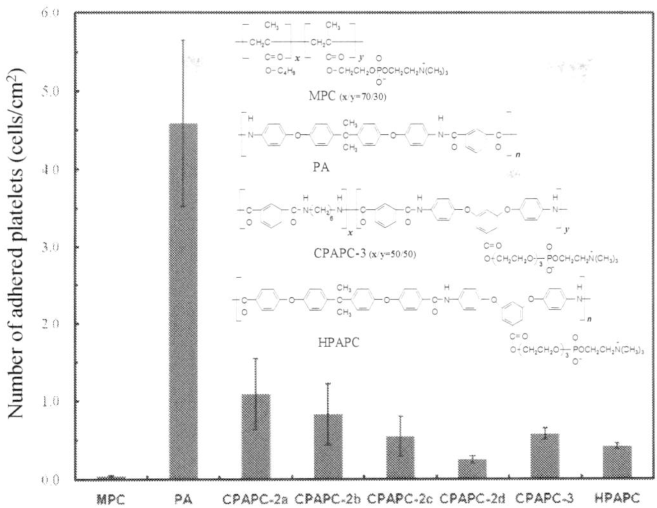

Fig. 3. Number of adhered platelets on the polymer films after contact with human PRP for 1 h.

The quantitative analysis of adhered platelets of each polymer film was also carried out to reveal the strict difference of thrombogenic property of these polymer films. Fig. 3 represents the difference of the number of platelets that adhered on each coated film. In this figure, the data of MPC polymer and other kinds of PC-containing polyamides, CPAPC-3 and HPAPC, are included to compare with PA and CPAPC-2 series. CPAPC-3 is a similar copolymer to CPAPC-2 series, the comonomer of which is 1,6-diaminohexane instead of BAP. HPAPC is a homopolyamide obtained from the polycondensation of BAPPC-2 with 4,4'-(4-carboxylphenoxy)-2,2-diphenylpropane, which has a good solubility in aprotic polar solvents. MPC polymer coated film has been also evaluated, because it is a good reference as the very high biocompatible material.

As shown in Fig. 3, it was obvious that PC-containing polyamides efficiently reduced the adhered platelets than polyamide without PC group (PA), where the number of adhered platelets of these polyamides was reduced in nearly one-tenth amount as compared with that of PA. These results indicate that the PC unit plays an important role for the blood compatibility of the polymers. Furthermore, the amount of adhered platelets decreased as the increase of the content of PC unit in CPAPC-2 series, therefore, the composition of the PC unit was a dominant factor in the reduction of the blood cell and platelet adhesion. For example, the amount of adhered platelets of CPAPC-2a (PC content: 28 mol%) was ten times larger than that of CPAPC-2d (PC content: 100 mol%). The similar tendency was observed for CPAPC-1 series (Horiguchi *et al.*, 2008). Therefore, the difference of the spacer structure of these copolyamides would not affect the biocompatibility. On the other hand, MPC polymer exhibited the extremely high nonthrombogenicity among the polymers evaluated in Fig. 3. Consequently, the improvement of nonthrombogenicity by introducing PC unit in such polyamide system would be limited, although the phospholipid moiety is effective to considerable extent for the reduction of the platelet and protein adhesion.

3.3 Physical property

The thermal property of PC-containing polyamides was evaluated by differential scanning calorimetry (DSC) and thermogravimetric analysis (TGA). The glass transition temperature (T_g) and the melting temperature (T_m) were not observed for CPAPC-1 and 2 series in the range between -100°C and 250°C of DSC thermograms, which suggested that these polyamides were glassy polymers. In general, aromatic polyamides are known to exhibit a crystalline state, however, bulky PC group in the side chain would prevent the crystallization of polyamide backbone.

Fig. 4 shows the TGA curves of PA and CPAPC-1b and 2b under N_2 flow. As seen in this figure, the thermal degradation of homopolyamide, PA, started at about 400°C, but the PC-containing copolyamides degraded at about 250°C. This would be due to the thermal degradation of polymer side chain, which consisted of the PC or spacer moiety. In nitrogen atmosphere, the aromatic backbone would be carbonized, which resulted in the residue more than 30 % at 1000°C. In the case of the copolyamides, the phosphate moiety would be incombustible, where the residue was a little higher, nearly 50 %. Anyhow, the heat resistance of these PC-containing polyamides until 250°C is enough to use for biomaterial devices, for example, for the thermal sterilization process over 150°C.

The very tough films could be obtained from PC-containing copolyamides by solvent casting method. Then, the mechanical properties of these copolyamides and MPC polymer films were quite different, where Young's moduli of the copolyamides, PA and MPC polymer films were 200-400, 642 and 15.2 MPa, respectively. Therefore, the physical properties of PC-containing copolyamides obviously depended on the aromatic polyamide backbone. Consequently, it is expected that the aromatic copolyamides containing PC group will be useful polymeric biomaterials to develop a new generation of biomedical devices, because of the durability to solvents, the high thermal stability and mechanical strength in addition to the good biocompatibility.

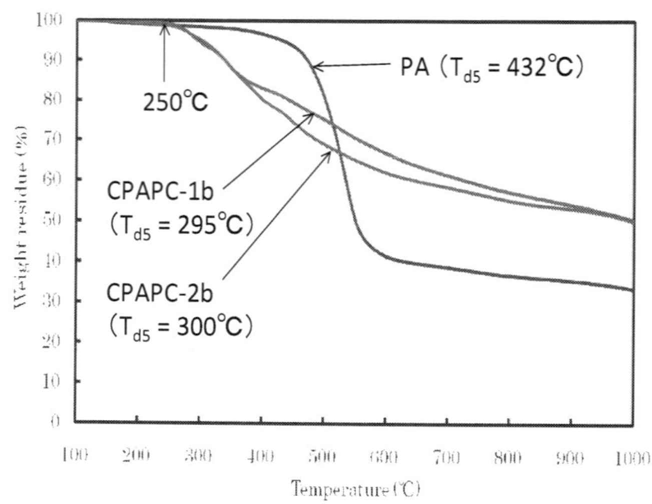

Fig. 4. TGA curves of polyamides at heating rate of 10°C/min in N_2 flow.

4. Segmented poly(urethane-urea) containing phospholipid moiety

Segmented polyurethanes have been widely used in the practical medical devices as elastomers (Lelah, 1986; Eisenbach, 1996) because of their suitable mechanical properties and biocompatibility, which consisted of short alternating blocks of soft and hard segments. The soft segment is typically a low glass transition temperature (*Tg*) polyether, polyester or polycarbonate, the molecular weights of which are 400-2000. The hard segment is usually a high *Tg* component, such as semicrystalline aromatic diisocyanate linked with a low molecular weight chain extender. The biocompatibility of segmented polyurethane is thought to be derived from the micro phase separation of soft and hard segments. However, the blood compatibility of segmented polyurethane is not enough to be applied for long-term implantation. It has been suggested that the biodegradation and cracking of polyurethane occurred *in vivo* due to the adsorption of proteins, the adhesion of macrophages and the peroxide formation (Zao *et al.*, 1991, 1993; Wu *et al.*, 1991), which resulted in the reduction of the mechanical strength of SPU. Moreover, it was reported that the soft segment of segmented polyurethane was degraded by the oxygen radicals produced from adherent macrophages (Stokes *et al.*, 1995). Therefore, several studies of the surface or chemical modification of segmented polyurethanes have been conducted to improve the blood compatibility through reducing the adhesion of cells and proteins (Kang *et al.*, 1997; Flemming *et al.*, 1999; Mathur *et al.*, 1997; Roh *et al.*, 1999; Lee *et al.*, 2000). The composite material of segmented polyurethane and MPC polymer has been also reported, which showed the high biocompatibility and the elasticity (Ishihara *et al.*, 2000).
In our study, as another approach to improve the biocompatibility of segmented polyurethane which has been widely used as a biomedical material, we attempted to prepare segmented poly(urethane-urea) containing PC group by using the PC-containing diamine monomer as a coupling reagent in the polyaddition of diols with diisocyanate, which was expected as new biocompatible polymers by combining the characteristics of segmented polyurethane and phospholipid moiety.

4.1 Preparation

As shown in Scheme 3, segmented polyurethane was first prepared by polyaddition of 4,4'-diphenylmethane diisocyanate (MDI) with 1,4-butanediol (BD) in NMP, followed by the addition of hydroxyl-terminated poly(tetramethylene glycol) (PTMG) as the soft segment.

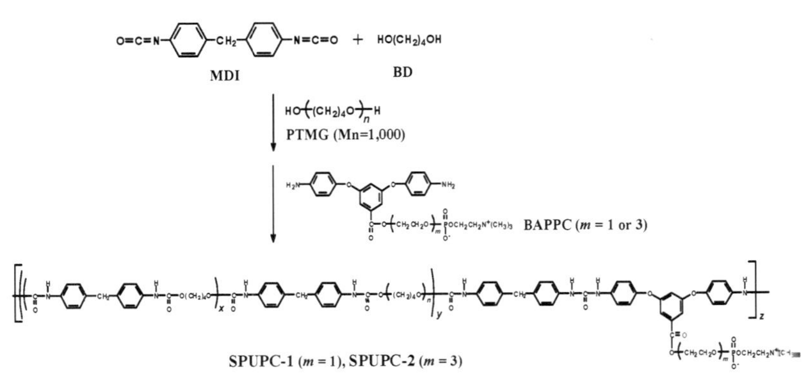

Scheme 3. Preparation of segmented poly(urethane-urea) containing PC moiety (SPUPC).

Next, in the polymerization vessel, PC-containing diamine monomer, BAPPC-1 or 2, was added to couple the polyurethane to obtain segmented poly(urethane-urea)s containing PC unit (SPUPC-1 and 2). These polymerization reactions proceeded smoothly without catalyst. By the way, dibutyltin dilaurate was necessary as a catalyst for the preparation of the similar segmented poly(urethane-urea) using DAPC in Scheme 1 (Nagase, *et al.*, 2008).
Table 2 summarizes the results of polymerizations. A few poly(urethane-urea)s with different contents of PC unit were prepared by changing the amount of BD, PTMG and BAPPC-1 or 2 in the polyaddition. The chemical structures of these polymers were confirmed by their ^{1}H-NMR and IR spectra. The compositions of PC unit in these copolymers were determined from the ratio of the peak intensities of the ammonium protons (3.10 - 3.15 ppm) of PC unit and methylene proton (3.78 - 3.80 ppm) of *p,p'*-diphenylmethane unit, which existed in every monomer components. In the gel permeation chromatography, bimodal peaks were observed in most of these copolymers. Thus, each two values were listed in Table 2 as the number-average molecular weights (*Mn*) of the obtained copolymers, which were in the range of 10^4 and 10^6. Probably, the higher molecular weight segments over 10^6 would be partly produced in the final coupling reaction with BAPPC-1 or 2. Anyhow, very high molecular weight poly(urethane-urea)s containing phospholipid moiety have been successfully prepared by polyaddition with PC-containing diamine monomers.

Code	*m*	BD/PTMG/BAPPC[a)]	PC content (mol%)	PC content (wt.%)	*Mn*[b)] ($\times 10^4$)	*Mw*/*Mn*[b)]
SPUUPC-1a	1	50 / 33 / 17	14	2.5	1.86	1.88
SPUUPC-1b	1	33 / 34 / 33	27	9.1	7.47, 254	1.85, 1.03
SPUUPC-1c	1	17 / 33 / 50	47	22	1.35, 99.0	1.78, 1.87
SPUUPC-2a	3	50 / 33 / 17	15	6.3	2.19, 210	1.74, 1.15
SPUUPC-2b	3	33 / 34 / 33	28	13	2.01, 120	1.51, 1.57
SPUUPC-2c	3	17 / 33 / 50	49	25	2.19, 111	1.82, 1.47
SPU	--	67 / 33 / 0	0	0	2.62	1.46

a) The molar ratio of monomers in the polyaddition.
b) Number-average and weight-average molecular weights (*Mn* and *Mw*) were estimated by gel permeation chromatgraphy using DMF as eluent.

Table 2. Results of polyadditions.

The obtained poly(urethane-urea)s exhibited a good solubility in aprotic polar solvents such as NMP, DMF and DMSO at room temperature, whereas it was insoluble in methanol, ethanol, acetone, chloroform and water. Such solubility in the specific solvents is advantageous in the processing for medical devices, and the insolubility in other solvents enables the material durable to these solvents. Actually, flexible and self-standing films could be prepared from these copolymers by a solvent casting method.

4.2 Biocompatibility

The blood compatibility of the poly(urethane-urea) films was evaluated by the similar procedure described in Section 3.2. For this experiment, the self-standing films prepared from each copolymer were used, not coating film. Fig. 5 shows the number of platelets adhered on the polymer films after contact with PRP for 1 h. It was found that the platelet adhesion was suppressed to a certain extent even on SPU film without PC unit, where the amount of adhered platelets was quite different from the values of polyamide (PA) shown in Fig. 3. Therefore, segmented polyurethane would have the higher non-thrombogenic efficiency than aromatic polyamide and other normal polymer materials. Furthermore, PC-containing poly(urethane-urea)s, SPUPC-2b and SPUPC-2c, efficiently reduced the platelet adhesion rather than SPU, and the number of adhered platelets of these copolymer films were almost same as that of MPC polymer film. Furthermore, the composition of PC unit was a dominant factor in the reduction of the blood cell and platelet adhesion, which was revealed from the result that the number of adhered platelets was much decreased on SPUPC-2c film rather than SPUPC-2a and SPUPC-2b films. Thus, the PC content of 25 wt.% in SPUPC-2c would be necessary to sufficiently reduce the platelet adhesion on the polymer surfaces, which would be an enough content of the PC unit located at the surface of the polymer film. The surface chemical structure of SPUPC-2c film was analyzed by X-ray photoelectron spectroscopy (XPS). The XPS signals was observed at 133, 398 and 402 eV in P_{2p} and N_{1s} regions, which were attributed to the phosphorus of the phosphate group, the nitrogen atoms in the urethane or urea bond (-NH-) and the ammonium group ($-N^{+}(CH_3)_3$), respectively. Then, PC group was clearly observed on the SPUPC-2c film surface. However, these peaks were not so clear on the surfaces of SPUPC-2a and 2b films. Therefore, in this poly(urethane-urea) system, PC content should be over *ca.* 25 wt.% to make the PC group clearly appear on the surface of polymer film. In addition, it was found from the surface analysis, that the PC group was easily rearranged by the immersion in water.

Moreover, such PC-containing poly(urethane-urea), SPUPC series, has the higher biocompatibility than PC-containing polyamide, CPAPC series, which would be due to the additive effect of PC unit to the potential biocompatibility of segmented polyurethane.

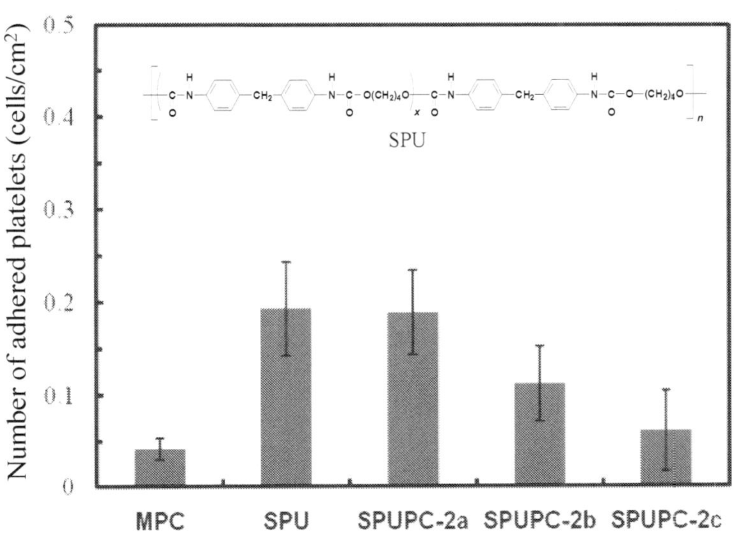

Fig. 5. Amount of adhered platelets on segmented polyurethane, poly(urethane-urea) and MPC polymer films after contact with human PRP for 1 h.

4.3 Mechanical property

From the results of DSC and TGA measurements, PC-containing poly(urethane-urea)s were glassy polymers, *Tg* of which was not observed in the range of -50°C - 250°C, and the thermal degradation temperature was confirmed at around 250°C. This is a similar thermal behavior as PC-containing polyamides. The characteristic property of such a polyurethane material is a mechanical strength and elasticity. Then, the stress-strain behaviors of PC-containing poly(urethane-urea) films were evaluated in order to reveal the effect of introduction of PC unit on the mechanical property of polyurethane backbone.

Fig. 6 shows the stress-strain behaviors of SPUPC-2a, 2b and 2c films, and the Young's modulus, the tensile strength and the elongation to break were summarized in the table as compared with those of SPU. The similar tendency of stress-strain curve was observed in SPU film, although the Young's moduli and elongations were different. Therefore, there was almost no change in such elastic stress-strain behaviors between SPU and SPUPC series. Young's moduli of SPUPC series increased with the increase of PC unit, as listed in the table of Fig. 6. It would be due to the increase of urea bond, which would enhance the molecular interaction in the hard segments rather than urethane bond. Consequently, the physical properties of these poly(urethane-urea)s obviously depended on the elastic segmented polyurethane backbone.

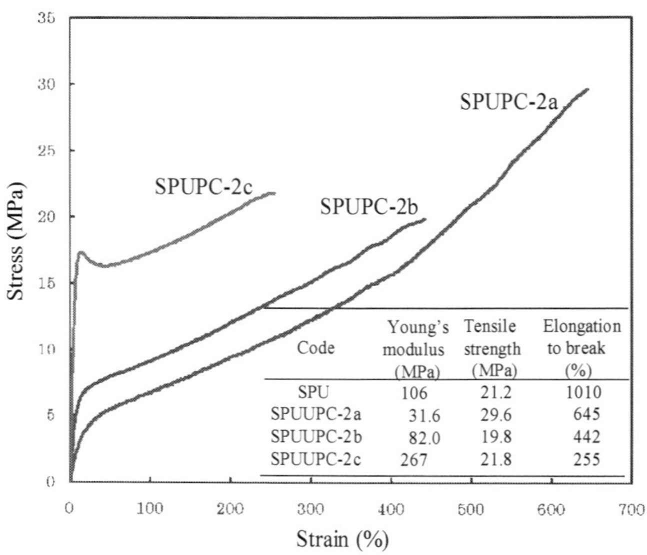

Code	Young's modulus (MPa)	Tensile strength (MPa)	Elongation to break (%)
SPU	106	21.2	1010
SPUUPC-2a	31.6	29.6	645
SPUUPC-2b	82.0	19.8	442
SPUUPC-2c	267	21.8	255

Fig. 6. Stress-strain behaviors of SPUPC films.

Taking such mechanical property into account, we have attempted to prepare the elastic tube from these polyurethane materials. A stainless steel stick (4 mmϕ) was dipped in 5 wt.% SPUPC-2c solution in NMP and dried at 70°C. This procedure was repeated six times, and the copolymer was coated on the stainless steel stick. Then, the coated stick was coated again with poly(carbonate urethane) (Bionate® 80A, Asahi Chemical Co.) by the same procedure. After dried, the stainless steel was pulled out carefully to obtain the flexible tube consisted of the composite polyurethanes. The picture of the obtained tube is shown in Fig.

7(a). Fig. 7(b) represents a cross section of the tube by the observation of SEM. In addition, the both side surfaces of the tube were analyzed by XPS, as shown in Fig. 7(c). The phosphorus of PC group was clearly observed inside of the tube at 133 eV, and the outside was confirmed to be coated by poly(carbonate urethane) without PC unit. Therefore, SPUPC-2c/poly(carbonate urethane) composite tube could be successfully prepared.

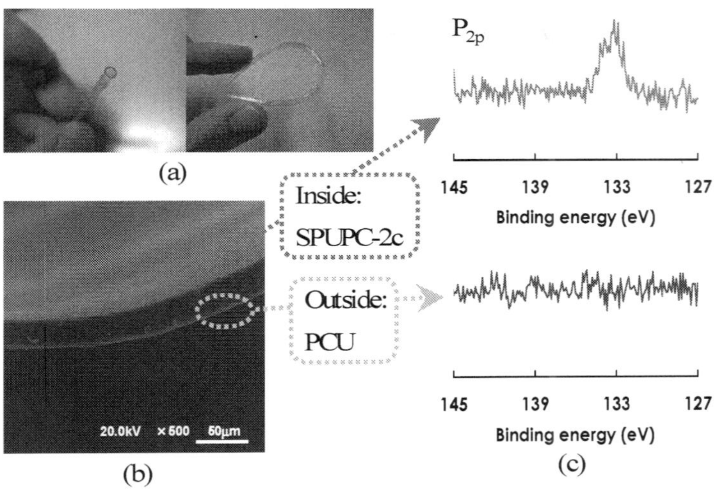

Fig. 7. Polyurethane composite tube made from SPUPC-2c and poly(carbonate urethane) (PCU). (a) Pictures of the tube. (b) SEM picture of the cross section of the tube. (c) XPS spectra of inside and outside of the tube.

The obtained tube has an elastic property derived from segmented polyurethane, and it is expected as artificial blood tube or catheter. The evaluations of this material for implant applications will be carried out in the future, although biomedical researchers are necessary as co-workers for the experiments.

5. Conclusion

This chapter covered the subject of our recent study to develop new biomaterials containing a phospholipid moiety. A novel aromatic diamine monomer containing PC group could be synthesized to prepare polycondensation or polyaddition type polymers. The PC-containing aromatic copolyamides and segmented poly(urethane-urea)s were successfully prepared from the monomer compound. Regarding the effect of PC group on the blood compatibility, the introduction of such a polar group of phospholipid was effective to appear the blood compatibility even in the aromatic copolyamides and segmented poly(urethane-urea)s. It is expected that these copolymers containing PC group will be useful polymeric biomaterials to develop a new generation of biomedical devices, because of the different solubility, the higher thermal stability and the similar biocompatibility as compared to MPC polymer. In addition, aromatic polyamides are hard materials, while segmented poly(urethane-urea)s are soft and elastic materials owing to the nature of main chain components. Therefore, we can add the several mechanical properties on PC-containing polymers according to any demands of medical applications. For example, the hard material is useful for artificial bone or joint, and the soft and elastic material will be used for artificial blood tube or catheter.

It has been also revealed that the biocompatibility is improved satisfactorily as the increase of PC content in the copolymer. However, in the case of these polycondensation or polyaddition type polymers, it is a problem that the solubility in organic solvents becomes poor as the PC content increases. It would be due to the high molecular interaction between side chain PC group and polar group in main chain, such as amide or urea bond. Furthermore, in the case of poly(urethane-urea) system, the increase of urea unit containing PC moiety let the polymer lose the elasticity owing to the aggregation between urea bonds.

To solve these problems, we have designed a new diol monomer containing PC moiety, which will be able to yield PC-containing polyurethanes or polyesters. By using the diol monomer, polyurethanes or polyesters with high content of PC unit will be developed, which is now in progress.

6. Acknowledgements

We express our sincere gratitude to Professor Kazuhiko Ishihara and Professor Yasuhiko Iwasaki, who belong to School of Engineering, the University of Tokyo, and Faculty of Chemistry, Materials and Bioengineering, Kansai University, respectively, for their scientific and technical supports. The authors also thank to Professor Takashi Asaka, Department of Applied Chemistry, Tokai University, for his help to conduct the stress-strain measurement. This work was partially supported by a Grant-in-Aid for Scientific Research from the Ministry of Education, Culture, Sports, Science and Technology, Japan (No. 15550110).

7. References

Chapman, D. (Ed.). (September 1968). *Biomedical Membranes,* Academic Press, ISBN-10: 0121685403, London

Eisenbach, C. D., Fischer, K., Hayen, H., Nefzger, H., Ribbe, A. and Stadler E. (1996), *Polymeric Materials Encyclopedia,* CRC Press, Boca Raton, Vol. 9, pp. 6957-6968

Flemming, R. G., Proctor, R. A. & Cooper, S. L. (1999). Bacterial adhesion to functionalized polyurethanes, *Journal of Biomaterials Science, Polymer Edition,* Vol. 10, No. 6, (June 1999), pp. 679-697, ISSN 1568-5624

Goda, T. & Ishihara, K. (2006). Novel Soft Contact Lens Biomaterials by Bioinspired Phospholipid Polymers, *Expert Review of Medical Devices,* Vol. 3, No. 2, (March 2006), pp. 167-174, ISSN 1743-4440

Gong, Y. K., Luo, L., Petit, A., Zukor, D. J., Huk, O. L., Antoniou, J., Winnik, F. M. & Mwale, F. (2005). Adhesion of human U937 macrophages to phosphorylcholine-coated surfaces, *Journal of Biomedical Materials Research,* Vol. 72A, No. 1, (January 2005), pp. 1-9, ISSN 1549-3296

Gregoriadis, G. & Allison, A. G. (Eds.). (April 1980). *Liposomes in Biological Systems,* Wiley, ISBN-10: 0471276081, New York

Hayward, J. A. & Chapman, D. (1984). Biomembrane surfaces as models for polymer design: the potential for haemocompatibility, *Biomaterials,* Vol. 5, No. 3, (May 1984), pp. 122-134, ISSN 0142-9612

Horiguchi K.; Shimoyamada N.; Nagawa D.; Nagase, Y.; Iwasaki, Y. & Ishihara, K. (2008). Syntheses of a novel diamine monomer and aromatic polyamides containing phosphorylcholine group. *Transactions of the Material Research Society of Japan.* Vol. 33, No. 4, (December 2008), pp. 1261-1264. ISSN 1382-3469

Ishihara, K.; Ueda, T. & Nakabayashi, N. (1990a). Preparation of phosphlipid polymers and their properties as polymer hydrogel membranes. *Polymer Journal,* Vol. 22, No. 5, (May 1990), pp. 355-360. ISSN 0032-3896

Ishihara, K., Aragaki, R., Ueda, T., Watanabe, A. & Nakabayashi, N. (1990b). Reduced thrombogenicity of polymers having phospholipid polar groups, *Journal of Biomedical Materials Research,* Vol. 24, No. 8, (August 1990), pp. 1069-1077, ISSN 0021-9304

Ishihara, K., Ziats, N. P., Tierney, B. P., Nakabayashi, N., Anderson, J. M. (1991). Protein adsorption from human plasma is reduced on phospholipid polymers, *Journal of Biomedical Materials Research,* Vol. 25, No. 11, (November 1991), pp. 1397-1407, ISSN 0021-9304

Ishihara, K. & Iwasaki, Y. (2000). Biocompatible elastomers composed of segmented polyurethane and 2-methacryloyloxyethyl phosphorilcholine polymer. *Polymers for Acvanced Technologies,,* Vol. 11, No. 8-12, (August-December 2000), pp. 626-634. ISSN 1042-7147

Iwasaki, Y., Mikami, A., Kurita, K. Yui, N., Ishihara, K. & Nakabayashi, N. (1997). "Reduction of surface-induced platelet activation on phospholipid polymer", *Journal of Biomedical Materials Research,* Vol. 36, No. 4 (December 1997), pp. 508-515, ISSN 0021-9304

Kang, I. K., Kwon, O. H., Kim, M. K., Lee, Y. M. & Sung, Y. K. (1997). *In vitro* blood compatibility of functional group-grafted and heparin-immobilized polyurethanes prepared by plasma glow discharge, *Biomaterials,* Vo. 18, No. 16, (August 1997), pp. 1099-1107, ISSN 0142-9612

Lee, J. H., Ju, Y. M. & Kim, D. M. (2000). Platelet adhesion onto segmented polyurethane film surfaces modified by addition and crosslinking of PEO-containing block copolymers, *Biomaterials,* Vol. 21, No. 7, (April 2000), pp. 683-691, ISSN 0142-9612

Lelah, M. D. & Cooper, S. L. (1986). *Polyurethanes in Medicine,* CRC Press, ISBN-10:0849363071, Boca Raton

Mathur, A. B., Collier, T. O., Kao, W. J., Wiggins, M., Schubert, M. A., Hiltner, A. & Anderson, J. M. (1997). *In vivo* biocompatibility and biostability of modified polyurethanes, *Journal of Biomedical Materials Research,* Vol. 36, No. 2, (August 1997), pp. 246-257, ISSN 0021-9304

Nagase, Y.; Oku, M.; Iwasaki, Y. & Ishihara, K. (2007). Preparations of aromatic diamine monomers and copolyamides containing phosphorylcholine moiety and the biocompatibility of copolyamides. *Polymer Journal,* Vol. 39, No. 7, (July 2007), pp. 712-721. ISSN 0032-3896

Nagase, Y.; Nakajima, S.; Oku, M.; Iwasaki, Y. & Ishihara, K. (2008). Synthesis and properties of segmented poly(urethane-urea)s containing phosphorylcholine moiety in the side-chain. *Polymer Journal,* Vol. 40, No. 12, (December 2008), pp. 1149 - 1156. ISSN 0032-3896

Ohishi, T., Fukuda, T., Uchiyama, H., Kondou, F., Ohe, H. & Tsutsumi, H. (1997). Synthesis and properties of poly(fumaramate) bearing a phosphorylcholine moiety, *Polymer,* Vol. 38, No. 12 (June 1997), pp. 3109-3115, ISSN 0032-3861

Patel, J., Iwasaki, Y., Ishihara, K. & Anderson, J. (2005). Phospholipid polymer surfaces reduce bacteria and leukocyte adhesion under dynamic flow conditions, *Journal of Biomedical Materials Research,* Vol. 73A, No. 3 (June 2005), pp. 359-366, ISSN 1549-3296

Roh, H. W., Song, M. J., Han, D. K., Lee, D. S., Ahn, J. H. & Kim, S. C. (1999). Effect of cross-link density and hydrophilicity of PU on blood compatibility of hydrophobic PS/hydrophilic PU IPNs, *Journal of Biomaterials Science, Polymer Edition*, Vol. 10, No. 1, (January 1999), 123-143, ISSN 1568-5624

Sawada, S., Iwasaki, Y., Nakabayashi, N. & Ishihara, K. (2006). Stress response of adherent cells on a polymer blend surface composed of a segmented polyurethane and MPC copolymers, *Journal of Biomedical Materials Research,* Vol. 79A, No. 3 (December 2006), pp. 476-484, ISSN 1549-3296

Snyder, T. A., Tsukui, H. Kihara, S., Akimoto, T., Litwak, K. N, Kameneva, M. V., Yamazaki, K. & Wagner, W. R. (2007). Preclinical biocompatibility assessment of the EVAHEART ventricular assist device: Coating comparison and platelet activation, *Journal of Biomedical Materials Research,* Vol. 81A, No. 1 (April 2007), pp. 85-92, ISSN 1549-3296

Stokes, K., McVenes, R. & Anderson, J. M. (1995). Polyurethane Elastomer Biostability, *Journal of Biomaterial Applications*, Vol. 9, No. 4, (April 1995), pp. 321-354

Sugiyama, K., Ohga, K., Aoki, H. & Amaya, N. (1995). Emulsion copolymerization of 2-(acryloyloxy)-ethylphosphorylcholine with vinyl monomers and protein adsorption at resultant copolymer microspheres, *Macromolecular Chemistry & Physics,* Vol. 196, No. 6, (June 1995), pp. 1907-1916, ISSN 1022-1352

Tadokoro, Y.; Nagase, Y.; Iwasaki, Y. & Ishihara, K. (2006). Synthesis of aromatic carboxylic acid compound containing phosphorylcholine moiety and the polymer reaction with ethyl cellulose, *Transactions of the Material Research Society of Japan*, Vol. 31, No. 4, (December 2006), pp. 1053-1056. ISSN 1382-3469

Ueda, T.; Oshida, H.; Kurita, K. Ishihara, K. & Nakabayashi, N. (1992). Preparation of 2-methacryloyloxyethyl phosphorilcholine copolymers with alkyl methacrylates and their blood compatibility. *Polymer Journal,* Vol. 24, No. 11, (November 1992), pp. 1259-1269. ISSN 0032-3896

Uchiyama, T., Watanabe, J. & Ishihara, K. (2002). Pressure-induced change in permeation of insulin through a polymer alloy membrane for an implantable insulin pump, *Journal of Membrane Science*, Vol. 210, No. 2, (December 2002), pp. 423-431, ISSN 0376-7388

Wu Y., Zhao Q., Anderson J. M., Hiltner A., London G. M. & Payet, C. R. (1991). Effect of some additives on the biostability of a poly(ether urethane) elastomer, *Journal of Biomedical Materials Research, Vol.* 25, No. 6, (June 1991), pp. 725-798, ISSN 0021-9304

Ye, S. H., Watanabe, J., Takai, M., Iwasaki, Y. & Ishihara, K. (2006). High functional hollow fiber membrane modified with phospholipid polymers for a liver assist bioreactor, *Biomaterials*, Vol. 27, No. 9, (March 2006), pp. 1955-1962, ISSN 0142-9612

Zhao Q., Topham N., Anderson J. M., Hiltner A., London G. & Payet C. R. (1991). Foreign-body giant cells and polyurethane biostability: *In vivo* correlation of cell adhesion and surface cracking, *Journal of Biomedical Materials Research,*, Vol. 25, No. 2, (February 1991), pp. 177-183, ISSN 0021-9304

Zhao, Q. H., McNally, A. K., Rubin, K. R., Renier, M. & Wu Y. V. (1993). Human plasma α_2-macroglobulin promotes *in vitro* oxidative stress cracking of pellethane 2363-80A: *In vivo* and *in vitro* correlations, *Journal of Biomedical Materials Research,* Vol. 27, No. 3, (March 1993), pp. 379-388, ISSN 0021-9304

12

Scalable Functional Bone Substitutes: Strategic Integration of Key Structural Elements of Bone in Synthetic Biomaterials

Tera M. Filion and Jie Song
Department of Orthopedics & Physical Rehabilitation, Department of Cell Biology, University of Massachusetts Medical School, Worcester, MA, USA

1. Introduction

Over 40% of the disabling medical conditions of persons aged 18 years and over are musculoskeletal related. This number is even higher within the older population (Weinstein, 2000). Surgical treatment for age-, trauma- or cancer-induced critical-size bone loss is particularly challenging. Current grafting material options for scaffold-assisted surgical repair of critical-size bone loss include autogenic bone grafts (autografts), allogenic bone grafts (allografts), and synthetic bone substitutes. Still considered as a golden standard, autografts, retrieved from patients' own skeleton, are used in approximately 50% of all orthopedic bone grafting procedures. Complications arising from possible donor-site morbidity and insufficient grafting materials are major drawbacks of autografting procedures (Bostrom & Seigerman, 2005). In addition, this option is highly limited within the aging population as the elderly are less likely to be qualified for such a procedure due to higher incidences of osteoporosis and metabolic diseases. Allografts, obtained from another human donor or animal cadaver, represent a useful alternate to autografts, and are used in approximately 40% of bone grafting surgeries. However, allografting procedures suffer from risks for rejection and disease transmission, and a significant structural failure rate due to poor tissue integration both structurally and biochemically (Blokhuis & Lindner, 2008; Bostrom & Seigerman, 2005; Eagan & McAllister, 2009; Goldberg & Stevenson, 1994). These limitations, along with the growing aging population, has led to an increasing need for viable synthetic bone substitute alternatives (Salgado et al., 2004). Current clinically used synthetic bone grafts such as brittle ceramics and weak gel foams are used in only ~10% of all bone grafting procedures (Bostrom & Seigerman, 2005), primarily due to their unstable graft fixation and insufficient tissue-graft interactions (Carson & Bostrom, 2007; Goldberg & Stevenson, 1994; Place et al., 2009; Stevens, 2008). In the past two decades, many new synthetic bone grafts designed to mimic key structural and biochemical properties of bone to enhance osteointegration and graft healing have emerged in literature. This rapidly evolving field has been extensively reviewed by others, including broad overviews of current requirements and techniques for preparing synthetic bone grafts (Burg et al., 2000; Salgado et al., 2004), calcium phosphate-based bone substitutes (De Long et al., 2007), polymeric bone substitutes (Seal et al., 2001), and biomimetic nanocomposite orthopedic biomaterials (Chan et al., 2006; Murugan & Ramakrishna, 2005). This chapter highlights the evolvement of non-metallic orthopedic biomaterials from bioinert, biodegradable/bioresorbable, bioactive to tissue-responsive, and emphasizes the strategic integration of key structural elements of bone in the design of organic-inorganic composite bone substitutes. Using FlexBone, an easy-to-fabricate elastomeric 3-dimensional hydrogel-nanocrystalline hydroxyapatite (nHA) composite exhibiting excellent structural integration, as an example, we illustrate the feasibility of accomplishing multifaceted functional requirements of a viable synthetic bone substitute by integrating the major bone mineral component with a hydrophilic 3-dimensional hydrogel matrix.

2. Brief overview of the evolvement of synthetic orthopedic biomaterials

Most synthetic polymers traditionally used in orthopedic care, including poly(ethylene terephthalate) (PET) as implant coating, polyetheretherketone (PEEK) as spacers for cervical fusion, maxillofacial defect repair, and hip prostheses (Eschbach, 2000; M. M. Kim, Boahene, & Byrne, 2009; Kulkarni, Hee, & Wong, 2007), poly(methyl methacrylate) (PMMA) as bone cements, ultra high molecular weight polyethylene (UHMWPE) as total joint replacement components, and polysulfone (PSU) as internal fracture fixators (De Long et al., 2007; Eschbach, 2000; Mano et al., 2004; M. Wang, 2003) are considered as bioinert. They are primarily used to provide structural or mechanical support without eliciting significant immune responses. The primary drawback of bioinert implant materials is that they lack the intrinsic ability to promote osteogenesis, thus are unable to structurally or biologically integrate with the host tissue. To overcome such limitations, physical modification (e.g. increasing porosity) or blending bioinert materials with bioceramics or biodegradable polymeric components have been attempted (Aparecida et al., 2008; Fini et al., 2002; Mano et al., 2004; Tan et al., 2003; Tanner 2010; K. Zhang et al., 2002).

Calcium phosphate-based bioceramics have long been used clinically as bioactive bone fillers (De Long et al., 2007; Nandi et al., 2010). They are known for good biocompatibility, osteoconductivity and easy surgical handling. However, these bone substitutes suffer from poor mechanical properties such as high brittleness and are often unsuitable for weight-bearing applications (De Long et al., 2007; Tanner, 2010). Their integration with the more compliant polymeric matrices, therefore, has been of intense investigations (Kim et al., 2006; Miranda et al., 2010; Rezwan et al., 2006; M. Wang & Bonfield, 2001).

Biodegradable synthetic polymers have great potential as resorbable orthopedic implants and tissue scaffolds. The *in situ* generated porosity of degradable polymers as a result of hydrolytic degradation is thought to be beneficial to tissue penetration / osteointegration. In addition, the gradual resorption of biodegradable polymer-based orthopedic fixation devices, if timed to match with the tissue integration rate, could ensure adequate mechanical integrity at the site of implantation while potentially eliminating the need for a second surgery for implant retrieval. Among all degradable synthetic polymers, poly(lactic acid) (PLA) (R. Y. Zhang & Ma, 1999), poly(glycolic acid) (PGA), poly(lactic-co-plycolic acid) (PLGA) (Ishaug et al., 1997; Lu et al., 2000; Ma & Choi, 2001; Mooney et al., 1996), polyhydroxybutyrate (PHB) (Y. W. Wang et al., 2004), polycaprolactone (PCL) (Yoshimoto et al., 2003), and their co-polymer blends (Tanner, 2010) have been the most investigated.

Blending biodegradable polyesters with weakly basic osteoconductive minerals such as tri-calcium phosphate (TCP) or hydroxyapatite (HA) have been widely pursued as a strategy for further enhancing scaffold osteoconductivity, drug retention capacity, and for neutralizing acidic degradation products and mitigating inflammatory tissue responses (Liao et al., 2007; Peter et al., 1999; Tanner, 2010; M. Wang, 2003). Achieving adequate structural integration between the organic matrix and the inorganic minerals, however, remains one of most significant challenges for the clinical translation of these polymer-mineral nanocomposites for orthopedic care as loosely integrated ceramic particles could not only lead to inferior mechanical properties of the composite, but also cause ectopic bone formation in nearby soft tissues. This is because most polyesters are hydrophobic in nature and exhibit an intrinsically low affinity to bioceramics. Recent development of high-affinity HA-surface mineralization strategies applicable to hydrophilic hydrogels such as poly(2-hydroxyethyl methacrylate) (pHEMA) and pHEMA-based copolymers (Song et al., 2005; Song et al., 2003a, 2003b), and identification of novel HA-binding/nucleating ligands, either small molecule-based (Licata, 2005; Yoshinari et al., 2001) or peptide-based (Bertozzi et al., 2006; Chung et al., 2011), could help address this challenge.

The past decade has witnessed an increasingly elaborated trend in the design of bioactive synthetic biomaterials (Bonzani et al., 2006). For bone tissue engineering applications, integrin-binding peptide sequences for promoting cellular adhesion, phosphorylated ligands for promoting HA-mineralization, heparin-mimicking motifs for drug retentions, and degradative enzyme substrate sequences have all been incorporated into multi-modality synthetic scaffold designs (Hartgerink et al., 2001; Jeon et al., 2007; M. P. Lutolf et al., 2003; M. R. Lutolf et al., 2003; Patterson & Hubbell, 2010). Of particular novelty is the design of self-assembling peptide-amphiphile (PA) gels by Stupp and coworkers for simultaneous presentation of cell adhesion peptide sequences, HA-mineral-nucleating sites, reversible crosslinking sites, and other therapeutic agents all within a single PA molecule (Cui et al., 2010; Hartgerink et al., 2001; Palmer et al., 2008; Palmer & Stupp, 2008) that self-assembles and dissembles in response to environmental perturbations. Likely limitations of these unique PA gels are their relatively high manufacturing cost and low mechanical modulus which could limit their use to treating smaller non-weight bearing skeletal lesions. Another innovative concept introduced by Hubbell and coworkers was to induce scaffold degradation by using peptide substrates of the degradative enzymes matrix metalloproteinases (MMPs) as the chemical crosslinker of a non-fouling crosslinked hydrogel system (M. P. Lutolf et al., 2003; M. R. Lutolf et al., 2003). Given the elevated expression of some MMPs within both degenerative bony defects and arthritic knee joints, such a hydrogel system could be useful for bone and cartilage repair as the *in situ* increase of scaffold porosity in response to tissue microenvironment-specific enzymatic degradation could promote cellular infiltration and matrix deposition. The selection of MMP substrates with proper degradation kinetics matching with those of the matrix deposition rate, however, is not a trivial task (Bahney et al., 2011).

Despite the many exciting orthopedic biomaterials emerging in the literature, successful clinical translations are rare. The challenge lies in the difficulty in accomplishing the functional sophistication of viable synthetic bone substitutes (e.g. physical properties enabling easy surgical handling and stable graft fixation, structural and biomechanical properties facilitating its osteointegration, biocompatibility ensuring long-term safety) within an easy-to-fabricate biomaterial that can be reproducibly manufactured at low cost. We, as well as some in the orthopedic biomaterials research community, believe that functional sophistication are not synonymous with complicated materials designs (Bonzani et al., 2006; Stevens, 2008). Instead, we believe that the key to meeting this challenge lies in the strategic integration of key structural elements of bone, which play multifaceted roles in defining the unique properties of the native tissue, in a low-cost biocompatible synthetic biomaterial.

3. Key structural elements of bone and their multifaceted functions

From a material's perspective, bone is an organic-inorganic composite comprising two major structural components that are hierarchically organized across various length scales: the calcium apatite crystals (primarily as substituted nanocrystalline hydroxyapatite nHA, but also as crystalline precursors) and the type I collagen matrix (Weiner et al., 1999). The quantity and quality of the hard calcium apatite crystals (crystal size, maturity and structural integration with the collagen matrices) influences the mechanical properties of bone (Tong et al., 2003). For instance, the bending and compression strength of bone is known to positively correlate to bone mineral content (Follet et al., 2004). In addition, bone minerals also support bone cell attachment, and serve as an important reservoir of calcium and phosphate ions, and help retain the secreted factors that are indispensable in defining the biochemical environment of the bony tissue. Thus, HA has long been recognized as an important design element for tissue-engineered bone substitutes (El-Ghannam, 2005). The intrinsic affinity of the dynamic apatite crystal surfaces for many acidic non-collagenous proteins widely found in calcified tissues (George et al., 1996; Gilbert et al., 2000; Stubbs et al., 1997) have also inspired the use of bioceramic scaffolds (Le Nihouannen et al., 2008) or polymer-bioceramics composite scaffolds (Abarrategi et al., 2008; Filion et al., 2011; Xu et al., 2009) to retain and deliver recombinant proteins for therapeutic uses. Overall, HA has been explored for bone tissue engineering applications more as a way to enhance the mechanical strength than as a tool to mediate the biochemical properties of the scaffold (Stevens, 2008; Tanner, 2010). In general, the potential of the large surface areas provided by nHA as opposed to micrometer-sized mineral particles for more efficient therapeutics delivery (e.g. higher retention capacity, more sustained release) has not been exploited to the fullest extent in the design of synthetic bone substitutes.

Type I collagen matrix of bone serves as a compliant template for the structural integration of the calcium apatite crystals, and, along with the mineral component, is responsible for defining the 3-demensional structure as well as the strong, tough, yet relatively compliant mechanical properties of bone (Scharnweber et al., 2004; Weiner et al., 1999). In addition, it also interacts with many non-collagenous proteins and mediates cellular adhesion and functions (Heino, 2000). The Gly-Pro-Hyp (Hyp: hydroxyproline) triplet repeats of type I collagen may also play an important role in template-driven biomineralization. Recent discovery of novel HA-binding oligopeptides using the combinatorial phage display technique reveals a [Pro-(OH)-X] tripeptide pattern (OH: hydroxylated amino acid residues (Ser, Thr, Tyr); X: any amino acid) among the dominant HA-binding motifs (Bertozzi et al., 2006; Chung et al., 2011). Such a hydroxylated tripeptide pattern resembles that of the type I collagen, underscoring the importance of hydroxylated residues in directing ligand-mineral interactions on a molecular level. These oligopeptides were shown to template the nucleation and growth of HA *in vitro* (Bertozzi et al., 2006; Chung et al., 2011), and may be useful in the design of synthetic polymer scaffolds enabling template-driven mineralization of HA or the preparation of bulk organic-inorganic bone-like composites with improved interfacial binding affinity. We also showed earlier that polymeric hydrogels displaying hydroxylated (e.g. pHEMA) and acidic residues could be used to template the surface mineralization of HA with excellent interfacial adhesion strength (Song et al., 2005; Song et al., 2003a, 2003b), further supporting the favorable interaction between the hydroxyls and the calcium ions. The strategy of modifying the surface of polymers or metallic substrates with hydroxylated or anionic coatings has also been pursued to facilitate the nucleation and growth of calcium apatite (Murphy & Mooney, 2002; H. L. Zhang et al., 2006).

4. FlexBone: A scalable functional bone substitute integrating key structural elements of bone

Inspired by the multifaceted roles of type I collagen matrix and nanocrystalline HA (nHA) in defining the unique structural, mechanical and biochemical properties of bone, we have developed a 3-dimensional synthetic bone substitute named FlexBone that integrates hydroxylated biocompatible pHEMA hydrogel with 50 wt% of nHA. This elastomeric structural composite exemplifies how multiple functional requirements for a viable bone substitute could be met with a scalable biomaterial that could be readily prepared at low cost. Here we focus our discussion on how the nHA component and its structural integration with the pHEMA matrix defines FlexBone's physical properties that enables its easy surgical insertion and stable fixation at the site of defect, its ability to retain and release protein therapeutics in a localized and sustained manner, its ability to enrich endogenous protein signals within the microenvironment of the tissue defect, and its ability to enable functional repair of critical long bone defect without exerting negative systemic side effects.

4.1 Preparation, microstructures and compressive behavior of FlexBone

FlexBone was prepared by crosslinking 2-hydroxyethyl methacrylate (HEMA) in the presence of up to 50 wt% nHA (Figs. 1A & B) in molds of any size and shape as previously described (Song et al., 2009). The choice of crosslinked pHEMA as the organic scaffold of FlexBone was inspired by its biocompatibility (Kost, 1987; Montheard et al., 1992), elasticity (enabling convenient surgical handling), potential high-affinity integration with the HA (providing long-term structural stability), and low manufacturing cost, all of which are critical considerations for bench-to-bedside translations. The choice of 50 wt% nHA as the inorganic component of FlexBone was inspired by the osteoconductive mineral content approximating that of human bone (An, 2000; Phelps et al., 2000) and the large surface areas of the nanocrystals enabling better integration with the hydroxylated hydrogel matrix and better retention of both endogenous protein signals and exogenous protein therapeutics.

The as-prepared FlexBone can be cut into any desired configuration matching with that of a potential defect, drilled with channels, and equilibrated with water to thoroughly remove radical initiators (Filion et al., 2011; Song et al., 2009). Upon freeze-drying, FlexBone can be stored long-term at room temperature, making it ideally suited as an "off-the-shelf" synthetic bone substitute for clinical applications.

Scanning electron microscopy (SEM) analysis revealed an even distribution of loose aggregates of nHA within the 3-dimensional pHEMA hydrogel matrix (Figs. 1A & B). As expected, the incorporation of 50 wt% of nHA in pHEMA resulted in an increase of the stiffness of the bulk material (Fig. 1C). Despite its high nHA content, however, FlexBone exhibited elastomeric properties in both as-prepared and fully hydrated states, showing excellent shape recovery after being subjected to repetitive moderate (MPa) compressive loadings under physiological conditions (in water, at body temperature). The excellent structural integration of nHA with the hydroxylated pHEMA matrix was reflected by the ability of freeze-dried FlexBone to withstand hundreds-of-megapascals compressive loadings and >80% compressive strains without exhibiting brittle fractures (Song et al., 2009). SEM examination of the cross-section of a freeze-dried FlexBone after it was being compressed to >80% did not reveal any microfractures (Fig. 1D). Instead, the spherical aggregates of nHA were compressed into plywood-like structures, suggesting that the rearrangement of nHA under the compressive loading provided an effective mechanism for energy dissipation, thereby contributing to the toughness of FlexBone. Such a fracture-resistant property could not be obtained with composites containing the same weight percentage of micrometer-sized HA particles, where crack propagations within the composite under the same compressive loading was observed (Song et al., 2009). These findings underscore the critical role that nHA plays in defining the microstructural and mechanical properties of FlexBone. The elastomeric and fracture-resistant properties of FlexBone will enable its surgical insertion into an area of defect by convenient press-fitting.

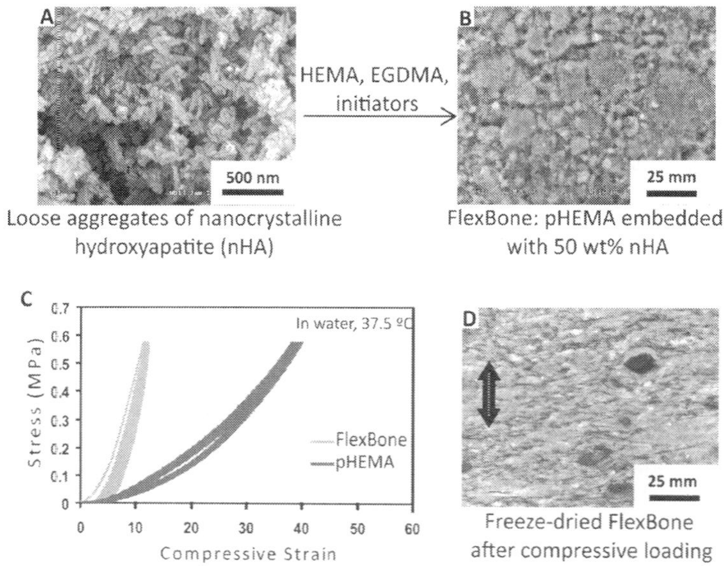

Fig. 1. Structural and mechanical properties of FlexBone. Cross-linking HEMA in the presence of 50 wt% nHA (A) generated FlexBone, where the spherical loose aggregates of nHA were well-distributed throughout the 3-dimensional pHEMA matrix (B) as revealed by SEM micrographs. (C) FlexBone, stiffer than pHEMA, withstood repetitive low-MPa compressive loadings with excellent shape recovery. The stress-strain curves were recorded on a dynamic mechanical analyzer equipped with a submersion compression fixture. Ten consecutive load-controlled loading-unloading cycles (3.0 N/min, 0.01 N to 10.0 N to 0.01 N) were applied to each specimen in water at body temperature. (D) SEM micrograph of the cross-section of a freeze-dried FlexBone after being compressed to >80% compressive strain revealed the rearrangement of nHA into plywood like structures upon compression. Arrow indicates the orientation of the applied compressive loading.

4.2 Retention and localized / sustained release of therapeutics from FlexBone

The large surface area of the nHA component of FlexBone, coupled with its good structural integration with the pHEMA hydrogel matrix, has enabled FlexBone to retain protein therapeutics and small molecule antibiotics and release them in a localized and sustained manner (Xu et al., 2009). Such a feature is attractive for clinical applications where a patient's tissue repair capacity is compromised by either age or metabolic conditions, or where the defect site is prone to infections (Hetrick & Schoenfisch, 2006).

Using a bone morphogenetic protein (BMP)-induced osteogenic trans-differentiation of myoblast C2C12 cell culture model (Katagiri et al., 1994), the ability of FlexBone to retain and release recombinant human bone morphogenetic protein-2/7 heterodimer (rhBMP-2/7) *in vitro* was evaluated. The pHEMA matrix enabled FlexBone to readily absorb an aqueous solution of rhBMP-2/7 and stably sequester these proteins, presumably on the surfaces of the nHA component. As shown in Figure 2, when a FlexBone carrier pre-absorbed with a single low dose of 40 ng of rhBMP-2/7 was placed in the culture of C2C12 cells, trans-differentiation of the myoblasts to alkaline phosphatase (ALP)-expressing (stained in red) osteoblastic cells was observed by 2-4 days. The highly localized ALP staining suggested that the rhBMP-2/7 was released from the FlexBone carrier in a highly localized manner. Further, when the FlexBone carrier retrieved from the 4-day culture was placed in a fresh culture of C2C12 cells, the continually released rhBMP-2 was able to induce osteogenic differentiation in 3.5 days, suggesting that the release was sustained over a period of >7 days. It is worth noting that the 40-ng/graft loading dose of rhBMP-2/7 on FlexBone for inducing trans-differentiation of C2C12 cells was 3 orders of magnitude lower than required for BMP-2 using a TCP-chitosan carrier (Abarrategi et al., 2008). This is likely a result of both the increased rhBMP-2/7 retention on the nHA surfaces and the relatively higher osteogenic potency (~10 fold) of rhBMP-2/7 as compared to rhBMP-2 (Israel et al., 1996; Zheng et al., 2010).

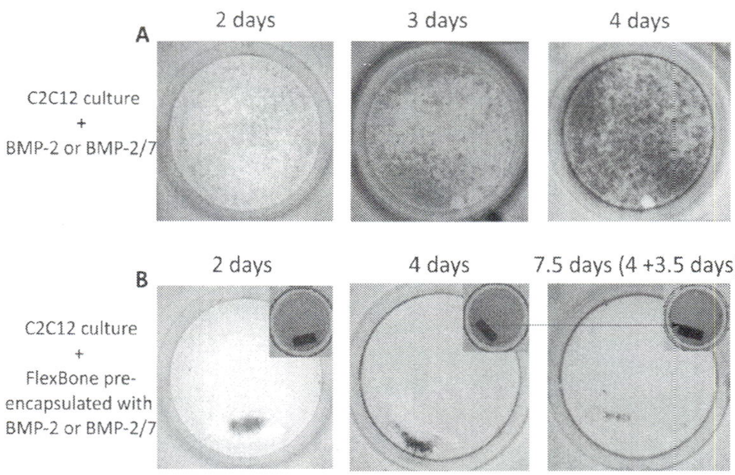

Fig. 2. FlexBone released pre-absorbed recombinant human bone morphogenetic proteins and induced osteogenic trans-differentiation of myoblast C2C12 cells in a localized and sustained manner. (A) Direct supplement of rhBMP-2/7 (40 ng/mL) or rhBMP-2 (300 ng/mL) in C2C12 culture media resulted in osteogenic trans-differentiation of C2C12 cells by 2-4 days as indicated by positive (red) ALP stains. (B) ALP stains were detected in C2C12 cultures in areas immediately adjacent to where the FlexBone carrier pre-absorbed with rhBMP-2/7 (40 ng/carrier) (Xu et al., 2009) or rhBMP-2 (300 ng/carrier) (Li et al., 2011) was placed. Continued detection of ALP stains induced by the BMPs released from FlexBone over 7 days suggests that the release was accomplished in a sustained manner. C2C12 seeding density: 10,000 cells/cm^2.

Similarly, FlexBone was also able to release pre-absorbed receptor activator of nuclear factor kappa-B ligand (RANKL, 10-ng/carrier) in a sustained manner over 7 days and induce the osteoclastogenesis of murine macrophage RAW264.7 cells in culture (Xu et al., 2009). By contrast, the un-mineralized pHEMA control carrier pre-loaded with 10-ng RANKL exhibited a burst-release of RANKL within the first 2 days of culture, and was not able to successfully induce the osteoclastogenesis of RAW264.7 cells over the course of 1 week under identical culture conditions. This observation underscores the critical role of nHA in achieving effective retention and sustained release of the recombinant protein. The low effective loading dose of 10-ng RANKL per carrier for inducing osteoclastogenesis of RAW264.7 accomplished with FlexBone was also significantly lower than that required using literature brushite cement carrier (600–800 ng RANKL per carrier required) using an identical cell culture model (Le Nihouannen et al., 2008). Overall, these findings suggest that FlexBone may be used to deliver protein therapeutics with significantly reduced loading doses that could lead to enhanced safety and reduced cost of growth factor-mediated clinical treatment of skeletal lesions.

Finally, 5 wt% of antibiotic tetracycline could be encapsulated in FlexBone without compromising the structural and compressive properties of FlexBone (Xu et al., 2009). The pre-encapsulated tetracycline was slowly released from FlexBone, with >80% of the tetracycline still retained on FlexBone after 1 week. By contrast, the un-mineralized pHEMA control released pre-encapsulated tetracycline much more rapidly, with only ~40% of tetracycline retained on the hydrogel scaffold after 7 days. We have also recently shown that the encapsulation and sustained release of vancomycin could also be accomplished using FlexBone as a carrier (Li et al., 2011).

4.3 FlexBone-mediated functional repair of rat critical-size femoral defects

Inspired by the elastomeric and fracture-resistant properties of FlexBone as well as its ability to deliver therapeutic agents in a localized and sustained manner, we recently evaluated the efficacy of FlexBone as a synthetic bone graft in mediating the repair of 5-mm critical-size femoral defects in rats with or without a single dose of 400-ng rhBMP-2/7 (Filion et al., 2011). The 5-mm femoral defects were stably press-fit with the elastomeric FlexBone with or without the absorption of 400-ng rhBMP-2/7 (Fig. 3). The grafts were predrilled with intersecting orthogonal drill holes to permit bone marrow access to expedite callus formations both within and surrounding the graft.

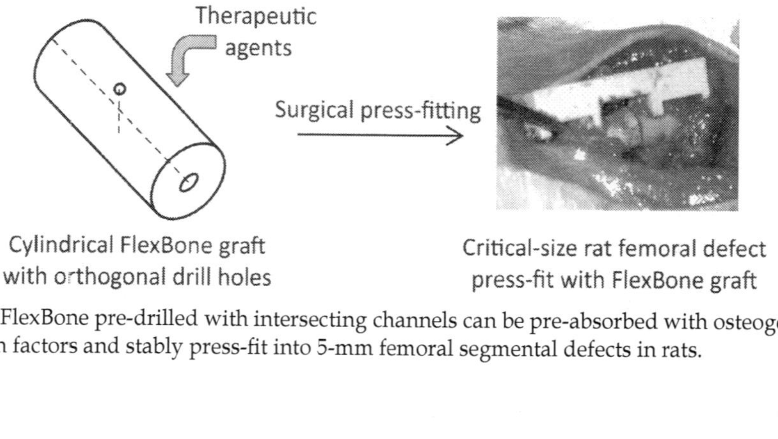

Fig. 3. FlexBone pre-drilled with intersecting channels can be pre-absorbed with osteogenic growth factors and stably press-fit into 5-mm femoral segmental defects in rats.

Histology, polarized light microscopy and microcomputed tomography (microCT) analyses showed that FlexBone enabled partial healing of the defect by 12 weeks in the absence of any exogenous growth factors (Filion et al., 2011). By 4 days post-operation, an internal callus emerged within the drill holes of FlexBone, which continued to mature and was recanalized by 6 weeks. The external callus bridging over the defect started to be mineralized at 2 weeks via the endochondral ossification mechanism. The partially mineralized external callus was matured and recanalized by 12 weeks, although it did not completely bridge over the entire defect. In a subset of experiments, we demonstrated by immunohistochemical staining that the partial healing enabled by FlexBone in the absence of any exogenous factors could be attributed to the ability of the nHA component to retain/sequester the endogenous protein signals present in the defect microenvironment. Specifically, FlexBone grafts retrieved from the surgical implantation site at different time points over the course of the first week of implantation revealed retained endogenously secreted transforming growth factor β (TGFβ), interleukin-1β (IL-1β), tumor necrosis factor α (TNFα), vascular endothelial growth

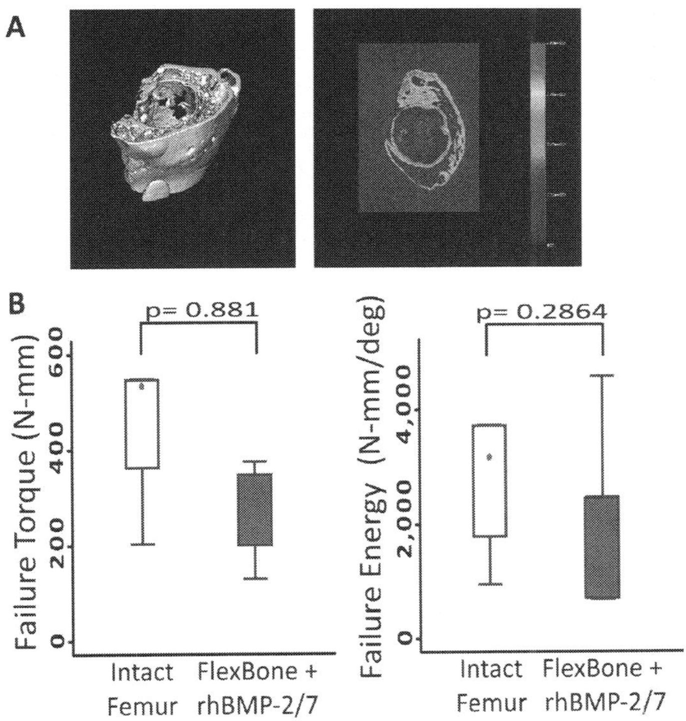

Fig. 4. FlexBone pre-absorbed with 400-ng rhBMP-2/7 led to functional repair of 5-mm segmental defects in rats as supported by the microCT analyses (A) and torsion tests (B) of 12-week explants. Effective voxel size of 18×18×18 μm^3 was applied to the reconstructed 3-D isosurface image and the 2-D color map of the center slice of the explant (red representing a higher degree of mineralization). No statistically significant difference was observed between the 12-week explant and the age-matched un-operated control femur.

factor (VEGF), RANKL, BMP-2, BMP-7 and stromal cell-derived factor-1 (SDF-1) in a temporally defined manner. These factors are known to play critical roles in initiating the inflammation / graft healing cascade and the recruitment of stem cells (Einhorn, 1998; Ito et al., 2005; Kitaori et al., 2009; Lieberman et al., 1999; Schindeler et al., 2008). The effective sequestering of these signals within FlexBone, but not the un-mineralized pHEMA control graft, supported the critical role of nHA in enabling the consequent partial repair of the defect.

With the absorption of a single dose of 400-ng rhBMP-2/7, FlexBone was able to enable the functional repair of the defect in 8-12 weeks (Filion et al., 2011). By 8 weeks, mature and recanalized external bony callus completely bridged over the defect as indicated by both histology and microCT analyses (Fig. 4A). More importantly, biomechanical testing revealed that the torsional strength of the repaired defects was restored to the level of age-matched un-operated femur controls (Fig. 4B). It is worth noting that such a functional repair of the defect was accomplished by FlexBone with a single low dose of rhBMP-2/7 that was 1-2 orders of magnitude lower than what has been required for treating similar defects using other scaffolds in combination with rhBMP-2 (Abarrategi et al., 2008; Kirker-Head et al., 2007). Such a feature of FlexBone could both reduce the cost and minimize negative systemic side-effects of scaffold-assisted BMP therapies. Indeed, the vital organs collected from the rats 12 weeks after receiving FlexBone-rhBMP-2/7 implants were pathologically indistinguishable from the age-matched un-operated controls.

In summary, FlexBone combines some of the best features of structural allografts (osteoconductivity and dimensional stability), desirable surgical compressibility, and the scalability of an easy-to-prepare synthetic biomaterial. The ability of FlexBone to locally deliver biological therapeutics in a significantly reduced effective dose to enable expedited functional repair of the critical defect opens the door to engineer the biochemical properties of the synthetic bone substitute based on individual patients' needs.

5. Conclusions

Many exciting orthopedic biomaterials have emerged in literature in the past 20 years, illustrating the shift of the focus in materials design from bioinert, biodegradable/bioresorbable, to bioactive and tissue-responsive. By recapitulating the multifaceted roles that key extracellular matrix components of bone play in defining bone-specific structural and biochemical properties, we show that easy-to-prepare biomaterials can be designed to facilitate the functional repair of critical-size bony defects. Our work supports the notion that functional sophistication of synthetic tissue grafts is not synonymous with complicated chemical/engineering designs.

6. References

Abarrategi, A., Moreno-Vicente, C., Ramos, V., Aranaz, I., Casado, J. V. S., & Lopez-Lacomba, J. L. (2008). Improvement of porous beta-TCP scaffolds with rhBMP-2 chitosan carrier film for bone tissue application. *Tissue Engineering Part A*, Vol.14, No.8, pp. 1305-1319, ISSN 1937-3341

An, Y. H. (2000). Mechanical properties of bone, In: *Mechanical Testing of Bone and the Bone-Implant Interface*, Y. H. An & R. A. Draughn (Eds.), 41-63, CRC Press, ISBN 0-8493-0266-8, Boca Raton

Aparecida, A. H., Guastaldi, A. C., & Fook, M. V. L. (2008). Development of Ultra High Molecular Weight Polyethylene (UHMWPE) Porous Supports for Use as Biomaterial in Osseous Replacement and Regeneration. *Polimeros-Ciencia E Tecnologia,* Vol.18, No.4, pp. 277-280, ISSN 0104-1428

Bahney, C. S., Hsu, C.-W., Yoo, J. U., West, J. L., & Johnstone, B. (2011). A bioresponsive hydrogel tuned to chondrogenesis of human mesenchymal stem cells. *Journal of the Federation of American Societies for Experimental Biology,* Vol.25, No. 5, pp. 1486-96. ISSN 0892-6638

Bertozzi, C. R., Song, J., & Lee, S.-W. (2006). Publication No. WO/2006/062776. World Intellectual Property Organization.

Blokhuis, T. J., & Lindner, T. (2008). Allograft and bone morphogenetic proteins: an overview. *Injury-International Journal of the Care of the Injured,* Vol.39, pp. S33-S36, ISSN 0020-1383

Bonzani, I. C., George, J. H., & Stevens, M. M. (2006). Novel materials for bone and cartilage regeneration. *Current Opinion in Chemical Biology,* Vol.10, No.6, pp. 568-575, ISSN 1367-5931

Bostrom, M. P., & Seigerman, D. A. (2005). The clinical use of allografts, demineralized bone matrices, synthetic bone graft substitutes and osteoinductive growth factors: a survey study. *Hospital for Special Surgery Journal,* Vol.1, No.1, pp. 9-18, ISSN 1556-3316

Burg, K. J. L., Porter, S., & Kellam, J. F. (2000). Biomaterial developments for bone tissue engineering. *Biomaterials,* Vol.21, No.23, pp. 2347-2359, ISSN 0142-9612

Carson, J. S., & Bostrom, M. P. G. (2007). Synthetic bone scaffolds and fracture repair. *Injury-International Journal of the Care of the Injured,* Vol.38, pp. S33-S37, ISSN 0020-1383

Chan, C. K., Kumar, T. S. S., Liao, S., Murugan, R., Ngiam, M., & Ramakrishman, S. (2006). Biomimetic nanocomposites for bone graft applications. *Nanomedicine,* Vol.1, No.2, pp. 177-188, ISSN 1743-5889

Chung, W. J., Kwon, K. Y., Song, J., & Lee, S. W. (2011). Evolutionary Screening of Collagen-like Peptides That Nucleate Hydroxyapatite Crystals. *Langmuir,* dx.doi.org/10.1021/la104757g

Cui, H. G., Webber, M. J., & Stupp, S. I. (2010). Self-Assembly of Peptide Amphiphiles: From Molecules to Nanostructures to Biomaterials. *Biopolymers,* Vol.94, No.1, pp. 1-18, ISSN 0006-3525

De Long, W. G., Einhorn, T. A., Koval, K., McKee, M., Smith, W., Sanders, R., & Watson, T. (2007). Bone, grafts and bone graft substitutes in orthopedic trauma surgery - A critical analysis. *Journal of Bone and Joint Surgery-American Volume,* Vol.89A, No.3, pp. 649-658, ISSN 0021-9355

Eagan, M. J., & McAllister, D. R. (2009). Biology of Allograft Incorporation. *Clinics in Sports Medicine,* Vol.28, No.2, pp. 203, ISSN 0278-5919

Einhorn, T. A. (1998). The cell and molecular biology of fracture healing. *Clinical Orthopaedics and Related Research,* No.355 Suppl, pp. S7-21, ISSN 0009-921X

El-Ghannam, A. (2005). Bone reconstruction: from bioceramics to tissue engineering. *Expert Review of Medical Devices,* Vol.2, No.1, pp. 87-101, ISSN 1743-4440

Eschbach, L. (2000). Nonresorbable polymers in bone surgery. *Injury,* Vol.31 Suppl 4, pp. 22-27, ISSN 0020-1383

Filion, T. M., Li, X., Mason-Savas, A., Kreider, J. M., Goldstein, S. A., Ayers, D. C., & Song, J. (2011). Elastomeric osteoconductive synthetic scaffolds with acquired osteoinductivity expedite the repair of critical femoral defects in rats. *Tissue Engineering Part A,* Vol.17, No.3-4, pp. 503-511, ISSN 1937-3341

Fini, M., Giavaresi, G., Aldini, N. N., Torricelli, P., Botter, R., Beruto, D., & Giardino, R. (2002). A bone substitute composed of polymethylmethacrylate and alpha-tricalcium phosphate: results in terms of osteoblast function and bone tissue formation. *Biomaterials,* Vol.23, No.23, pp. 4523-4531, ISSN 0142-9612

Follet, H., Boivin, G., Rumelhart, C., & Meunier, P. J. (2004). The degree of mineralization is a determinant of bone strength: a study on human calcanei. *Bone,* Vol.34, No.5, pp. 783-789, ISSN 8756-3282

George, A., Bannon, L., Sabsay, B., Dillon, J. W., Malone, J., Veis, A., Jenkins, N. A., Gilbert, D. J., & Copeland, N. G. (1996). The carboxyl-terminal domain of phosphophoryn contains unique extended triplet amino acid repeat sequences forming ordered carboxyl-phosphate interaction ridges that may be essential in the biomineralization process. *Journal of Biological Chemistry,* Vol.271, No.51, pp. 32869-32873, ISSN 0021-9258

Gilbert, M., Shaw, W. J., Long, J. R., Nelson, K., Drobny, G. P., Giachelli, C. M., & Stayton, P. S. (2000). Chimeric peptides of statherin and osteopontin that bind hydroxyapatite and mediate cell adhesion. *Journal of Biological Chemistry,* Vol.275, No.21, pp. 16213-16218, ISSN 0021-9258

Goldberg, V. M., & Stevenson, S. (1994). Bone-Graft Options - Fact and Fancy. *Orthopedics,* Vol.17, No.9, pp. 809, ISSN 0147-7447

Hartgerink, J. D., Beniash, E., & Stupp, S. I. (2001). Self-assembly and mineralization of peptide-amphiphile nanofibers. *Science,* Vol.294, No.5547, pp. 1684-1688, ISSN 0036-8075

Heino, J. (2000). The collagen receptor integrins have distinct ligand recognition and signaling functions. *Matrix Biology,* Vol.19, No.4, pp. 319-323, ISSN 0945-053X

Hetrick, E. M., & Schoenfisch, M. H. (2006). Reducing implant-related infections: active release strategies. *Chemical Society Reviews,* Vol.35, No.9, pp. 780-789, ISSN 0306-0012

Ishaug, S. L., Crane, G. M., Miller, M. J., Yasko, A. W., Yaszemski, M. J., & Mikos, A. G. (1997). Bone formation by three-dimensional stromal osteoblast culture in biodegradable polymer scaffolds. *Journal of Biomedical Materials Research,* Vol.36, No.1, pp. 17-28, ISSN 0021-9304

Israel, D. I., Nove, J., Kerns, K. M., Kaufman, R. J., Rosen, V., Cox, K. A., & Wozney, J. M. (1996). Heterodimeric bone morphogenetic proteins show enhanced activity in vitro and in vivo. *Growth Factors,* Vol.13, No.3-4, pp. 291-300, ISSN 0897-7194

Ito, H., Koefoed, M., Tiyapatanaputi, P., Gromov, K., Goater, J. J., Carmouche, J., Zhang, X. P., Rubery, P. T., Rabinowitz, J., Samulski, R. J., Nakamura, T., Soballe, K., O'Keefe, R. J., Boyce, B. F., & Schwarz, E. M. (2005). Remodeling of cortical bone allografts mediated by adherent rAAV-RANKL and VEGF gene therapy. *Nature Medicine,* Vol.11, No.3, pp. 291-297, ISSN 1078-8956

Jeon, O., Song, S. J., Kang, S. W., Putnam, A. J., & Kim, B. S. (2007). Enhancement of ectopic bone formation by bone morphogenetic protein-2 released from a heparin-conjugated poly(L-lactic-co-glycolic acid) scaffold. *Biomaterials,* Vol.28, No.17, pp. 2763-2771, ISSN 0142-9612

Katagiri, T., Yamaguchi, A., Komaki, M., Abe, E., Takahashi, N., Ikeda, T., Rosen, V., Wozney, J. M., Fujisawasehara, A., & Suda, T. (1994). Bone Morphogenetic Protein-2 Converts the Differentiation Pathway of C2c12 Myoblasts into the Osteoblast Lineage. *Journal of Cell Biology,* Vol.127, No.6, pp. 1755-1766, ISSN 0021-9525

Kim, S. S., Park, M. S., Jeon, O., Choi, C. Y., & Kim, B. S. (2006). Poly(lactide-co-glycolide)/hydroxyapatite composite scaffolds for bone tissue engineering. *Biomaterials,* Vol.27, No.8, pp. 1399-1409, ISSN 0142-9612

Kirker-Head, C., Karageorgiou, V., Hofmann, S., Fajardo, R., Betz, O., Merkle, H. P., Hilbe, M., von Rechenberg, B., McCool, J., Abrahamsen, L., Nazarian, A., Cory, E., Curtis, M., Kaplan, D., & Meinel, L. (2007). BMP-silk composite matrices heal critically sized femoral defects. *Bone,* Vol.41, No.2, pp. 247-255, ISSN 8756-3282

Kitaori, T., Ito, H., Schwarz, E. M., Tsutsumi, R., Yoshitomi, H., Oishi, S., Nakano, M., Fujii, N., Nagasawa, T., & Nakamura, T. (2009). Stromal cell-derived factor 1/CXCR4 signaling is critical for the recruitment of mesenchymal stem cells to the fracture site during skeletal repair in a mouse model. *Arthritis & Rheumatism,* Vol.60, No.3, pp. 813-823, ISSN 0004-3591

Kost, J. & Langer, R. (1987). *Hydrogels in Medicine and Pharmacy,* N. Peppas(Ed.), 95, CRC Press, ISBN 9780849355486, Boca Raton

Le Nihouannen, D., Hacking, S. A., Gbureck, U., Komarova, S. V., & Barralet, J. E. (2008). The use of RANKL-coated brushite cement to stimulate bone remodelling. *Biomaterials,* Vol.29, No.22, pp. 3253-3259, ISSN 0142-9612

Li, X., Xu J., Smit J., Filion, TM., Ayers, DC., Song, J. (2011). Sustained and Localized *In Vitro* Release of Vancomycin and rhBMP-2 from an Elastomeric Osteoconductive Synthetic Bone Graft Substitute, *57th Annual Meeting of the Orthopedics Research Society,* Long Beach, CA, Jan. 13-16, 2011

Liao, S., Watari, F., Zhu, Y., Uo, M., Akasaka, T., Wang, W., Xu, G., & Cui, F. (2007). The degradation of the three layered nano-carbonated hydroxyapatite/collagen/PLGA composite membrane in vitro. *Dental Materials,* Vol.23, No.9, pp. 1120-1128, ISSN 0109-5641

Licata, A. A. (2005). Discovery, clinical development, and therapeutic uses of bisphosphonates. *Annals of Pharmacotherapy,* Vol.39, No.4, pp. 668-677, ISSN 1060-0280

Lieberman, J. R., Daluiski, A., Stevenson, S., Wu, L., McAllister, P., Lee, Y. P., Kabo, J. M., Finerman, G. A., Berk, A. J., & Witte, O. N. (1999). The effect of regional gene therapy with bone morphogenetic protein-2-producing bone-marrow cells on the repair of segmental femoral defects in rats. *Journal of Bone and Joint Surgery American Volume,* Vol.81, No.7, pp. 905-917, ISSN 0021-9355

Lu, L., Peter, S. J., Lyman, M. D., Lai, H. L., Leite, S. M., Tamada, J. A., Uyama, S., Vacanti, J. P., Langer, R., & Mikos, A. G. (2000). In vitro and in vivo degradation of porous poly(DL-lactic-co-glycolic acid) foams. *Biomaterials,* Vol.21, No.18, pp. 1837-1845, ISSN 0142-9612

Lutolf, M. P., Lauer-Fields, J. L., Schmoekel, H. G., Metters, A. T., Weber, F. E., Fields, G. B., & Hubbell, J. A. (2003). Synthetic matrix metalloproteinase-sensitive hydrogels for the conduction of tissue regeneration: Engineering cell-invasion characteristics.

Proceedings of the National Academy of Sciences of the United States of America, Vol.100, No.9, pp. 5413-5418, ISSN 0027-8424

Lutolf, M. R., Weber, F. E., Schmoekel, H. G., Schense, J. C., Kohler, T., Muller, R., & Hubbell, J. A. (2003). Repair of bone defects using synthetic mimetics of collagenous extracellular matrices. *Nature Biotechnology,* Vol.21, No.5, pp. 513-518, ISSN 1087-0156

Ma, P. X., & Choi, J. W. (2001). Biodegradable polymer scaffolds with well-defined interconnected spherical pore network. *Tissue Engineering,* Vol.7, No.1, pp. 23-33, ISSN 1076-3279

Mano, J. F., Sousa, R. A., Boesel, L. F., Neves, N. M., & Reis, R. L. (2004). Bloinert, biodegradable and injectable polymeric matrix composites for hard tissue replacement: state of the art and recent developments. *Composites Science and Technology,* Vol.64, No.6, pp. 789-817, ISSN 0266-3538

Miranda, P., Martinez-Vazquez, F. J., Perera, F. H., Pajares, A., & Guiberteau, F. (2010). Improving the compressive strength of bioceramic robocast scaffolds by polymer infiltration. *Acta Biomaterialia,* Vol.6, No.11, pp. 4361-4368, ISSN 1742-7061

Montheard, J. P., Chatzopoulos, M., & Chappard, D. (1992). 2-Hydroxyethyl Methacrylate (Hema) - Chemical-Properties and Applications in Biomedical Fields. *Journal of Macromolecular Science-Reviews in Macromolecular Chemistry and Physics,* Vol.C32, No.1, pp. 1-34, ISSN 0736-6574

Mooney, D. T., Mazzoni, C. L., Breuer, C., McNamara, K., Hern, D., Vacanti, J. P., & Langer, R. (1996). Stabilized polyglycolic acid fibre based tubes for tissue engineering. *Biomaterials,* Vol.17, No.2, pp. 115-124, ISSN 0142-9612

Murphy, W. L., & Mooney, D. J. (2002). Bioinspired growth of crystalline carbonate apatite on biodegradable polymer substrata. *Journal of the American Chemical Society,* Vol.124, No.9, pp. 1910-1917, ISSN 0002-7863

Murugan, R., & Ramakrishna, S. (2005). Development of nanocomposites for bone grafting. *Composites Science and Technology,* Vol.65, No.15-16, pp. 2385-2406, ISSN 0266-3538

Nandi, S. K., Roy, S., Mukherjee, P., Kundu, B., De, D. K., & Basu, D. (2010). Orthopaedic applications of bone graft & graft substitutes: a review. *Indian Journal of Medical Research,* Vol.132, No.1, pp. 15-30, ISSN 0971-5916

Palmer, L. C., Newcomb, C. J., Kaltz, S. R., Spoerke, E. D., & Stupp, S. I. (2008). Biomimetic Systems for Hydroxyapatite Mineralization Inspired By Bone and Enamel. *Chemical Reviews,* Vol.108, No.11, pp. 4754-4783, ISSN 0009-2665

Palmer, L. C., & Stupp, S. I. (2008). Molecular Self-Assembly into One-Dimensional Nanostructures. *Accounts of Chemical Research,* Vol.41, No.12, pp. 1674-1684, ISSN 0001-4842

Patterson, J., & Hubbell, J. A. (2010). Enhanced proteolytic degradation of molecularly engineered PEG hydrogels in response to MMP-1 and MMP-2. *Biomaterials,* Vol.31, No.30, pp. 7836-7845, ISSN 0142-9612

Peter, S. J., Kim, P., Yasko, A. W., Yaszemski, M. J., & Mikos, A. G. (1999). Crosslinking characteristics of an injectable poly(propylene fumarate)/beta-tricalcium phosphate paste and mechanical properties of the crosslinked composite for use as a biodegradable bone cement. *Journal of Biomedical Materials Research,* Vol.44, No.3, pp. 314-321, ISSN 0021-9304

Phelps, J. B., Hubbard, G. B., Wang, X., & Agrawal, C. M. (2000). Microstructural heterogeneity and the fracture toughness of bone. *J. Biomed. Mater. Res.*, Vol.51, pp. 735-741, ISSN 0021-9304

Place, E. S., Evans, N. D., & Stevens, M. M. (2009). Complexity in biomaterials for tissue engineering. *Nature Materials*, Vol.8, No.6, pp. 457-470, ISSN 1476-1122

Rezwan, K., Chen, Q. Z., Blaker, J. J., & Boccaccini, A. R. (2006). Biodegradable and bioactive porous polymer/inorganic composite scaffolds for bone tissue engineering. *Biomaterials*, Vol.27, No.18, pp. 3413-3431, ISSN 0142-9612

Salgado, A. J., Coutinho, O. P., & Reis, R. L. (2004). Bone tissue engineering: State of the art and future trends. *Macromolecular Bioscience*, Vol.4, No.8, pp. 743-765, ISSN 1616-5187

Scharnweber, D., Born, R., Flade, K., Roessler, S., Stoelzel, M., & Worch, H. (2004). Mineralization behaviour of collagen type I immobilized on different substrates. *Biomaterials*, Vol.25, No.12, pp. 2371-2380, ISSN 0142-9612

Schindeler, A., McDonald, M. M., Bokko, P., & Little, D. G. (2008). Bone remodeling during fracture repair: The cellular picture. *Seminars in Cell and Developmental Biology*, Vol.19, No.5, pp. 459-466, ISSN 1084-9521

Seal, B. L., Otero, T. C., & Panitch, A. (2001). Polymeric biomaterials for tissue and organ regeneration. *Materials Science & Engineering R-Reports*, Vol.34, No.4-5, pp. 147-230, ISSN 0927-796X

Song, J., Malathong, V., & Bertozzi, C. R. (2005). Mineralization of synthetic polymer scaffolds: A bottom-up approach for the development of artificial bone. *Journal of the American Chemical Society*, Vol.127, No.10, pp. 3366-3372, ISSN 0002-7863

Song, J., Saiz, E., & Bertozzi, C. R. (2003a). A new approach to mineralization of biocompatible hydrogel scaffolds: An efficient process toward 3-dimensional bonelike composites. *Journal of the American Chemical Society*, Vol.125, No.5, pp. 1236-1243, ISSN 0002-7863

Song, J., Saiz, E., & Bertozzi, C. R. (2003b). Preparation of pHEMA-CP composites with high interfacial adhesion via template-driven mineralization. *Journal of the European Ceramic Society*, Vol.23, No.15, pp. 2905-2919, ISSN 0955-2219

Song, J., Xu, J. W., Filion, T., Saiz, E., Tomsia, A. P., Lian, J. B., Stein, G. S., Ayers, D. C., & Bertozzi, C. R. (2009). Elastomeric high-mineral content hydrogel-hydroxyapatite composites for orthopedic applications. *Journal of Biomedical Materials Research Part A*, Vol.89A, No.4, pp. 1098-1107, ISSN 1549-3296

Stevens, M. M. (2008). Biomaterials for bone tissue engineering. *Materials Today*, Vol.11, No.5, pp. 18-25, ISSN 1369-7021

Stubbs, J. T., 3rd, Mintz, K. P., Eanes, E. D., Torchia, D. A., & Fisher, L. W. (1997). Characterization of native and recombinant bone sialoprotein: delineation of the mineral-binding and cell adhesion domains and structural analysis of the RGD domain. *J Bone Miner Res*, Vol.12, No.8, pp. 1210-1222, ISSN 0884-0431

Tan, K. H., Chua, C. K., Leong, K. F., Cheah, C. M., Cheang, P., Abu Bakar, M. S., & Cha, S. W. (2003). Scaffold development using selective laser sintering of polyetheretherketone-hydroxyapatite biocomposite blends. *Biomaterials*, Vol.24, No.18, pp. 3115-3123, ISSN 0142-9612

Tanner, K. E. (2010). Bioactive ceramic-reinforced composites for bone augmentation. *Journal of the Royal Society Interface*, Vol.7, pp. S541-S557, ISSN 1742-5689

Tanner, K. E. (2010). Bioactive composites for bone tissue engineering. *Proceedings of the Institution of Mechanical Engineers Part H-Journal of Engineering in Medicine,* Vol.224, No.H12, pp. 1359-1372, ISSN 0954-4119

Tong, W., Glimcher, M. J., Katz, J. L., Kuhn, L., & Eppell, S. J. (2003). Size and shape of mineralites in young bovine bone measured by atomic force microscopy. *Calcified Tissue International,* Vol.72, No.5, pp. 592-598, ISSN 0171-967X

Wang, M. (2003). Developing bioactive composite materials for tissue replacement. *Biomaterials,* Vol.24, No.13, pp. 2133-2151, ISSN 0142-9612

Wang, M., & Bonfield, W. (2001). Chemically coupled hydroxyapatite-polyethylene composites: structure and properties. *Biomaterials,* Vol.22, No.11, pp. 1311-1320, ISSN 0142-9612

Wang, Y. W., Wu, Q. O., & Chen, G. Q. (2004). Attachment, proliferation and differentiation of osteoblasts on random biopolyester poly(3-hydroxybutyrate-co-3-hydroxyhexanoate) scaffolds. *Biomaterials,* Vol.25, No.4, pp. 669-675, ISSN 0142-9612

Weiner, S., Traub, W., & Wagner, H. D. (1999). Lamellar bone: Structure-function relations. *Journal of Structural Biology,* Vol.126, No.3, pp. 241-255, ISSN 1047-8477

Weinstein, S. (2000). 2000-2010: The Bone and Joint Decade. *Journal of Bone and Joint Surgery American Volume,* Vol.82, pp. 1-3, ISSN 0021-9355

Xu, J., Li, X., Lian, J. B., Ayers, D. C., & Song, J. (2009). Sustained and localized in vitro release of BMP-2/7, RANKL, and tetracycline from FlexBone, an elastomeric osteoconductive bone substitute. *Journal of Orthopaedic Research,* Vol.27, No.10, pp. 1306-1311, ISSN 0736-0266

Yoshimoto, H., Shin, Y. M., Terai, H., & Vacanti, J. P. (2003). A biodegradable nanofiber scaffold by electrospinning and its potential for bone tissue engineering. *Biomaterials,* Vol.24, No.12, pp. 2077-2082, ISSN 0142-9612, ISSN 0142-9612

Yoshinari, M., Oda, Y., Ueki, H., & Yokose, S. (2001). Immobilization of bisphosphonates on surface modified titanium. *Biomaterials,* Vol.22, No.7, pp. 709-715, ISSN 0142-9612

Zhang, H. L., Simpson, D., Kumar, S., & Smart, R. S. C. (2006). Interaction of hydroxylated PACVD silica coatings on titanium with simulated body fluid. *Colloids and Surfaces a-Physicochemical and Engineering Aspects,* Vol.291, No.1-3, pp. 128-138, ISSN 0927-7757

Zhang, K., Ma, Y., & Francis, L. F. (2002). Porous polymer/bioactive glass composites for soft-to-hard tissue interfaces. *Journal of Biomedical Materials Research,* Vol.61, No.4, pp. 551-563, ISSN 0021-9304

Zhang, R. Y., & Ma, P. X. (1999). Poly(alpha-hydroxyl acids) hydroxyapatite porous composites for bone-tissue engineering. I. Preparation and morphology. *Journal of Biomedical Materials Research,* Vol.44, No.4, pp. 446-455, ISSN 0021-9304

Zheng, Y. N., Wu, G., Zhao, J., Wang, L. H., Sun, P., & Gu, Z. Y. (2010). rhBMP2/7 Heterodimer: An Osteoblastogenesis Inducer of Not Higher Potency but Lower Effective Concentration Compared with rhBMP2 and rhBMP7 Homodimers. *Tissue Engineering Part A,* Vol.16, No.3, pp. 879-887, ISSN 1937-3341

13

Bacterial Cellulose for Skin Repair Materials

Fu Lina[1,2], Zhang Yue[1], Zhang Jin[1,2] and Yang Guang[1,2]
[1]*College of Life Science and Technology,*
Huazhong University of Science and Technology, Wuhan
[2]*National Engineering Research Center for Nano-Medicine,*
Huazhong University of Science and Technology, Wuhan,
China

1. Introduction

As is well-known, cellulose is one of the most abundant biodegradable materials in nature and has been the topic of extensive investigations in macromolecular chemistry. It is of great importance to explore renewable natural polymeric materials to solve problems such as population growth, the energy crisis, environment polution, etc. Presently, human beings can produce cellulose by four means. Two of these are by natural synthesis procedures including plant photosynthesis and microbial synthesis. The other two methods are synthetic and enzymatic synthesis from cellobiose fluoride *in vitro* and the ring-opening polymerization of new carbonyl derivatives such as nitralin. Over the past 30 years, with the development of molecular biology and the application of cell systems *in vitro*, the mechanism underlying the biosynthesis of cellulose in nature has been extensively explored. Recently, environmental standards have been enhanced for every product and process. Employing new technologies or redesigning products is thus necessary to meet these new environmental standards (El-Saied et al., 2004).

Bacterial cellulose (BC, also known as microbial cellulose, MC) is a promising natural polymer synthesized by certain bacteria. Because of its unique structural and mechanical properties as compared to higher plant cellulose, BC is expected to become a commodity material in various fields. The BC fibers have a high aspect ratio with a diameter of 20-100 nm. As a result, BC has a very high surface area per unit mass. This property, combined with its highly hydrophilic nature, results in a very high liquid loading capacity. Morever, biocompatibility makes it an attractive candidate for a wide range of applications in different fields, especially those related to biomedical and biotechnology applications (Dahman, 2009). The fibrous structure of BC consists of a three-dimensional non-woven network of nanofibrils, sharing the same chemical structure as plant cellulose, which is held together by inter- and intra-fibrilar hydrogen bonding resulting in a never-dry hydrogel state with high strength.

The biosynthetic pathways of BC, including those involving enzymes and precursors, have been described (Chawla et al., 2009). These cellulosic materials are particularly attractive because of their relatively low cost and plentiful supply. Thus, BC utilization is responsible for one of the largest material flows in the biosphere and is of interest in relation to the analysis of carbon flux at both local and global scales (Lynd et al., 2002). Plenty of work has been devoted to designing ideal biomedical devices from BC. Such devices are advantageous in terms of their high paper-like reflectivity, flexibility, contrast, and biodegradability (Iguchi et al., 2000, Klemm, 2006). Besides, BC has proven to be a remarkably versatile biomaterial and can be used in a wide variety of products such as paper, electronics, acoustics and so on. Cellulose has always been the prime medium for displaying information in our society and is far better than the various existing display technologies. The BC device has the potential to be extended to countless other applications such as e-book tablets, e-newspapers, dynamic wall papers, rewritable maps, and learning tools (Shah, 2005). Olsson et al. used freeze-dried bacterial cellulose nanofibril aerogels as templates to make lightweight porous magnetic aerogels, which can be compacted into a stiff magnetic nanopaper (Olsson et al., 2010). As intuitionistic introduction, the biomedical applications of BC are shown in Figure 1.

However, in most practical applications, BC may not be of perfect quality and its cost may not be suituable for industrialization either. For economical mass production, it is essential to design a culture aeration and agitation process (Yoshinaga, 1997; Yamanaka, 1998). This chapter will discuss the biosynthesis of BC and its application as skin tissue repair material. The skin tissue materials derived from BC may create a luciferous future.

In this chapter, we focus on the applications of BC as skin tissue repair materials. Specifically, we summarize the basic properties, different types of BC, and research on BC for the purpose of applying BC to skin tissue engineering. Experimental results and clinical treatments have demonstrated good performance of BC-based wound healing materials. Further, all the results indicate that BC as skin tissue material in the biomedical field will continue to be important in the future.

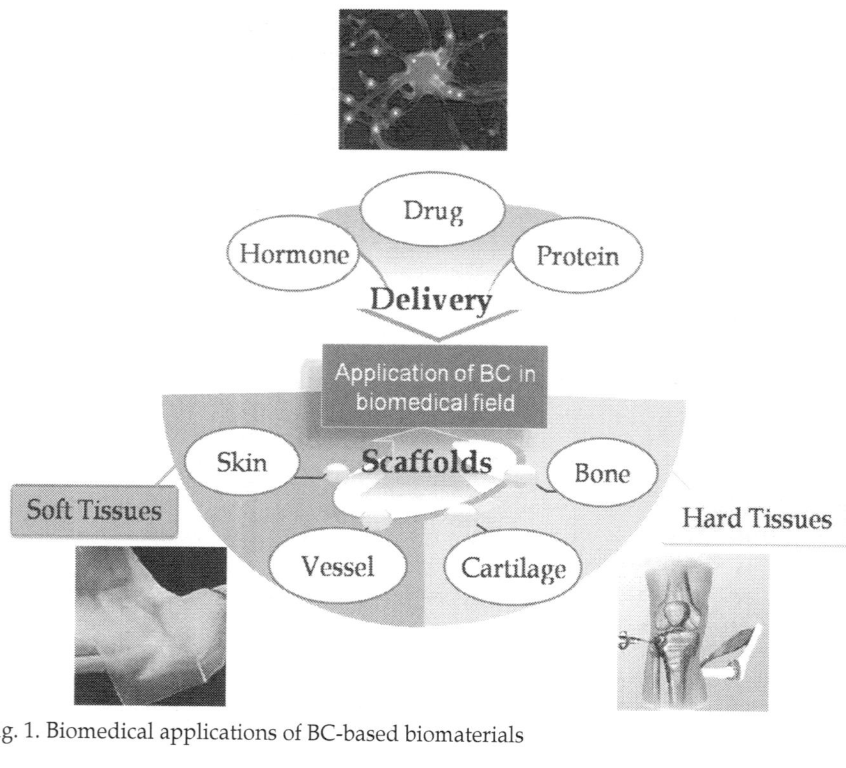

Fig. 1. Biomedical applications of BC-based biomaterials

2. Structure and properties of Bacterial Cellulose

2.1 Structure of BC

Based on X-ray investigations, the orientational state of polymers in general can be defined. BC membranes exhibit uniplanar orientation and an additional axial orientational component that depends on the drying procedure. It is possible to produce uniplanar-axial orientation by drawing, the degree of uniplanar and especially uniaxial orientation depending on the drawing conditions (Bohn et al., 2000). In 1984, VanderHart & Atalla investigated various cellulose samples by Nuclear Magnetic Resonance (NMR) spectroscopy and found that all natural cellulose was a complex of both I_{α} and I_{β} forms, and the content of I_{α} was about 65% in BC (VanderHart & Atalla, 1984). The study of Hirai et al. showed that decreased I_{α}-cellulose content led to smaller microfibrils in BC (Hirai et al., 1998). Generally, a uniplanar texture with the $(1\bar{1}0)$ planes parallel to the fiber surface and an axial component in the drawing direction were found. As compared to wet aqueous samples, a higher coherent deformation of BC can be achieved by soaking the samples in NaOH solutions with concentration ranging from 8 to 10 wt %. In the presence of lye, significant improvement (up to 100%) in axial chain orientation can be obtained, resulting in a maximum strength of 580 MPa. Improved orientability is likely due to a NaOH-induced reduction in the number of inter-fibrillar bridging points formed by H-bonds (Bohn et al., 2000).

The analysis based on the simple spin diffusion theory for the process experimentally observed reveals that the upfield carbons may be located at a distance less than about 1 nm from the downfield carbons in ^{13}C spin diffusion measurements. It was found that the downfield and upfield carbons were almost equally subjected to ^{1}H spin diffusion from the poly (vinyl alcohol) phase, indicating that the upfield carbons were not localized in some limited area, e.g. in the surfacial region, but were distributed throughout the whole area in the microfibrils. These experimental results suggested that the C4U carbons might exist as structural defects, probably due to conformational irregularity associated with disordered hydrogen bonding of the CH_2OH groups in the microfibrils (Masuda et al., 2003).

2.2 Characterization of bound water

BC is a gel containing 99% of water by weight, mainly due to its amorphous structure. Unfortunately, comparing the water holding capacities of different BC samples is difficult because different methods have been used. Drying under vacuum (10 mm H_2O or 98 Pa) was found to be preferable to stabilize the sample prior to determining its wet weight. This simple method lowered the standard deviation on the measurements by 50% or more as compared to other methods (Schrecker & Gostomski, 2005). According to dielectric spectroscopy and electron microscopy, the majority of the water molecules is tightly bound to BC, while only 10% out of the 99 wt% water presenting in BC gels behaves like free bulk water (Gelin et al., 2007).

The sorption properties of BC gel films were studied by Baklagina et al. The crystal structure of BC remained unchanged when polyvinylpyrrolidone or its complex with silver nanoparticles was incorporated into its matrix. By washing with distilled water, polyvinylpyrrolidone was readily removed from composite gel films of BC and polyvinylpyrrolidone or Poviargol without causing any changes in the cellulose structure and the amount of the adsorbed silver (Baklagina et al., 2005).

2.3 Mechanical properties

Recent studies have shown that atomic force microscopy can be used to measure the elastic modulus of suspended fibers by performing a nanoscale three-point bending test, in which the center of the fiber is deflected by a known force. By calculating the displacement with respect to the applied strain, it was shown that the stiffness of a single fibril of BC could be estimated. To demonstrate this concept, Guhados et al. have measured Young modulus of BC fibers with diameters ranging from 35 to 90 nm at a value of 78 ± 17 Gpa. This value was considerably higher than previous estimates obtained from the mechanical strength of individual cellulose fibers (Guhados et al., 2005). The modulus was also predicted from a calibration curve for a Raman band shift against modulus, based on previously published data, and by using Krenchel analysis to back-calculate the modulus of a single fibril. The value obtained (114 GPa) was higher than those reported previously, but lower than estimates from the modulus of crystalline cellulose-I (130-145 GPa) (Hsieh et al., 2008).
The fermentation time had a large effect on both the number of bacteria and the cellulose yield, but only minor effects on the mechanical properties, indicating that the fermentation technique is a robust method for the production of cellulose with predictable properties. A study by McKenna et al. showed that an increase in the fermentation time could led to a decrease in mechanical strength, Young's modulus first increasing and then decreasing after 96 h. Treatment with NaOH had minimal effects on the mechanical properties. The failure zone in uniaxial tension was shown to be associated with large-scale fibre alignment, this being a major determinant of mechanical properties. As was expected, the elastic modulus and failure stress under uniaxial tension were one order of magnitude lower than the values obtained under biaxial tension, since a fibre alignment mechanism is not available under biaxial tension. BC behaves like a viscoelastic material, brittle failure being reached at approximately 20% strain and 1.5 MPa stress under uniaxial tension (McKenna et al., 2009).
Compression pressure has been found to be an important parameter controlling the final mechanical properties of BC films: Slightly enhanced tensile strength and deformation at break were obtained by increasing the molding compression pressure, while the modulus also decreased nearly linearly with increasing film porosity. This behavior was related to higher densification under the increased mold compression pressure which reduced the interfibrillar space, thus increasing the probability of interfibrillar bonding (Retegi et al., 2010).

2.4 Rheology properties

Rheological analysis was developed to evaluate the fibril width and length of disintegrated BC. During the early stage of the disintegration process, the BC particles formed loose fibrous aggregates, followed by cutting of the disintegrated fibrils that produced short fibrils. On the other hand, the fibril width decreased steadily throughout the disintegration process. The relationships between fibril structure and suspension properties were analyzed. The thinner and longer the disintegrated bacterial cellulose fibrils were, the higher the viscosity and water-holding capacity became (Ougiya et al., 1998).
To characterize the mixing of BC culture broth, which can affect the productivity of BC, non-Newtonian behavior during mixing of a 1% BC suspension was studied using an image processor capable of detecting color changes for a pH indicator and was compared with that of a 2% carboxy methyl cellulose (CMC) solution. The CMC solution was mixed homogeneously within the measured range of agitation speeds, while the BC suspension was not homogeneously mixed at agitation speeds lower than 15 rps because mixing was

delayed in some areas of the vessel. A possible reason for the inhomogeneity of the BC suspension at low agitation speeds is the non-Newtonian behavior which increases viscosity at low shear rates (Kouda et al., 1996).
For the three kinds of cellulose solutions, the values of $\eta_0 - \eta_s$ (η_0: zero-shear viscosity of the solution, η_s: solvent viscosity) were in proportion to the weight fraction of polymer, φ_w, in the dilute solution regime. The plateau modulus, G_N, was proportional to φ_w^2 for Cotton linter solutions, signifying that an entangled network structure was formed in the cotton linter solution, as is often observed for solutions of flexible synthetic polymers. On the other hand, the concentrated solution of BC typically displayed small-angle X-ray scattering (SAXS) profiles typical of two-phase systems (Tamai et al., 2003).

3. Bio-fabrication of Bacterial Cellulose

Biodegradable composites made entirely from renewable resources are urgently sought after to improve material recyclability. Many biobased polymers and natural fibers usually display poor interfacial adhesion in composite materials. To modify the surface of natural fibers, BC was utilized as substrates for bacteria during fermentation of BC (Pommet et al., 2008).
The fabrication of a BC network sheet was attempted by heat-pressing in metal molds with a micro pattern to open a pathway to potentially versatile materials. A structural hydrophobic similar to the "Lotus effect" on this sheet was thus examined by introducing a micro-lattice pattern onto its surface. Indeed, the surface of the sheet was found to be more hydrophobic when the structural hydrophobic effect and the synergistic effects of heating and micro-patterning were combined (Tomita et al., 2009).

3.1 Self-assembled and oriented Bacterial Cellulose

Potato and corn starch were added to the culture medium and partially gelatinized in order to allow BC nanofibrils to grow in the presence of a starch phase. The BC-starch gels were hot pressed into sheets with a BC volume fraction higher than 90%. During this step, starch was forced to further penetrate the BC network. The self-assembled BC-starch nanocomposites displayed coherent morphologies (Grande et al., 2009).
Since the oxygen produced by the electrolysis of water in the culture media is far from the liquid-air boundary, aerobic cellulose production into 3D structures is readily achievable. Five separate sets of experiments were conducted to demonstrate the assembly of nanocellulose by *A. xylinum* (*G. Xylinus*) in the presence of electric fields in micro-and macro-environments, which demonstrated a new concept of bottom up material synthesis through a biological assembly process (Sano et al., 2010).
The effect of agar plates on BC production in a static culture medium was investigated in order to reveal the role of the agar component as a surface-modifying agent. The maximum water holding capacity value 92.21 g/g was measured for BC formed in reactors modified with 3.0% of agar. The maximum production rate was observed after the second day of cultivation as compared to the third day of cultivation in the case of the control experiment without agar (Shah et al., 2010).
BC with an unoriented microfibril network forms at the air-liquid interface (BC-air), while BC gel can be produced on an oxygen-permeable substrate such as polydimethylsiloxane (PDMS). The gel thus obtained shows strong birefringence with colorful images in polarized light microscopy, which is typical of liquid crystal-like structures. The optimum ridge size of

4.5 μm was related to the contour length of the bacteria cells. The fracture stress (σ) of uniaxially oriented BC gel under elongation was 4.6 MPa, which was 2.3 times higher than that of the BC-air material (σ = 2 MPa) (Putra et al., 2008).

The extraction and refinement of high-strength crystalline microfibril bundles (15-20 nm thick) from BC networks was investigated, as well as their morphology prior to and post electrospinning. The diameter of the fibers decreased significantly with increasing cellulose contents from about 1.8 μm (1 wt %) to about 100 nm (20 wt %). The nominal content of cellulose in the fibers was assessed by Lorentzian profile fit assignment of the crystalline phase, and the results showed significantly improved thermal stability for the composite material. The fibers were aligned into an anisotropic nanocomposite during spinning (Olsson et al., 2010).

3.2 Magnetic Bacterial Cellulose

Uniform magnetic membranes can be obtained from microfibrillar bacterial cellulose suspensions loaded with nanosized ferrites (mainly magnetite). The cellulose microfibrils act as a nucleation site for the growing ferrites (Sourty et al., 1998). Ferrites were thus synthetized in situ in two different neutral cellulose gels: a never-dried bacterial cellulose membrane and a never-dried film cast from N-methylmorpholine-N-oxide. The results showed the presence of ferrites in two different shapes, acicular and equiaxial, respectively corresponding to hydrated ferric oxides (FeOOH) and the spinel oxides (maghemite, γ-Fe_2O_3, or magnetite, Fe_3O_4). Thin sections of bacterial cellulose showed that these particles were located along the cellulose microfibrils, which were assumed to provide sites for the nucleation of these particles. Room temperature magnetization curves showed that all the samples were superparamagnetic (Sourty et al., 1998). Bacterial cellulose, with its porous network structure, was also used as an accelerator to precipitate Ni nanoparticles by the room temperature chemical reduction of $NiCl_2$ hexahydrate. Interestingly, BC did not undergo any change and retained its crystal structure even after the chemical reduction reaction. The fraction of isolated superparamagnetic nanoparticles present in the composite was estimated from the saturation magnetization and found to be around 88% (Vitta et al., 2010).

3.3 Modification of Bacterial Cellulose

The process of modifying large quantities of natural fibers with BC was investigated, and the adhesion between the modified fibers and renewable polymers such as cellulose acetate butyrate and poly(L-lactic acid) was quantified by employing the single fiber pullout test (Bodin, 2010), providing new ideas for the modification of BC. Natural fibers have been modified for the reinforcement of polymers, for example by producing a diblock copolymer of BC and poly(methyl methacrylate) (BC-block-PMMA) through the mechanical fracture of BC with MMA (methyl methacrylate) in vacuum at 77 K. The radical polymerization of MMA was initiated by the mechanoradicals located on the BC surface, which was fully covered with the PMMA chains of the BC-block-PMMA (Sakaguchi et al., 2010).

A novel copolymer of polylactide and glycidyl methacrylate (PLA-co-PGMA) was prepared and used to modify the BC surface. PLA-co-PGMA was efficient at modifying the surface of BC nanofibrils and improving the compatibility of PLA/cellulose composites (Li et al., 2010). Moreover, polylactide-graft-methacryloxypropyltrimethoxysilane (PLA-g-MPS) was prepared by grafting MPS onto PLA, and then used to modify BC. The results revealed that the modified BC possessed a much more hydrophobic nature than virgin BC (Li et al., 2010).

3.4 Multiform Bacterial Cellulose

The field of application of BC synthesized by *A. xylinum* under agitated culture conditions is narrower than for cellulose produced statically. This is mainly due to the smaller crystallite size of the microfibrils produced in agitated cultures. A mechanism was proposed to explain BC sphere formation from the microfibrils and cell arrangement in agitated cultures. During agitation, the cells were stacked in organized groups around the outer surface of the cellulose spheres (Czaja et al., 2004). Spherelike BC formaion has been investigated as a function of agitation speed and flask size. The analysis of lyophilized spherelike cellulose particles indicated that the agitation speed of the culture had an impact on the internal structure of the spherelike particles. The smaller spherelike particles produced at 150 rpm were hollow and their cellulose shell exhibited a layered structure. The larger particles produced at 125 rpm, and the cellulose in the central region did not exhibit a layered structure, while the outer layer was similar in structure to the particles produced at 150 rpm (Hu et al., 2010).

Phase separation phenomena in aqueous suspensions of BC nanocrystals obtained by sulfuric acid hydrolysis have been studied. Suspensions at concentration above 0.42 wt % separated into isotropic and chiral nematic phases with a clear phase boundary. The size of the ordered domains in the anisotropic phase decreased with NaCl concentrations in the range from 0 to 2.75 mM. At 2.75 mM only tactoids were observed in the entire region, while at 5.0 mM, chiral nematic domains were no longer observed. The chiral nematic pitch decreased as the concentration of NaCl incvreased, reaching a minimum value at approximately 0.75 mM, and then increased sharply with the NaCl concentration up to 2.0 mM (Hirai et al., 2009). Obtaining a well-dispersed suspension is a prerequisite when preparing smooth model surfaces based on neutral bacterial cellulose nanocrystals (BCNs). However, neutral nanocrystal suspensions suffer from pronounced particle aggregation. Carboxymethyl cellulose (CMC) or xyloglucan (XG) were added to the aggregated BCN suspensions to minimize this problem. CMC enhanced the dispersion of BCN above a concentration ratio of 0.05. In the case of XG, enhanced colloidal stability was observed above a concentration ratio of 0.5. The results obtained demonstrated that cellulose-based model surfaces obtained by spin-coating from CMC/BCN or XG/BCN solutions exhibited a more uniform topography and less surface roughness than the reference unmodified BCN model surface (Winter et al., 2010).

4. Skin tissue repair materials from Bacterial Cellulose

Owing to its unique nano-scaled three-dimensional network structure, BC has a high water retention, high mechanical strength, and outstanding biocompatibility, which enable it to serve as a natural scaffold material for the regeneration of a wide variety of tissues (MacNeil, 2007; Siró, 2010; Klemm, 2006; Czaja, 2006). For most repair materials, important characteristic are their ability to lock exudate during the dressing process, as well as their removal from a wound surface after recovery. Traditionally, skin tissue repair materials have been absorbent, permeable materials. For example gauze, a traditional dressing material, can adhere to desiccated wound surfaces and induce trauma on removal of the dressing. Recently, interest in cellulose produced by bacteria from surface cultures has increased steadily because of its potential for application in medicine and cosmetics (Hornung et al., 2009). On one hand, its potential lies in the unique properties (such as the high mechanical strength) of the never-dried BC membrane; on the other hand, its high liquid absorbency, biocompatibility and hygienic nature perfectly cater to the specific demands for skin tissue repairing. Thus, considering the properties of BC as well as its clinical performance, the commercialization of BC for wound care is very promising (Czaja et al., 2006).

4.1 Basic properties of skin tissue repair materials

Compared to plant cellulose, BC has features such as a high crystallinity, tensile strength and water absorption capacity; good permeability; biocompatibility; resistance to degradation and a low solubility that may be advantageous features for skin tissue materials. The BC pellicle has an asymmetric structure composed of a fine network of nanofibrils similar to a collagen network. The shape of the stress-strain response curve of BC is reminiscent of the stress-strain response of the carotid artery, most probably due to the similar architecture of both types of nanofibrill networks (Backdahl et al., 2006). The freezable bound water behaves like water confined within pores rather than a typical polymer solvent, and it is possible to use the Gibbs-Thomson equation based on thermoporosimetry to obtain information on the pore structure of BC. In comparison with nitrogen adsorption, it was found that thermoporosimetry underestimated the porosity of BC, which may be due to a large non-freezable water fraction interacting with cellulose (Kaewnopparat et al., 2008).

The water vapor permeability of air-dried BC is quite excellent because of the presence of a large number of hydroxyl groups. BC membranes are highly selective to water; the highest selectivity observed [$\alpha(p) = 186$] was obtained for a mixture of trihydric alcohol viz. glycerol (Gly) with 40% (v/v) water. The binary system of monohydric alcohol viz. ethanol (EtOH) and water (40% (v/v)) showed the lowest selectivity [$\alpha(p) = 12$] but the highest pervaporative flux of 614 $g{\cdot}m^{-2}{\cdot}h$ at 35 °C, which further increased to 1429 $g{\cdot}m^{-2}{\cdot}h$ at 75 °C. However, the selectivity also decreased to 1.3 with the increase in temperature. The pervaporation behaviour was interpreted in terms of sorption and diffusivity of the organics, which in turn was influenced by the extent of their hydrogen bonding with the cellulose units in the membrane and the plasticization induced by the permeating water present in the binary mixture (Pandey et al., 2005).

4.2 Biocompatibility of skin tissue repair materials

BC is advantageous as engineered skin tissue material. However, little information is available concerning the potential toxicity of BC-based biomaterials. The toxicity of BC nanofibers was evaluated *in vitro* through cell viability and flow cytometric assays and *in vivo* using C57/B16 mice surgeries. The microscopic morphology of the human umbilical vein endothelial cells (HUVEC) was also examined following culture in the absence of the cellulose nanofibers and with nanofibers for 24 h and 48 h. No obvious difference in morphology was observed (Jeong et al., 2010).

After co-culture with fibroblasts (FB) and chondrocytes, respectively, BC compositions were implanted into nude mice. The BC co-culture composition was well integrated into the skin of nude mice. Thus, it is natural to conclude that BC was beneficial to cell attachment and proliferation under these conditions (Wang et al., 2009).

Helenius et al. implanted BC subcutaneously into rats and evaluated the implants with respect to chronic inflammation, foreign body responses, cell ingrowth, and angiogenesis through histology, immunohistochemistry, and electron microscopy. There were no macroscopic signs of inflammation around the implants: No fibrotic capsule or giant cells were present. Fibroblasts infiltrated BC, which was well integrated into the host tissue and did not elicit any chronic inflammatory reactions (Helenius et al., 2006). The *in vitro* evaluation of the interactions between cells and BC was performed through viability staining analysis on the cells grown on the biomaterial, and showed that 95% of the mesenchymal stem cells aggregating to the cellulose membrane were alive and that 5% were necrotic. Scanning electron microscopy showed that mesenchymal stem cells were morphologically normal and attached to the cellulose membrane surface (Mendes et al., 2009).
The attachment of cells to biomedical materials can be improved by utilizing adhesive amino acid sequences, such as Arg-Gly-Asp (RGD), found in several extracellular matrix proteins. To improve the cell biocompatibility of BC, Andrade et al. grafted RGD onto BC films that exhibited improved biocompatibility (Andrade et al., 2010). In order to enhance cell affinity, BC was also modified with nitrogen plasma. The treatment did not increase the wettability of the material, but increased its porosity and modified its surface chemistry, as demonstrated by the presence of nitrogen. The potential of plasma treatment for the surface modification of BC was demonstrated by Pertile et al. (Pertile et al., 2010). Specially, microporous BC scaffolds were seeded with urine-derived stem cells, which were induced to differentiate into urothelial and smooth muscle cells (Bodin, 2010).

4.3 Composites of Bacterial Cellulose

While BC can be used as skin tissue repair material, it has no significant influence on the biochemical state of chronic wounds. To improve the positive features of BC as wound dressing material, it was modified by the incorporation of collagen type I into a cellulose pellicle. The modified biomaterial was able to reduce the adsorbed amounts of certainproteases and interleukins significantly and possessed a distinct antioxidant capacity as well (Wiegand et al., 2006).
Double-network (DN) hydrogels with high mechanical strength were synthesized from BC and gelatin. The fracture strength and elastic modulus of a BC-gelatin DN gel under compressive stress were on the order of megapascals, which is several orders of magnitude higher than for a gelatin gel, and almost equivalent to articular cartilage. Similar enhancement in the mechanical strength was also observed for a combination of BC with polysaccharides such as sodium alginate, gellan gum, and i-carrageenan (Nakayama et al., 2004). For example, the membrane with 80 wt % BC/20 wt % alginate displayed a homogeneous structure and exhibited enhanced water adsorption capacity and water vapor transmission rate. Supercritical carbon dioxide drying was used for the formation of a nanoporous structure. However, the tensile strength and elongation at break of a film with a thickness of 0.09 mm decreased to 3.38 MPa and 31.60%, respectively. The average pore size of the blend membrane was 10.6 Å with a 19.5 m^2/g specific surface area (Phisalaphong et al., 2008). Beside the composite with alginate, BC and gelatin were also selected to prepare membranes and the morphology of Swiss mouse embryo fibroblast NIH/3T3 cells grown on the surface of these membranes was examined to select the best material for the development of a biodegradable skin tissue regeneration template. Membranes derived cow bone gelatin and fish skin gelatin were stronger and more flexible than those prepared from pork skin gelatin in their wet forms (New et al., 2010).

To develop functional property, a freeze-dried BC film was immersed in a benzalkonium chloride solution, a cationic surfactant and antimicrobial agent, followed by another freeze-drying step. It was showed that the drug-loading capacity of the BC dry film was about 0.116 mg/cm^2 when soaked in 0.102% benzalkonium chloride solution (Fig. 2). As to the antimicrobial activity, a stable and prolonged activity was observed for at least 24 h, especially against *Staphylococcus aureus* and *Bacillus subtilis*, two Gram-positive bacteria generally found on contaminated wounds (Wei et al., 2011).

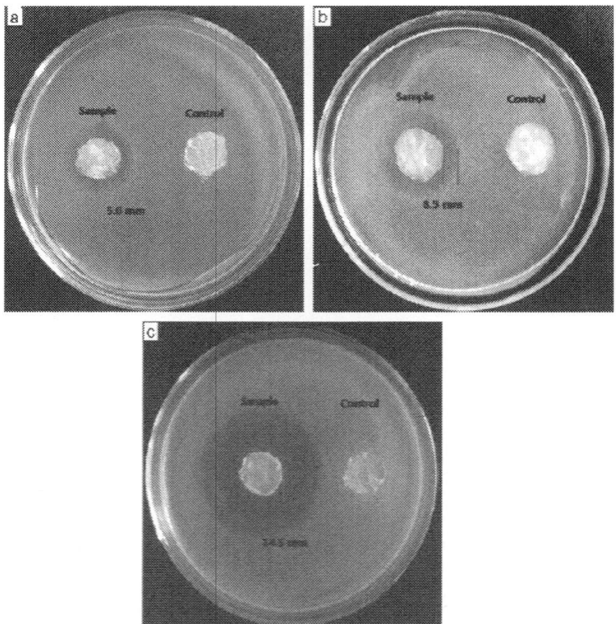

Fig. 2. Comparison of the antibacterial activity of benzalkonium chloride-containing BC dry films and BC without drug as control against (a) *Escherichia coli*, (b) *Staphylococcus aureus*, and (c) *Bacillus subtilis*. (Reproduced with the permission from Wei, B. et al. (2011). Preparation and evaluation of a kind of bacterial cellulose dry films with antibacterial properties, Carbohydrate Polymers, Vol. 84, No.1, pp.536. Copyright (2011) Elsevier)

BC was formed and coated on cotton gauze samples during its biosynthesis. The composite obtained displayed more than 30% increase in water absorbency and wicking ability, and a 33% reduction in drying time as compared to untreated gauze (Meftahi et al., 2010).
The interactions between BC fibrils and aloe vera gel were investigated by Saibuatong et al. With a 30% v/v aloe gel supplement in the culture medium, the fibre-reinforced bio-polymer film obtained displayed significantly improved properties in terms of mechanical strength, crystallinity, water absorption capacity, and water vapor permeability in comparison to unmodified BC films. The average pore size of the modified films either in the dry or re-swollen form was decreased to approximately 1/5 of the unmodified BC films, while a narrow pore size distribution was maintained (Saibuatong et al., 2010).

BC/poly (ethylene glycol) (PEG) composites were prepared by immersing wet BC pellicle in PEG aqueous solutions followed by freeze-drying. Scanning electron microscope (SEM) images showed that the PEG molecules not only coated on the BC fibrils surface but also penetrated into the BC fiber network. It was found that PEG affected the preferential orientation of the $(1\bar{1}0)$ plane during drying of the BC pellicle, which in turn decreased the crystallinity of the dried BC film. Thermogravimetric analysis (TGA) results showed that the thermal stability was improved from 263 to 293 degrees C, which may be associated with strong interactions between BC and PEG. Biocompatibility of the composite was preliminarily evaluated by cell adhesion studies using 3T3 fibroblast cells. Incubation of the cells with the BC/PEG scaffolds accelerated cell adhesion and proliferation (Cai et al., 2010). Various BC composites have displayed enhanced applicability as skin tissue repair materials (Table 1).

Component	Effect	References
Collagen	Reduced sorption of proteases and interleukins	Wiegand et al., 2006
DN gelatin hydrogels	Enhanced mechanical strength	Nakayama et al., 2004
Alginate	Changed tensile strength and elongation at break	Phisalaphong et al., 2008; New et al., 2010
Benzalkonium chloride	Stable and prolonged antimicrobial activity	Wei et al., 2011
PEG	Decreased crystallinity, improved thermal stability	Cai et al., 2010
Cotton gauze	Increased water absorbency, wicking and water retention ability	Meftahi et al., 2010
Aloe vera gel	Improved mechanical strength, crystallinity, water sorption capacity, and water vapor permeability	Saibuatong et al., 2010

Table 1. Composites of Bacterial cellulose

4.4 Nano-composites of Bacterial Cellulose and Ag

BC is an optimal material for skin tissue repair since it provides a moist environment to a wound, which is beneficial to healing. Unfortunately, BC itself has no antimicrobial activity to prevent wound infection. To achieve antimicrobial activity, silver nanoparticles and chitosan were combined with BC. Due to the electron-rich oxygen atoms in the BC macromolecules and the large surface area of nanoporous BC effective as nanoreactor, the *in situ* metallization technique was successfully applied to the synthesis of Ag and BC nano-composites, which could serve as antimicrobial skin tissue repair materials.

The composite was obtained by immersing BC in a silver nitrate solution, and sodium borohydride was used to reduce the absorbed silver ions (Ag^+) inside of BC to metallic silver nanoparticles (Fig.3). A red-shift and broadening of the optical absorption band was observed. The freeze-dried silver nanoparticle-impregnated BC exhibited strong antimicrobial activity against *Escherichia coli* (Gram-negative) and *Staphylococcus aureus* (Gram-positive) (Maneerung et al., 2008).

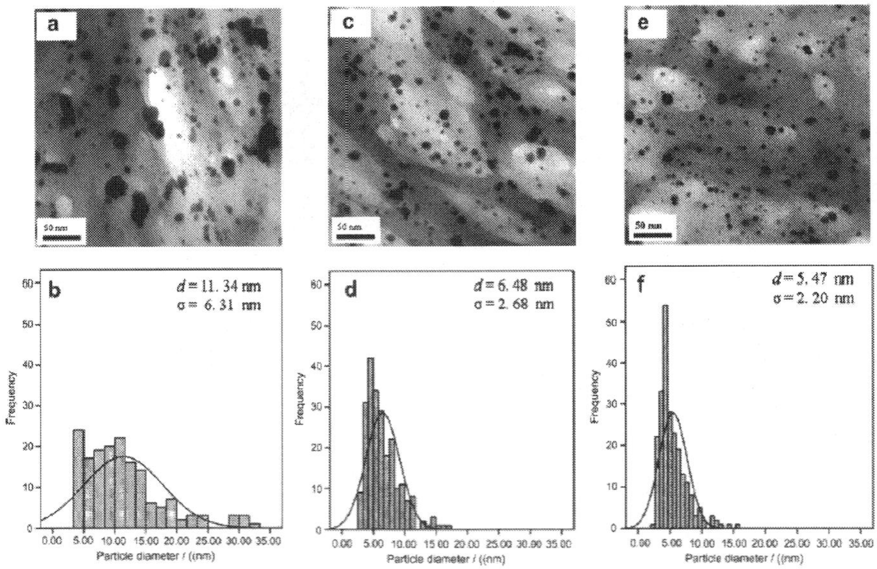

Fig. 3. TEM images and histograms of freeze-dried silver nanoparticle-impregnated bacterial cellulose prepared from a $NaBH_4$:$AgNO_3$ molar ratio of 1:1 (a and b), 10:1 (c and d) and 100:1 (e and f) (Reproduced with the permission from Maneerung, T et al. (2008) . Impregnation of silver nanoparticles into bacterial cellulose for antimicrobial wound dressing, Carbohydrate Polymers, Vol.72 , No. 1, pp. 48. Copyright (2008) Elsevier)

With absorbed silver nanoparticles and stabilized by N-polyvinylpyrrolidone, inhomogeneous nanoparticle in the BC gel film were synthesized. The dried composite had large particles located on the layer surface of cellulose (Volkov et al., 2009). Colloidal submicron Ag particles were prepared on BC *in situ*. Different reducing agents were compared (hydrazine, hydroxylamine or ascorbic acid) in combination with gelatin or polyvinylpyrrolidone employed as colloid protectors. The Ag cubic phase deposited oil to BC, which resulted in a high efficiency of silver loading (Maria et al., 2009).
To obtain the composite of BC and Ag, an ion exchange of the sodium to the silver salt was performed in an $AgNO_3$ solution, followed by thermal reduction. By using oxidized BC nanofibers as a reaction template, stable silver nanoparticles were prepared with a narrow size distribution and a high density, through strong ion interactions between the host carboxylate groups from BC and guest silver cations (Ifuku et al., 2009). The *in situ* synthesis of silver chloride (AgCl) nanoparticles was carried out under ambient condition by employing nanoporous BC membranes as nanoreactors. Growth of the nanoparticles was readily achieved by alternating dipping of BC membranes in solutions of silver nitrate and sodium chloride, followed by a rinsing step. The AgCl nanoparticle-impregnated BC membranes exhibited a high hydrophilicity and strong antimicrobial activity against *Escherichia coli* (Gram-negative) and *Staphylococcus aureus* (Gram-positive) (Hu et al., 2009). A

simple method was also developed to load a large amount of silver nanoparticles into BC. These composite fibers showed nearly 100% antibacterial activities against *Escherichia coli* (Maria et al., 2010).

A facile method was developed to prepare a magnetic Ag nanocomposite. The 3D nanofibrous structure of BC was first homogenized with a ferric and ferrous salt mixture on a high speed blender. The magnetite nanoparticles were precipitated and incorporated into the BC nanostructures by adjusting the homogenate to alkaline pH. The magnetic BC nanofiber, when soaked in dopamine solution, can be coated with an adherent self-polymerized polydopamine layer. Since the polydopamine surface is very effective for reducing the silver ion, Ag nanoparticles were incorporated into the dopamine-treated magnetic BC by soaking in silver nitrate solution. The magnetization of the as-prepared Ag nanocomposite was maintained, and the magnetic Ag nanocomposite possessed a high antimicrobial activity against the model microbes *Escherichia coli* and *Bacillus subtilis* (Sureshkumar et al., 2010).

4.5 Nano-composite of Bacterial Cellulose and chitosan

Nanocomposite films based on different chitosan matrices (chitosans with two different degrees of polymerization and one water-soluble derivative) and BC were prepared by casting the water-based suspension of chitosan and BC nanofibrils, which is a fully "green" procedure. The films were highly transparent, flexible, and displayed better mechanical properties than the corresponding unfilled chitosan films (Fernandes et al., 2009). BC/chitosan composite materials showed a high sensitivity to enzymatic degradation and bioactivity. This innovatively modified BC nevertheless represents a good value for biomedical applications (Ciechanska, 2004). The potential of chitosan/BC was compared with that of the parent polymers and with chitosan/poly(vinyl alcohol) blends (Dubey et al., 2005).

By varying the chitosan concentration and immersion time, a foam-like structure was obtained. With increasing chitosan content, the crystalline structure remained unchanged, but the crystallinity index tended to decrease. The tensile strength and Young's modulus of the composites tended to decrease with increasing chitosan content but the values were much higher than for pure chitosan (Cai et al., 2009). A family of polysaccharide-based BC/chitosan porous scaffold materials with various weight ratios (from 20/80 to 50/40 w/w %) were prepared by freezing (-30 and -80 degrees C) and lyophilization of a mixture of microfibrillated BC suspension and chitosan solution. The microfibrillated BC (MFC) was subjected to 2,2,6,6-tetramethylpyperidine-1-oxyl radical (TEMPO)-mediated oxidation to introduce surface carboxyl groups before mixing. The composite scaffolds had a three-dimensional open pore microstructure with pore sizes ranging from 120 to 280 µm with enhanced compressive moduli and strength (Nge et al., 2010).

4.6 Clinical treatment

Following standard care, nonhealing lower extremity (LE) ulcers were treated with a BC wound dressing, Dermafill ™, (AMD/Ritmed, Tonawanda, NY). The time required for 75% reduction in wound size was compared for 11 chronic wounds without and with the application of BC. The mean period of observation without the application of BC was 315 days; (95% CI: 239-392 days). With the application of BC to these chronic wounds, the mean time for 75% epithelization was reduced to 81 days (95% CI 50-111 days) with a median

value of 79 days. When applied to nonhealing LE ulcers, a BC wound dressing clearly shortens the time to wound closure over standard care (Portal et al., 2009).
Clinical trials were conducted on 34 patients suffered from severe thermal burns (second-degree A/B) covering 9-18% of the total body surface area (TBSA), 22 of the patients received the BC as testing group. The adherence of BC membrane to the wound surface was excellent to avoid any dead spaces because of its high conformability, and none of the patients using BC wound dressing during the trial developed any kind of hypersensitive reactions. By the tenth day of the treatment period, the process of reepithelialization had begun in 7 patients from the testing group (58.3%) in comparison with 4 patients (33.3%) from the control group. These results show that the application of BC dressing in the treatment of partial thickness burns promotes the creation of a favorable environment for fast wound cleansing, and consequently its rapid healing. It is worth mentioning that the release of the dressing from the wound was an entirely painless operation, due to the moisture still present in the never-dried cellulose structure (Czaja et al., 2007) .
The conformability and elastic properties of BC dressing allowed a high degree of adherence to the wound sites, even to the moving parts like hands (Fig. 4), torso, faces (Fig. 5) and so on. A complete closure of the wounded face with a single sheet of BC in which the holes for eyes, nose, and mouth were made after placement has been applied to a patient with the severe deep second-degree burns of the facial surface. After 44 days, the wounded face was entirely healed with no need for skin grafting and no significant signs of extensive scarring (Czaja et al., 2007).

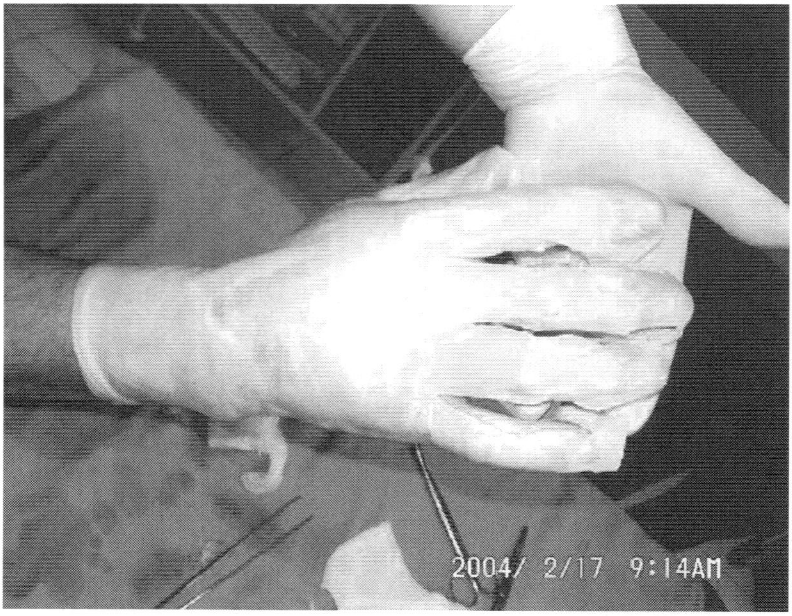

Fig. 4. Bacterial cellulose dressing applied on a wounded hand. (Reproduced with the permission from Czaja, W. et al . (2006). Microbial cellulose – the natural power to heal wounds, Biomaterials, Vol.27, No. 2, 149. Copyright (2006) Elsevier)

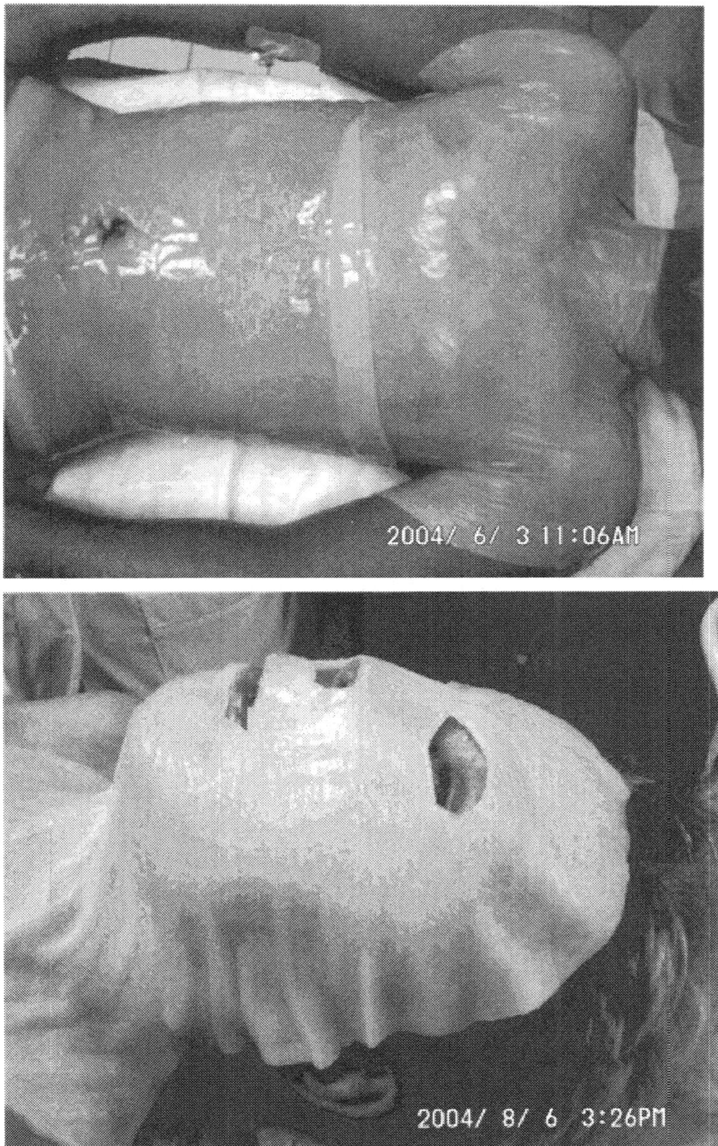

Fig. 5. Bacterial cellulose dressing applied on wounded torso and face. (Reprinted with permission from Czaja, W. K. et al. (2007). The future prospects of microbial cellulose in biomedical applications, Biomacromolecules, Vol.8, No.1, pp. 4. Copyright (2007) American Chemical Society)

In a randomized trial on predominantly category II and III skin tears in a population of frail elderly nursing home residents, standard wound care (24 residents) with Xeroform™ and a secondary dressing (Tegaderm™) was compared with a single application of BC Dermafill (27 residents). Outcomes included a decrease in the time to wound closure, pain reduction, and ease of use. Even though the wound area was slightly larger in the BC-treated group, the healing time was equivalent to the controls. However pain control, ease of use, and patient and nursing staff satisfaction were superior to the control experiments with the use of the BC skin tissue repair materials (Solway et al., 2010). Another test compared the rate of wound healing in diabetic foot ulcers (DFU) using either BC wound dressing or Xeroform™ Petrolatum gauze. In a parallel, open-label trial in which the primary outcome was the rate of wound healing and the time to wound closure, 15 ulcers in type II diabetic patients received a BC dressing. Wounds in 19 control patients with type II diabetes were treated with a Xeroform™ gauze dressing. All wounds were non infected Wagner stage II or III and received standard care including debridement, non-weight bearing limb support and weekly wound evaluation. With the provision of current care standards, the application of a BC dressing to a diabetic ulcer enhanced the rate of wound healing and shortened the epithelisation time (Solway et al., 2011). All treatments showed that using BC dressings or films was easy to manage because the patients exhibited a rapid rate of closure with the treatment. Therefore, clinical treatment with BC skin tissue repair materials can be considered an efficient method to treat acute and chronic wounds.

5. Patents

Since 1988, the interest in applications of BC has grown rapidly (Bielecki et al., 2005). Some patents concerning different aspects are presented in Table 2.

Material	Applications	Patents
Bacterial cellulose hydrogel	cold pack	[ZL 201020239963.4] (Li et al, 2011)
Bacterial cellulose-nano silver	Mask	[ZL 200910149665.8] (Zhong, 2011)
bacterial cellulose membrane	Membrane electrode	[ZL 200810022130.X] (Xu et al, 2011)
Metalized bacterial cellulose	Construction of fuel cells, electronic devices	[US 7,803,477 B2] (Evans et al., 2010), [US 2011 / 0014525 A1] [85] (Evans et al., 2011)
Bacterial cellulose network, cationic polymer	Personal cleansing compositions	[US 2011 / 0039744 A1] (Heath et al., 2011)
Bacterial cellulose	Cultural relics conservation	[ZL 200810246345.X] (Wu et al, 2011)
Bacterial cellulose	Skin tissue repair materials	[ZL 200810047793.7] (Yang et al., 2010)

Patterned bacterial cellulose	Smart materials	[ZL 200810047875.1] (Yang et al., 2010)
Novel bacterial cellulose	Food industry	[US 2010 / 0016575 A1] (Yang et al., 2010)
Poly(vinyl alcohol)- bacterial cellulose	Artificial dura mater	[ZL 200710015537.5] (Ma et al, 2010)
Palladized bacterial cellulose	Reductive conversion reactions	[US 2010 / 0126945 A1] (Patel & Suresh, 2010)
Bacterial cellulose network	Liquid detergent composition	[US 2010 / 0210501 A1] (Caggioni et al., 2010)
modified bacterium cellulose	Food wrap	[ZL 200810051298.3] (Yu et al, 2010)
Bacterial cellulose	Carbon nanotube-like thin films, cathode material, batteries	[US 2009 / 0309072 A1] (Hwang et al., 2009)
bacterial cellulose membrane	face mask	[ZL 200610075040.8] (Zhong, 2008)
Bacterial cellulose	Viscosity modifier	[US 2007 / 0197779 A1] (Yang et al., 2007)
Novel bacterial cellulose	Viscosity modifier	[US 2007 / 0027108 A1] (Yang et al., 2007)
Poly(vinyl alcohol)- bacterial cellulose nanocomposite	Soft tissue replacement, medical devices	[US 2005 / 0037082 A1] (Wan. & Millon, 2005)
Bacterial cellulose	Industry, clothes, medical supplies, food, functional materials	[US RE38,792 E] (Iguchi et al., 1988), [US 2004/ 0091978 A1] (Ishihara & Yamanaka, 2004), [US 2002/ 0065409 A1] (Ishihara & Yamanaka, 2002)
Bacterial cellulose	Yield improvement in BC production	[6,132,998] (Naritomi et al., 2000)
Bacterial cellulose	Improvement of the properties of paper	[6,069,136] (Tahara et al., 2000)
Bacterial cellulose	In creased BC production rate and yield	[6,017,740] (Kouda et al., 2000)
Bacterial cellulose	Increased BC production rate	[6,013,490] (Kouda et al., 2000)
Enzymatic detergent drain cleaners	Removal or prevention of BC growth	[5,975,095] (Ahmed et al., 1999)
Gelationous bacterial cellulose	Production of soft and light fibers	[5,962,676] (Tammarate, 1999)
Reticulated bacterial cellulose	Coating on a substantially continuous basis, coated products	[5,637,197] (Watt et al., 1997)

Reticulated bacterial cellulose	Reinforced elastomeric articles, pneumatic tires	[5,290,830] (Tung et al., 1994)
Bacterial cellulose	Banding agent	[5,207,826] (Westland et al., 1993)
Purified bacterial cellulose	Binding- suspended cholesterol or cholesterol esters	[4,960,763] (Stephen et al., 1990)
Bacterial cellulose	Replacement for latex binders	[4,919,753] (Johnson & Neon, 1990)
Bacterial cellulose	Printing materials	[4,861,427] (Johnson et al., 1989)
Bacterial cellulose	Molding material	[4,742,164](Iguchi et al., 1988)

Table 2. Applications of Bacterial Cellulose

6. Conclusions

Bacterial cellulose (BC) is a promising natural polymer with many applications, especially for skin tissue repairing. Many advantages of BC give it great potential in wound healing system, such as biocompatible, conformability, elasticity, transparency, ability to maintain a moist environment in the wound and absorb exudates during inflammatory phase, and so on. This chapter discussed the most recent developments in BC-based skin tissue repair materials, including their biosynthesis, methods of treatment, properties, and frontier research on BC skin tissue repair materials. The structure of native and modified BC having been studied intensively and biocompatibility having been evaluated, suggested that BC could function as a skin tissue repair material well. Different BC products having been successfully applied as skin tissue repair and wound dressing materials, confirmed this. In addition, BC could have other applications in wound healing and regenerative medicine, such as guided tissue regeneration, periodontal treatments, or as a replacement for dura mater (the membrane surrounding brain tissue). Last but not least, BC is valuable in tissue engineering applications including bone, cartilage, blood vessel engineering, and so on. In a conclusion, if BC can be successfully mass-produced, it will eventually become a vital biomaterial used in the creation of a wide variety of medical devices and consumer products.

7. Acknowledgments

It was supported by National Natural Science Foundation of China (20774033, 21074041), the Fundamental Research Funds for the Central Universities, Huazhong University of Science and Technology (2010JC016), and the Natural Science of Hubei Province for Distinguished Young Scholars (2008CDB279). The authors are also grateful Professor Mario Gauthier (University of Waterloo, Canada) and Mr. Bo Wang (University of Tennessee, USA) for their valuable suggestions during the preparation of this manuscript.

8. References

Ahmed, F. U.; Goldschmidt, J. E. & La Cosse, G. E. (1999). Enzymatic detergent composition and method degrading and removing bacterial cellulose and glycerides, *US Patent* 5,975,095

Andrade, F. K.; Moreira, S. M. G.; Domingues, L. & Gama, F. M. P. (2010). Improving the affinity of fibroblasts for bacterial cellulose using carbohydrate-binding modules fused to RGD, *Journal of Biomedical Materials Research Part A*, Vol. 92A, No.1, pp. 9-17

Backdahl, H.; Helenius, G.; Bodin, A.; Nannmark, U.; Johansson, B. R.; Risberg, B. & Gatenholm, P.(2006). Mechanical properties of bacterial cellulose and interactions with smooth muscle cells, *Biomaterials*, Vol. 27, No.9, pp. 2141-2149

Baklagina, Y. G.; Khripunov, A. K.; Tkachenko, A. A; Kopeikin, V. V; Matveeva, N. A.; Lavrent'ev, V. K.; Nilova, V. K.; Sukhanova, T. E.; Smyslov, R. Y.; Zanaveskina, I. S.; Klechkovskaya, V. V. & Feigin, L. A. (2005). Sorption properties of gel films of bacterial cellulose, *Russian Journal of Applied Chemistry*, Vol. 78, No. 7, pp. 1176-1181

Bielecki, S.; Krystynowicz, A.; Turkiewicz, M. & Kalinowska H. (2005). Bacterial Cellulose, *Biopolymers Online - Polysaccharides I : Polysaccharides from Prokaryotes*, 15 JAN, Vol.5, pp. 37-85

Bodin A.; Bharadwaj, S.; Wu S.; Gatenholm P.; Atala A. & Zhang Y. (2010) . Tissue-engineered conduit using urine-derived stem cells seeded bacterial cellulose polymer in urinary reconstruction and diversion, *Biomaterials*, Vol. 31, No.34, pp. 8889-8901

Bohn, A.; Fink, H. P.; Ganster, J. & Pinnow, M. (2000). X-ray texture investigations of bacterial cellulose, *Macromolecular Chemistry and Physics*, Vol. 201, No. 15, pp. 1913-1921

Bohn, A.; Fink, H. P.; Ganster, J. & Pinnow, M. (2005). Measurement of the elastic modulus of single bacterial cellulose fibers using atomic force microscopy, *Langmuir*, Vol.21 , No. 14, pp. 6642-6646

Caggioni, M.; Ortiz, R.; Barnabas, F. A.; Nunes, R. V.; Flood, J. A.& Corominas, F. (2010) Liquid detergent composition comprising an external structuring system comprising a bacterial cellulose network, *US Patent* 2010 / 0210501 A1

Cai, Z. & Kim, J. (2010). Bacterial cellulose/poly (ethylene glycol) composite: characterization and first evaluation of biocompatibility, *Cellulose*, Vol.17, No. 1, pp.83-91

Cai, Z.; Chen, P.; Jin, H. J. & Kim, J. (2009). The effect of chitosan content on the crystallinity, thermal stability, and mechanical properties of bacterial cellulose-chitosan composites, *Proceedings of the Institution of Mechanical Engineers Part C-Journal of Mechanical Engineering Science*, Vol.223, No.10, pp. 2225-2230

Chawla, P. R.; Bajaj, I. B.; Survase, S. A.; Singhal, R. S. (2009).Microbial Cellulose: Fermentative Production and Applications, *Food Technology And Biotechnology*, Vol.47, No.2, pp.107-124

Ciechanska, D. (2004). Multifunctional bacterial cellulose/chitosan composite materials for medical applications, *Fibres & Textiles in Eastern Europe*, Vol.12, No.4, pp.69-72

Czaja, W. K.; Young, D. J.; Kawecki, M. & Brown, R. M. (2007).The future prospects of microbial cellulose in biomedical applications, *Biomacromolecules*, Vol.8, No.1, pp.1-12

Czaja, W.; Krystynowicz, A.; Bielecki, S. & Brown, R. J. (2006) . Microbial cellulose – the natural power to heal wounds, *Biomaterials*, Vol.27, No. 2, 145-151

Czaja, W.; Krystynowicz, A.; Kawecki, M.; Wysota, K.; Sakiel, S.; Wróblewski, P.; Glik, J.; Nowak, M.; Bielecki, S. Biomedical Applications of Microbial Cellulose in Burn

Wound Recovery. Brown, R. M.; Jr. and I.M. Saxena (2007). *Cellulose: Molecular and Structural Biology*, Springer, 307–321

Czaja, W.; Romanovicz, D. & Brown, R. M. (2004). Structural investigations of microbial cellulose produced in stationary and agitated culture , *Cellulose*, Vol. 11, No.3-4, pp. 403-411

Dahman, Y. (2009). .Nanostructured Biomaterials and Biocomposites from Bacterial Cellulose Nanofibers, *Journal of Nanoscience and Nanotechnology*, Vol. 9, No. 9, pp.5105-5122

Dubey, V.; Pandey, L. K. & Saxena, C. (2005). Pervaporative separation of ethanol/water azeotrope using a novel chitosan-impregnated bacterial cellulose membrane and chitosan-poly (vinyl alcohol) blends, *Journal of Membrane Science*, Vol.251, No.1-2, pp. 131-136

El-Saied, H.; Basta, A. H. & Gobran, R. H. (2004). Research progress in friendly environmental technology for the production of cellulose products (bacterial cellulose and its application), *Polymer-Plastics Technology and Engineering*, Vol.43, No. 3, pp.797-820

Evans, B. R.; O'Neill, H. M.; Jansen, V. M.; Woodward, J. (2010). Metalization of bacterial cellulose for electrical and electronic device manufacture, *US Patent* 7,803,477 B2.

Evans, B. R.; O'Neill, H. M.; Jansen, V. M.; Woodward, J. (2011). Metalization of bacterial cellulose for electrical and electronic device manufacture, *US Patent* 2011 / 0014525 A1

Fernandes, S. C. M.; Oliveira, L.; Freire, C. S. R.; Silvestre, A. J. D.; Neto, C. P .; Gandini, A .; Desbrieres, J. (2009). Novel transparent nanocomposite films based on chitosan and bacterial cellulose, *Green Chemistry*, Vol.11, No. 12, pp.2023-2029

Gelin, K.; Bodin, A.; Gatenholm, P.; Mihranyan, A.; Edwards, K.; Stromme, M. (2007). Characterization of water in bacterial cellulose, *Polymer*, Vol.48, No.26, pp.7623-7631

Grande, C. J.; Torres, F. G.; Gomez, C. M.; Troncoso, O. P.; Canet-Ferrer, J. & Martinez-Pastor, J. (2009). Development of self-assembled bacterial cellulose-starch nanocomposites, *Materials Science & Engineering C-Biomimetic and Supramolecular Systems*, Vol.29, No. 4, pp.1098-1104

Heath, B. P.; Coffindaffer, T. W.; Kyte, K. E.; Smith, E. D. & McConaughy, S. D. (2011). Personal cleansing compositions comprising a bacterial cellulose network and cationic polymer, *US Patent* 2011 / 0039744 A1

Helenius, G.; Backdahl, H.; Bodin, A.; Nannmark, U.; Gatenholm, P. & Risberg, B. (2006). In vivo biocompatibility of bacterial cellulose, *Journal of Biomedical Materials Research Part A*, Vol. 76A, No.2, pp.431-438

Hirai, A.; Inui, O.; Horii, F. & Tsuji, M. (2009). Phase Separation Behavior in Aqueous Suspensions of Bacterial Cellulose Nanocrystals Prepared by Sulfuric Acid Treatment, *Langmuir*, Vol. 25, No. 1, pp. 497-502

Hornung, M.; Biener, R. & Schmauder, H. P. (2009). Dynamic modelling of bacterial cellulose formation, *Engineering in Life Sciences*, Vol. 9, No. 4, pp.342-347

Hsieh, Y. C.; Yano, H.; Nogi, M. & Eichhorn, S. J. (2008).An estimation of the Young's modulus of bacterial cellulose filaments, *Cellulose*, Vol.15, No. 4, pp. 507-513

Hu, W. L.; Chen, S. Y.; Li, X.; Shi, S. A. K.; Shen, W.; Zhang, X.; Wang, H. P. (2009). In situ synthesis of silver chloride nanoparticles into bacterial cellulose membranes,

Materials Science & Engineering C-Biomimetic and Supramolecular Systems, Vol.29, No. 4, pp.1216-1219

Hu, Y. & Catchmark, J. M. (2010). Formation and Characterization of Spherelike Bacterial Cellulose Particles Produced by *Acetobacter xylinum* JCM 9730 Strain, *Biomacromolecules*, Vol.11, No. 7, pp.1727-1734

Hwang, S.; Chen, H. & Hwang, B. (2009). Bacterial cellulose film and Carbon nanotubes-like thin film structures developed from bacterial cellulose, *US Patent* 2009 / 0309072 A1

Ifuku, S.; Tsuji, M.; Morimoto, M.; Saimoto, H. & Yano, H. (2009). Synthesis of Silver Nanoparticles Templated by TEMPO-Mediated Oxidized Bacterial Cellulose Nanofibers, *Biomacromolecules*, Vol.10 9, pp.2714-2717 SEP

Iguchi, M.; Mitsuhashi, S.; Ichimura, K.; Nishi, Y.; Uryu, M.; Yamanaka, S. & Watanabe, K. (1988). Bacterial cellulose-containing molding material having high dynamic strength, *US Patent* 4,742,164

Iguchi, M.; Mitsuhashi, S.; Ichimura, K.; Nishi, Y.; Uryu, M.; Yamanaka, S. & Watanabe, K. (1988). Bacterial cellulose-containing molding material, *US Patent* RE38,792 E.

Iguchi, M; Yamanaka, S; Budhiono, A. (2000). Bacterial cellulose - a masterpiece of nature's arts, *Journal of Materials Science*, Vol.35, No.2, pp. 261-270

Ishihara, M. & Yamanaka, S. (2002). Modified bacterial cellulose, *US Patent* 2002/ 0065409 A1

Ishihara, M. & Yamanaka, S. (2004). Modified bacterial cellulose, *US Patent* 2004 / 0091978 A1

Jeong, S. I.; Lee, S. E.; Yang, H.; Jin, Y. H.; Park, C. S. ; Park, Y. S. (2010). Toxicologic evaluation of bacterial synthesized cellulose in endothelial cells and animals, *Molecular & Cellular Toxicology*, Vol.6, No.4, pp. 373-380

Johnson, D. C. & Neon, A. N. & LeBlanc, H. A. (1989). Bacterial cellulose as surface treatment foe fibrous web, *US Patent* 4,861,427

Johnson, D. C. & Neon, A. N. (1990). Nonwoven fabric-like product using a bacterial cellulose binder and method for its preparation, *US Patent* 4,919,753

Kaewnopparat, S.; Sansernluk, K. & Faroongsarng, D. (2008). Behavior of freezable bound water in the bacterial cellulose produced by Acetobacter xylinum: An approach using thermoporosimetry, *Aaps PharmSciTech*, Vol. 9, No. 2, pp, 701-707

Klemm, D.; Heublein, B.; Fink, H.-P. & Bohn, A . (2005). Cellulose: fascinating biopolymer and sustainable raw material, *J Angew Chem Int Ed*, Vol. 44, pp. 3358-3393

Klemm, D.; Schumann D.; Kramer, F.; Hessler, N.; Hornung, M.; Schmauder, H. P. & Marsch, S. (2006). Nanocelluloses as innovative polymers in research and application, *Polysaccharides*, Vol.205, pp. 49–96

Kouda, T.; Naritomi, T.; Yano, H. & Yoshinaga, F. (2000). Method for cultivation apparatus for the production of bacterial cellulose in an aerated and agitated culture, *US Patent* 6,013,490

Kouda, T.; Naritomi, T.; Yano, H. & Yoshinaga, F. (2000). Process for the production of Bacterial cellulose-containing molding material, *US Patent* 6,017,740

Kouda, T.; Yano, H.; Yoshinaga, F.; Kaminoyama, M. & Kamiwano, M. (1996). Characterization of non-Newtonian behavior during mixing of bacterial cellulose in a bioreactor, *Journal of Fermentation and Bioengineering*, Vol.82, No. 4, pp.382-386

Li Z.; Zhu B. J.; Yang J. X.; Peng K.; Zhou B. H.; Xu R. Q.; Hu W. L.; Chen S. Y.; Wang H. P. (2011). Method for manufacture of bacterial cellulose hydrogel cold pack, *CN Patent*, 201020239963.4

Li, Z. Q.; Zhou, X. D. & Pei, C. H. (2010). Synthesis and Characterization of MPS-g-PLA Copolymer and its Application in Surface Modification of Bacterial Cellulose , *International Journal of Polymer Analysis and Characterization*, Vol.15, No.4, pp. 199-209

Li, Z. Q.; Zhou, X. D. & Pei, C. H. (2010). Synthesis of PLA-co-PGMA Copolymer and its Application in the Surface Modification of Bacterial Cellulose, *International Journal of Polymeric Materials*, Vol. 59, No. 9, pp. 725-737

Lynd, L. R.; Weimer, P. J.; van Zyl, W. H. & Pretorius, I. S. (2002). Microbial cellulose utilization: Fundamentals and biotechnology, *Microbiology and Molecular Biology Reviews*, Vol.66, No.3, pp. 506

Ma X.; Wang R. M.; Guan F. M.; Wang T. F. (2010) . Artificial dura mater made from bacterial cellulose and polyvinyl alcohol, *CN Patent*, 200710015537.5

MacNeil, S. (2007). Progress and opportunities for tissue-engineered skin. *Nature*, Vol.445, pp. 874-880

Maneerung, T.; Tokura, S. & Rujiravanit, R. (2008). Impregnation of silver nanoparticles into bacterial cellulose for antimicrobial wound dressing, *Carbohydrate Polymers*, Vol.72 , No. 1, pp. 43-51

Maria, L. C. D.; Santos, A. L. C.; Oliveira, P. C.; Barud, H .S.; Messaddeq, Y.; Ribeiro, S. J. L . (2009). Synthesis and characterization of silver nanoparticles impregnated into bacterial cellulose, *Materials Letters*, Vol.63, No. 9-10, pp. 797-799

Maria, L. C. S.; Santos, A. L. C.; Oliveira, P. C.; Valle, A. S. S.; Barud, H. S.; Messaddeq, Y. & Ribeiro, S. J. L. (2010).Preparation and Antibacterial Activity of Silver Nanoparticles Impregnated in Bacterial Cellulose. *Polimeros-Ciencia E Tecnologia*, Vol.20, No.1, pp. 72-77

Masuda, K.; Adachi, M.; Hirai, A.; Yamamoto, H.; Kaji, H. & Horii, F . (2003). Solid-state ^{13}C and ^{1}H spin diffusion NMR analyses of the microfibril structure for bacterial cellulose, *Solid State Nuclear Magnetic Resonance*, Vol.23, No. 4, pp.198-212

McKenna, B. A.; Mikkelsen, D.; Wehr, J. B.; Gidley, M. J. & Menzies, N. W. (2009). Mechanical and structural properties of native and alkali-treated bacterial cellulose produced by *Gluconacetobacter xylinus* strain ATCC 53524, *Cellulose*, Vol.16, No.6, pp. 1047-1055

Meftahi, A.; Khajavi, R.; Rashidi, A.; Sattari, M.; Yazdanshenas, M. E. &Torabi, M. (2010). The effects of cotton gauze coating with microbial cellulose, *Cellulose*, Vol.17, No. 1, pp.199-204

Mendes, P. N.; Rahal, S. C.; Pereira-Junior, O. C. M.; Fabris, V. E.; Lenharo, S. L. R.; de Lima-Neto, J. F. & Landim-Alvarenga, F. D. (2009). In vivo and in vitro evaluation of an *Acetobacter xylinum* synthesized microbial cellulose membrane intended for guided tissue repair, *Acta Veterinaria Scandinavica*, Vol.51, No. 12

Nakayama, A.; Kakugo, A.; Gong, J.P.; Osada, Y.; Takai, M.; Erata, T. &Kawano, S. (2004). High mechanical strength double-network hydrogel with bacterial cellulose, *Advanced Functional Materials*, Vol.14, No. 11, pp.1124-1128

Naritomi, T.; Kouda, T.; Naritomi, M.; Yano, H.; Yoshinaga, F. (2000) .Process for continuously preparing bacterial cellulose, *US Patent* 6,132,998

Nge, T. T.; Nogi, M.; Yano, H. & Sugiyama, J. (2010). Microstructure and mechanical properties of bacterial cellulose/chitosan porous scaffold, *Cellulose*, Vol.17, No. 2, pp. 349-363

Nwe, N.; Furuike, T. & Tamura, H. (2010). Selection of a biopolymer based on attachment, morphology and proliferation of fibroblast NIH/3T3 cells for the development of a biodegradable tissue regeneration template: Alginate, bacterial cellulose and gelatin, *Process Biochemistry*, Vol.45, No. 4, pp.457-466

Olsson, R. T.; Kraemer, R.; Lopez-Rubio, A.; Torres-Giner, S.; Ocio, M. J. & Lagaron, J. M. (2010). Extraction of Microfibrils from Bacterial Cellulose Networks for Electrospinning of Anisotropic Biohybrid Fiber Yarns, *Macromolecules*, Vol.43, No.9, pp.4201-4209

Olsson, R. T.; Azizi Samir, M. A. S.; Salazar-Alvarez, G.; Belova, L.; StrÖm, V.; Berglund, L. A.; Ikkala, O.; Nogués, J.; Gedde, U. W. (2010). Making flexible magnetic aerogels and stiff magnetic nanopaper using cellulose nanofibrils as templates, *Nature Nanotechnology*, Vol. 5, pp. 584-588

Ougiya, H.; Watanabe, K.; Matsumura, T. & Yoshinaga, F. (1998). Relationship between suspension properties and fibril structure of disintegrated bacterial cellulose, *Bioscience, Biotechnology and Biochemistry*, Vol. 62, No.9, pp. 1714-1719

Pandey, L. K.; Saxena, C. & Dubey, V. (2005). Studies on pervaporative characteristics of bacterial cellulose membrane, *Separation and Purification Technology*, Vol .42, No. 3,pp. 213-218

Patel, U. & Suresh, S. (2010). Reactor for reductive conversion reactions using palladized bacterial cellulose, *US Patent* 2010 / 0126945 A1

Pertile, R.A. N.; Andrade, F. K.; Alves, C & Gama, M. (2010). Surface modification of bacterial cellulose by nitrogen-containing plasma for improved interaction with cells, *Carbohydrate Polymers*, Vol.82, No. 3, pp.692-698

Phisalaphong, M.; Suwanmajo, T. & Tammarate, P. (2008). Synthesis and characterization of bacterial cellulose/alginate blend membranes, *Journal of Applied Polymer Science*. Vol .107, No. 5, pp.3419-3424

Pommet, M.; Juntaro, J.; Heng, J. Y. Y; Mantalaris, A.; Lee, A. F.; Wilson, K.; Kalinka, G.; Shaffer, M. S. P. ; Bismarck, A. (2008). Surface modification of natural fibers using bacteria: Depositing bacterial cellulose onto natural fibers to create hierarchical fiber reinforced nanocomposites, *Biomacromolecules*, Vol.9, No.6, pp. 1643-1651

Portal, O.; Clark, W. A. & Levinson, D. J. (2009). Microbial Cellulose Wound Dressing in the Treatment of Nonhealing Lower Extremity Ulcers, *Wounds-A Compendium of Clinical Research and Practice*, Vol .21, No.1, pp. 1-3

Putra, A.; Kakugo, A. Furukawa, H.; Gong, J. P.; Osada, Y.; Uemura, T. & Yamamoto, M. (2008). Production of bacterial cellulose with well oriented fibril on PDMS substrate, *Polymer Journal*, Vol .40, No.2, pp. 137-142

Retegi, A.; Gabilondo, N.; Pena, C.; Zuluaga, R.; Castro, C.; Ganan, P.; de la Caba, K. & Mondragon, I. (2010). Bacterial cellulose films with controlled microstructure-mechanical property relationships, *Cellulose*, Vol.17, No.3, pp. 661-669

Saibuatong, O. A. & Phisalaphong, M. (2010). Novo aloe vera-bacterial cellulose composite film from biosynthesis, *Carbohydrate Polymers*, Vol .79, No.2, pp. 455-460

Sakaguchi, M.; Ohura, T.; Iwata, T.; Takahashi, S.; Akai, S.; Kan, T.; Murai, H.; Fujiwara, M .; Watanabe, O. & Narita, M. (2010). Diblock Copolymer of Bacterial Cellulose and

Poly(methyl methacrylate) Initiated by Chain-End-Type Radicals Produced by Mechanical Scission of Glycosidic Linkages of Bacterial Cellulose, *Biomacromolecules*, Vol.11, No.11, pp. 3059-3066

Sano, M. B.; Rojas, A.D.; Gatenholm, P. & Davalos, R. V. (2010). Electromagnetically Controlled Biological Assembly of Aligned Bacterial Cellulose Nanofibers, *Annals of Biomedical Engineering*, Vol .38, No. 8, pp. 2475-2484

Schrecker, S. T.; Gostomski, P. A. (2005). Determining the water holding capacity of microbial cellulose, *Biotechnology Letters*, Vol .27, No.19, pp.1435-1438

Shah, J. & Brown, R. M. (2005) .Towards electronic paper displays made from microbial cellulose, *Applied Microbiology and Biotechnology*, Vol .66, No.4, pp.352-355

Shah, N.; Ha, J. H. & Park, J. K. (2010). Effect of Reactor Surface on Production of Bacterial Cellulose and Water Soluble Oligosaccharides by *Gluconacetobacter hansenii* PJK, *Biotechnology And Bioprocess Engineering*, Vol.15, No.1, pp. 110-118

Siró I. & Plackett D. (2010). Microfibrillated cellulose and new nanocomposite materials: a review, *Cellulose*, Vol .17, No. 3, pp.459-494

Solway, D. R.; Clark, W. A. & Levinson, D. J. (2011). A parallel open-label trial to evaluate microbial cellulose wound dressing in the treatment of diabetic foot ulcers, *International Wound Journal*, Vol .8, No.1, pp. 69-73

Solway, D. R.; Consalter, M. & Levinson, D. J. (2010). Microbial Cellulose Wound Dressing in the Treatment of Skin Tears in the Frail Elderly, *Wounds-A Compendium of Clinical Research and Practice*, Vol. 22, No.1, pp. 17-19

Sourty, E.; Ryan, D. H.; Marchessault, R. H. (1998). Ferrite-loaded membranes of microfibrillar bacterial cellulose prepared by in situ precipitation, *Chemistry of Materials*, Vol.10, No.7, pp. 1755

Sourty, E.; Ryan, D. H.; Marchessault, R. H. (1998). Characterization of magnetic membranes based on bacterial and man-made cellulose , *Cellulose*, Vol.5, No.1, pp. 5-17

Stephen, R.S.; Westland, J. A. & Neogi, A.N. (1990). Method of using bacterial cellulose as a dietary fiber component, *US Patent* 4,960,763

Sureshkumar, M.; Siswanto, D. Y. & Lee, C. K. (2010). Magnetic antimicrobial nanocomposite based on bacterial cellulose and silver nanoparticles, *Journal of Materials Chemistry*, Vol. 20, No. 33, pp. 6948-6955

Tahara, N.; Watanabe, K.; Hioki, N.; Morinaga, Y.; Hajouda, T.; Miyashita, H.; Shibata ,A. & Ougiya, H. (2000). Bacterial cellulose concentrate and method for the treatment of the concentrate, *US Patent* 6,069,136

Tamai, N.; Aono, H.; Tatsumi, D. & Matsumoto, T. (2003). Differences in rheological properties of solutions of plant and bacterial cellulose in LiCl/N,N-dimethylacetamide, *Journal of the Society of Rheology Japan*, Vol. 31, No. 3, pp.119-130

Tammarate, P. (1999). Method for the modification and utilization of bacterial cellulose, *US Patent* 5,962,676

Tomita, Y.; Tsuji, T. & Kondo, T. (2009). Fabrication of Microbial Cellulose Nanofiber Network Sheets Hydrophobically Enhanced by Introduction of a Heat-printed Surface, *Sen-I Gakkaishi*, Vol. 65 , No.2, pp.73-79

Tung, W. C.; Tung, D. A.; Callandei, D. D.; Bauer, R. G. (1994). Reticulated bacterial cellulose reinforcement for elastomers, *US Patent* 5,290,830

VanderHart, D. L. & Atalla, R. H. (1984). Studies of Microstructure in Native Celluloses Using Solid-state13C NMR, *Macromolecules*, Vol.17, pp. 1465-1472

Vitta, S.; Drillon, M. & Derory, A. (2010). Magnetically responsive bacterial cellulose: Synthesis and magnetic studies, *Journal of Applied Physics*, Vol. 108, No.5

Volkov, V. V.; Klechkovskaya, V. V.; Shtykova, E. V.; Dembo, K. A.; Arkharova, N. A. (; Ivakin, G. I. & Smyslov, R. Y. (2009). Determination of the size and phase composition of silver nanoparticles in a gel film of bacterial cellulose by small-angle X-ray scattering, electron diffraction, and electron microscopy, *Crystallography Reports*, Vol. 54 , No.2, pp.169-173

Wan, W. & Millon, L. (2005). Poly (vinyl alcohol) - bacterial cellulose nanocomposite, *US Patent* 2005 / 0037082 A1

Wang, Z. L.; Jia, Y. Y.; Shi, Y.; Cong, D. L.; Chen, Y. Y.; Jia, S. R.; Zhou, Y. L. (2009). Research on Characterization and Biocompatibility of Nano-bacterial Cellulose Membrane, *Chemical Journal of Chinese Universities-Chinese*, Vol.30, No.8, pp. 1553-1558

Watt, W. D.; Adams, T. N.; Peterson, G. D.; Stephens, R. S. & Askew, J. M. (1997). Process of coating a substrate with reticulated bacterial cellulose, *US Patent* 5,637,197

Wei, B.; Yang, G. A. & Hong, F. (2011). Preparation and evaluation of a kind of bacterial cellulose dry films with antibacterial properties, *Carbohydrate Polymers*, Vol. 84, No.1, pp.533-538

Westland, J. A.; Stephens, R. S.; Johaston, W. C. & Rosenkrans, H. J. (1993). Bacterial cellulose binding agent, *US Patent* 5,207,826

Wiegand, C.; Elsner, P.; Hipler, U. C. & Klemm, D. (2006). Protease and ROS activities influenced by a composite of bacterial cellulose and collagen type I in vitro, *Cellulose*, Vol.13, No.6, pp. 689-696

Winter, H. T.; Cerclier, C.; Delorme, N.; Bizot, H.; Quemener, B. & Cathala, B. (2010). Improved Colloidal Stability of Bacterial Cellulose Nanocrystal Suspensions for the Elaboration of Spin-Coated Cellulose-Based Model Surfaces, *Biomacromolecules*, Vol. 11, No.11, pp.3144-3151

Wu S. Q.; Yang Z. W.; Chen G. L.; Fang B. S.; Wang K. M.; Chen H.; Zhou R. H.; Wan Z. Y.; Wu H.; Wei Y. F.; Min Y.; Jiang A. B.; Liu C. J.; Liang Y.; Zhang Z. G.; Liu F.; Qiu Z. M. (2011). Method for utilizing bacterial cellulose in protecting silk cultural relic, *CN Patent*, 200810246345.X

Xu C. Y.; Sun D. P. (2011). Manufacture of membrane electrode of proton exchange fuel cell using bacterial fibers, *CN Patent*, 200810022130.X

Yamanaka, S.; Watanabe, K.; Iguchi, M. &Nishi, Y. (1998) .Production, property, and application of bacterial cellulose, *Nippon Nogeikagaku Kaishi-Journal of the Japan Society for Bioscience Biotechnology and Agrochemistry*, Vol.72, No.9, pp.1039-1044

Yang G.; Fu L. N.; He F.; Zhou P.; Yu L. J. (2010). *Acetobacter xylinum* Y05 and bio-fabrication of nano-cellulose material for skin tissue repairment, *CN Patent*, 200810047793.7

Yang G.; Wang G.; Liu B. F.; Shi X. D.; Chen X. F.(2010) · A new approach for controllable bio-fabrication of patterned cellulose nano-fibers via micro-fluidic techniques, *CN Patent*, 200810047875.1

Yang, Z. F.; Raczkjowski, R.; Rubic, L. B; Mazyck, M. J. & Deely, K.M. (2007). Bacterial cellulose-containing formulations, *US Patent* 2007 / 0197779 A1

Yang, Z. F.; Raczkjowski, R.; Rubic, L. B; Mazyck, M. J. & Deely, K.M. (2007). Method for producing effective bacterial cellulose-containing formulations, *US Patent* 2007 / 0027108 A1

Yang, Z. F.; Raczkjowski, R.; Rubic, L. B; Mazyck, M. J. & Deely, K.M. (2010). Bacterial cellulose-containing formulations lacking a carboxymethyl cellulose component, *US Patent* 2010 / 0016575 A1

Yoshinaga, F.; Tonouchi, N. & Watanabe, K. (1997). Research progress in production of bacterial cellulose by aeration and agitation culture and its application as a new industrial material, *Bioscience, Biotechnology and Biochemistry*, Vol.61, No.2, pp.219-224

Yu D. Y.; Qiao N.; Zhang J. B.; Guan X. H.; Zhang J.; Liu W. C.; Yu J. (2010). Method of preparing bacterium cellulose food-preserving film, *CN Patent*, 200810051298.3

Zhong C. Y. (2008). Bacterial cellulose gel face mask, *CN Patent*, 200610075040.8

Zhong C. Y. (2011). Method for manufacturing air-filtering bacterial cellulose face mask, *CN Patent*, 200910149665.8

14

Hydrogel Biomaterials

Alpesh Patel and Kibret Mequanint
Department of Chemical and Biochemical Engineering, University of Western Ontario, London Ontario, Canada

1. Introduction

A staggering number of medical devices, diagnostic and therapeutic products that are designed to improve the health of mankind have exploited biomaterials as platform technologies (Peppas et al., 2006). Defined as natural or synthetic materials (other than drugs) to treat, augment, or replace any tissues, organ, or function of living tissues, biomaterials design requires both materials and biological considerations. In addition to the mechanical requirements, biomaterials have to accomplish some specific requirements, such as non-toxicity, desired functionality, sterilizability and biocompatibility (Rosiak & Yoshii, 1999). Despite the widespread use of biomaterials in medicine, most biomaterials do not provide all of the desired requirements to interact with biological systems. Therefore, there is a significant progress to redesign current biomaterials or to develop new materials in order to overcome limitations associated with fulfilling the above-mentioned requirements. Although the term biomaterial includes metals and ceramics, polymers account for the vast majority. In this last group, hydrogels, having considerable biocompatibility and similarity with tissue components of the body, have demonstrated great potential as one of the most promising groups of biomaterials (Rosiak & Yoshii, 1999; Rogero et al., 2003).
Hydrogels are three-dimensional (3D) materials with the ability to absorb large amounts of water while maintaining their dimensional stability. The 3D integrity of hydrogels in their swollen state is maintained either by physical or chemical crosslinking. Lower interfacial tension, soft and tissue-like physical properties, higher permeability to undersized molecules and release of entrapped molecules in a controlled manner made hydrogels to be explored in different biomedical fields (Yaszemski et al., 2004; Slaughter, 2009). In the absence of crosslinking points, hydrophilic linear polymer chains dissolve in water due to the thermodynamic compatibility of the polymer chains and water. However, in the presence of crosslinking points, solubility is counter-balanced by the retractive force of elasticity, induced by crosslinking points of the network. Swelling reaches at an equilibrium point as these forces becomes equal (Peppas et al., 2000). The amount of water absorbed in hydrogels is related to the presence of specific groups such as -COOH, -OH, $-CONH_2$, -CONH-, and $-SO_3H$. Capillary effect and osmotic pressure are other variables that also influence the equilibrium water uptake of hydrogels (Dergunov & Mun, 2009).
The presence of chemical or physical crosslinking points within the network maintains the three-dimensional integrity of hydrogels in their swollen state. In chemically crosslinked hydrogels, the linear polymer chains are covalently bonded with each other via crosslinking

agents. Their usage is limited as the resulting network cannot be reshaped and/or resized since the polymer is no longer soluble in solvents and heating to melt-process can only degrade the polymer once crosslinking takes place. Moreover, the crosslinking agents applied to develop strong hydrogel network systems are mainly toxic. Thus, any unreacted crosslinking agents have to be leached out before the final application. However, partially reacted toxic crosslinking agents have no possibility to be completely leached out. In contrast, physically crosslinked hydrogels possess physical junction domains associated with chain entanglements, hydrophobic interaction, hydrogen bonding, crystallinity, and/or ionic complexation (Park & Bae 2002). The presence of these reversible crosslinking points allows solvent casting and/or thermal processing. The interest for physically crosslinked hydrogel is obvious since the use of crosslinking agents is avoided and they are beneficial for post-process bulk modification and ease of fabrication (Hennink & van Nostrum 2002; Li et al., 2002; Adams et al., 2003; Kubo et al., 2005; Liu et al., 2009). Hydrophobic - hydrophilic block copolymers are one of the well-explored and applied physically crosslinked polymers for various biomedical applications. The major disadvantage of physically crosslinked hydrogels, however, is their weak mechanical properties in the swollen state. This can be improved by using polyurethane as a hydrophobic segment into hydrophobic-hydrophilic block copolymers. Due to the excellent mechanical properties of polyurethanes(Lamba et al., 1998), hydrogels based on their chemistry are appealing for biomedical applications. Polyurethane-based hydrogels can form strongly hydrogen bonded structures, allowing linear polymer systems to be designed with tunable swelling and mechanical properties. Thus, along with the hydrophobic interaction and chain entanglements, the presence of strong H-bonding between the ether/ester and urethane groups into polyurethane can help to improve mechanical properties(Lamba et al., 1998; Mequanint et al., 2006). Following the pioneering work of Wichtrle (de Groot et al., 2003) on crosslinked PHEMA hydrogels as contact lenses, hydrogels have been of great interest as potential biomaterial for cell encapsulation, drug delivery system, contact lenses, wound dressing, immunoisolation, tissue engineering scaffolds, soft tissue replacement and other related applications (Hoffman 2002; Kashyap et al., 2005).

2. Classifications of hydrogels

Depending on the preparation methods, ionic charges, sources, nature of swelling with changes in the environment, rate of biodegradation or the nature of crosslinking, hydrogels can be classified in several ways. A detailed classification of hydrogels is presented in Figure 1 (Dumitriu, 2002; Hin, 2004; Ratner et al., 2004). Among all, one of the important classifications is based on their crosslinking nature (Figure 1). The network stability of hydrogels in their swollen state is due to the presence of either chemical or physical crosslinking. Chemically crosslinked hydrogels are also known as thermosetting hydrogels or permanent gels. They cannot be dissolved in any solvents unless the covalent crosslink points are cleaved. Moreover, they cannot be reshaped through heat melting. They can be prepared using any of these methods:

- Copolymerizing hydrophilic monomers with crosslinkers.
- Crosslinking of water-soluble polymer segments with di and/or multi functional crosslinkers or using irradiation method (UV, microwave, γ–irradiation and electron beam).

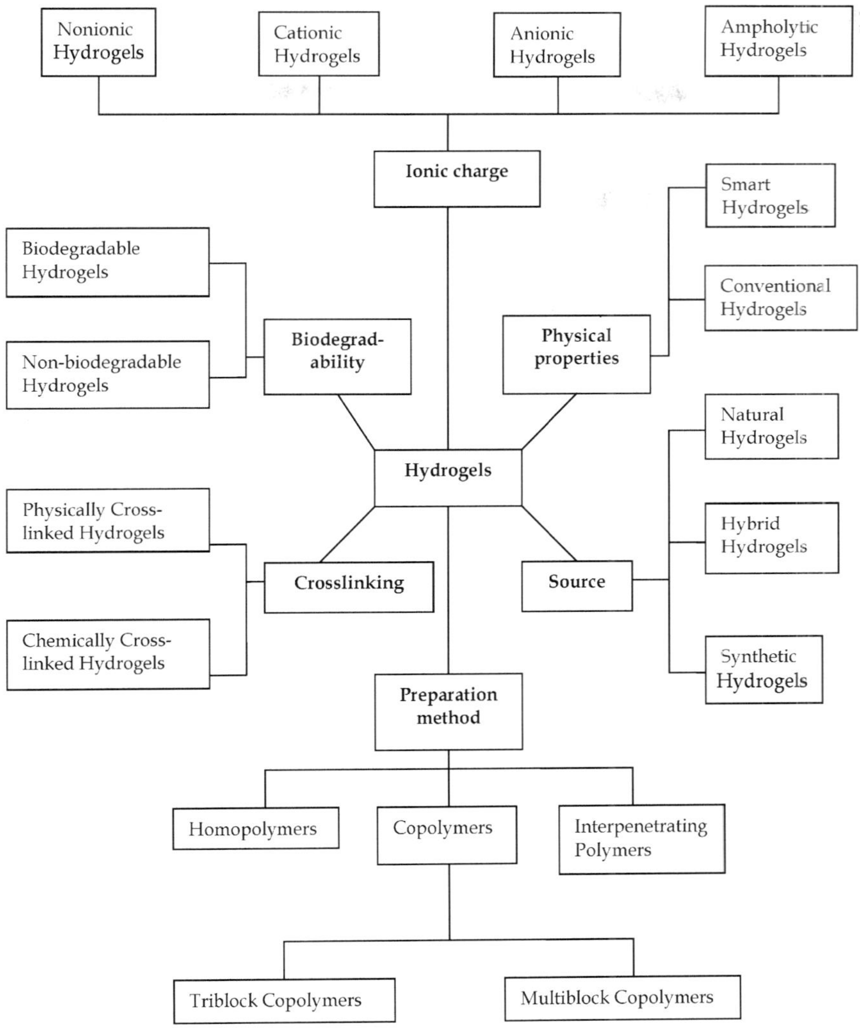

Fig. 1. Classifications of hydrogels.

The utility of chemically crosslinked hydrogels is often limited by the lack of processability and post-process modifications. Because of this, shaping is carried out along with their polymerization reaction step. Moreover the crosslinking agents used to prepare hydrogels are highly toxic and the residues must be completely removed before their use as biomaterials. Physically crosslinked hydrogels, on the other hand, maintain their physical stability due to the presence of reversible physical junction domains associated with hydrogen bonding, hydrophobic interaction, chain entanglements, crystallinity, and/or ionic complexation (Bae et al., 2000; Qu et al., 2000; Park & Bae 2002). Physically crosslinked hydrogels are also known as thermoplastic hydrogels or temporary gels. Swelling of these hydrogels is mostly dependent on the thermodynamic parameters such as temperature, pH, salt type and/or ionic strength. Changes in such parameters may increase or decrease their swelling. The presence of reversible crosslinking points in physically crosslinked hydrogels allows solvent casting and/or thermal processing. In the preparation of these hydrogels, the use of toxic crosslinkers can also be avoided. Physically crosslinked hydrogels possess higher compressive strength compared with the corresponding chemically crosslinked hydrogels since the mechanical load can be more uniformly distributed through the crystallites of the three-dimensional structure (Devine & Higginbotham 2003).

2.1 Stimuli responsive hydrogels

Stimuli responsive hydrogels are defined as hydrogels that undergo relatively large and abrupt changes in their swelling behavior, network structure, permeability and/or mechanical strength in response to small environmental changes. Stimuli responsive hydrogels are also called intelligent, smart, or environmentally sensitive hydrogels (Peppas et al., 2000; Gil & Hudson 2004). Stimuli responsive hydrogels could be further classified as either physical or chemical stimuli responsive hydrogels as shown in Figure 2.

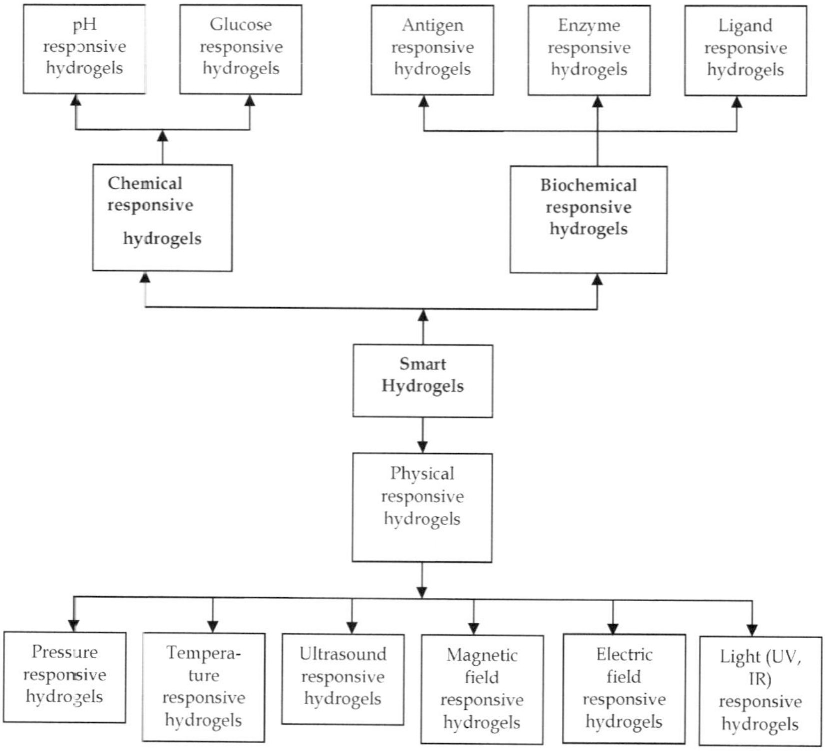

Fig. 2. Classifications of smart hydrogels.

Chemical stimuli, such as pH, ionic factors and chemical agents, will change the interactions between polymer chains or between polymer chains and solvent at the molecular level. The physical stimuli, such as temperature, electric or magnetic fields, and mechanical stress, will affect the level of various energy sources and alter molecular interactions at critical onset points. Some systems have been developed to combine two stimuli-responsive mechanisms into one polymer system, in the so-called dual responsive polymer systems. Polyacrylic acid-co-polyvinyl sulfonic acid is an example of dual responsive polymer system(Kim et al., 2004). Recently, biochemical stimuli have been considered as another category, which involves the responses to antigen, enzyme, ligand, and other biochemical agents (Peppas, et al. 2000; Gil & Hudson 2004). Thus stimuli-responsive hydrogels are appealing biomaterials for pharmaceutical, biotechnological and biomedical applications (Kashyap et al., 2004).

2.2 pH responsive hydrogels

pH responsive hydrogels are made of polymeric backbones with ionic pendant groups that can accept and/or donate protons in response to an environmental pH change (Bushetti et al., 2009). As the environmental pH changes, the degree of ionization in pH responsive hydrogel is dramatically changed at specific pH known as pKa or pKb. This rapid change in the net charge of ionized pendant groups causes abrupt volume transition by generating electrostatic repulsive forces between ionized groups, which creates large osmotic swelling force. There are two types of pH responsive hydrogels: anionic and cationic hydrogels. In anionic hydrogels having pendent groups such as carboxylic (Ende & Peppas 1996; Ying et al., 1998; Jabbari & Nozari 1999; Jianqi & Lixia 2002; Wang et al. 2006) or sulfonic acid, deprotonation occurs when the environmental pH is above the pKa leading to the ionization of the pendent groups. This, in turn, increases swelling of the hydrogel. On the other hand, in cationic hydrogels containing pendent groups such as amine groups(Baker et al., 1992), ionization takes place below the pKb and this increases the swelling due to an increase in electrostatic repulsions (Gupta et al., 2002). Two major factors control the degree of swelling of ionic hydrogels. The first factor is the properties of the polymers such as ionic charge, concentration and pKa or pKb of the ionizable groups, degree of ionization, crosslink density as well as hydrophilicity or hydrophobicity. The second factor is the properties of the swelling medium like pH, ionic strength and the counterion and its valence (Gupta et al., 2002). Polyvinyl sulfonic acid (PVSA)(Kim et al., 2005), polymethacrylic acid (PMAA),(Eichenbaum et al., 1998; Kozlovskaya et al., 2006) polydiethylaminoethyl methacrylate (PDEAEMA)(Vamvakaki et al., 2006) and polydimethylaminoethyl methacrylate (PDMAEMA)(Sen & Sari, 2005; Bossard et al., 2006) and their copolymers are other examples of pH responsive hydrogels.

2.3 Temperature responsive hydrogels

Temperature responsive hydrogels have gained considerable attention in the biomedical field. Numerous researchers studied various applications of these hydrogels, in the area of smart drug delivery system, injectable scaffolds, biosensors and intelligent cell culture dishes(Peppas et al., 2000; Schmaljohann et al., 2003; He et al., 2008). Temperature responsive hydrogels can be classified as positive or negative temperature responsive systems. Physically crosslinked thermo sensitive hydrogels may undergo sol-gel phase transitions instead of volume change at a critical solution temperature (Peppas et al., 2000; Kashyap et al., 2004). Positive temperature responsive hydrogels show phase transition at critical temperature called the upper critical solution temperature (UCST). Hydrogels made from polymers with UCST shrink when cooled below their UCST. Negative temperature responsive hydrogels have a lower critical solution temperature (LCST). These hydrogels shrink upon heating above their LCST. Chemically crosslinked thermo sensitive hydrogels undergo volume change rather than sol-gel transitions. Certain molecular interactions, such as hydrophobic associations and hydrogen bonds play vital role in the abrupt volume change of these hydrogels at the critical solution temperature (CST). In the swollen state, water molecules form hydrogen bonds with polar groups of polymer backbone within the hydrogels and organize around hydrophobic groups as iceberg water. At the CST, hydrogen bonding between the polymer and water, compared to polymer–polymer and water–water interactions, becomes unfavorable. This forces the quick dehydration of the system and water is released out of the hydrogel with a large gain in entropy, resulting in shrinkage of the polymeric structure (Kopecek, 2003; Ruel-Gariepy & Leroux 2004). The mostly studied temperature responsive hydrogels are methylcellulose (Stabenfeldt et al. 2006), hydroxypropyl methylcellulose (Vinatier et al., 2005), chitosan (Zan et al., 2006), *N*-isopropylacrylamide (NIPAAm) based copolymers (Lu et al., 2000; Kim et al., 2002; Schmaljohann, 2005; Lee et al., 2006; Qiao et al., 2006) and other *N*-alkylacrylamide polymers (Hirokawa & Tanaka, 1984), poly(vinyl methyl ether) (PVME) (Kabra et al., 1992; Arndt, Schmidt et al. 2001; Theiss et al. 2004), poly(*N*-vinylisobutyramide) (PNVIBA) (Akashi et al., 1996; Kunugi et al., 1997; Suwa et al., 1997; Suwa et al., 1997), poly(ethylene oxide-*b*-propylene oxide-*b*-ethylene oxide) (PEO-PPO-PEO) (Bohorquez et al., 1999; Song, Lee et al., 2000), and poly(ethylene oxide)/(D,L-lactic acid-co-glycolic acid) (PEO-PLLA-PLGA)(Jeong et al., 1997) copolymers. Poly(*N*-isopropylacrylamide) (PNIPAAm) is the most popular temperature-responsive polymer since it exhibits a sharp phase transition in water at 34.3°C which is close to physiological temperature(Peppas et al., 2000). Its LCST can be controlled by copolymerizing with other monomers. The LCST increases with the addition of hydrophilic monomers whereas it decreases with the incorporation of hydrophobic monomers. Grafting of hydrophilic or hydrophobic monomers does not show any significant changes in LCST (Ruel-Gariepy & Leroux, 2004).

2.4 Glucose responsive hydrogels

For the treatment of diabetes, desirable insulin delivery hydrogel systems could be developed having glucose-sensing carrier to trigger the release of required amounts of insulin. Glucose sensitive hydrogels have been attractive for this particular application. Cationic hydrogels as a carrier for insulin and glucose oxidase mixture are the most extensively studied glucose sensor systems (Podual et al., 2000; Podual et al., 2000; Traitel et al., 2000; Brahim et al., 2002). In the presence of oxygen, glucose oxidase converts glucose to gluconic acid and reduces the local pH; which increases the swelling of cationic hydrogels and releases insulin. To improve controlled loading of insulin, glucose oxidase has been covalently tethered on the hydrogel system that reduces its fast diffusion out of the system (Kang & Bae 2003). Other mechanisms including the use of concanavalin-A as a crosslinker(Obaidat & Park 1996), use of phenylboronic acid (Shiino et al., 1995) or glucose dehydrogenase (Kashyap et al., 2004) as a biosensor have been also investigated to fabricate glucose responsive hydrogels.

2.5 Protein-based hydrogels

Protein-based hydrogels have been studied for drug delivery and tissue engineering applications(Wang et al., 1999; Xu et al., 2005). These protein-based hydrogels are precisely designed with defined compositions, sequences, stereochemistry, and molecular weights using recombinant DNA technology. Coiled-coil is an attractive approach for protein-based hydrogels. The hydrophobic amino acid residues of coiled-coil proteins are used as physical crosslinkers in protein-based polymer hydrogels. Tri-block copolymers with coiled-coil domains at the end and water-soluble polypeptide domain at the centre have been designed as physically crosslinked protein-based hydrogels (Wright & Conticello 2002; Wright et al., 2002). Consequently, temperature and/or pH-responsiveness may be achieved by manipulating the amino acid sequences of the coiled-coil domains (Kopecek, 2003; Xu et al., 2005). Addition of RGD sequence within the hydrophilic polypeptide sequence also improves cell interactions. Moreover, coiled-coil proteins are used as crosslinkers with water soluble linear synthetic polymers to prepare 3D structure of hydrogels (Wang et al., 1999).

2.6 Antigen-responsive hydrogels

Antigen-responsive hydrogels have been designed to deliver biomolecules at a specific targeted site (Miyata et al., 1999; Lu et al., 2003). In these hydrogels, antigens are grafted on hydrophilic polymeric backbones. They can also be mixed with antibody-grafted crosslinked hydrophilic polymeric backbones. In the absence of a free antigen, the hydrogel structure shrinks due to the intra-chain antigen-antibody binding in the polymer network. Specific molecular recognition is a remarkable feature of the antigen-sensitive hydrogels that made them useful biomaterials to fabricate an antigen sensing device for biomolecules, protein or drug delivery at desired sites (Miyata et al., 2002).

3. Water in hydrogels

Swelling behavior of hydrogel systems is an important parameter governing their applications specifically in pharmaceutical, ophthalmology and tissue engineering. The presence of water at the surface of hydrogels reduces the interfacial free energy in a physiological environment and thus improves their biological properties(Jhon & Andrade 1973). The final water content of hydrogels depends on both kinetics and thermodynamics parameters. During the swelling process, the first water molecules hydrate the most polar, hydrophilic groups, and this portion of water is called 'primary bound water'. As the hydration of polar and hydrophilic groups is completed, the network swells, and exposes hydrophobic groups, which start interacting with water through hydrophobic interaction called secondary bound water molecules. Together, primary and secondary bound water molecules are often called the total bound water (Hoffman, 2002). After the water has interacted with both hydrophilic and hydrophobic sites, the osmotic driving force of the network chains allows the network to absorb more water. This additional swelling is opposed by the presence of covalent or physical crosslinking junctions through an elastic network retraction force. Finally, the balance of the retraction force and the infinite dilution force establish an equilibrium swelling level. The additional water absorbed beyond the total bound water is defined as 'free water' or 'bulk water'(Hoffman, 2002).

3.1 Thermodynamics of hydrogel swelling

Hydrophilic polymer networks show high affinity to water and, in the presence of water, the polymer-water interaction is preferred to the inter-polymer chains interactions. Thus, the hydrophilic network allows large water absorption and proceeds towards infinite dilution.

However, the presence of crosslinking junctions resists the infinite dilution by the retractive force of elasticity. In the absence of ionic moieties in the polymer chains, the counter balance of these forces decides the water uptake of hydrogels. The Flory-Huggins theory can be used to calculate the thermodynamic behavior of hydrogel swelling (Flory, 1953; Peppas et al., 2000; Ratner 2004). Considering an isotropic crosslinked structure of hydrogel, the total Gibbs free energy change of the system, upon swelling, can be written as:

$$\Delta G = \Delta G_{\text{mixture}} + \Delta G_{\text{elastic}} \tag{1}$$

Where,

$\Delta G_{\text{mixture}}$ = the free energy of mixing due to water affinity of hydrophilic polymers.

$\Delta G_{\text{elastic}}$ = the elastic free energy as a result of the network expansion.

In order to express the chemical potential change of water in terms of elastic and mixing contributions at any time of swelling, differentiating equation (1) with respect to the water molecules in the system gives:

$$\mu_{\text{wh}} - \mu_{\text{pw}} = \Delta\mu_{\text{mixture}} + \Delta\mu_{\text{elastic}} \tag{2}$$

Where,

μ_{wh} = the chemical potential of water within the hydrogel.

μ_{pw} = the chemical potential of pure water.

$\Delta\mu_{mixture}$ = the change in chemical potential due to mixing.

$\Delta\mu_{elastic}$ = the change in chemical potential as a result of the network expansion.

The chemical potential change on mixing can be obtained using Flory-Huggins theory that is applied to the fundamentals of the thermodynamics of polymer solution.

3.1.1 Determination of $\Delta\mu_{\text{mixure}}$ –the entropy of mixing

In the absence of crosslinkages, the ideal entropy of mixing can be given by the Boltzmann relation, $\Delta S_m = k \times \ln\Omega$. Here k represents the Boltzmann constant and Ω represents the probability of arrangements of polymer chains within the solvent. By considering that the polymer molecules have the same size, the Lattice Model can be used to find the possibility of such arrangements. The formation of the polymer solution can be thought to happen in two steps: disorientation of the polymer chains and mixing of the disoriented polymer with solvent. The entropy change related to both steps and the overall entropy change is given as:

$$\Delta S_m = -k\left(n_1 \ln \text{v}_1 + n_2 \ln \text{v}_2\right) \tag{3}$$

Where,

v_1 = volume fraction of water

v_2 = volume fraction of polymer

n_1, n_2 = moles of water and polymer respectively.

3.1.2 Determination of $\Delta\mu_{\text{mixure}}$ – the heat of mixing

According to the Lattice Model, three types of first neighbor contacts are possible: [1,1], [2,2] and [1,2]. The solution is prepared by having the chemical reaction in which bonds of [1,2] types are formed at the expense of an equal number of [1,1] and [2,2] as per the following stoichiometric balance:

$$\frac{1}{2}[1,1]+\frac{1}{2}[2,2]=[1,2]$$

If w_{11}, w_{22} and w_{12} are the energies associated with these respective bonds, the change in energy due to the formation of unlike pairs is given as:

$$\Delta w_{12} = w_{12}-\frac{1}{2}(w_{11}+w_{22})$$

The overall heat of mixing is then given as:

$$\Delta H_m = \Delta w_{12}\times p_{12} = z\Delta w_{12}x_1 n_1 v_2 \quad (4)$$

Where,

p_{12} = probability that the sites adjacent to a polymer segment is occupied by a solvent molecule = $zx_1n_1v_2$.

z = the lattice coordination number which equals the number of cells which are first neighbors to a given cell.

x_1 = the segments of water molecule.

The quantity $z\Delta w_{12}x_1$ represents the change in the internal energy of a solvent molecule immersed in the pure polymer compared with the one surrounded by molecules of its own kind, i.e., in the pure solvent. Another parameter is introduced to define this energy difference and is called water-polymer interaction parameter (χ). It is the dimensionless quantity, which is defined as $\frac{z\Delta w_{12}x_1}{kT}$. Using this interaction parameter into the equation (4) gives:

$$\Delta H_m = kT\chi n_1 v_2 \quad (5)$$

3.1.3 The chemical potential change on mixing

The Gibbs free energy of the mixing is simply given by combining equations (3) and (5). That is,

$$\Delta G_m = \Delta H_m - T\Delta S_m = kT\chi n_1 v_2 + kT(n_1 \ln v_1 + n_2 \ln v_2)$$

$$\Delta G_m = \Delta H_m - T\Delta S_m = kT(\chi n_1 v_2 + n_1 \ln v_1 + n_2 \ln v_2) \quad (6)$$

Now, in the case of hydrogels, the number n_2 of polymer molecules is to be equated to zero owing to the absence of individual polymer molecules in the network structure. Thus

$$\Delta G_m = kT(\chi n_1 v_2 + n_1 \ln v_1) \quad (7)$$

Differentiation of the above equation with respect to the number water molecules, n_1, at constant temperature and pressure (bearing in mind that v_1 and v_2 are functions of n_1) into the system gives,

$$\Delta\mu_{\text{mixture}} = \frac{\partial \Delta G_m}{\partial n_1} = kT\left(\ln v_1 + v_2 + \chi v_2^2\right) \quad (8)$$

3.1.4 Determination of $\Delta\mu_{elastic}$

The presence of crosslinks induces a retractive force as the dry hydrogel expand into the water. This retractive force can be explained by using the theories of rubber elasticity. Rubbers are materials that respond to stresses with nearly instantaneous and fully reversible deformation up to 1000% elongation. Rubbers are crosslinked networks possessing large free volume that makes them capable to respond to external stresses by rearranging the polymer chains. In the swollen state, most hydrogels satisfy this phenomenon of rubber. To derive the relationship for the chemical potential change of water during swelling, statistical thermodynamics have been used[69]. The expansion of hydrogel is considered to be isotropic. So the developed strain related to the expansion of structure (say α_s) can also be considered the same in all direction. The entropy change involved in expansion of hydrogels, obtained by using statistical thermodynamics and by applying the Boltzmann expression (Flory, 1953) is:

$$\Delta S_{el} = -\frac{kv_e}{2}\left[\alpha_x^{\,2} + \alpha_y^{\,2} + \alpha_z^{\,2} - 3 - \ln\left(\alpha_x\alpha_y\alpha_z\right)\right] \quad (9)$$

Using $\alpha_s = \alpha_x = \alpha_y = \alpha_z$, for isotropic expansion, we get

$$\Delta S_{el} = -\frac{kv_e}{2}\left[3\alpha_s^{\,2} - 3 - \ln\left(\alpha_s^{\,3}\right)\right] \quad (10)$$

The extensibility of a rubber is driven by entropic change rather than enthalpic changes. For ideal elastic behavior, the extension takes place due to the rearrangement of polymer chains and bonds are not stretched with change in length. This behavior is not true for most other materials (e.g. metals) where changes in length cause internal energy driven retractive force. For elastomeric materials, an increase in length is counter-balanced by decreasing the entropy only, which is due to the changes in the end-to-end distances of the network chains. The extensibility of hydrogels during swelling can be considered in the same way. The enthalpy change is ideally zero and practically very small in the case of swelling. By neglecting the enthalpy change during swelling, the free energy of elasticity for swelling is given as:

$$\Delta G_{\text{elastic}} = \Delta H_{\text{elastic}} - T\Delta S_{\text{elastic}} = \frac{kTv_e}{2}\left[3\alpha_s^{\,2} - 3 - \ln\left(\alpha_s^{\,3}\right)\right] \quad (11)$$

Differentiation of the above equation with respect to the number water molecules, n_1, at constant temperature and pressure (having in mind that α_s is the function of n_1) into the system gives,

$$\frac{\partial \Delta G_{\text{elastic}}}{\partial n_1} = kTv_e V_1\left[v_2^{\,1/3} - \frac{v_2}{2}\right] \quad (12)$$

Where,

V_1 = molar volume of water

v_2 = volume fraction of unswollen polymer in swollen hydrogel

υ_e = effective crosslinking density = $\frac{\upsilon_n}{V_o}$

υ_n = effective number of polymer chains in the network

V_0 = volume of unswollen polymer

This equation assumes that the network is ideal and all chains in the network are elastically active to contribute to the elastic stress. In hydrogels, free chain ends represent gel network "defects" that do not contribute to the elasticity of the network. Other network defects are chain "loops" and entanglements, which also do not contribute to the permanent network elasticity. These network imperfections such as chain entanglements, and chain ends are not taken into account. The corrected equation for these imperfections is:

$$\frac{\partial \Delta G_{el}}{\partial n_1} = kT\left(\frac{V_1}{v_a M_c}\right)\left(1-\frac{2M_c}{M_n}\right)\left({v_2}^{1/3}-\frac{v_2}{2f}\right) \tag{13}$$

Where,

v_a = specific volume of unswollen polymer

M_c = the number average molecular weight between cross-link points

M_n = the number average molecular weight of linear polymer chains prepared at the same conditions without crosslinking.

f = functionality of crosslinking agent.

Now, the overall chemical potential change of water in swollen hydrogel is

$$\mu_{wh} - \mu_{pw} = \Delta\mu_{mixture} + \Delta\mu_{elastic}$$

$$\Delta\mu = N_A\left[\frac{\partial \Delta G_m}{\partial n_1} + \frac{\partial \Delta G_{el}}{\partial n_1}\right]$$

$$\Delta\mu = N_A\left[kT\left(\ln v_1 + v_2 + \chi v_2^2\right) + kT\upsilon_e V_1\left({v_2}^{1/3} - \frac{v_2}{2}\right)\right]$$

$$\Delta\mu = RT\left[\ln v_1 + v_2 + \chi v_2^2 + \upsilon_e V_1\left({v_2}^{1/3} - \frac{v_2}{2}\right)\right] \tag{14}$$

Here, N_A is the Avogadro's number and form the definition; $k = R/N_A$.

At equilibrium, the chemical potential of the water within hydrogel must be the same as that of pure water. The term at the right hand side of the equation (14) should be zero at equilibrium. At the equilibrium we can write:

$$\Delta\mu = RT\left[\ln v_1 + v_2 + \chi {v_2}^2 + \upsilon_e V_1\left({v_2}^{1/3} - \frac{v_2}{2}\right)\right] = 0 \tag{15}$$

v_1 can be eliminate in favor of v_2 since $v_1 = 1 - v_2$. This equation is used to calculate the number average molecular weight between crosslinks:

$$\chi = -\frac{\ln(1-v_2)+v_2+\upsilon_e v_1\left(v_2^{1/3}-\frac{v_2}{2}\right)}{v_2^{\;2}} \tag{16}$$

3.2 Kinetics of hydrogel swelling

The kinetic behavior of hydrogel swelling is mainly due to diffusion and capillary rise of water into the hydrogel. Water uptake through capillary rise is much faster than the diffusion process. 1-cm rise of fluid in a narrow capillary (~100 μm) takes place in the order of milliseconds(Yui et al., 2004). The presence of small pore size (100 μm to 300 μm), good pore size distribution and extensive interconnected capillary channels in super porous hydrogel systems, make them fast swelling systems that are advantageous for specific applications such as sanitary adsorbants. Following capillary rise, diffusion of water into the polymer network takes place. The network relaxation, limited by the water-polymer interaction, plays a major role during the water diffusion process. To determine the nature of water diffusion into the hydrogels, the swelling data over the time intervals has been fitted into the Fickian diffusion equation (Ritger & Peppas 1987):

$$f = \frac{W_t}{W_\infty} = Kt^n \tag{17}$$

Where, f is the fractional water uptake at time t, W_t and W_∞ are the mass of the hydrogel at time t and at equilibrium swelling respectively, K is a characteristic rate constant that rely on the hydrogel structure and, n is a transport number that indicates whether diffusion and/or network relaxation controls the swelling. For one-dimensional slab geometry, the swelling is diffusion controlled for $n \le 0.50$, known as Fickian diffusion, where the rate of network relaxation is faster than the rate of diffusion. For $n = 1.00$, water transport is controlled by the rate of relaxation of the polymer network where the rate of diffusion is faster than rate of network relaxation and is known as non-Fickian diffusion. For the value of n between 0.50 and 1.00, both rates affect considerably on the swelling rate and none of their effect can be neglected. Such transport is called anomalous diffusion. For non-Fickian behavior of hydrogels, the deviation from Fickian behavior is due to the finite rates at which the polymer structure may change or reorient in response to the sorption or desorption of water molecules. In such polymers, a sorption process will be affected through the segmental motion that occurs at about the same rate or slower than the diffusion process. Thus, non-Fickian behavior is polymer structure dependant, and based on the polymer composition, wide range of relaxation times associated with structural changes can be observed. A number of mathematical models have been proposed for non-Fickian behavior of polymers(Ritger & Peppas 1987), however no single model successfully predicts all experimental observations.

For diffusion controlled swelling kinetics, the diffusion coefficient (D) is used to describe the rate of swelling. The flux, J, of a diffusing substance through the unit area of a section can be expressed by Fick´s first law(Ritger & Peppas 1987):

$$J = -D\left(\frac{\partial C}{\partial x}\right) \tag{18}$$

Where, $\left(\frac{\partial C}{\partial x}\right)$ is the concentration gradient which is the driving force for diffusion, and D is the diffusion coefficient. The diffusion coefficient is a constant and independent of x, C, and time, t. When the concentration gradient varies with time, the rate of change of concentration in one-dimension is given by Fick´s second law (Ritger and Peppas 1987):

$$\left(\frac{\partial C}{\partial t}\right) = D\left(\frac{\partial^2 C}{\partial x^2}\right) \tag{19}$$

Several solutions for equation 19 that depend on the boundary conditions were developed by Crank (Ritger & Peppas 1987). Using the time-dependent swelling data on thin films, the following equation can be used to calculate diffusion coefficient of water considering unsteady state diffusion and using planner geometry(Ritger & Peppas 1987):

$$\frac{W_t}{W_\infty} = \left(\frac{16D}{\pi L^2}\right)^{0.50} \times t^{0.50} \tag{20}$$

Where, L is the initial section thickness and D is the diffusion coefficient of water. Thus, the slope of the plot of $\frac{W_t}{W_\infty}$ against $t^{0.50}$ provides the diffusion coefficient of water for a given hydrogel system. Equation 20 is a good approximation for the solution obtained when the surface concentration is constant at both sides of the film for values of $\frac{W_t}{W_\infty}$ less than 0.6. Thus, when fractional swelling, $\frac{W_t}{W_\infty}$, is linear with the square root of time, the swelling profiles fit Fick's law, allowing the determination of diffusion coefficients.

4. Applications of hydrogels as biomaterials

Certain important properties of hydrogels for their applications as biomaterials can be tabulated as follows:

- Superior biocompatibility
- Good oxygen permeability
- Low protein adsorption and cell adhesion
- Aqueous surface environment to protect cells and therapeutic drugs (peptides, proteins, oligonucleotides, DNA)
- Minimal frictional irritation within the surrounding tissues upon implantation
- Soft and tissue-like physical properties
- Micro-porous structure for additional transport channels
- Ease of surface modification with specific biomolecules
- Can be injected in vivo as a solution that gels at body temperature

These properties of hydrogels made them ideal biomaterials for applications in drug delivery system, cell encapsulation, contact lenses, scaffolds for tissue engineering, biosensors, intelligent cell culture substrates, wound dressing, soft tissue replacement and many more.

4.1 Hydrogels for drug delivery applications

Well-designed drug delivery systems must control solute release over time. Various biomaterials have been investigated to control drug release; however, among them, hydrogels show two distinct advantages. (i) Drugs can easily diffuse out through the hydrogels. The rate of drug release can be controlled in many ways such as by changing the crosslinking density, preparing the hydrogel with monomers of controlled hydrophilicity and/or controlling the ratio of hydrophilic to hydrophobic monomers. (ii) Compared with hydrophobic materials, hydrogels may interact less strongly with drugs; consequently, a larger fraction of active molecules of drug, especially proteins and peptides, can be released through hydrogel carriers (Silva et al., 2009).

4.2 Hydrogels for cell encapsulation

Cell encapsulation technology provides a promising therapeutic modality for diabetes, hemophilia, cancer and renal failure (Orive et al., 2003; Orive et al., 2004). The selection of a suitable biomaterial as a membrane for encapsulating cells is the major challenge towards the success of cell encapsulation therapy. Biocompatibility, microporous structure and minimal surface irritation within the surrounding tissues of hydrogels attracted them for this application. They can be designed with required porosity that resists any entrance of immune cells and allows stimuli, oxygen, nutrients and/or waste transfer through the pores. Genetically modified alginates (King et al., 2003) and polyethylene oxide based hydrogels (Miura et al., 2006) have been studied as cell encapsulation systems.

4.3 Hydrogels for tissue engineering scaffolds

Tissue engineering has emerged as a promising technology for the design of an ideal, responsive, living substitute with properties similar to that of the native tissue (Lee & Mooney 2001). To date, it has focused mainly on restoration, maintenance and/or improvement of the functions of bone, cartilage, tendon, ligament, skin, blood vessels and heart valves. Scaffolds play an important role in scaffold-guided in vitro tissue engineering. Scaffolds are basically 3D structural templates which support cell adhesion, migration, differentiation, proliferation and provide guidance for neo tissue formation. The chosen scaffold material should be biocompatible and reproducible without any batch-property variation with high porosity and well organized inter-connectivity (Patel et al., 2006). Hydrogels in particular emerged as useful scaffolding biomaterials as they most closely resemble the natural tissues. Moreover, an aqueous environment provided by hydrogels mimics those of cells in the body. They are porous for nutrient and waste diffusion, and as discussed before they are usually considered to be biocompatible. However, the possibility of batch to batch variation is an issue with natural hydrogels which can be overcome using biologically modified synthetic hydrogels. Both synthetic and natural hydrogels are used as scaffolds for tissue engineering in order to repair cartilage, tendon, ligament, skin, blood vessels and heart valves(Drury & Mooney 2003; Patel et al., 2006). Synthetic hydrogels focused as scaffolds are polyurethanes (PU), poly(ethylene oxide) (PEO), poly(*N*-isopropylacrylamide) (PNIPAAm), poly(vinyl alcohol) (PVA), poly(acrylic acid) (PAA) and poly(propylene furmarate-*co*-ethylene glycol) (P(PF-*co*-EG)) whereas, naturally derived hydrogels are agarose, alginate, chitosan, collagen, fibrin, gelatin, and hyaluronic acid (HA) (Peppas et al., 2006).

4.4 Hydrogels for contact lens application

The cornea of the eye is a precisely formed transparent structure of protein fibers containing about 80% water and 20% formed materials making it a natural hydrogel (Merrett et al., 2009). Synthetic hydrogels have found to be suitable in contact lens applications when the refractive power of cornea is compromised. In addition to their biocompatibility and softness, inter-connected microstructures of hydrogels help oxygen diffusivity to the epithelial layer of the cornea. Certain hydrogels possess high refractive index, modulus, and transparency, required to fit for this application. Poly(HEMA) was the first hydrogel used as a contact lens in 1960 (Wichterle & Lim 1960). Since no single hydrophilic polymer structure provides all required properties, copolymers developed from a group of hydrophilic monomers like dimethylacrylamide (DMAAm), N-vinyl pyrrolidone (NVP) and methacrylic acid (MAA) and hydrophobic monomers like perfluoro polyethers (PFPE), methyl methacrylate (MMA) and silicon-containing monomers are utilized to design contact lenses(Nicolson & Vogt 2001; de Groot et al., 2003).

Moreover, hydrogels have also been studied as potential biomaterials for biosensors (Miyata et al., 2002), intelligent cell culture dish (Schmaljohann et al., 2003), wound-dressing (Sen & Avci 2005), injectable scaffolds (Stile & Healy 2001), and soft tissue replacement (Millon & Wan 2006).

5. Conclusions

Hydrogels are important classes of biomaterials with attractive properties. The review presented in this chapter highlights some aspects of hydrogel properties and applications. It is expected that hydrogels will continue to play significant roles in biomaedical engineering applications.

6. References

Adams, M.; Lavasanifar A. & Kwon, G. (2003). Amphiphilic block copolymers for drug delivery. *Journal of Pharmaceutical Sciences*. Vol. 92, No. 7, (July 2003), pp. 1343-1355, ISSN: 0022-3549.

Akashi, M., Nakano, S. & Kishida, A. (1996). Synthesis of poly(N-vinylisobutyramide) from poly(N-vinylacetamide) and its thermosensitive property. *Journal of Polymer Science Part A-Polymer Chemistry*. Vol. 34, No. 2, (January 1996), pp. 301-303, ISSN: 1099-0518

Arndt, K.; Schmidt, T. & Menge, H. (2001). Poly (vinyl methyl ether) hydrogel formed by high energy irradiation. *Macromolecular Symposia*. Vol. 164, No. 1, (February 2001), pp. 313-322.

Bae, Y.; Huh, K.; Kim, Y. & Park, K. (2000). Biodegradable amphiphilic multiblock copolymers and their implications for biomedical applications. *Journal of Controlled Release*. Vol. 64 No.1-3 (February 2000), pp. 3-13, ISSN: 0168-3659.

Baker, J.; Stephens, D., Blanch, H. & Prausnitz, J. (1992). Swelling Equilibria for Acrylamide-Based Polyampholyte Hydrogels. *Macromolecules*. Vol 25, No.7, (February 1992), pp. 1955-1958, ISSN 0024-9297.

Bohorquez, M.; Koch, C., Trygstad, T. & Pandit, N. (1999). A study of the temperature-dependent micellization of pluronic F127. *Journal of Colloid and Interface Science* Vol. 216, No. 1, (August 1999), pp.34-40, ISSN:1095-7103.

Bossard, F; Aubry, T., Gotzamanis, G. & Tsitsilianis, C. (2006). pH-Tunable rheological properties of a telechelic cationic polyelectrolyte reversible hydrogel. *Soft Matter*. Vol. 2, No. 6, (May 2006), pp. 510-516, ISSN 1292-8941.

Brahim, S.; Narinesingh, D. & Guiseppi-Elie, A. (2002). Bio-smart hydrogels: co-joined molecular recognition and signal transduction in biosensor fabrication and drug delivery. *Biosensors & Bioelectronics*. Vol. 17, No. 11-12, (December 2002), pp. 973-981. ISSN: 09565663.

Bushetti, S; Singh, V., Raju, S., Atharjaved & Veermaram (2009). Stimuli sensitive hydrogels: A review. *Indian Journal of Pharmaceutical Education and Research*. Vol. 43, No. 3, (July -September 2009), pp.241-250, ISSN: 0019-5464

de Groot, J; Spaans, C., van Calck, R., van Beijma, F., Norrby, S. & Pennings, A. (2003). Hydrogels for an accommodating intraocular lens. An explorative study. *Biomacromolecules*. Vol. 4 No. 3, (May-June 2003), pp. 608-616, *ISSN:* 1525-7797.

Dergunov, S. & Mun, G. (2009). Gamma-irradiated chitosan-polyvinyl pyrrolidone hydrogels as pH-sensitive protein delivery system. *Radiation Physics and Chemistry*. Vol. 78, No. 1, (January 2009), pp. 65-68. ISSN: 0969-806X.

Devine, D. & Higginbotham, C. (2003). The synthesis of a physically crosslinked NVP based hydrogel. *Polymer*. Vol. 44, No. 26, (December 2003), pp. 7851-7860, ISSN: 0032-3861

Drury, J., & Mooney, D. (2003). Hydrogels for tissue engineering: scaffold design variables and applications. Biomaterials. Vol. 24, No. 24, pp.4337-4351, (November 2003), ISSN 0142-9612.

Dumitriu, S. (Ed.). (2002). Polymeric Biomatrials, Marcel Dekker, Inc., SBN: 0824705696, New York.

Eichenbaum, G.; Kiser, P., Simon, S. & Needham, D. (1998). pH and ion-triggered volume response of anionic hydrogel microspheres. Macromolecules. Vol. 31, No. 15 (July 1998), pp. 5084-5093, ISSN 0024-9297

Ende, M. & Peppas, N. (1996). Transport of ionizable drugs and proteins in crosslinked poly(acrylic acid) and poly(acrylic acid-co-2-hydroxyethyl methacrylate) hydrogels .1. Polymer characterization. *Journal of Applied Polymer Science*. Vol. 59 No. 4, (January 1996), pp.673-685, ISSN: 0021-8995.

Flory, P. (1953). *Principles of polymer chemistry*, Cornell University Press. ISBN 0-8014-0134-8 Ithaca, NY.

Gil, E. & Hudson, S. (2004). Stimuli-reponsive polymers and their bioconjugates. *Progress in Polymer Science. Vol.* 29 No. 12, (December 2004), pp. 1173-1222, *ISSN*: 0079-6700.

Gupta, P.; Vermani, K. & Garg, S. (2002). Hydrogels: from controlled release to pH-responsive drug delivery. *Drug Discovery Today*. Vol. 7, No. 10, (15 May 2002), pp. 569-579, ISSN: 1359-6446.

He, C.; Kim, S. & Lee, D. (2008). In situ gelling stimuli-sensitive block copolymer hydrogels for drug delivery. *Journal of Controlled Release*. Vol. 127, No. 3, (May 2008), pp.189-207. ISSN: 0168-3659

Hennink, W. & van Nostrum, C. (2002). Novel crosslinking methods to design hydrogels. *Advanced Drug Delivery Reviews*. Vol. 54, No. 1 (January 2002), pp.13-36, ISSN 0169-409X

Hin, T. (2004). *Engineering Materials for Biomedical Applications*. World Scientific Publishing, Singapore, ISBN: 981-256-061-0.

Hirokawa, Y. & Tanaka, T. (1984). Volume Phase-Transition in a Nonionic Gel. *Journal of Chemical Physics.* Vol. 81, No. 12, pp.6379-6380. ISSN: 0021-9606

Hoffman, A. S. (2002). Hydrogels for biomedical applications. Advanced Drug Delivery Reviews. Vol. 54, No. 1, (January 2002), pp.3-12, ISSN 0169-409X.

Jabbari, E. & Nozari, S. (1999). Synthesis of Acrylic Acid Hydrogel by γ-Irradiation Cross-linking of Polyacrylic Acid in Aqueous Solution. *Iranian Polymer Journal.* Vol. 8, No. 4, pp. 264-270,ISSN 1735-5265.

Jeong, B., Y. H. Bae, et al. (1997). Biodegradable block copolymers as injectable drug-delivery systems. *Nature.* Vol. 388, No. 6645, (August 1997), pp.860-862, ISSN: 0028-0836

Jhon, M. & Andrade, J. (1973). Water and Hydrogels. *Journal of Biomedical Materials Research* Vol. 7, No. 6, pp. 509-522, ISSN 1097-4636.

Jianqi, F.& Lixia. G. (2002). PVA/PAA thermo-crosslinking hydrogel fiber: preparation and pH-sensitive properties in electrolyte solution. *European Polymer Journal.* Vol. 38, No. 8, (August 2002), pp.1653-1658, ISSN: 0014-3057

Kabra, B.; Akhtar, M. & Gehrke, S. (1992). Volume Change Kinetics of Temperature-Sensitive Poly(Vinyl Methyl-Ether) Gel. *Polymer.* Vol. 33, No. 5, pp. 990-995. ISSN: 0032-3861

Kang, S. & Bae, Y. (2003). A sulfonamide based glucose-responsive hydrogel with covalently immobilized glucose oxidase and catalase. *Journal of Controlled Release. Vol.* 86, No. 1, (January 2003), pp.115-121. ISSN: 0168-3659

Kashyap, N.; Kumar, N, & Ravi Kumar, M. (2005). Hydrogels for pharmaceutical and biomedical applications. *Critical Reviews in Therapeutic Drug Carrier Systems. Vol.* 22, No. 2, pp. 107-149. *ISSN*: 0743-4863

Kashyap, N., Kumar, N. & Ravi Kumar (2004). Smart gels for drug delivery applications. *Drug Development and Delivery. Vol.* 4, No. 7 (Sept 2004), pp. 32-39.

Kim, J.; Lee, S., Kim, S. & Lee, Y. (2002). Rapid temperature/pH response of porous alginate-g-poly(N-isopropylacrylamide) hydrogels. Polymer. Vol. 43, No. 26, (December 2002), pp. 7549-7558. ISSN: 0032-3861

Kim, S.; Kim, H.; Park, S.; Ki,. I.; Lee, S.; Lee, T. & Kim, S. (2005). Behavior in electric fields of smart hydrogels with potential application as bio-inspired actuators. *Smart Materials & Structures. Vol.* 14, No. 4, pp.511-514, ISSN 1361-665X

Kim, S.; Park, S. & Kim, S. (2004). Properties of smart hydrogels composed of polyacrylic acid/poly(vinyl sulfonic acid) responsive to external stimuli. *Smart Materials & Structures. Vol.* 13, No. 2, pp.317-322, ISSN 1361-665X.

King, A., B. Strand, et al. (2003). Improvement of the biocompatibility of alginate/poly-L-lysine/alginate microcapsules by the use of epimerized alginate as a coating. *J Biomed Mater Res* A. Vol. 64, No. 3, (March 2003),pp.533-539.ISSN 1549-3296.

Kopecek, J. (2003). Smart and genetically engineered biomaterials and drug delivery systems. *European Journal of Pharmaceutical Sciences.* Vol. 20, No. 1, pp.1-16, ISSN: 1530-9932.

Kozlovskaya, V.; Kharlampieva, E., Mansfield, M. & Sukhishvili, S. (2006). Poly(methacrylic acid) hydrogel films and capsules: Response to pH and ionic strength, and encapsulation of macromolecules. *Chemistry of Materials.* Vol. 18, No. 2, pp.328-336, ISSN 0897-4756.

Kubo, M.; Matsuura, T.; Morimoto, H.; Uno, T. & Itoh, T. (2005). Preparation and polymerization of a water-soluble, nonbonding crosslinking agent for a mechanically crosslinked hydrogel. *Journal of Polymer Science Part A-Polymer Chemistry*. Vol. 43, No. 21, pp.5032-5040, ISSN 0887-624X.

Kunugi, S.; Takano, K, Tanaka, N.; Suwa, K. &Akashi, M. (1997). Effects of pressure on the behavior of the thermoresponsive polymer poly(N-vinylisobutyramide) (PNVIBA). *Macromolecules*. Vol. 30, No. 15, pp.4499-4501, ISSN 0024-9297.

Lamba, N.; Woodhouse, K. & Cooper, S. (1998). *Polyurethanes in Biomedical Applications.*, CRC Press, ISBN 0849345170, New York.

Lee, B.; West, B.,McLemore, R., Pauken, C. & Vernon, B. (2006). In-situ injectable physically and chemically gelling NIPAAm-based copolymer system for embolization. *Biomacromolecules*. Vol. 7, No. 6, pp.2059-2064. ISSN 1525-7797.

Lee, K. & Mooney, D. (2001). Hydrogels for tissue engineering. *Chemical Reviews*. Vol. 101, No. 7, pp. 1869-1879, ISSN:0009-2665

Li, S.; Molina, I.; Martinez, M. & Vert, M. (2002). Hydrolytic and enzymatic degradations of physically crosslinked hydrogels prepared from PLA/PEO/PLA triblock copolymers. *Journal of Materials Science-Materials in Medicine*. Vol. 13, No. 1, pp. 81-86, ISSN: 0957-4530.

Liu, Y.; Vrana, N. & McGuinness, G. (2009). Physically Crosslinked Composite Hydrogels of PVA With Natural Macromolecules: Structure, Mechanical Properties, and Endothelial Cell Compatibility. *Journal of Biomedical Materials Research Part B-Applied Biomaterials*. Vol. 90B, No. 2, pp. 492-502, ISSN: 1552-4981

Xuequan, L.; Maolin, Z.; Jiuqiang, L. & Hongfei, H. (2000). Radiation preparation and thermo-response swelling of interpenetrating polymer network hydrogel composed of PNIPAAm and PMMA. *Radiation Physics and Chemistry*. Vol. 57, No. 3-6, (March 2000), pp.477-480, ISSN: 0969-806X.

Lu, Z.; Kopeckova, P. & Kopecek, J. (2003). Antigen responsive hydrogels based on polymerizable antibody Fab ' fragment. *Macromolecular Bioscience*. Vol. 3, No. 6, pp. 296-300, ISSN 1616-5195

Mequanint, K.; Patel, A.; Bezuidenhout, D. (2006). Synthesis, swelling behavior, and biocompatibility of novel physically cross-linked polyurethane-block-poly(glycerol methacrylate) hydrogels. *Biomacromolecules*. Vol. 7, No. 3, pp. 883-891. ISSN 1525-7797.

Merrett, K.; Liu, W.; Mitra, D.; Camm, K.; McLaughlin, C.; Liu, Y.; Watsky, M.; Li, F.; Griffith, M. & Fogg, D. (2009). Synthetic neoglycopolymer-recombinant human collagen hybrids as biomimetic crosslinking agents in corneal tissue engineering. Biomaterials. Vol. 30, No. 29, pp.5403-5408, ISSN: 0142-9612

Millon, L. & Wan, W. (2006). The polyvinyl alcohol-bacterial cellulose system as a new nanocomposite for biomedical applications. *Journal of Biomedical Materials Research Part B-Applied Biomaterials*. Vol. 79B, No. 2, pp.245-253. ISSN: 1552-4981

Miura, S.; Teramura, Y. & Iwata, H. (2006). Encapsulation of islets with ultra-thin polyion complex membrane through poly(ethylene glycol)-phospholipids anchored to cell membrane. *Biomaterials*. Vol. 27, No. 34, (December 2006), pp. 5828-5835. ISSN: 0142-9612

Miyata, T.; Asami, N. & Uragami, T. (1999). A reversibly antigen-responsive hydrogel. *Nature*. Vol. 399, No. 6738, pp.766-769. ISSN: 0028-0836

Miyata, T., Uragami, Nakamae, K (2002). Biomolecule-sensitive hydrogels. *Advanced Drug Delivery Reviews*. Vol. 54, No. 1, (January 2002), pp.79-98, ISSN 0169-409X.

Nicolson, P. & Vogt, J. (2001). Soft contact lens polymers: an evolution. *Biomaterials*. Vol. 22, No. 24, pp.3273-3283, ISSN: 0142-9612.

Obaidat, A. & Park, K. (1996). Characterization of glucose dependent gel-sol phase transition of the polymeric glucose-concanavalin A hydrogel system. *Pharmaceutical Research* Vol. 13, No. 7, pp.989-995. ISSN: 0724-8741

Orive, G.; Hernández, R.; Gascón, A.; Calafiore, R.; Chang, T.; De Vos, P.; Hortelano, G.; Hunkeler, D.; Lacík, I.; Shapiro, J. & Pedraz, J. (2003). Cell encapsulation: promise and progress. *Nature Medicine*. Vol. 9, No. 1, pp.104-107, ISSN: 1078-8956.

Orive, G.; Hernández, R.; Gascón, A.; Calafiore, R.; Chang, T.; De Vos, P.; Hortelano, G.; Hunkeler, D.; Lacík, I.& & Pedraz, J. (2004). History, challenges and perspectives of cell microencapsulation. *Trends in Biotechnology*. Vol. 22, No. 2, (February 2004), pp. 87-92, ISSN: 0167-9430

Park, J. & Bae, Y. (2002). Hydrogels based on poly(ethylene oxide) and poly(tetramethylene oxide) or poly(dimethyl siloxane): synthesis, characterization, in vitro protein adsorption and platelet adhesion. *Biomaterials*. Vol. 23, No. 8: 1797-1808. ISSN: 0142-9612

Patel, A.; Fine, B., Sandig, M. & Mequanint, K. (2006). Elastin biosynthesis: The missing link in tissue-engineered blood vessels. *Cardiovascular Research*. Vol. 71. No. 1, pp. 40-49, ISSN 2151-920X.

Peppas, N.; Bures, P.; Leobandung, W. & Ichikawa, H. (2000). Hydrogels in pharmaceutical formulations. *European Journal of Pharmaceutics and Biopharmaceutics*. Vol. 50, No. 1, pp. 27-46, ISSN 0939-6411.

Peppas, N.; Hilt, J.; Khademhosseini, A. & Langer, R. (2006). Hydrogels in biology and medicine: From molecular principles to bionanotechnology. *Advanced Materials*. Vol. 18, No, 11, (May 2006), pp. 1345-1360, ISSN: 1521-4095

Peppas, N.; Huang, Y.; Torres-Lugo, M.; Ward, J. & Zhang J. (2000). Physicochemical, foundations and structural design of hydrogels in medicine and biology. *Annual Review of Biomedical Engineering*. Vol. 2, (August 2000), pp.9-29, ISSN:1523-9829.

Podual, K.; Doyle, F. & Peppas, N. (2000). Glucose-sensitivity of glucose oxidase-containing cationic copolymer hydrogels having poly(ethylene glycol) grafts. *Journal of Controlled Release*. Vol. 67, No. 1, (June 2000), pp. 9-17, ISSN: 0168-3659

Podual, K.; Doyle, F. & Peppas, N. (2000). Preparation and dynamic response of cationic copolymer hydrogels containing glucose oxidase. *Polymer. Vol.* 41, No. 11, (May 2000), pp. 3975-3983, ISSN: 0032-3861.

Xiangli, Q.; Zhenjia, Z. & Side, Y. (2006). Preparation of initiator and cross-linker-free poly (N-isopropylacrylamide) nanogels by photopolymerization. *Journal of Photochemistry and Photobiology A-Chemistry*. Vol. 177, No. 2-3, (January 2006), pp. 191-196, ISSN: 1010-6030.

Qu, X.; Wirsen, A. & Albertsson (2000). Novel pH-sensitive chitosan hydrogels: swelling behavior and states of water. *Polymer*. Vol. 41, No. 12, (June 2000), 4589-4598. ISSN: 0032-3861.

Ratner, B.; Hoffman, A.; Schoen, F. & Lemons, J. (2004). Biomaterials Science: An Introduction to Materials in Medicine, Elsevier Academic Press, ISBN 0-12-582463-7, San Diego, CA.

Ritger, P. & Peppas, N. (1987). A simple equation for description of solute release I. Fickian and non-fickian release from non-swellable devices in the form of slabs, spheres, cylinders or discs. Journal of Controlled Release. Vol. 5, No. 1, (June 1987), pp. 23-36, ISSN: 0168-3659

Rogero, S.; Malmonge, S.; Lugao, A.; Ikeda, T.; Miyamaru, L. & Cruz, A. (2003). Biocompatibility study of polymeric biomaterials. *Artificial Organs.* Vol. 27, No. 5, (May 2003), pp. 424-427, ISSN: 1525-1594.

Rosiak, J. & Yoshii, F. (1999). Hydrogels and their medical applications. *Nuclear Instruments & Methods in Physics Research Section B-Beam Interactions with Materials and Atoms.* Vol. 151, No. 1-4, pp.56-64, ISSN: 0168-583X

Ruel-Gariepy, E. & Leroux, J. (2004). In situ-forming hydrogels - review of temperature-sensitive systems. *European Journal of Pharmaceutics and Biopharmaceutics.* Vol. 58, No. 2, pp. 409-426. ISSN: 0939-6411

Schmaljohann, D. (2005). Thermo-responsive polymers and hydrogels in tissue engineering. *e-Polymers.* No. 021, pp. 1-17, ISSN 1618-7229

Schmaljohann, D.; Oswald, J.; Jørgensen, B.; Nitschke, M.; Beyerlein, D. & Werner, C. (2003). Thermo-responsive PNiAAm-g-PEG films for controlled cell detachment. Biomacromolecules. Vol. 4, No. 6, (August 2003), pp.1733-1739. ISSN 1525-7797

Sen, M. & Avci, E. (2005). Radiation synthesis of poly(N-vinyl-2-pyrrolidone)-kappa-carrageenan hydrogels and their use in wound dressing applications. I. Preliminary laboratory tests. *Journal of Biomedical Materials Research Part A.* Vol. 74A, No. 2, pp.187-196 ISSN: 1549-3296.

Sen, M. & Sari M. (2005). Radiation synthesis and characterization of poly(N,N-dimethylaminoethyl methaerylate-co-N-vinyl 2-pyrrolidone) hydrogels. *European Polymer Journal.* Vol. 41, No. 6, pp.1304-1314. ISSN 0014-3057

Shiino, D.; Murata, Y.; Kubo, A.; Kim, Y.; Kataoka, K.;Koyama, ; Y.; Kikuchi, A.; Yokoyama, M.; Sakurai, Y. & Okano, T. (1995). Amine containing phenylboronic acid gel for glucose-responsive insulin release under physiological pH. *Journal of Controlled Release. Vol.* 37, No. 3, pp. 269-276, ISSN: 0168-3659

Silva, A.; Richard, C.; Bessodes, M.; Scherman, D. & Merten, O. (2009). Growth factor delivery approaches in hydrogels. *Biomacromolecules.* Vol. 10, No.1 (November 26, 2008) pp.9-18. ISSN 1525-7797

Slaughter, B.; Khurshid, S. Fisher, O.; Khademhosseini, A.& Peppas, N. (2009). Hydrogels in regenerative medicine. *Advanced Materials.* Vol. 21, pp. 3307-3329. ISSN: 1521-4095

Song, M.; Lee, D.; Ahn, J.; Kim, D. & Kim, S. (2000). Dielectric behavior during sol-gel transition of PEO-PPO-PEO triblock copolymer aqueous solution. *Polymer Bulletin* Vol. 43, No. 6, pp. 497-504, ISSN 1436-2449.

Stabenfeldt, S.; Gacia, A. & LaPlaca, M. (2006). Thermoreversible laminin-functionalized hydrogel for neural tissue engineering. *Journal of Biomedical Materials Research Part A.* Vol. 77A, No. 4, pp. 718-725. ISSN 1549-3296.

Stile, R. & Healy, K. (2001). Thermo-responsive peptide-modified hydrogels for tissue regeneration. *Biomacromolecules.* Vol. 2, No. 1, pp.185-194. ISSN 1525-7797

Suwa, K.; Morishita, K.; Kishida, A. & Akashi, M. (1997). Synthesis and functionalities of Poly(N-vinylalkylamide) .5. Control of a lower critical solution temperature of poly(N-vinylalkylamide). *Journal of Polymer Science Part A-Polymer Chemistry.* Vol. 35, No. 15, pp. 3087-3094. ISSN: 1099-0518

Suwa, K.; Wada, Y. & Akashi, M. (1997). Synthesis and functionalities of poly(N-vinylalkylamide) .6. A novel thermosensitive hydrogel crosslinked poly(N-vinylisobutyramide). *Journal of Polymer Science Part A-Polymer Chemistry. Vol.*35, No. 16, pp.3377-3384, ISSN: 0887-624X.

Theiss, D.; Schmidt, T. & Arndt K-F. (2004). Temperature-sensitive poly(vinyl methyl ether) hydrogel beads. *Macromolecular Symposia.* Vol. 210, No. 1, (March 2004), pp.465-474, ISSN:1521-3900

Traitel, T.; Cohen, Y. & Kost, J. (2000). Characterization of glucose-sensitive insulin release systems in simulated in vivo conditions. *Biomaterials. Vol.* 21, No. 16, pp. 1679-1687. ISSN: 0142-9612

Vamvakaki, M.; Palioura, D.; Spyros, A.; Armes, S. & Anastasiadis, S. (2006). Dynamic light scattering vs H-1 NMR investigation of pH-responsive diblock copolymers in water. *Macromolecules. Vol.* 39, No. 15, (July 2006), pp.5106-5112. ISSN 1525-7797

Vinatier, C.; Magne, D.; Weiss, P.; Trojani, C.; Rochet, N.; Carle, G.; Vignes-Colombeix, C.; Chadjichristos, C.; Galera, P.; Daculsi, G. & Guicheux, J. (2005). A silanized hydroxypropyl methylcellulose hydrogel for the three-dimensional culture of chondrocytes. *Biomaterials.* Vol. 26, No. 33, (November 2005) pp 6643-6651. ISSN: 0142-9612

Wang, C.; Stewart, R. & Kopecek, J. (1999). Hybrid hydrogels assembled from synthetic polymers and coiled-coil protein domains. *Nature* Vol. 397, No. 6718, (February 1999), pp. 417-420, ISSN : 0028-0836

Wang, Y.; Shen, Y.; Zhang,Y.; Yue, B. & Wu, C. (2006). pH-sensitive polyacrylic acid (PAA) hydrogels trapped with polysodium-p-styrenesulfonate (PSS). *Journal of Macromolecular Science Part B-Physics.* Vol. 45, No. 4, pp.563-571. ISSN 1525-609X

Wichterle, O. & Lim, D. (1960). Hydrophilic Gels for Biological Use. *Nature.* Vol. 185, No. 4706, pp.117-118, ISSN : 0028-0836.

Wright, E. & Conticello, V. (2002). Self-assembly of block copolymers derived from elastin-mimetic polypeptide sequences. *Advanced Drug Delivery Reviews.* Vol. 54, No. 8, pp. 1057-1073, ISSN 0169-409X.

Wright, E. R., R. A. McMillan, et al. (2002). Thermoplastic elastomer hydrogels via self-assembly of an elastin-mimetic triblock polypeptide. *Advanced Functional Materials* Vol. 12, No. 2, pp.149-154, ISSN: 1616-3028.

Xu, C.; Breedveld, V. & Kopecˇek, J. (2005). Reversible hydrogels from self-assembling genetically engineered protein block copolymers. *Biomacromolecules.* Vol. 6, No. 3, (April 2005), pp.1739-1749, ISSN 1525-7797.

Yaszemski, M.; Trntolo, D.; Lewandrowski, K-U.; Hasirci, V.; Altobelli, D. &, Wise, D. (Eds.), (2004). *Tissue Engineering and Novel Delivery Systems,* CRC Press, ISBN-13: 978-0824747862

Ying, Y.; Gu, X. & Yang, C. (1998). Abnormal pH sensitivity of polyacrylate-polyurethane hydrogels. *Journal of Applied Polymer Science. Vol.* 70, No. 6, (November 1998). pp. 1047-1052. ISSN: 0021-8995.

Yui, N.; Mrsny, R. & Park, K. (Eds.), (2004). *Reflexive Polymers and Hydrogels: Understanding and Designing Fast Responsive Polymeric Systems,* CRC Press, ISBN: 978-0-8493-1487-2, New York.

Zan, J.; Chen, H.; Jiang, G.; Lin, Y. & Ding F. (2006). Preparation and properties of crosslinked chitosan thermosensitive hydrogel for injectable drug delivery systems. *Journal of Applied Polymer Science*. Vol. 101, No. 3, pp.1892-1898. ISSN: 0021-8995.

15

On the Application of Gas Discharge Plasmas for the Immobilization of Bioactive Molecules for Biomedical and Bioengineering Applications

Frank Hempel et al.*
Leibniz Institute for Plasma Science and Technology e.V. (INP), Greifswald, Germany

1. Introduction

Biomedical and biotechnological applications of polymeric materials often require specific interactions of the substrate surface with the biochemical or biological milieu. However, the standard surface properties of polymers like polystyrene (PS), polycarbonate (PC), polypropylene (PP), fluorinated ethylene polypropylene (FEP) or cyclic olefin copolymers (COC) do not meet these requirements. Therefore, the creation of functional surfaces is a very important topic to meet the requirements of advanced applications in bioengineering.

For this purpose, gas-discharge plasmas offer some unique possibilities (Ohl & Schröder. 2008; Schröder et al., 2010a). They can lead to surface activation and functionalization, often not obtainable with conventional, solvent-based chemical methods. In addition, the superior chemical reactivity of plasmas allows surface activation of inert materials down to the nanoscale range including the creation of covalently bound functional groups in such small structures (Meyer-Plath et al., 2003). While it is possible to implant substances into the substrate and to etch surface structures by gas discharges, properly operated plasma processes might as well neither affect bulk materials characteristics nor produce undesirable substances and cause only minor thermal load to substrates (Schröder et al., 2011).

Plasma processes are especially suitable for the equipment of polymer surfaces with chemical functional groups. Plasma functionalizations as well as depositions of nanometer-thick coatings with chemical groups can be used to receive the required biological response, for instance to control the cell density, distribution, adhesion and differentiation (Wende et al., 2006). Furthermore, plasma based processes can be combined with lateral pattern generation. Common mask techniques are suitable to create

* Hartmut Steffen[1], Benedikt Busse[2], Birgit Finke[1], J. Barbara Nebe[3], Antje Quade[1], Henrike Rebl[3], Claudia Bergemann[3], Klaus-Dieter Weltmann[1] and Karsten Schröder[1].
1 Leibniz Institute for Plasma Science and Technology e.V. (INP), Greifswald, Germany,
2 zell-kontakt GmbH, Nörten-Hardenberg, Germany,
3 University of Rostock, Medical Faculty, Dept. of Cell Biology, Rostock, Germany.

lateral chemical structures with different dimensions and interface properties. Sometimes, e.g. for multi-spot arrays in consumables used in high throughput screening (HTS), micro structures are required if such surfaces should be applied. Plasma processes are especially suitable for the functionalization of fine morphological 3D-structures with complex shapes like for instance cavities and trenches in HTS platforms, holes in textiles and membranes, and pores in foams (Schröder et al., 2005). Another aspect is localized chemical (micro) pattern for lateral array structures. Applications of such micro-patterned polymer surfaces could be tissue-like cell culture systems as well as neuronal networks, bioartificial organs, implants, biosensors, DNA and protein biochips or further tools for pharmaceutical screening.

For the optimization of the plasma and patterning processes it is necessary to analyze the surfaces for their physicochemical properties and cell compatibility in an appropriate way. In particular different surface chemistries have to be analyzed in direct neighbourhood. Often highly resolved XPS analysis and imaging is applied for the chemical characterization of surface microstructures. Using XPS analysis, well-defined chemical functionalizations, good homogeneities, and sharp edges can be verified allowing a high density of such patterns.

Both, plasmas at atmospheric pressure and low pressure can be applied for surface modification. While atmospheric pressure plasmas offer advantages in terms of investment cost and process integrability, low pressure plasmas excel by their superior chemical selectivity. Therefore, in this article examples of low pressure plasma-assisted immobilization strategies will be given for cell-adhesion molecules for biomaterials surfaces and enzyme-carriers for white biotechnology.

2. Plasma enhanced micro structuring of cell-based RNA arrays

2.1 Background

The investigations and analyses of surface modifications to control cell adhesion are an important topic of biomaterials research. Chemical micro patterns consisting of cell-adhesive and cell-repulsive regions can be applied to additionally influence cell position, migration, proliferation, phenotype, membrane integrity and finally live and death (Chen et al., 1997; Ohl & Schröder, 1999). Gas-discharge plasma processes can be used to create functional groups or ultra thin functional coatings, which are covalently fixed to the substrate. They could be interesting for DNA- and protein chips in high-throughput-screening (HTS), too (Müller et al. 2003).

Prospective applications of chemically patterned polymer surfaces are cell-based RNA arrays. Cell-based arrays usually are made of polymers as substrate material. For this reason their surface is very heat sensitive and has to become chemically inert before it will come in contact with aqueous liquids. In addition, for bio-applications it must be biocompatible and so it needs a defined surface treatment for controlled modification of these material parameters. Plasma processing meets all these requirements (Ohl, 1999).

Plasma-assisted chemical surface functionalization is a frequently-used processing step for the preparation of chemical micro patterns on polymeric surfaces (Schröder et al., 2002). Plasma processes were also applied for the treatment of interior surfaces of small trench structures (Besch et al., 2008) and for the creation of localized chemical structures for a cell-based high content screening system (Steffen et al., 2007). In the present chapter we present a special pattern which consists of an arrangement with three different chemical zones for a cell-based array for reverse siRNA transfection.

The discovery of a ribonucleic interference (RNAi) (Fire et al., 1998) opened up new possibilities for functional genome research in particular by cell transfection with small interfering RNA (siRNA). In such a reverse transcription assay, the siRNA is immobilized in a gel-forming matrix like gelatine or alginate (Zlauddin & Sabatini, 2001). Arrays of similar gel spots with very small volumes have to be created on a carrier chip for high-throughput-screening (HTS) (Szili et al., 2004). To guarantee optimum transfection, the siRNA should be spotted in direct neighbourhood to the growing cells. For multiple analyses, the single cell spots have to be separated by barriers to prevent cell migration and siRNA cross-talk between the different assays. Many eukaryotic cells do not grow on untreated polymers which are typically applied as base materials for HTS labware such as polystyrene (PS), polycarbonate (PC), polypropylene (PP), cyclic olefin polymers- and copolymers (CCP and COC), or poly(methyl methacrylate) (PMMA). For this reason, untreated polymers could act as barriers regions. But, γ- and e-beam sterilization methods introduce oxygen-containing functional groups (Fire et al., 1998) at the polymer's surface and lead to an undesired cell migration. Ideally, a small round spot of immobilized siRNA is surrounded by a cell layer in intimate contact. Obviously, specific surface structures of the chip have to be analyzed to verify the successful modification procedure.
On this account, a triple contrast has to be visualized for cell-based RNA arrays. A high local definition of chemical contrasts is required. For the development of such arrays, chemical surface properties have to be known with high spatial resolution. Obviously, quantifications of transfection effect need defined borderlines. Thus, the investigation of borders in chemical microstructures on polymer surfaces is of special importance with respect to accuracy of dimensions and geometry as well as the correlation with large-area treatments. The characterization of the quantitative chemical composition inside the micro pattern is important for the miniaturization of diagnostic tools (Schröder et al., 2009). The chemical structures can be visualized by fluorescence microscopy after labelling of functional groups with fluorescence dyes or by atomic force microscopy (AFM) by modification of the tips with specific molecules. Quantitative chemical analyses of such micro pattern can be performed with Auger electron spectroscopy (AES), time-of-flight secondary ion mass spectrometry (TOF-SIMS), and X-ray photoelectron spectroscopy (XPS). XPS is advantageous according to the absolute values without calibration (Schröder et al., 2004).
So, three surface zones with different physicochemical properties on optical clear substrates had to be produced: a cellophobic border (zone 1), cellophilic marrow area (zone 2) and a spotting zone (zone 3) for the siRNA.

2.2 Materials and methods

Cell array chambers (CAC) (Fig. 1) were applied as substrates for plasma modification. They were provided by zell-kontakt (Nörten-Hardenberg, Germany). These disposables contain four rectangular chambers, every chamber with the dimensions of a microscope slide (75 mm x 26 mm). They are injection-moulded from extremely clean polymers (PS, PC, COC) and have a very smooth surface necessary for pattern generation by mask processes.
Fig. 1 shows a medium-scaled array of 3x8 zones for siRNA immobilisation. The central analytical zones (zone 3) are surrounded by ring-shaped areas (zone 2) which support in this case the growth of adherence-dependent mammalian cells. The surrounding third zone (zone 1) fills the rest of the surface to prevent the cross-talk between different spots.

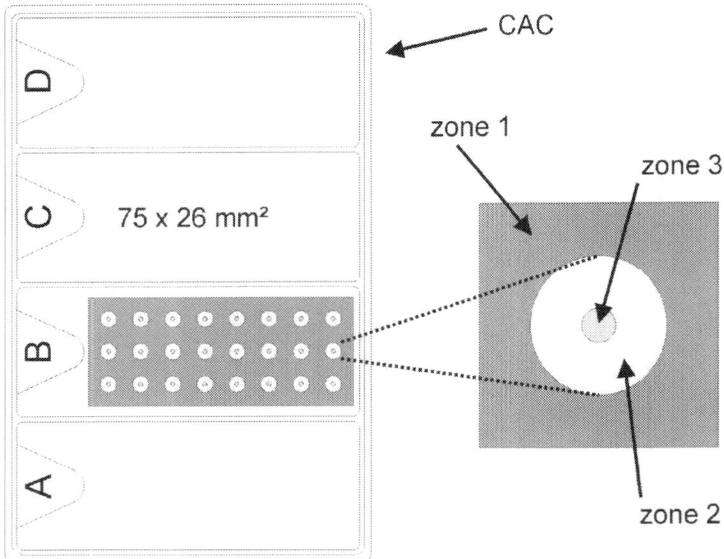

Fig. 1. Schematic view of a single element (right) and arrangement (left) of the cell-based RNA array in a cell array chamber (CAC) (Schröder et al., 2009).

Zone 1 prevents the cross-talk between the elements of the array. That way, many different experiments can be performed in interaction with one and the same cell culture on one array. For this purpose, surface properties of this zone have to suppress adhesion of cells reliably.

Zone 2 is the cell growth area. It needs a functionalization, which supports the growth of sensitive adherent cells. The contact angle should be between 40° and 60°. The attachment of more than 10-15 spread cells should be possible. This gives a lower limit of about 500 µm for the width.

The siRNA will be spotted onto zone 3. This zone should guarantee the immobilization of the siRNA and the interfacial interaction with the cells. The cells grow over the spotted area and absorb the siRNA. Zone 3 has to be remarkably more hydrophilic than zone 2 to keep the siRNA at this area.

All modified surfaces mentioned in this article can be generated with microwave plasmas. The plasma treatments were performed with a V55G plasma reactor (PLASMA-finish, Schwedt, Germany) (Fig. 2). The reactor consists of an aluminium process chamber which has the dimensions 40 x 45 x 34 cm³ (width x depth x high). Microwaves (2.45 GHz) were coupled top down into the chamber. A parabolic reflector was used to spread microwave power over the whole area of a 200 mm in diameter quartz window in the top wall of the chamber. Thus, a relatively high lateral homogeneity of large area surface treatments can be achieved in certain cases (van Wachem, 1985).

NH_3 (40 sccm) was used as process gas for NH_3 plasma treatment at 20 Pa and 500 W. The distance to the microwave window was 5 cm and the treatment duration was 5 s.

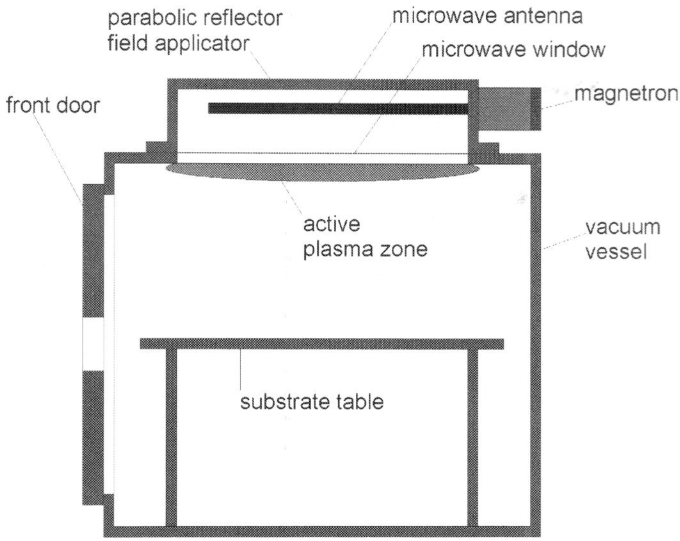

Fig. 2. Schematic view of the plasma reactor VG55 used for the three plasma modifications.

For the plasma polymerization, a mixture of allylamine and Ar (50 sccm) was used. The plasma was pulsed (0.1 s / 1.5 s, on/off) with a power of 500 W at a pressure of 25 Pa. The samples were placed 9 cm below the microwave window and treated for 288 s.
The fluorinated hydrocarbon surface was functionalized by pure NH_3 as well as H_2/NH_3 cw microwave plasma. In both cases the treatment time was varied between 1 and 60 s. The other conditions for the NH_3 plasma treatment were the same as mentioned above.
The chemical composition of the modified polymer surfaces was analyzed with high resolution XPS (Axis Ultra, DLD, Kratos, Manchester GB). For spectroscopic measurements, the spot size was 250 µm in diameter. All elements were quantified after measurement with low energy resolution (pass energy was (PE) of 80 eV) and calculated with atomic sensitivity factors given by a XPS-instrument-specific RSF data library. The C1s peak was measured with high energy resolution with a PE of 10 eV. Moreover, the chemical differences within the 3 zones were visualized with XPS images. The XPS measurements were evaluated with CasaXPS 2.3 (Casa Software Ltd) mainly (Fairley et al., 2005).
Contact angles were measured using the sessile drop method with ultra pure water at room temperature with a Digidrop contact angle meter (GBX Instrumentation Scientifique, Romance, France). At least five measurements were performed on different positions of the sample and averaged.
Cell culture experiments were carried out with Human Embryonic Kidney (HEK) cells in untreated and plasma modified CAC's. This cell line is a frequently used model. The HEK cells were seeded into the CAC's with a density of 200 cells/mm^2 and grown for 24 h (37 °C, 5 % CO_2). PC12HEK cells were cultured in RPMI 1640 Dulbecco's Modified Eagle's Medium (DMEM) with 7 % fetal calf serum (FCS). Microphotographic images were taken with an IX70 microscope (Olympus, Germany) to estimate cell density and morphology.

2.3 Results and discussion

The surface modification processes have to fulfil numerous requirements in such applications. Not any of the modifications may have a cytotoxic effect neither in direct nor in indirect contact with cells. This requires preventing solvent-based processes, which often leave small molecules (solvents or short-chain molecules). In contrast, gas-discharge plasma processes are advantageous to create functional groups or ultra thin functional coatings, which are covalently fixed to the substrate. This means, they can withstand rinsing procedures. Minimum coating thickness is mandatory to avoid interference with optical measurements in detailed optical or fluorescence cell observation in high content screening (HCS). A transparent organic coating with a thickness of about 100 nm can already interfere with optical and fluorescence signals at 400 nm wavelength. Cold processes are necessary to avoid thermal load in subsequent plasma processes with masks. Sufficient contrasts have to be created between different surface zones.
The structure was prepared by a bottom-up method. This method requires the compatibility of subsequent plasma steps among each other and the selection of adequate masks. Several materials were tested for the mask. These experiments advised us to use materials with reduced stiffness. Finally, biaxial oriented polypropylene (BOPP) was the material chosen. This material was able to have a tight contact with the PS surface because this flexible material could huddle against PS (Schröder et al., 2009).
Several versions of surface combinations were tested. The surface combinations which where under investigation are listed in Fig. 3. Because of these large number of surface combinations the structures can be generated on several substrates and customized for specific cell lines and assays.

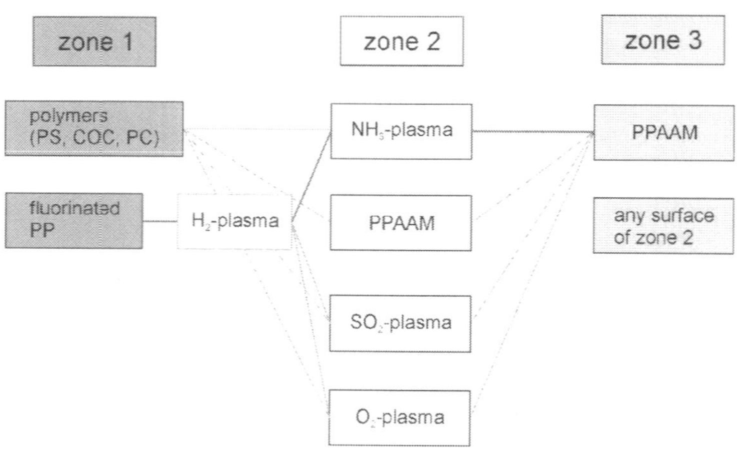

Fig. 3. Possible surface combinations for zones 1 to 3.

In principle for zone 1 untreated polymer surfaces can be used. A rather simple version comprised untreated polymer (e.g. PS) for zone 1, NH_2-funtionalized polymer for zone 2, and an allylamine plasma polymer (PPAAm) for zone 3. Two plasma processes and two different masks were applied to generate this structure. The production process is schematic shown in Fig. 4.

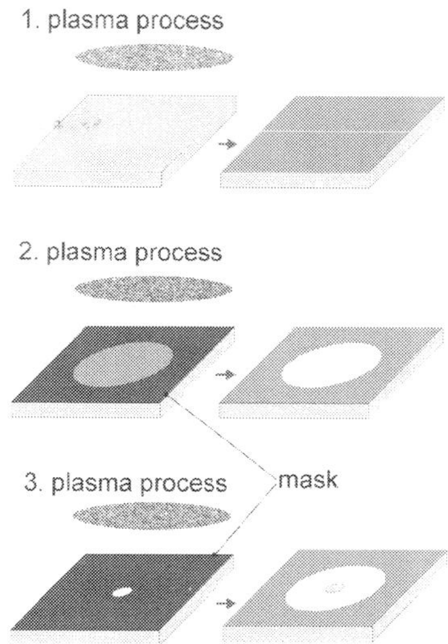

Fig. 4. Steps for the generation of the chemically structured surface.

In case of untreated surface for zone 1 the production starts with the generation (e.g. NH_2-funtionalization) of zone 2. The parts of the CAC which should not be functionalized were protected by a mask. The next plasma process is the deposition of allylamine plasma polymer in zone 3 using another mask. In case of a clean PS for zone 1 the cell- repulsive properties are sufficient. Unfortunately, the practical usefulness of this first version of micro pattern is limited, because subsequent γ- or e-beam sterilisation will introduce oxygen-containing functional groups reducing cell-repulsive properties of zone 1.
Therefore, cell-repulsive materials or modifications have to be used for zone 1, which do not lose their properties during sterilisation. Poly(ethylene oxide) (PEO) or PEO-like surfaces would be the best choice, because they are already highly oxidized and prevent protein and cell adhesion very well. But it is not recommended to modify their surfaces using subsequent plasma processing steps. Therefore, we tried to apply fluorinated polymer surfaces for zone 1. Plasma polymerized fluorinated hydrocarbons are convenient for forming inert hydrophobic surfaces. Moreover, this surface minimizes the cell adhesion too. The water contact angle was above 115°, which is considerable higher than the contact angle of untreated PS (90°). A fundamental advantage of the application of a plasma polymer for zone 1 is the large number of possible substrates e.g. glass with excellent optical properties.
It is known that plasma assisted functionalization of fluorocarbons with amino groups leads to better cell culture supports than standard tissue culture polystyrene (TCPS). Nevertheless, the functionalization of this layer with NH_2-groups is a technological problem. While PS surfaces can be functionalized with superior cell adhesion characteristics using ammonia plasma for several seconds, it takes remarkable longer treatment times to obtain similar effects on fluorinated surfaces. A pure ammonia plasma treatment reduces the water contact angle of the fluoropolymer to about 60° after long treatments times of more than 60 s. To avoid overheating of the polymer substrate, hydrogen plasma activation was applied before ammonia plasma treatment. A 60 s hydrogen plasma pre-treatment

allows a water contact angle lower than 60° after an ammonia plasma treatment of less than 30 s. This reduces the treatment time by a factor of three and water contact angles lower 60° can be obtained which are useful for cell culture.

For zone 3 any surface of zone 2 is possible. However, a good choice is a thin plasma polymerized allylamine (PPAAm) layer. A PPAAm layer with a thickness of some nm only is not closed. That means the surface is rough in the nanometer range. According to the Wenzel equation the contact angle of a hydrophilic surface will be reduced (Marmur et al., 2003).

A structure version comprised a fluorinated hydrocarbon layer for zone 1, NH_2-funtionalized fluorinated hydrocarbon for zone 2, and a thin PPAAm for zone 3 will be described in more detail. Three low-pressure plasma processes and two different masks were applied to generate this structure (Fig. 4).

Fig. 5 shows a XPS line scan over one single element of the assay. The figure clearly demonstrates the contrasting chemical properties between the different zones, the fluorinated hydrocarbon for zone 1, NH_2-funtionalized hydrocarbon for zone 2, and a thin allylamine plasma polymer for zone 3.

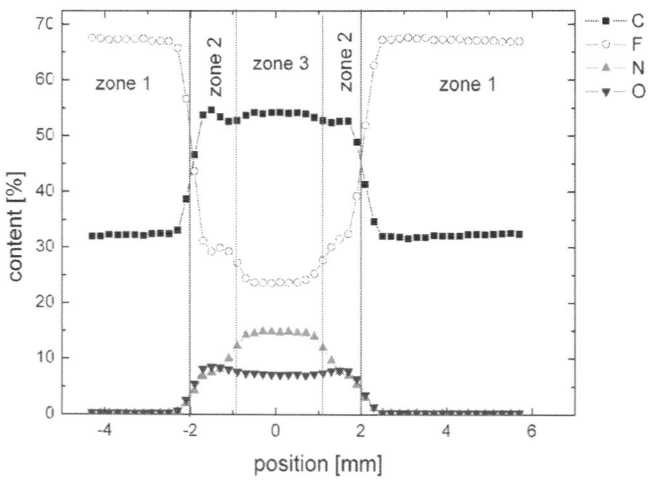

Fig. 5. Line scan across a single element of the cell-based RNA array (spectra with 250 µm spot size).

The fluorinated hydrocarbon layer consists mainly of C and F. The oxygen and nitrogen content is lower then 0.3 %. The ratio F/C is about 2.0 suggesting a teflon like structure. This assumption will be approved by the analysis of the highly resolved C1s peak (Fig. 6a). The CF_2 component was adjusted to 291.7 eV. The C 1s peak shows mainly CF_2 chain groups and CF_3 end groups. A small part of C is bonded in cross links (CF-CF).

By the H_2/NH_2--functionalization, the fluorine content was essentially reduced to about 30 % and moreover nitrogen was incorporated into the surfaces. The highly resolved C 1s peak shows drastically changes of the bond relations at the surface (Fig. 6b). There is still the bond group which belongs to the fluorinated plasma polymer. However, the peak structure is dominated by aliphatic (C-C/C-H), N and O containing groups. Nitrogen is bonded to C as amines (C-N) and amides (N-C=O).

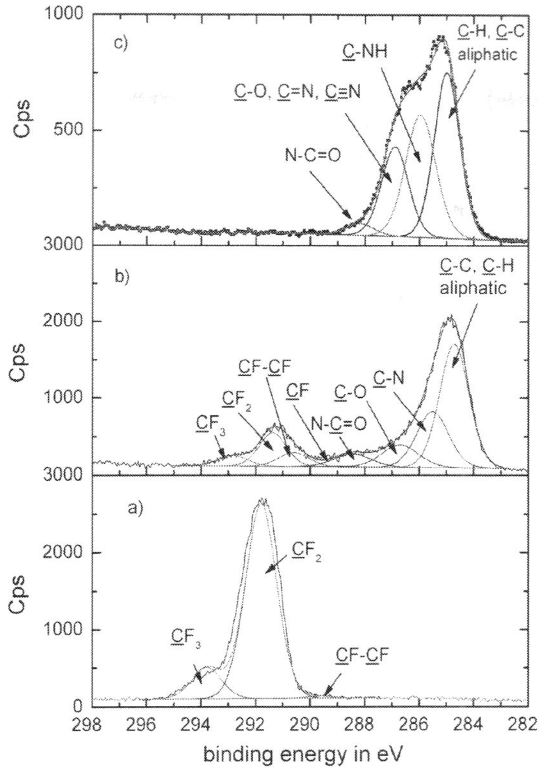

Fig. 6. Highly resolved C 1s peaks for a) the fluorinated plasma polymer, b) the H_2/NH_2 functionalized fluorinated plasma polymer and c) PPAAm.

The plasma polymer in zone 3 yields a further reduction of the fluorine content and the nitrogen content increases to 15 %. Because of the large amount of fluorine we can conclude that this layer is not really closed. The C 1s peak is dominated by aliphatic and N containing groups (Fig. 6c)). The C-C/C-H peak was adjusted to 285 eV. The other components of the C 1s peak can be assigned to: amines (C-N), imines and nitriles (C=N, C≡N) and amides (N-C=O). Nitriles have been found in FTIR measurements, too. The C-O bond which occurs most likely can not be separated from imines and nitriles (Finke et al., 2011).

The allylamine plasma polymer is quiet rough and has got a gel-like structure. These properties are important for the immobilization of the siRNA. The contact angle for water on zone 3 is remarkable lower than on zone 2. On zone 2 the contact angle for water is about 60°. This is well qualified for cell culture. After coating with an allylamine plasma polymer, the water contact angle was reduced to 25°. This is still reasonable for cell growth. On the other hand, the difference of contact angles is sufficient for retaining spotted siRNA on zone 3. About 10 nl of the solved siRNA will be spotted at one single element of the array. The diameter of the drop will be mainly determined by the contact angle for water of the spotting zone 3. It is about 600 µm for the allylamine plasma polymer surface. Hence, the diameter of zone 3 should not be less than about 800 µm. This requirement was met by the here investigated arrays.

Zone 2 and zone 3 contain about 10 % oxygen. This concomitant oxygen functionalization cannot be avoided. One very possible reason for this oxygen contamination is the reaction of metastable carbon surface radicals with molecular oxygen upon contact with air. Moreover, zone 2 and 3 contain a large amount of fluorine. Because of this reason, a reliable quantification of amino group density by derivatisation with TFBA was not possible (Schröder et al., 2009).

The sharpness of the borders between the three zones is another feature which might influence the function of the assay. However, Fig. 5 displays the borders wrong. The reason is the spot size of 250 µm which was used during the measurements. This means, that about 68 % of the signal was generated from an area with the diameter of 250 µm (Gauss function with a width of 250 µm). Actually, a three times greater diameter has to be considered. In case of the Axis ultra, the spot size can be reduced to 15 µm to increase the spatial resolution. Unfortunately, this is often not practicable, because the intensity of the signal will be reduced remarkable and the resolution is still not high enough. On the other hand, the spatial resolution of the XPS device is much better in the imaging mode than in spectroscopy mode. In case of the Axis Ultra the spatial resolution can reach less than 2 µm. With the Axis Ultra stitched images (up to 10x10 single images) can be taken. By this technique a whole single element can be pictured in one XPS image. The edges can be analyzed by line scans from such XPS images. With this method the width of the transitions between the several zones were estimated to be between 30 µm and 70 µm. These values are in the order of the thickness of the masks (50 µm) (Steffen et al., 2011).

Cell culture tests with microstructures obtained by this version of processing and modification revealed a vey good pattern reproduction. Fig. 7 shows a typical example. Actually, cells growing on zone 2 could detect the borderline between zone 1 and zone 2.

A special effect was observed at this borderline, namely a concentration of cells near the borderline compared to the inner regions of zone 2. The forces for this accumulation are not yet clear. Perhaps there is a migration of cells from the cell-repulsive to cell-adhesive areas where they are captured. This hypothesis is supported by the observation that cells are able to build up clusters on zone 1. This accumulation of cells influences cell morphology. It makes additional cells available for the assay. But it could be seen that cell morphology was partially influenced. This indicates different cell function which could falsify the results of the assay. Also, the high cell density will complicate the analyses. So, it is suggested to restrict the analysis to the inner parts of the adhesion zones.

2.4 Summary

Arrays of chemical micro patterns in CAC's were tested for the purpose of cell-based siRNA assays. Basically, the micro patterns consist of three surface zones with different adhesion properties. A central spot-like region with very good wetting properties and sufficient cell adhesion is surrounded by a ring-like area exhibiting excellent cell adhesion. These regions are embedded in a background area which is highly repulsive for cells. A version of such a structure comprises a plasma polymerized allylamine coating, ammonia plasma functionalized fluorinated hydrocarbon and a fluorinated hydrocarbon layer. Results of surface analysis and cell culture tests are reported.

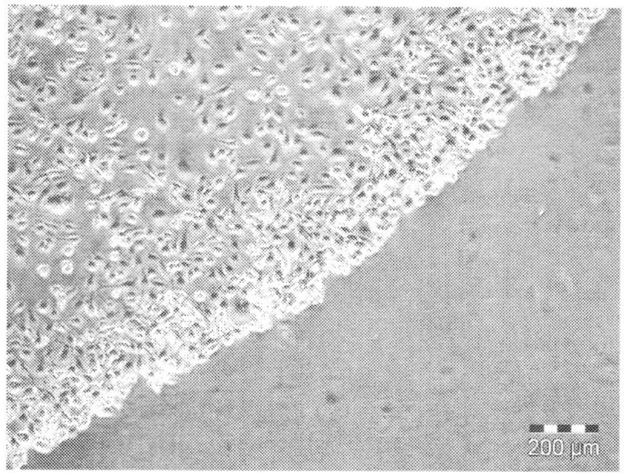

Fig. 7. Transition between zone 2 (NH_2-funtionalized polymer, left) and zone 1 (untreated polymer, right). HEK cells growing on zone 2, only.

3. Plasma-based bioequivalent coatings of biomaterial surfaces for an improved cell physiology

3.1 Background

The biologization of medical devices and in particular of implants is increasingly in the focus of research and development all over the world. For optimal adaptation of implants to the human surrounding tissue, the main focus of investigations is on molecular regeneration technologies and on improvements in material- and nanotechnology. The combination of these two technologies is the key for the realization of innovative implants.

Reliable first adhesion and spreading of cells on surfaces plays an important role for the success of implant applications. Typically, the adhesion of biomolecules on untreated biomaterial surfaces, e.g. synthetic polymers, ceramics or metals is only poor. A successful bioactivation of such surfaces can be achieved by different coupling strategies as for instance wet-chemical application of silane chemistry to bind amino group carrying silanes (Puleo, 1997). But properties of this silane-linker as their deliquescence and their tendency to polymerize and to form island-like domains gave rise to search for other coupling strategies (Falconnet et al., 2006).

Plasma polymerization is a convenient alternative method to prepare polymeric-like thin coatings not only on metals or ceramics (Morra et al., 2003) but also on inert synthetic polymer substrates, e.g. poly-ether-ether-ketone (PEEK) (Schröder et al., 2010b) or polylactid (PLA). PLA is a suitable biodegradable polymer for the improvement of the mechanical strength of calcium phosphate scaffolds (Ma et al., 2001). Low osteoconductivity of PLA surfaces is known but can be eliminated by plasma treatment (Wang et al., 2005). Due to plasma processes the number of hydroxyl groups on biomaterial surfaces can be increased and reactive functional amino- or carboxyl groups can be deposited (Schröder et al., 2010b, 2010c). Plasma polymerized allylamine (PPAAm) coatings induce strong cell-adhesive effects (Nebe et al., 2010; Nebe et al., 2007; Finke et al., 2007). Decisive for plasma applications on biomaterial surfaces is if cell physiology can be stimulated by the deposited functional groups of its own or, if additional immobilization of biorelevant molecules is necessary.

3.2 Improvement of osteoblast adhesion: comparision of a plasma polymer nanolayer vs. collagen-coating

Basically, cell adhesion to surfaces is mediated via integrins to the extracellular matrix (ECM) and has considerable influence on many cell functions. Thus, the properties of the artificial surface affect the cellular response *in vivo* and coatings which exhibit similarities of this surface to the extracellular matrix are in widespread use. Typically, immobilized proteins and peptides are used for the improvement of the interface (Rammelt et al., 2006; Schuler et al. 2006; Rychly and Nebe, 2009). Immobilized proteins may contain RGD sequences (arginine-glycin-aspartat) which are binding sites for cellular integrin receptors. Also our own adhesion experiments with human bone cells demonstrate the adhesive effect of collagen (COL) coated surfaces (Fig. 8).

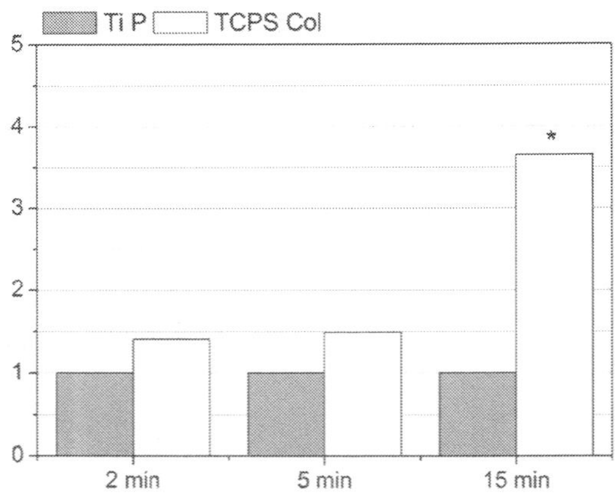

Fig. 8. Cell adherence in the initial phase is significantly enhanced on a COL-coated tissue culture polystyrene surface (TCPS Col) vs. pure polished titanium (Ti P). Human MG-63 osteoblastic cells, 1x10^4/Ø 30mm, adherent cells related to Ti_P=1, flow-cytometry, BD FACSCalibur, n = 6, T-test, *p<0.005.

In contrast to conventional methods, plasma polymers offer a greater versatility for binding biomolecules using different immobilization chemistries. Unfortunately, knowledge of the bonding mechanisms between the TiO_2-surface and deposited polymers is rather poor up to now (Possart, 1998). For plasma polymers it has been shown that swelling and dissolution of unbound material may be a problem in aqueous environments (Chu et al., 2006; Friedrich et al., 2003).

Therefore we studied the characteristics of an extremely thin, homogeneous plasma polymer film on titanium oxide, which is also sufficiently adherent in aqueous medium (Fig. 9). The polymer deposition process based on pulsed low pressure micro wave discharge plasmas has some advantages over radio frequency excitation (Hamerli et al., 2003). Allylamine is a well-suited molecular precursor for film deposition since it gives good retention of amino groups (Finke et al., 2006; Förch et al., 2005; Tang et al., 1998; Kühn et al., 2001). Films were characterized by advanced surface analytical techniques, such as high resolution scanning XPS, attenuated total reflectance Fourier transform infrared spectroscopy (ATR FT-IR), water contact angle measurements and zeta-potential measurements. More information on these

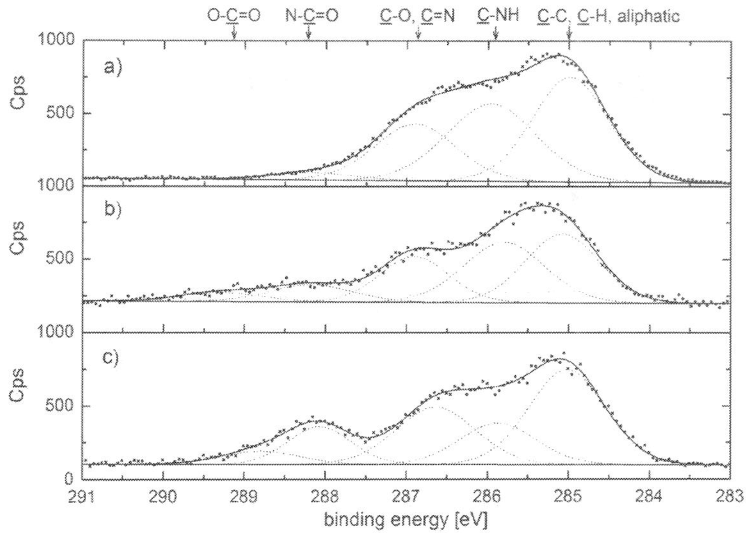

Fig. 9. High-resolution XPS-analysis of C1s spectra of PPAAm (a), the immobilization of polyethylene glycol diacid (PEG DA, b) in the first and the following coupling of collagen I (COL, c) in the second step.

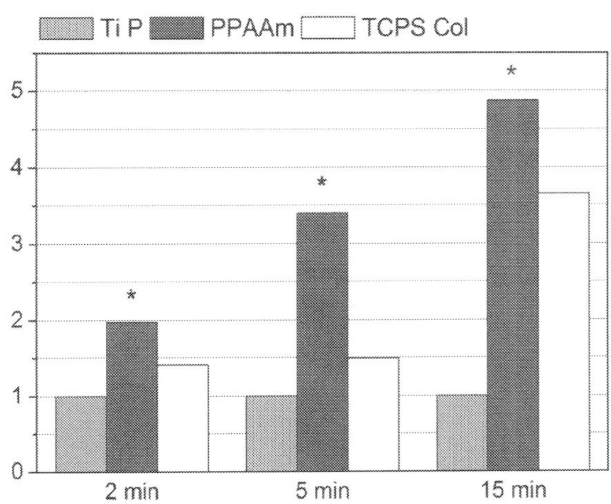

Fig. 10. Comparison of the initial osteoblast adhesion on titanium biofunctionalized with PPAAm vs. a COL-treated surface. Note that already after 2 min cell adhesion is impressively improved on PPAAm which is significant, but not for cell adhesion on COL (details see Nebe et al., 2007). Human MG-63 cells, adherent cells related to Ti_P=1, flow cytometric approach, T-test paired, *p<0.01.

experiments can be found elsewhere (Finke et al., 2007; Nebe et al., 2007; Rebl et al., 2010a). Furthermore, covalent coupling reactions of the plasma generated amino groups with collagen I (COL) were carried out to compare the cell adhesion between solely surface charges received by PPAAm and additionally immobilized COL. For the immobilization of collagen I the bifunctional spacer polyethylene glycol diacid (PEG DA) catalyzed by carbodiimide, was used. Collagen I is a main component of the extracellular matrix whose usefulness for the improvement of implant surfaces was already shown (e.g. Yang et al., 2009).

Although many studies apply the technique of the bioactivation of material surfaces with immobilized proteins and peptides, our results indicated that bioequivalent functionalization of titanium with the positively charged amino-groups (PPAAm) is sufficiently enough to significantly improve initial steps of the osteoblast's contact to the titanium surface (Fig. 10). Not only short time adhesion was impressively improved but also cell functions, e.g. spreading characterized by the time-dependent increase of the cell area as well as the organization of the actin cytoskeleton (Fig. 11) (Finke et al., 2007; Nebe et al., 2007). The induced development of the actin cytoskeleton on PPAAm was accompanied by longer actin filaments and a higher number of stress fibres per cell.

Finally, this PPAAm nanolayer was able to stimulate the cell occupation of the biomaterial surface by cells.

In our studies MG-63 osteoblastic cells (human osteoblastic cell line, ATCC, CRL-1427) were used and cultured in serum-free Dulbecco's modified Eagle medium (DMEM, Invitrogen) to investigate cell behavior on PPAAm deposited, polished titanium substrates (roughness average 0.19 µm, Lüthen et al., 2005) in comparison to untreated titanium substrates (grade 2) and to collagen I (COL) coated tissue culture polystyrene (TCPS). The improvement of adhesion and spreading of osteoblasts on plasma polymer deposited thin films of PPAAm was more increased as found on COL coated surfaces or on Ti-PPAAm additional immobilized with COL via the spacer PEG-DA (Finke et al., 2007).

To engineer the direction of a cell response to implant surfaces, it is essential to gain clear insights in how cell adhesion mechanisms contribute to cell-material interactions at the interface of plasma modified surfaces. Earlier in our cell studies we recognized hyaluronan (HA) - a large linear glycosaminoglycan with carboxyl groups in the molecule - as to be responsible for osteoblast attachment in the first phase of the material surface occupation (Nebe and Lüthen, 2008; Nebe et al., 2007). Because of the net negative charge of HA the strong adhesion capacity of the positively charged PPAAm is explainable based on electrostatic power. Cells get a growth advantage due to this very early strong adhesion. Although these plasma-based surfaces are non-protein coated surfaces without any ligands for integrin receptors cell's development is pushed as lot of our experiments could demonstrate: the spreading was increased, the formation of adhesion components (paxillin, vinculin) was pronounced (Finke et al., 2007; Nebe et al., 2007) and an increase in long term adhesion of living cells could be observed, accompanied by enhanced cell migration (Rebl et al., 2010a; Rebl et al. 2010b).

The cell physiology of cells on plasma polymerized allylamine is altered in a positive manner - signalling molecules in the downstream signal cascade become stimulated intracellularly or are faster in their phosphorylation process (Fig. 12).

Further interdisciplinary research is required to find out new possibilities of low temperature plasmas to optimize titanium implants because plasma processes are preeminently suitable for the goal-directed finishing of their surfaces.

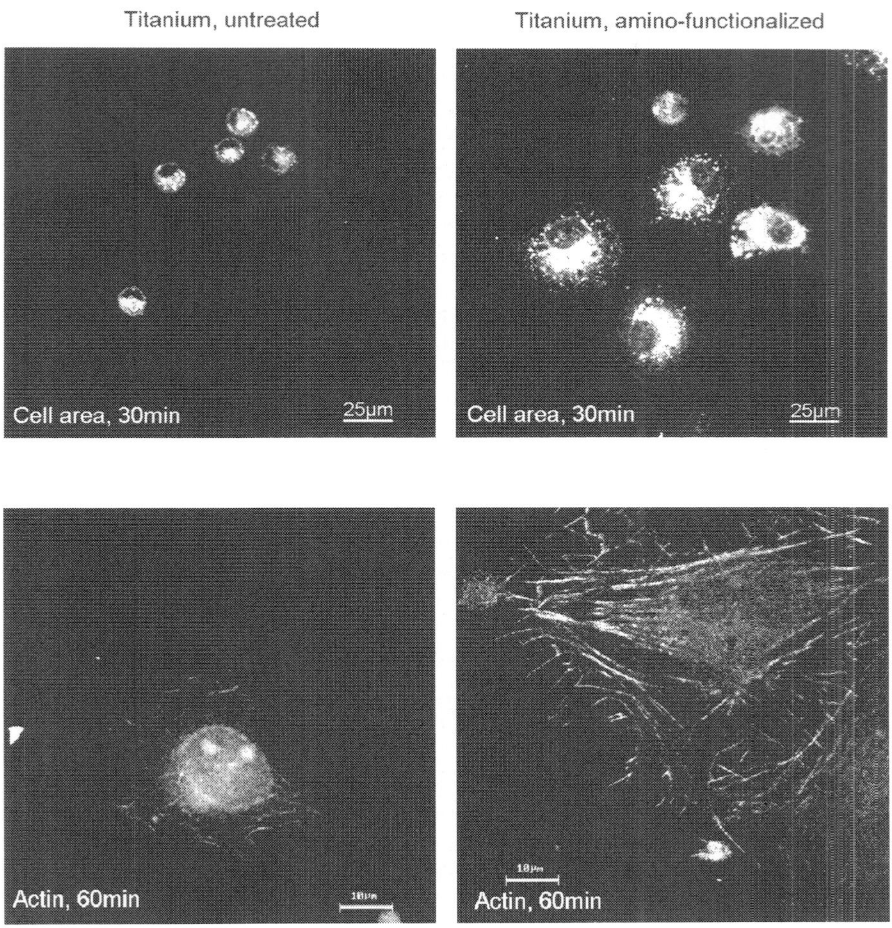

Fig. 11. Positive charges due to the deposition of plasma polymerized allylamine (PPAAm) induce cell spreading (above) as well as the development of the actin cytoskeleton (below). The cell area is increased 6 fold already after 30 min and many of the actin filaments are impressively formed as stress fibres after 60 min of cell culture.
Human MG-63 osteoblasts; cell staining: PKH-26 for spreading, phallacidine BODYPI for actin; confocal microscopy, LSM 410, Carl Zeiss, 63x oil immersion objectives 1.25 oil/0.17.

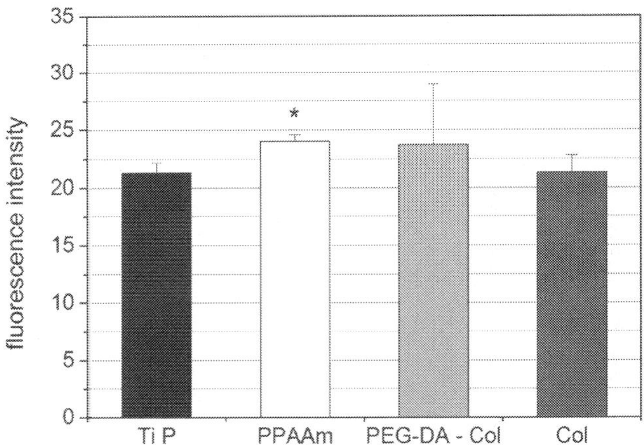

Fig. 12. The plasma deposition of PPAAm on titanium stimulate the cell physiology compared to the pure polished titanium surface (Ti P) to the same extent as an additional COL immobilization via the spacer PEG DA. The phosphorylated signal protein IkappaB (p-IκB-a), responsible for the activation of NFkappaB in the downstream signalling process in cells, is significantly enhanced in human osteoblasts due to PPAAm. Human MG-63, Bio-Plex analysis, BioRad, n=3, T-test, *$p < 0.05$.

3.3 Surface functionalization by plasma deposition of functional groups for regulation of stem cell behavior

Surface functionalization for bioengineering applications may have several different goals. By the plasma-based deposition of functional groups like -OH, -COOH, -CHO, Epoxide or $-NH_2$ the surface-bound of spacer molecule for cell immobilization, containing hydrocarbon chains, cyclic compounds or ethylene oxide chains may be improved. In addition the covalent fixation of bioactive molecules and the immobilization by self-assembly (by van-der Waals interactions, hydrogen bridges or ionic interaction, hydrophobic-hydrophobic interaction and thiols on gold) determines the bioactivity of the surface and the surface-bound of bioactive molecules as well. These effects can be used to achieve the immobilization of proteins, DNA, sugars and fatty acids or even bacteria. On the other hand the repulsion of biomolecules can be utilized for instance for antifouling applications. Similiar immobilization strategies are used as well for the covalent collagen immobilization for stem cell adhesion. The adhesive and cell stimulatory properties of plasma modified surfaces were investigated using human stem cells important for orthopedic and dental implantology and are described here.

The gas discharge-based processing of the substrate material first applied an ultrathin plasma polymer allylamine (PPAAm) coating on the plasma-activated titanium surface to modify the water contact angle from a typical value of $77° \pm 3°$ of pure titanium to $48° \pm 3°$. Then, a spacer substance, as for example polyethylene glycol diacid (PEG-DA), was deposited on the PPAAm to achieve a covalent immobilization of collagen I (COL). The chemistry and length of the spacer determines the physico-chemical properties of the surface and so the efficiency of the collagen coupling.

In Fig. 13 the bonding components in the C1s peak of PPAAm- and PPAAc-prepared surfaces are demonstrated.

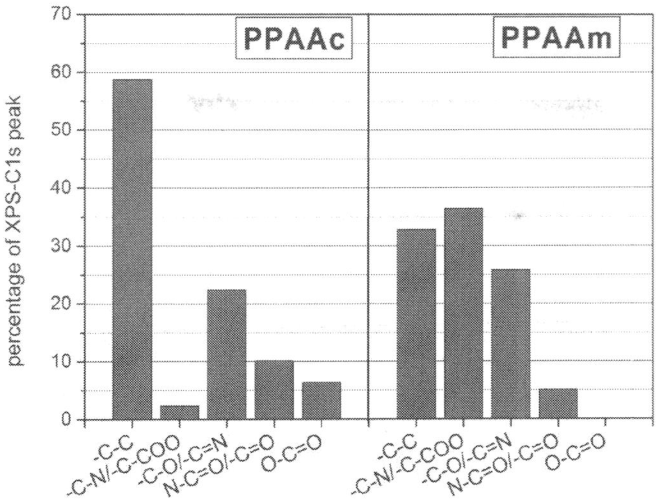

Fig. 13. Percentages of bonding components in C1s peak after film preparation on polished titanium for PPAAm (right) and PPAAc (left).

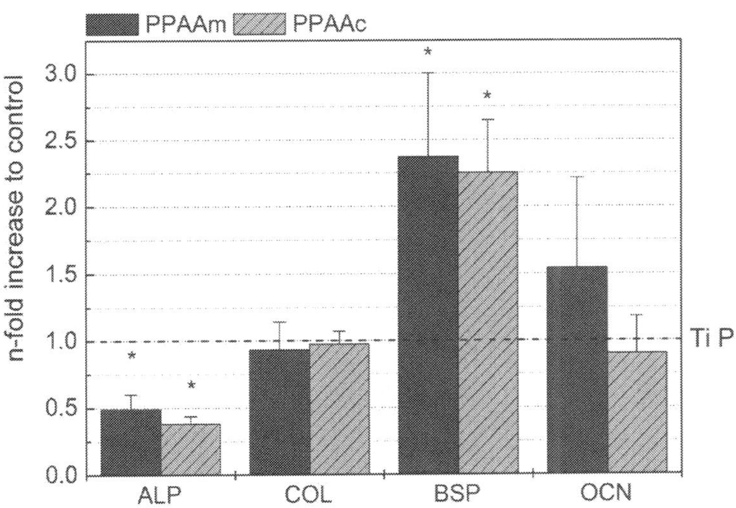

Fig. 14. mRNA expression for the osteogenic marker proteins ALP, COL, BSP, and OCN in stem cells hMSC on PPAAm and PPAAc in osteogenic medium for 3 days, compared to cells on Ti P (as control). Note the increase of BSP and OCN on PPAAm and PPAAc in osteogenic medium (details see Schröder et al., 2010c). The influence of the medium seems to be dominant. Cells: hMSC (Lonza), quantitative real-time RT-PCR, ABI PRISM 7500, Applied Biosystems, calculated by the comparative ΔΔCT-method and normalized to Ti_P (control), n=3 (3 measurements each), U-test, $^*p < 0.1$.

Different surface functional groups are reported to induce various differentiation of stem cells manifesting in discret gene expression. According to a human osteoblast differentiation model, alkaline phosphatase (ALP) and collagen 1 (COL) mRNA´s are early differentiation markers in the osteoblast lineage and decline again during osteoblast maturation. On the other hand, bone sialo protein (BSP) and osteocalcin (OCN) mRNA´s are expressed at very low levels in the early osteoblast differentiation stage, but transcription is enhanced during later differentiation stages (Billiard et al., 2003). In our studies (Schröder et al., 2010d) we

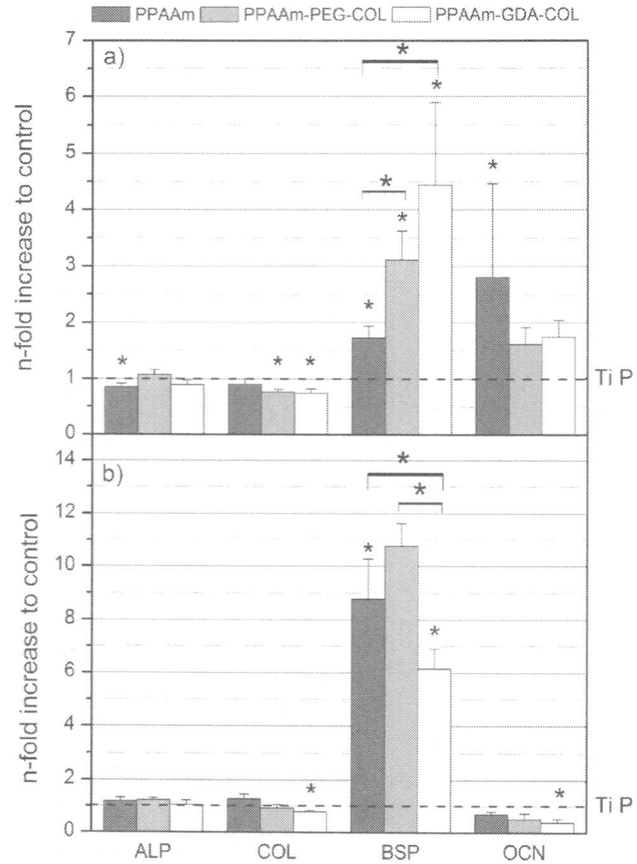

Fig. 15. mRNA expression for the osteogenic marker proteins ALP, COL, BSP, and OCN in stem cells hMSC on PPAAm, PPAAm-PEG-COL and PPAAm-GDA-COL after 14 days of culture in basal (A) and osteogenic medium (B), compared to cells on Ti P (control). Note the huge increase of BSP as late stage diffentiation marker after 14 days of culture. Cells: hMSC (Lonza), quantitative real-time RT-PCR, ABI PRISM 7500, Applied Biosystems, calculated by the comparative ΔΔCT-method and normalized to Ti P (control), n=3 (3 measurements each), U-test, *$p < 0.1$.

investigated the influence of positivly and negatively charged plasma deposited polymers e.g. PPAAm and plasma polymerized acrylic acid (PPAAc). We could observe that BSP late-stage differentiation-related mRNA expression was enhanced in human stem cells (hMSC, Lonza) cultivated on PPAAm and PPAAc in osteogenic medium for three days relatively to Ti_P, whereas OCN is upregulated on PPAAm only (Fig. 13). Concerted with the increase of late-stage differentiation markers the downregulation of ALP and COL is understandable as a sign of maturation. These results show that both positively and negatively charged surfaces facilitate osteogenic differentiation controlled by the osteogenic medium used. The osteogenic medium may have the dominant effect on cell behavior in these approaches, but additional charges at the surfaces due to functional groups suppose differentation. Apart from that the spreading of hMSCs on PPAAm surfaces in basal cell culture medium without osteogenic factors was significantly enhanced, but reduced on PPAAc (data not demonstrated). The positively charged PPAAm on Ti surfaces can promote differentiation of hMSC´s independently of osteogenic supplements in the culture media, but not a PPAAc deposition.

The positive influence of PPAAm surfaces on the differentiation of hMSC could be further improved by covalent immobilization of COL through spacers e.g. polyethylene glycol diacid (PEG) and glutardialdehyde (GDA). After 14 days of culture on these surfaces hMSC´s showed a significantly enhanced BSP mRNA expression under basal culture conditions (Fig. 15A). Here a significant impact due to covalent coupling of COL could be observed for both coupling methods, which reached its peak for PPAAm-GDA-COL. But a significant influence was detectable also for PPAAm alone.The increase of BSP mRNA expression on PPAAm surfaces relativly to non treated Ti P was further developed using osteogenic medium (Fig. 15B). Osteogene stimulation obliterated differences resulting from COL coupling. Thus PPAAm treatment of Ti seems to be sufficant for surface optimation in respect of diffentiation of hMSC´s under osteogenic conditions.

4. Acknowledgments

We would like to thank U. Kellner, U. Lindemann, G. Friedrichs (INP), I. Mardi (Zell-Kontakt) and A. Peters, J. Wetzel (University of Rostock) for the excellent technical accomplishment of the experiments. We appreciate technical support of G. Fulda of the Electron Microscopic Center of the Medical Faculty of the University of Rostock. This study was supported by the Federal State of Mecklenburg-Vorpommern and the Helmholtz Association of German Research Centres (UR 0402210), by the Federal Ministry of Education and Research (Campus PlasmaMed, grant No. 13N9779 and 13N11188) and by AIF (FKZ: KF0086501UL4).

5. References

Besch, W., Foest, R., Schröder, K. & Ohl, A (2008). Allylamine Plasma Polymer Coatings of Interior Surfaes in Small Trench Structures, *Plasma Process. Polym.* 5: 105-112s.

Billiard, J., Moran, R.A., Whitley, M.Z., Chatterjee-Kishore, M., Gillis, K., Brown, E.L., Komm, B.S. & Bodine P.V. (2003) Transcriptional profiling of human osteoblast differentiation, *J Cell Biochem* 89(2): 389-400.

Callen, B.W. , Sodhi, R.N.S., Shelton, R. M. & Davies, J.E. (1993). Behavior Of Primary Bone-Cells On Characterized Polystyrene Surfaces, *J. Biomed. Mater. Res.* 27: 851-859.

Chen, C.S., Mrksich, M., Huang, S., Whitesides, G.M. & Ingber, D.E. (1997) Geometric control of cell life and death, *Science* 276: 1425.

Chu, L., Knoll, W. & Förch, R. (2006). Biologically Multifunctional Surfaces Using Plasma Polymerization Methods, *Plasma Process Polym* 3:498–505.

Fairley, N. & Carrick, A. (2005). The Casa Cookbook, Acolyte Science:Kinderton Close.

Falconnet, D., Csucs, G., Grandin, H.M. & Textor, M. (2006). Surface engineering approaches to micropattern surfaces for cell-based assays, *Biomaterials*, 27(16): 3044-3063.

Finke, B., Schröder, K., Lüthen, F., Nebe, B. Rychly, J. & Ohl, A. (2006) Chemical Functionalization of Titanium Surfaces by Plasma Assisted Polymerization, *BIOmaterialien* 7(S1):69.

Finke, B., Luethen, F., Schroeder, K., Mueller, P.D., Bergemann, C., Frant, M., Ohl, A. & Nebe, B.J. (2007). The effect of positively charged plasma polymerization on initial osteoblastic focal adhesion on titanium surfaces, *Biomaterials*, 28(30): 4521-4534.

Finke, B., Hempel, F., Testrich, H., Artemenko, A., Rebel, H., Kylian, O., Meichsner, J., Biedermann, H., Nebe, B., Weltmann, K.-D., Schröder, K. (2011) Plasma processes for cell-adhesive titanium surfaces based on nitrogen-containing coatings, *Surf. Coat. Technol.*, in press., doi: 10.1016/j.surfcoat.2010.12.044

Fire, A., Xu, S.Q., Montgomery, M.K., Kostas, S.A., Driver, S.E. & Mello, C.C. (1998). Potent and specific genetic interference by double-stranded RNA in Caenorhabditis elegans, *Nature*, 391(6669): 806-811.

Förch, R., Zhang, Z. & Knoll, W. (2005). Soft Plasma Treated Surfaces: Tailoring of Structure and Properties for Biomaterial Application, *Plasma Process Polym* 2:351–72.

Friedrich, J., Kühn, G., Mix, R., Fritz, A. & Schönhals, A. (2003). Polymer surface modification with monofuctional groups of variable types and densities, *J Adhes Sci Technol* 17:1591–617.

Hamerli, P., Weigel, T., Groth, T. & Paul, D. (2003). Enhanced tissue-compatibility of polyethylenterephtalat membranes by plasma aminofunctionalisation, *Biomaterials* 24:3989–99.

Kühn, G., Retzko, I., Lippitz, A., Unger, W. & Friedrich (2001). Homofunctionalized polymer surfaces formed by selective plasma processes, *J. Surf Coat Technol* 42:494–500.

Lüthen, F., Lange, R., Becker, P., Rychly, J., Beck, U. & Nebe, J.B. (2005) The influence of surface roughness of titanium on beta1- and beta3-integrin adhesion and the organization of fibronectin in human osteoblastic cells. *Biomaterials* 26:2423-2440.

Ma, P.X., Zhang, R.Y., Xiao G.Z. & Franceschi, R. (2001). Engineering new bone tissue in vitro on highly porous poly(alpha-hydroxyl acids)/hydroxyapatite composite scaffolds. *J. Biomed. Mater. Res.* 54(2):284-293.

Marmur, A. (2003). Wetting on hydrophobic rough surfaces: To be heterogeneous or not to be?, *Langmuir* 19: 8343–8348.

Morra, M., Cassinelli, C., Cascardo, G., Cahalan, P., Cahalan, L., Fini, M. & Giardino, R. (2003). Surface engineering of titanium by collagen immobilization. Surface characterization and in vitro and in vivo studies, *Biomaterials* 24(25):. 4639-4654.

Müller, M., Sciarratta, V. & Oehr, C. (2003). Plasmachemical microstructuring of polymeric surfaces for pharmacology and medical diagnostics, *Vak. Forsch. Prax.* 15:19.

Meyer-Plath, A.A., Schröder, K., Finke, B. & Ohl, A. (2003) Current trends in biomaterial surface functionalization - nitrogen-containing plasma assisted processes with enhanced selectivity, *Vacuum* 71/3:391-406.

Nebe, B., Finke, B., Lüthen, F., Bergemann, C., Schröder, K., Rychly, J., Liefeith, K. & Ohl, A. (2007). Improved initial osteoblast functions on amino-functionalized titanium surfaces, *Biomolecular Engineering* 24(5): 447-454.

Nebe, J.B. & Lüthen F (2008) Integrin- and Hyaluronan-mediated cell adhesion on titanium – Hyaluronan-mediated adhesion. In: Metallic Biomaterial Interactions, Eds.: J. Breme, C.J. Kirkpatrick, R. Thull, WILEY-VCH, ISBN 978-3-527-31860-5, 2008, p. 179-182.

Nebe, J.B., Jesswein, H., Weidmann, A., Finke, B., Lange, R., Beck, U., Staehlke, S. & Schroeder, K. (2010) Osteoblast's sensitivity to topographical and chemical features of titanium. *Mater Sci Forum* 638-642:652-657.

Ohl, A., Schröder, K., Keller, D., Meyer-Plath, A., Bienert, H., Husen, B. & Rune, G.M. (1999) Chemical micropatterning of polymeric cell culturing substrates using low pressure hydrogen gas discharge plasmas *J. Mater. Sci. Mater. Med.* 10:747-754.

Ohl, A. & Schröder, K. (1999) Plasma induced chemical micropatterning for cell culturing applications: a brief review. *Surface and Coatings Technology* 116-119:820-830.

Ohl, A. & Schröder, K. (2008) Plasma assisted surface modification of biointerfaces, In: *Low temperature plasma physics*, R. Hippler, H. Kersten, M. Schmidt & K. H. Schoenbach (Ed.), VCH Wiley, Berlin, 803-819.

Possart W. (1998). Adhesion of polymers. in: Helsen J.H. & Breme, H.J. (ed), *Metals as biomaterials*, Wiley, Chichester, New York.

Puleo, D.A. (1997). Retention of enzymatic activity immobilized on silanized Co-Cr-Mo and Ti-6Al-4V, *Journal of Biomedical Materials Research* 37(2): 222–228.

Rammelt, S., Illert, T., Bierbaum, S., Scharnweber, D., Zwipp, H. & Schneiders, W. (2006). Coating of titanium implants with collagen, RGD peptide and chondroitin sulfate, *Biomaterials* 27:5561-71.

Rebl, H., Finke, B., Rychly, J., Schröder, K. & Nebe, J.B. (2010a), Positively charged material surfaces generated by plasma polymerized allylamine enhance vinculin mobility in vital human osteoblasts, *Advanced Biomat.* 12/8:356-364.

Rebl, H., Finke, B., Schröder, K. & Nebe, J.B. (2010b), Time-dependent metabolic activity and adhesion of human osteoblast-like cells on sensor chips with a plasma polymer nanolayer, *Int. J. Artif. Organs* 33:738-748.

Rychly, J. & Nebe, B. (2009) Meeting report: Interface biology of implants. Cell adhesion & Migration 3:4 1-5.

Schröder, K., Meyer-Plath, A., Keller, D. & Ohl, A. (2002). On the Applicability of Plasma Assisted Chemical Micropatterning to Different Polymeric Biomaterials, *Plasmas and Polymers* 7(2): 103-125.

Schröder, K., Babucke, G. & Ohl, A. (2004). Visualization of a plasma-gnerated chemical micro-pattern on polystyrene by XPS ,*Surf. Interface Anal.* 36:702-705.

Schröder, K., Finke, B. & Ohl, A. (2005) Improved low-pressure microwave plasma-assisted amino functionalization of polymers, In *Plasma Processes and Polymers*, R.d'Agostino, P. Favia, C. Oehr, M.R. Wertheimer (Ed.), pp. 333-349, Wiley VCH, Weinheim.

Schröder K., Busse, B., Steffen, H., Ohl, A., Quade, A. & Weltmann, K.-D. (2009). Configuratuion of Plasma Processes for the Generation of a Chemical Triple Pattern for Cell-Based RNA Arrays *Plasma Processes and Polymers* 6(S1): S46-S50.

Schröder, K., Ohl, A. & Nitschke, M. (2010a) Plasmaprozesse zur Beeinflussung der Biokompatibilität von Oberflächen, In: *Vakuum-Plasma-Technologien Beschichtung und Modifizierung von Oberflächen*, G. Blasek, G. Bräuer (Ed.), 1106-1124, ISBN 978-3-87480-257-4, Saulgau, Germany, Eugen G. Leuze Verlag

Schröder, K., Finke, B., Jesswein, H., Lüthen, F., Diener, A., Ihrke, R., Ohl, A., Weltmann, K.-D., Rychly, J. & Nebe, J.B. (2010b). Similarities between Plasma Amino Functionalized PEEK and Titanium Surfaces Concerning Enhancement of Osteoblast Cell Adhesion, *Journal of Adhesion Science and Technology* 24(5): 905-923.

Schröder, K., Finke, B., Polak, M., Lüthen, F., Nebe, J.B., Rychly, J., Bader, R., Lukowski, G., Walschus, U., Schlosser, M., Ohl, A. & Weltmann, K.-D. (2010c) Gas-discharge plasma-assisted functionalization of titanium implant surfaces. *Mater. Sci. Forum* 638-642:700-705.

Schröder, K., Finke, B., Ohl, A., Lüthen, F., Bergemann, C., Nebe, B., Rychly, J., Walschus, U., Schlosser, M., Liefeith, K., Neumann, H.-G. & Weltmann, K.-D. (2010d) Capability of differently charged plasma polymer coatings for control of tissue interactions with titanium surfaces. *J Adh Sci Technol* 24:1191–1205.

Schröder, K., Foest, R. & Ohl, A. (2011) Biomedical applications of plasmachemical surface functionalization, In *Non-thermal Plasma Chemistry and Physics"*, J.Meichsner, M.Schmidt, H.E. Wagner (Ed.), Taylor&Francis, Oxon, submitted.

Schuler, M., Owen, G.R., Hamilton, D.W., de Wild, M., Textor, M., Brunette, D.M. & Tosatti, S.G.P. (2006) Biomimetic modification of titanium dental implant model surfaces using the RGDSP-peptide sequence: a cell morphology study. *Biomaterials* 27(21):4003–15.

Steffen, H., Schröder, K., Busse, B., Ohl, A. & Weltmann, K.D. (2007). Functionalization of COC Surfaces by Microwave Plasmas, *Plasma Processes and Polymers* 4(S1): S392-S396.

Steffen, H., Busse, B., Schröder, K., Quade, A., Ohl, A. & Weltmann, K.D. (2011).Analysis of plasma enhanced generated chemical micro structures for cell-based RNA arrays, *Plasma Processes and Polymers*, submitted.

Szili, E., Thissen, H., Hayes, J.P. & Voelcker, N. (2004). A biochip platform for cell transfection assays, *Biosens. Bioelectron.* 19:1395.

Tang, L., Wu, Y. & Timmons, R.B. (1998). Fibrinogen adsorption and host tissue responses to plasma functionalized surfaces, *J Biomed Mater Res* 42:156.

van Wachem, P.B., Beugeling, T., Feijen, J.J., Bantjes, A., Detmers, J.P. & van Aken, W.G. (1985). Interaction of Cultured Human-Endothelial Cells with Polymeric Surfaces of Different Wettabilities, *Biomaterials* 6: 403-408.

Wang, S.G., Cui, W.J. & and Bei, J.Z. (2005) Bulk and surface modifications of polylactide. *Anal. Bioanal. Chem.* 381(3):547-556.

Wende, K., Schröder, K., Lindequist, U. & Ohl, A. (2006) Plasma-based modification of polystyrene surfaces for serum-free culture of osteoblastic cell lines, *Plasma Process. Polymer* 3 :516-523.

Yang, X., Jiang, B., Huang, Y., Tian, Y., Chen, H., Chen, J. & Yang, B. (2009) Collagen nanofilm immobilized on at surfaces by electrodeposition method. *J. Biomed. Mater. Res. B. Appl. Biomater.* 90(2):608-13.

Ziauddin, J. & Sabatini, D.M. (2001). Microarrays of cells expressing defined cDNAs, *Nature* 411:107.

16

The Application of Biomolecules in the Preparation of Nanomaterials

Zhuang Li[1] and Tao Yang[2]
[1]*State Key Lab. of Electroanalytical Chemistry, Changchun Institute of Applied Chemistry, Chinese Academy of Sciences; Changchun, Jilin,*
[2]*Key Laboratory of Medicinal Chemistry and Molecular Diagnosis, Ministry of Education, College of Chemistry and Environmental Science, Hebei University; Baoding, Hebei, China*

1. Introduction

1.1 Using ascorbic acid or amino acids as reducing agent to synthesize nanomaterials of special morphology

Recently, preparation of nanomaterial by the use of the spectial propertities of biomolecules has gained more and more research interest. These strategies usually utilize the environmentally benign and "green" experimental condition, not the harsh condition used in the traditional chemical synthesis. And, preparation of nanomaterials with the use of biomolecules can often has some control on the morphology and size of the final products.

It is well-known that ascorbic acid has the mild reducing ability, which made it very appealing in the fabrication of nanomaterial with unusual morphology. Using the mild reducing ability of ascorbic acid, Murphy's group and Huang's group have synthesized silver nanowirs and gold nanorods of controllable aspect ratio via seed-mediated growth approach (Jana et al., 2001; Gole et al., 2004; Wu et al., 2007). In the presence of trisodium citrate, nanoparticle seeds with the size about 4 nm were obtained via the reduction of the aqueous solution of $AgNO_3$ or $HAuCl_4$ by $NaBH_4$. The growth solution includes $AgNO_3$ (or $HAuCl_4$), the reducing agent ascorbic acid and surfactant cetyltrimethylammonium bromide (CTAB). After the seeds were added into the growth solution, silver nanowire or gold nanorod will be produced by reducing the corresponding metal salts with ascorbic acid for a period of time.

Some amino acids also have the reduction ability and can be used as reducing agent to prepare nanomaterials of special structure. For example, Shao and his coworkers have prepared the hexagonal single crystal gold nanoplate in one-step by aspartate reduction of $HAuCl_4$ (Figure 1). Their experimental procedure is as following: mix the aqueous solution of $HAuCl_4$ and aspartate directly at room temperature, slowly stirring the mixture for 12 hours, then the nanoplate structure of gold can be produced (Shao et al., 2004). Electron diffraction results suggests that these nanoplates are single crystals grown mainly along the Au{111} facets. In the formation process of the gold nanoplates, aspartate not only acts as the reducing agent, but also has some control on the morphology of the gold nanostructures formed. Synthesis of gold nanomaterials with the use of amino acids is a "green" synthesis method for gold nanomaterials, since it does not need additional reducing agents or surfactants.

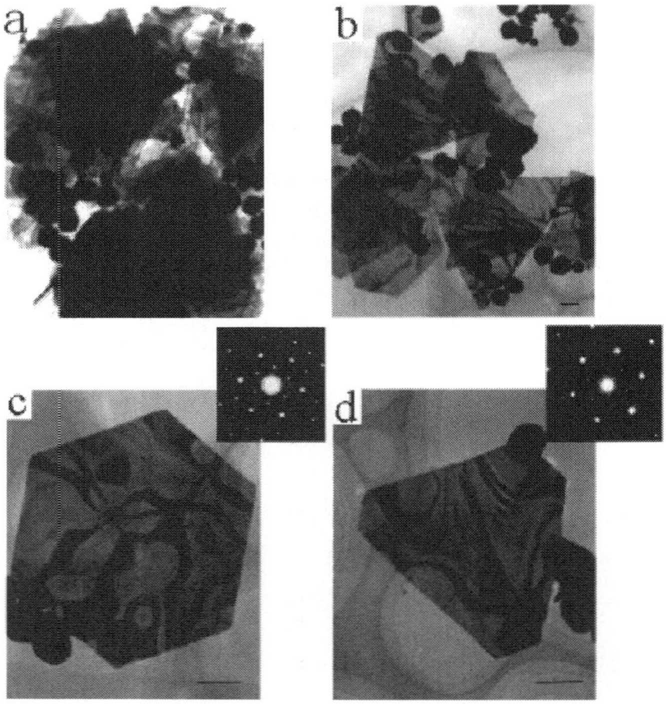

Fig. 1. TEM imags of the gold nanoplates. (a) and (b) are the images of high and low degree aggregated nanoplates. The images of the hexagonal and truncated triangular nanoplates are shown in (c) and (d). The insets are the electron diffraction patterns. The scale bar is 200 nm.

1.2 Preparation of nanomaterials with amino acids as protecting agents

There are mainly two methods that nanoparticles can be synthesized by using amino acids as protecting agents. The first method is that: first prepare the nanoparicles, then conjugate amino acids onto the nanoparticles to protect the nanoparticles from aggregation. For example, using lysine as the capping agent, Sastry's group has prepared gold nanoparticles with good dispersibility in water (Selvakannan et al., 2003). In their experiment, gold nanoparticles were first produced by reducing the aqueous solution of $HAuCl_4$ with $NaBH_4$. Lysine protected gold nanoparticles were obtanined after mixing gold nanoparticles with lysine aqueous solution for 12 hours. The lysine capped gold nanoparticles show good dispersibility in water. Sastry et al. have also found that the dispersibility of lysine capped gold nanoparticles depends on the pH value of the aqueous solution. Under acidic condition (pH=3), the lysine capped gold nanoparticle are well dispersed from each other and the network of gold nanoparticles can be formed via the hydrogen bonding. In the basic environment, the gold nanoparticles aggregate into large superstructure in which the individual gold particles are difficult to be distinguished. The pH depended self-assembly of lysine capped gold nanoparticles was related to the formation of hydrogen bonding among the amino acids on the surfaces of the adjacent gold particles.

The second method for preparation of amino acid protected gold nanoparticles is that the amino acid protected gold nanostructures were produced in one step via reducing the corresponding noble metal salts directly by reducing agent in the presence of amino acids. For example, Zhong et al. have directly utilized lysine as protecting agent to prepare gold nanowires through reduction of $HAuCl_4$ by $NaBH_4$ (Zhong et al., 2004). Their preparation method is: First, mix the aqueous solution of $HAuCl_4$ and lysine at a certain molar ratio. Then, adjust the pH value of the mixture solution with aqueous NaOH to the suitable range. Finally, lysine protected gold nanowire structure was obtained directly by reducing $HAuCl_4$ with the addition of $NaBH_4$ under vigourous stirring. Lysine acts as capping and bridging agent in the formation process of the gold nanowire. There are two factors, the pH value and the molar ratio of lysine to gold, which influence the formation of the gold narowire structure. Zhong et al. found that linear structures of gold, with the diameter of ca. 5 nm and length in the range of 80-200 nm, can be produced when the molar ratio of lysine to gold is 0.5 and the pH value is in the range of 8.4-9.5. At the low pH value, the mian products of the reaction are some aggregates without uniform morphology. Under the basic conditon (pH=11.1), the reaction products consist of the gold nanowire which are short and thickly bound with each other. Additionaly, ultrasound also has influence on the formation of the gold nanowire structure. Gold nanoparticles with good dispersibility will be the products when heavy ultrasound was applied in the preparation process of the gold nanowire structure.

2. The application of biomacromolecules in the preparation of nanomaterials

2.1 The application of sugar in the synthesis of nanomaterials

Recently, the preparation of sugar modified metal nanoparticles has attracted a wide research interest. There are two methods that can be used to prepare sugar modified nanoparticles. The first method uses the biomolecules, such as glucose (Raveendran et al., 2003), chitosan (Huang et al., 2004), and amino-dextran (Ma et al., 2005), directly as reducing agent to reduce metal salts to produce metal nanoparticles. For example, Raveendran et al. have prepared the starch stabilized silver nanoparticles which were almost monodispersed by gentle heating the mixture aqueous solution of $AgNO_3$, glucose and starch (Raveendran et al., 2003). In their experiment, glucose was used as the "green" reducing agent and starch was used as the stabilizer of the nanoparticle. Additionaly, Ma et al. have utilized a similar method to prepare the amino-dextran protected gold and silver nanoparticles via heating the mixture solution of amino-dextran and $HAuCl_4$ or $AgNO_3$. The amino-dextran was used directly as reducing and protecting agent. The size of the obtained nanoparticles can be adjusted by changing the molar ratio of amino-dextran to metal salts. These amino-dextran protected gold and silver nanoparticles can be used as biosensor for the detection of concanavalin A.

The second method utilizes the sugar, such as mannose and dextran, to modify the as-prepared nanoparticles (Zhang et al., 2004; Aslan et al., 2004; Lyu et al., 2008). These sugar modified nanoparticles can be used as biosensor for the detection of concanavalin A and glucose. Recently, Lyu and his co-workers have prepared the mannose-stabilized gold nanoparticles by the displacement self-assembly of citrate-capped gold nanoparticles solution with thiol-modified mannoside. The mannose-stabilized gold nanoparticles were also monodispersed as that of the original citrate-capped particles. These mannose-stabilized gold nanoparticles can be used as the signal amplifier in the determination of concanavalin A by quartz crystal microbalance (QCM).

2.2 The application of lipids in the preparation of nanomaterials

Recently, lipid bilayer modified nanomaterials, such as noble metal nanoparticles (He et al., 2005; Takahashi., 2006; Zhang et al., 2006, 2008), semiconductor quantum dots (Geissbuchler et al., 2005; Gopalakrishnan et al., 2006), silica nanoparticles (Mornet et al., 2005) and carbon nanotubes (Zhou et al., 2007; He et al., 2005; Artyuklin et al., 2005), have gained a wide research attention due to their water solubility, biocompatibility and their potential application in many fields. It is believed that the lipid bilayers capped on the nanomaterials act in the same way as biomembranes to a certain extent. This may lead people to use lipid bilayers as biomembrane models to study a wide variety of biological functions, such as membrane fusion, the interaction between protein and cell membranes, and other processes in the fields of biophysics, chemistry, and medicine (Mornet et al., 2005; Zhou et al., 2007).

The representative example of the lipid bilayer-coated nanomaterial is the didodecyldimethylammonium bromide (DDAB) lipid bilayer-protected gold nanoparticles prepared by Zhang et al (Zhang et al., 2006, 2008). Their preparation method is: *in situ* reduce $HAuCl_4$ with $NaBH_4$ in the aqueous solution of DDAB to directly form the DDAB lipid bilayer-capped gold nanoparticles. The scheme of the lipid bilayer-protected gold nanoparticle and its TEM image were shown in Figure 2. In addition, the research carried out by Li et al. has shown that capping of DDAB on the surface of gold nanoparticle can notably enhance the stability of the DDAB-DNA complex in the blood serum, which is crucial to the efficiency of gen delivery (Li et al., 2008). The other work of Li et al. further showed that lipid bilayer-capped gold nanoparticles can effectively transfer the plasmid DNA into human cells in the presence of blood serum (Li et al., 2008). Therefore, it can be seen that lipid bilayer-coated nanomaterials possess enormous application potential in biomedical field, especially the gen transfer area, due to their biocompatible surface.

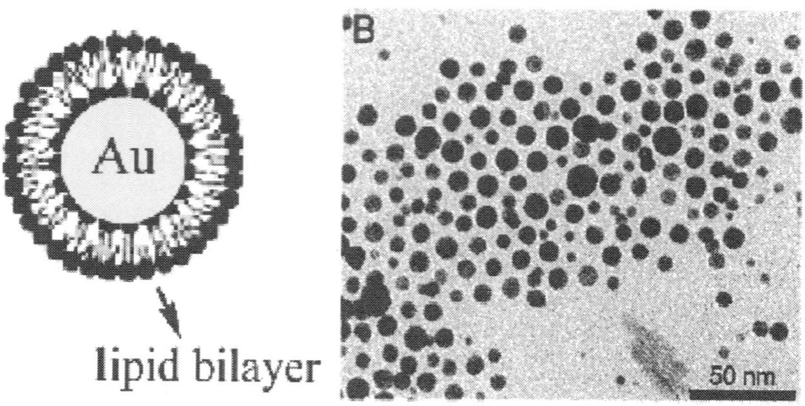

Fig. 2. The scheme of the DDAB lipid bilayer protected gold nanoparticle and its TEM image.

2.3 The application of DNA in the fabrication of nanostructures

The biomacromolecule, DNA, demonstrates huge application potential in the fabrication of nanostructures and nanodevices (Nalwa, 2005). DNA molecules can be used in the assembly of device as well as its connecting wires (Strohoff et al., 1999). Fabrication of nanostructure using DNA as building blocks has three advantages: (1) The intramolecule interaction of DNA can be programbly designed and controlled. Ther is a simple base-pairing theory between the components of DNA. Adeine (A) pairs thymine (T) via forming two hydrogen bonds. Guaine (G) pairs cytosine (C) via forming three hydrogen bonds. This unique property makes DNA not only an effective genetic substance but also a programble building block in self-assembly. (2) The DNA sequence can be synthesized by chemical method. Many DNA derivatives, such as biotin or fluorescein labeled DNA fragments and some DNA linkers, have also been chemically synthesized due to the demand in biological science & technology. (3) DNA can be manipulated or modified by many enzymes, such as DNA polymerases, restriction endonucleases and kinases.

2.3.1 The application of oligonucleotides in the self-assembly of metal nanoparticles

In 1996, Mirkin's research group in the Northwestern University of USA first reported that gold nanoparticles can be self-assembled into microscale aggregates by using DNA molecules as the linker (Mirkin et al., 1996). Two different thiol-derivated noncomplementary oligonucleotides were first used to modify the gold nanoparticles. Then, these two kinds of gold nanoparticles were mixed and the DNA linker was added. The fragments on the two ends of the DNA linker can complement with the oligonucleotides on the gold nanoparticles. The gold nanoparticles can self-assemble into aggregates when the hybridization process proceeds. This process is reversible. When the temperature was elevated, the DNA double strands would dissociate and the gold nanoparticles became monodispersed again. The DNA linkers possess special recognition property. By changing the composition of the DNA linker, the structure and property of the nanoparticle aggregates, such as the distance between the particles and the strength of the linking between the particles, can be effectively controlled. In the same year, Alivisators et al. also reported that gold nanoparticles can be self-assembled based on DNA hybridization (Alivisators et al., 1996). In their work, the 3′ or 5′ ends of a 19 nucleotides single strand DNA was first connected with gold nanoaprticle by thiol. Then, a 37 nucleotides single strand DNA template was added into the gold nanoparticles solution. Gold nanoparticles were assembled onto the DNA template through hybridization into two kinds of dimer: parallel and antiparallel patterns.

2.3.2 DNA templated self-assembly of metal nanoparticles

The basic principle of DNA templated self-assembly of nanoparticle is: First, monodispersed nanoparticles with uniform size should be prepared. Then, the nanoparticles were assembled onto the DNA molecule via certain interactions between DNA and the particles. Based on the electrostatic interaction between the negatively charged DNA and the positively charged nanoparticles, gold nanoaprticles (Nakao et al., 2003), silver nanoparticles (Wei et al., 2005; Sun et al., 2006), Fe_3O_4 nanoparticles (Nyamjav et al., 2005) have been self-assembled onto DNA. The representative work in this area is the self-assembly of aniline-capped gold nanoparticles on λ-DNA carried out by Nakao et al. Aniline was first used to reduce $HAuCl_4$ to produce the aniline-capped gold nanoparticles in one step. Two different assembly methods were used to prepare the highly ordered gold nanoparticles assemblies. In method (I), the DNA template was first stretched and fixed on the substrate, gold nanoparticles were then assembled on the DNA chains to form the continuous linear structure of gold nanoparticles. In method (II), gold nanoparticles were first bound onto DNA in solution. The DNA-gold nanoparticle complex was then stretched and fixed onto the substrate. Gold nanoparticles assemblies prepared by the method (II) were loosely deposited, like the necklace.

Our group has also carried out some works on the DNA-templated self-assembly of metal nanoparticles and the *in situ* formation of metal nanostructures on the DNA assemblies. Based on the electrostatic interaction, 4-aminothiophenol capped silver nanoparticles have been successfully assembled on the predefined circular plasmid pBR322 DNA to form the silver nanoparticles ring (Sun et al., 2006), as shown in Figure 3. Another work from our group further showed that silver nanostructures can be generated on the DNA network by reduction of the silver ions that adsorbed on the DNA network with $NaBH_4$ solution (Wei et al., 2005). In this work, silver nanoparticles, nanorods, and nanowires can be formed by controlling the size of the DNA network. AFM images of the DNA network and the silver nanoparticles generated after different reducing time were shown in Figure 4.

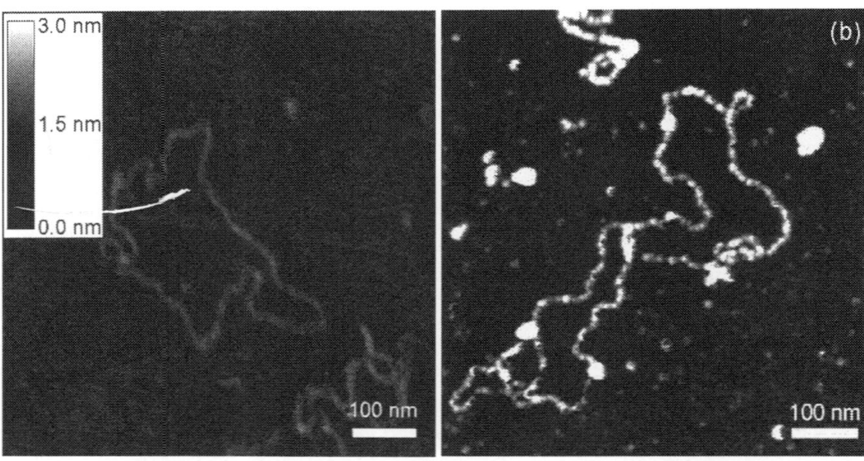

Fig. 3. AFM images of the pBR322 DNA template (left) and the DNA templated silver nanoparticles assemblies (right).

In addition to the electrostatic interaction, other interactions can also be used to assemble nanoparticles onto the DNA template. Harnack et al. reported the self-assembly of tris(hydroxymethl) phophine-capped gold nanoparticles on DNA template (Harnack etal., 2002). It should be noted that the tris(hydroxymethyl) phosphine-capped gold particles are negatively charged. So, the electrostatic interaction between DNA and the nanoparticle can be excluded. The reason that the negatively charged gold nanoparticles can still bind onto the DNA chain is because the formation of the DNA-nanoparticle conjugates. These DNA-gold nanoparticle conjugate can be used as precursors of the gold nanowires. Electroless plating the DNA-gold nanoparticle conjugates with gold leads to the formation of gold nanowires as narrow as ca.30-40 nm in width and longer than 2 μm showing ohmic behavior and resistivity of ca.10^{-5} Ωm.

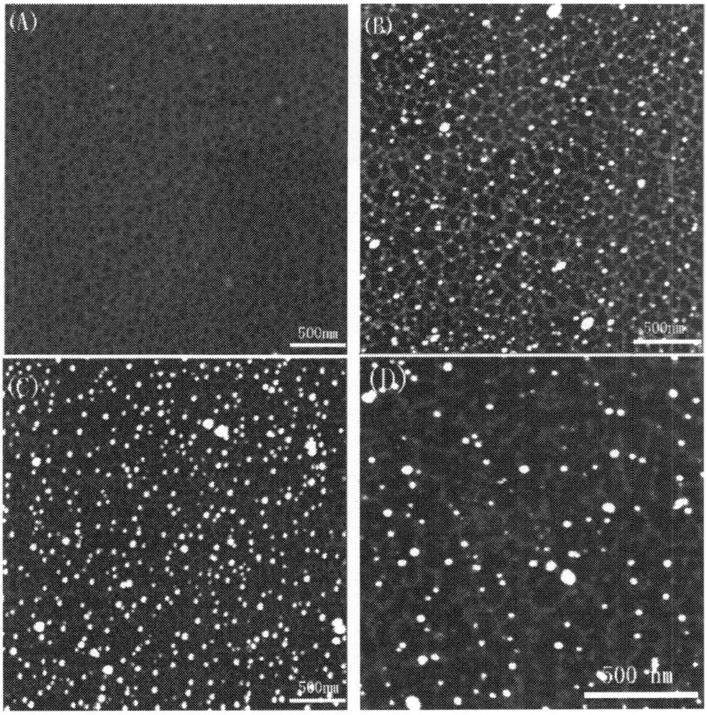

Fig. 4. AFM images of the DNA network template (A) and the silver nanoparticles generated on the DNA network after different reducing time: 1 min (B), 5min (C) and 10 min (D).

2.3.3 DNA templated nanowire formation

DNA molecules can further be used as templates to fabricate metal or conducting polymer nanowires. For example, DNA has been used as templates for the fabrication of conductire silver nanowires (Braun etal., 1998). Positively charged Ag^+ was first absorbed onto the negatively charged λ-DNA molecules. The absorbed Ag^+ was then reduced on the DNA template and the silver nanoparticles coated DNA nanowire was formed. The as-formed silver nanowires, with the width of ca.100 nm and length on the order of micrometer, connected two gold electrodes. The conductivity of the DNA-templated silver nanowire was also measured by Braun etal. The current-voltage (I-V) characteristic of the silver nanowire showed that no current was flowed through the nanowire when the bias voltage was low (10 V). These results suggested that the resistivity of silver wire was high. The silver nanowire can become conductive at very high bias voltage. Deposition of more silver onto the DNA-templated silver nanowire can produce thicker silver nanowire and the non-conducting area can be decreased from 10 V to 0.5 V, which showed that the electronic property of this system is controllable. Moreover, in the control experiment, no electrical current will be detected when any components of the system, such as DNA or silver, was removed. This showed that all the components are necessary to the conductivity of the DNA-templated silver nanowire.

The above DNA-templated nanowire formation method reported by Braumn et al. can also be introduced to fabricate other metal nanowires. By using DNA molecule as template, many metal nanowires and polymer nanowires, such as Pd nanowires (Deng et al., 2003; Richter et al., 2000, 2001), Pt nanowires (Ford et al., 2001; Seidel et al., 2004), Cu nanowires (Monson etal., 2003) and polynailine nanowires (Ma et al., 2004), have been produced by reducing the metal ions or polymerizing the monomers that bound on the DNA template. For example, Deng et al. have fabricated the parallel arrays or crossed arrays of Pd nanowire (Deng et al., 2003). Their experiment consisted of three steps: First, "molecule combing" method was used to stretch the DNA molecules into 1D parallel or 2D crossed patterns. Then, the Pd^{2+} ions were quickly absorbed onto the negatively charged DNA back-bone. Finally, chemical reduction of the Pd^{2+} ions on the DNA templates forms the Pd nanowires.
With the similar strategy, DNA-templated polyaniline nanowires have been fabricated (Ma et al., 2004). In the experiment, DNA molecules were first stretched and fixed on the silicon substrate via the "molecule combing" method. Then, the protonated aniline solution was incubated with the DNA tenplates for some time to let aniline absorb onto DNA. The aniline was finally polymerized on the DNA template to form the polyaniline nanowires. It was also found that the DNA-templated polyaniline nanowires can be used as the sensors of chemical gases.
Our group has also used a solution method to fabricate the DNA-aniline complex nanowire as well as the DNA templated polyaniline nanowire (Yang et al., 2006). With DNA as templates, linear aniline-DNA complex nanowires have been produced in solution. Gas flow was used to stretch the obtained aniline-DNA complex nanowires onto mica substrate. The ordered aniline-DNA complex nanowires can be directly observed from the AFM images. We propose that DNA molecular in solution were enwraped by aniline monomers via a self-assembled process (Figure 5). Moreover, we obtained the polyaniline (PANI) nanowires based on the precursor of aniline-DNA complex nanowires through further chemical oxidative polymerization. The aniline-DNA complex and the PANI-DNA nanowires exhibit a low background on the unmodified mica substrates (Figure 6).

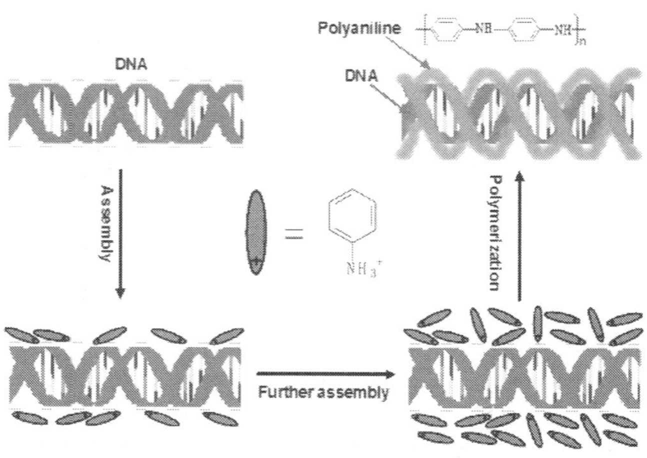

Fig. 5. Schematic representing the formation of the aniline-DNA complex nanowire and the DNA-templated nanowire

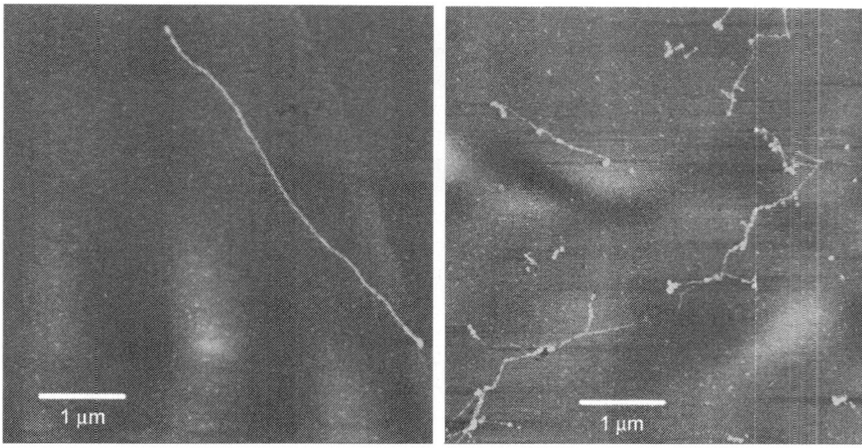

Fig. 6. Representative AFM images of the aniline-DNA complex nanowire (left) and the DNA-templated polyaniline nanowires (right).

2.4 The application of peptides and proteins in the preparation of nanoparticles

In the past few years, the preparation of bioactive or biocompatible nanomaterials has attracted more and more research attention due to the demand of various practical applications. It was believed that bioactive or biocompatible nanomaterials have wide application potential in biomedical field and bioanalysis. There are mainly two strategies that can be used to prepare bioactive and biocompatible nanomaterials: (1) conjugate biomolecules with nanomaterials via a linker agent or the protecting agent on the nanomaterial; (2) conjugate the biomolecules directly onto nanomaterials by chemical interaction or biological method.

The conjugates of biomolecules and nanoparticles were usually prepared by mixing biomolecules and the modified nanoparticles in solution. Before mixing, the nanoparticles were usually functionalized by a linker agent, which can not only recognize the biomolecule but also stabilize the nanoparticles and prevent the nanoparticles from uncontrollable growth or aggregation (Niemeyer et al., 2001). For example, inorganic nanocrystals and nanoparticles have been bioconjugated by modification with various peptides (Dameron et al., 1989; Whaley et al., 2000) or proteins (Donglas et al., 1998; Chan et al., 1998; Mamedova et al., 2001). Protein transferrin and immunoglobulin G (IgG) have been conjugated onto the ZnS capped CdSe quantun dots by Chan et al. and the bioconjugated quantum dots were used in the ultrahigh sensitive biological detection. These quantum dot-protein conjugates are water soluble and biocompatible. The transferrin conjugated quantum dots can be transferred into Hela cells and IgG conjugated quantum dots can recognize certain antigen or antibody.

It can be proposed that direct conjugation of biomolecules onto nanomaterials will produce many advantages, but the direct conjugation was not usual. The reason is that usually the harsh experiment condition used in the chemical synethesis of nanomaterilas was not suitable for the biological samples. Direct conjugation of biomolecules on nanomaterials can eliminate the use of the linker agents or the passivation of nanomaterial with capping agents. Therefore, the direct conjugation of biomolecule and nanomaterial is more simple and effective for the preparation of bioactive and biocompatible nanomaterials than the first method. In the past, water soluble and biocompatible gold nanoparticles with the diameter less than 2 nm have been produced by using peptides, such as triopronin (Templeton et al., 1999) and glutathione (Schaaff et al., 1998), to directly stabilize the gold nanoparticles. Recently, biomacromolecules, such as proteins, have been used to conjugate nanoparticles directly. Sun's group has prepared the bovine serum albumin (BSA) directly conjugated Ag_2S nanoparticles from rapid expansion of supercritical fluid solution into aqueous solution (Meziani et al., 2003). The Ag_2S nanoparticles produced by this method are monodispersed and well coated by BSA molecules. Because the protein BSA undergoes solution pH-dependent association and dissociation, the BSA-nanoparticle conjugates also assemble and disassemble with the change in solution in a reversible fashion.

Later, a more direct and convenient strategy for direct conjugation of BSA and gold nanoparticles was reported (Burt et al., 2004). With protein BSA directly as protecting agent, the BSA directly stabilized gold nanoaprticles were prepared by reducing $HAuCl_4$ with $NaBH_4$ in the aqueous solution of BSA. TEM revealed that the obtained gold nanoparticles were well dispersed with an average diameter less than 2 nm. Infrared spectroscopy confirmed that the polypeptide backbone of BSA remianed intact after BSA was conjugated with the gold particles. The conjugation of BSA onto gold nanoparticle was realized by the break of the disulfid bonds in the conjugated protein and thus available for interaction with the gold surface.

Enzymes have intrinsic ability to catalyze the formation of metal nanoparicles. It has been reported that α-amylase can be used to synthesize and stabilize gold nanoparticles in aqueous solution via mixing the aqueous solution of α-amylase and $HAuCl_4$ (Rangnekar et al., 2007). The activity of α-amylase was retained in the enzyme-gold nanoparticle complex after the nanoparticles were synthesized. The α-amylase in the enzyme-gold nanoparticle complex also showed its ability to digest starch.

We have also utilized proteins as stabilizer to prepare the protein-conjugated gold nanoparticles. Lysozyme monolayer-protected gold nanoparticles which are hydrophilic and biocompatible were synthesized in aqueous solution by chemical reduction of $HAuCl_4$ with $NaBH_4$ in the presence of lysozyme (Yang et al., 2007). The formation of a lysozyme monolayer on gold was achieved by the chemisorption of the free amino group or carboxylic group of lysozyme to the gold. The use of protein lysozyme as the capping agent gives the particles a biocompatible and hydrophilic surface, which allows their potential applications in biological and medical fields. The formation mechanism of the lysozyme monolayer-stabilized gold nanoparticles and the TEM image of obtained gold particles were shown in Figure 7.

Before aging under ambient conditions, the lysozyme-Au NPs aqueous solution is wine-colored and transparent, as shown in the photo 1 of Figure 8A. Interestingly, after the lysozyme-Au NPs aqueous solution was aged at room temperature for about 1 week, some red flocculent, fibrous material formed at the bottom of the solution, and could be seen with the naked eye (photo 2 of Figure 8A). Analysis of the red floccules by Field-emission scanning electron microscopy revealed that the wirelike products were tubular in nature, as observed by the clear contrast between the light periphery and the darker central part (Figure 8B). Hydrogen bonding between the carboxylic groups of lysozymes plays a key role in the self-assembly of lysozyme molecules and the formation of lysozyme microtubes. It is likely that partially unfolded lysozyme molecules on the Au NPs seed the formation of lysozyme microtubes. Moreover, the unusual formation of lysozyme microtubes in the lysozyme-Au NPs aqueous solution implies that bare Au NPs may be dangerous to organisms if they are present in organisms for a relative longer time because there is a possibility that they might induce the aggregation of proteins in the organisms, which is often associated with a range of human diseases including Parkinson's disease, Alzheimer's disease, and type 2 diabetes. So, special care should be taken when bare Au NPs are introduced in physiological environments. It is obvious that the spontaneous formation of lysozyme microtubes via the self-assembly process is a facile, effective, and economic method to produce protein microtube structure, which may not only have potential applications in biomedical fields but also provide new inspiration for protein study.

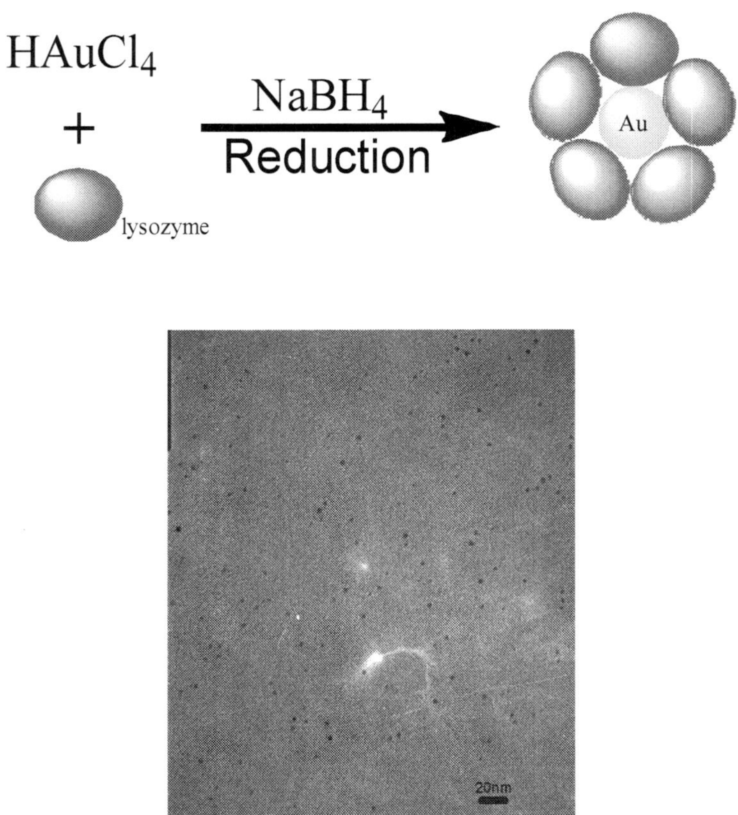

Fig. 7. The scheme of the formation of lysozyme-stabilized gold nanoparticle (up) and the TEM image of the as-formed gold particles (bottom).

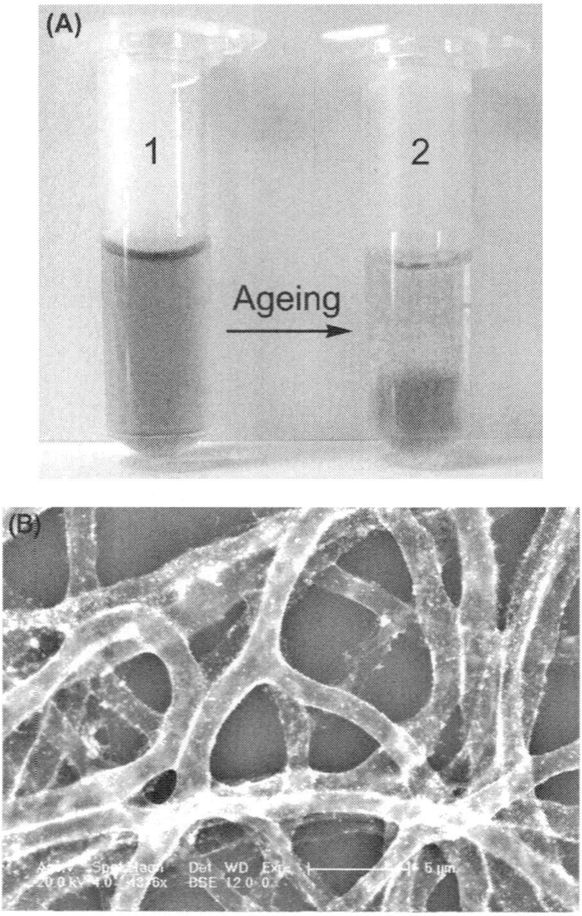

Fig. 8. (A) The photographs of the lysozyme-Au NPs aqueous solution before aging (1) as well as after 1 week of aging under ambient conditions (2), some red fibrous materials formed at the bottom of sample 2; (B) Field-emission scanning electron microscopy images of the lysozyme microtubes on a silicon wafer.

3. References

Alivisatos, A. P.; Johnsson, K. P.; Peng, X.; Wilson, T. E.; Loweth, C. J.; Bruchez, M. P.; Schultz, P. G. Organization of 'nanocrystal molecules' using DNA . *Nature* 1996, *382*, 609-611.

Artyukhin, A. B.; Shestakov, A.; Harper, J.; Bakajin, O.; Stroeve, P.; Noy, A. Functional One-Dimensional Lipid Bilayers on Carbon Nanotube Templates. *J. Am. Chem. Soc.* 2005, *127*, 7538-7542.

Aslan, K.; Lakowicz, J. R.; Geddes, C. D. Tunable plasmonic glucose sensing based on the dissociation of Con A-aggregated dextran-coated gold colloids. *Anal. Chim. Acta* 2004, *517*, 139-144.

Braun, E.; Eichen, Y.; Sivan, U.; Ben-Yoseph, G. DNA-templated assembly and electrode attachment of a conducting silver wire. *Nature* 1998, *391*, 775-778.

Burt, J. L.; Gutierrez-Wing, C.; Miki-Yoshida, M.; Jose-Yacaman, M. Noble-Metal Nanoparticles Directly Conjugated to Globular Proteins. *Langmuir* 2004, *20*, 11778-11783.

Chan, W. C. W.; Nie, S. Quantum Dot Bioconjugates for Ultrasensitive Nonisotopic Detection. *Science* 1998, *281*, 2016-2018.

Dameron, C. T.; Reese, R. N.; Mehra, R. K.; Kortan, A. R.; Carroll, P. J.; Steigerwald, M. L.; Brus, L. E.; Winge, D. R. Biosynthesis of cadmium sulphide quantum semiconductor crystallites. *Nature* 1989, *338*, 596-597.

Deng, Z.; Mao, C. DNA-Templated Fabrication of 1D Parallel and 2D Crossed Metallic Nanowire Arrays. *Nano Lett.* 2003, 3(11), 1545-1548.

Douglas, T.; Young, M. Host?guest encapsulation of materials by assembled virus protein cages. *Nature* 1998, *393*, 152-155.

Ford, W. E.; Harnack, O.; Yasuda, A.; Wessels, J. M. Platinated DNA as precursors to templated chains of metal nanoparticles. *Adv. Mater.* 2001, *13*, 1793-1797.

Geissbuchler, I.; Hovius, R.; Marinez, K. L.; Adrian, M.; Thampi, K. R.; Vogel, H. Lipid-Coated Nanocrystals as Multifunctionalized Luminescent Scaffolds for Supramolecular Biological Assemblies. *Angew. Chem., Int. Ed.* 2005, *44*, 1388-1392.

Gopalakrishnan, G.; Danelon, C.; Izewska, P.; Prummer, M.; Bolinger, P. Y.; Geissbuchler, I.; Demurtas, D.; Dubochet, J.; Vogel, H. Multifunctional Lipid/Quantum Dot Hybrid Nanocontainers for Controlled Targeting of Live Cells. *Angew. Chem., Int. Ed.* 2006, *45*, 5478-5483.

Gole, A.; Murphy, C. J. Seed-mediated synthesis of gold nanorods: role of the size and nature of the seed. *Chem. Mater.* 2004, *16*, 3633-3640.

Harnack, O.; Ford, W. E.; Yasuda, A.; Wessels, J. M. Tris(hydroxymethyl)phosphine-capped gold particles templeated by DNA as nanowire precursors. *Nano Lett.* 2002, *2*, 919-923.

He, P.; Urban, M. W. Controlled Phospholipid Functionalization of Single-Walled Carbon Nanotubes. *Biomacromolecules* 2005, *6*, 2455-2457.

He, P.; Urban, M. W. Phospholipid-Stabilized Au-Nanoparticles. *Biomacromolecules* 2005, *6*, 1224-1225.

Huang, H.; Yang, X. Synthesis of Chitosan-Stabilized Gold Nanoparticles in the Absence/Presence of Tripolyphosphate. *Biomacromolecules* 2004, *5*, 2340-2346.

Jana, N. R.; Gearheart, L. & Murphy, C. J. (2001) Wet chemical synthesis of silver nanorods and nanowires of controllable aspect ratio. *Chem. Commun.*, 617-618.

Jana, N. R.; Gearheart, L.; Murphy, C. J. Wet chemical synthesis of high aspect ratio cylindrical gold nanorods. *J. Phys. Chem. B* 2001, *105*, 4065-4067.

Jana, N. R.; Gearheart, L.; Murphy, C. J. Seed-mediated growth approach for shape-controlled synthesis of spheroidal and rod-like gold nanoparticles using a surfactant template. *Adv. Mater.* 2001, *13*, 1389-1393.

Li, P.; Li, D.; Zhang, L.; Li, G.; Wang, E. Cationic lipid bilayer coated gold nanoparticles-mediated transfection of mammalian cells. *Biomaterials* 2008, *29*, 3617-3624.

Li, P.; Zhang, L.; Ai, K.; Li, D.; Liu, X.; Wang, E. Coating didodecyldimethylammonium bromide onto Au nanoparticles increases the stability of its complex with DNA. *J. Control. Release* 2008, *129*, 128-134.

Lyu, Y-K.; Lim, K-R.; Lee, B. Y.; Kim, K. S.; Lee, W-Y. Microgravimetric lectin biosensor based on signal amplification using carbohydrate-stabilized gold nanoparticles. *Chem. Commun.* 2008, 4771-4773.

Ma, Y.; Li, N.; Yang, X. One-step synthesis of amino-dextran-protected gold and silver nanoparticles and its application in biosensors. *Anal. Bioanal. Chem.* 2005, 382, 1044-1048.

Mamedova, N. N.; Kotov, N. A.; Rogach, A. L.; Studer, J. Albumin-CdTe Nanoparticle Bioconjugates: Preparation, Structure, and Interunit Energy Transfer with Antenna Effect. *Nano Lett.* 2001, 1, 281-286.

Ma, Y.; Zhang, J.; Zhang, G.; He, H. Polyaniline nanowires on Si surfaces fabricated with DNA templates. *J. Am. Chem. Soc.* 2004, *126*, 7097-7101.

Meziani, M. J.; Sun, Y.-P. Protein-Conjugated Nanoparticles from Rapid Expansion of Supercritical Fluid Solution into Aqueous Solution. *J. Am. Chem. Soc.* 2003, *125*, 8015-8018.

Mirkin, C. A.; Letsinger, R. L.; Mucic, R. C.; Storhoff, J. J. A DNA-based method for rationally assembling nanoparticles into macroscopic materials. *Nature*, 1996, *382*, 607-609.

Monson, C. F.; Woolley, A. T. DNA-templated construction of copper nanowires. *Nano Lett.* 2003, *3*, 359-363.

Mornet, S.; Lambert, O.; Duguet, E.; Brisson, A. The Formation of Supported Lipid Bilayers on Silica Nanoparticles Revealed by Cryoelectron Microscopy. *Nano Lett.* 2005, 5, 281-285.

Nakao, H.; Shiigi, H.; Yamamoto, Y.; Tokonami, S.; Nagaoka, T.; Sugiyama, S.; Ohtani, T. Highly ordered assemblies of Au nanoparticles organized on DNA. *Nano Lett.* 2003, 3, 1391-1394.

Nalwa. Handbook of nanostructured biomaterials and their applications in nanotechnology. Chapter VII, "DNA-based artificial nanostructures:fabrication, properties and applications". American Scientific Publishers, 2005, pp 224-246.

Niemeyer, C. M. Nanoparticles, Proteins, and Nucleic Acids: Biotechnology Meets Materials Science. *Angew. Chem. Int. Ed.* 2001, *40*, 4128-4158.

Nyamjav, D.; Ivanisevic, A. Templates for DNA-templated Fe_3O_4 nanoparticles. *Biomaterials* 2005, *26*, 2 749-2757.

Rangnekar, A.; Sarma, T. K.; Singh, A. K.; Deka, J.; Ramesh, A.; Chattopadhyay, A. Retention of Enzymatic Activity of α-Amylase in the Reductive Synthesis of Gold Nanoparticles. *Langmuir* 2007, *23*, 5700-5706.

Raveendran, P.; Fu, J.; Wallen, S. L. Completely "Green" Synthesis and Stabilization of Metal Nanoparticles. *J. Am. Chem. Soc.* 2003, *125*, 13940-13941.

Richter, J.; Seidel, R.; Kirsch, R.; Mertig, M.; Pompe, W.; Plaschke, J.; Schackert, H. K. Nanoscale palladium metallization of DNA. *Adv. Mater.* 2000, *12*, 507-510.

Richter, J.; Mertig, M.; Pompe, W.; Monch, I.; Schackert, H. K. Construction of highly conductive nanowires on a DNA template. *Appl. Phys. Lett.* 2001, *78*, 536-538.

Schaaff, T. G.; Knight, G.; Shafigullin, M. N.; Borkman, R. F.; Whetten, R. L. Isolation and Selected Properties of a 10.4 kDa Gold:Glutathione Cluster Compound. *J. Phys. Chem. B.* 1998, *102*, 10643-10646.

Seidel, R.; Ciacchi, L. C.; Weigel, M.; Pompe, W.; Mertig, M. Synthesis of platinum cluster chains on DNA templates: conditions for a template-controlled cluster growth. *J. Phys. Chem. B* 2004, *108*, 10801-10811.

Selvakannan, PR.; Mandal, S.; Phadtare, S.; Pasricha, R.; Sastry, M. Capping of Gold Nanoparticles by the Amino Acid Lysine Renders Them Water-Dispersible. *Langmuir* 2003, 19, 3545-3549.

Shao, Y.; Jin, Y.; Dong, S. Synthesis of gold nanoplates by aspartate reduction of gold chloride. *Chem. Commun.* 2004, 1104-1105.

Strohoff, J. J.; Mirkin, C. A. Programmed materials synthesis with DNA. *Chem. Rev.* 1999, *99*, 1849-1862.

Sun, L.; Wei, G.; Song, Y.; Liu, Z.; Wang, L.; Li, Z. Fabrication of silver nanoparticles ring templated by plasmid DNA. *Appl. Sur. Sci.* 2006, *252*, 4969-4974.

Takahashi, H.; Niidome, Y.; Niidome, T.; Kaneko, K.; Kawasaki, H.; Yamada, S. Modification of Gold Nanorods Using Phosphatidylcholine to Reduce Cytotoxicity. *Langmuir* 2006, 22, 2-5.

Templeton, A. C.; Chen, S.; Gross, S. M.; Murray, R. W. Water-Soluble, Isolable Gold Clusters Protected by Tiopronin and Coenzyme A Monolayers. *Langmuir* 1999, 15, 66-76.

Wei, G.; Wang, L.; Zhou, H.; Liu, Z.; Song, Y.; Li, Z. Electrostatic assembly of CTAB-capped silver nanoparticles along predefined λ-DNA template. *Appl. Sur. Sci.* 2005, *252*, 1189-1196.

Wei, G.; Zhou, H.; Liu, Z.; Song, Y.; Wang, L.; Sun, L.; Li, Z. One-step synthesis of silver nanoparticles, nanorods, and nanowires on the surface of DNA network. *J. Phys. Chem. B* 2005, *109*, 8738-8743.

Whaley, S. R.; English, D. S.; Hu, E. L.; Barbara, P. F.; Belcher, A. M. Selection of peptides with semiconductor binding specificity for directed nanocrystal assembly. *Nature* 2000, *405*, 665-668.

Wu, H.-Y.; Huang, W.-L.; Huang, M. H. Direct high-yield synthesis of high aspect ratio gold nanorods. *Cryst. Growth Des.* 2007, *7*, 831-835.

Yang, T.; Li, Z.; Wang, L.; Guo, C. L.; Sun, Y. J. Synthesis, Characterization and Self-Assembly of Protein Lysozyme Monolayer-Stabilized Gold Nanoparticles *Langmuir* 2007, *23*, 10533-10538.

Yang, T.; Wei, G.; Niu, L.; Li, Z. Fabrication of linear aniline-DNA complex nanowires and DNA-templated polyaniline nanowires. *Chemical Journal of Chinese Universities-Chinese* 2006, *27*, 1126-1130.

Zhang, L. X.; Sun, X. P.; Song, Y. H.; Jiang, X. E.; Dong, S. J.; Wang, E. K. Didodecyldimethylammonium Bromide Lipid Bilayer-Protected Gold Nanoparticles: Synthesis, Characterization, and Self-Assembly. *Langmuir* 2006, 22, 2838-2843.

Zhang, L.; Li, P.; Li, D.; Guo, S.; Wang, E. Effect of Freeze-Thawing on Lipid Bilayer-Protected Gold Nanoparticles. *Langmuir* 2008, *24*, 3407-3411.

Zhang, J.; Roll, D.; Geddes, C. D.; Lakowicz, J. R. Aggregation of Silver Nanoparticle-Dextran Adducts with Concanavalin A and Competitive Complexation with Glucose. *J. Phys. Chem. B.* 2004, *108,* 12210-12214.

Zhong, Z.; Luo, J.; Ang, T. P.; Highfield, J.; Lin, J.; Gedanken, A. Controlled Organization of Au Colloids into Linear Assemblies. *J. Phys. Chem. B.* 2004, *108,* 18119-18123.

Zhou, X.; Moran-Mirabal, J. M.; Craighead, H. G.; McEuen, P. L. Supported lipid bilayer/carbon nanotube hybrids. *Nat. Nanotechnol.* 2007, *2,* 185-190.

17

Dielectrophoresis for Manipulation of Bioparticles

Naga Siva K. Gunda and Sushanta K. Mitra
University of Alberta
Canada

1. Introduction

The objective of the present chapter is to provide a comprehensive description of dielectrophoresis (DEP), an electrokinetic technique, which has immense capability to manipulate bioparticles from micro- to nano-scale range. DEP is the movement of dielectric particles due to polarization effects in nonuniform electric fields (Pohl, 1978). The usual way of applying this technique is by flowing/placing the suspended particle solution on the planar microelectrode structures. The advancements in micro/nano fabrication techniques help in the development of such micro/nano electrode structures to generate the nonuniform electric field in DEP channels (Hughes, 2003). DEP assisted by such miniaturized electrodes have been used for separating, sorting, positioning, trapping, concentrating, and mixing (Gunda et al., 2009) of biomolecules such as cells, bacteria, virus, DNA and proteins (Basuray & Chang, 2010; Bunthawin et al., 2010; Church et al., 2009; Du et al., 2008; Ferrier et al., 2008; Gagnon et al., 2009; Hughes, 2003; Hwang et al., 2009; Jones, 1995; Lewpiriyawong et al., 2008; Lin & Yeow, 2007; Nguyen & Werely, 2006; Parikesit et al., 2008; Pohl, 1978; Wei et al., 2009; Yang et al., 2010; Zhu et al., 2010). These applications of DEP for manipulating such bioparticles has been further exploited in different fields namely drug delivery, food diagnostics, point of care analysis, biomedical, etc (Hughes, 2003).
The present chapter begins with brief description of DEP theory and mathematical modeling of DEP force field and spatial concentration distribution of particles inside the microchannel embedded with array of rectangular microelectrodes at the bottom. Then fabrication and experimental details of such DEP microfluidic device to manipulate bioparticles is discussed.

2. DEP Theory

DEP is manipulation of dielectric particles because of polarization effects under nonuniform direct current (DC) or alternating current (AC) electric fields (Pohl, 1978). The net force created with DEP generates momentum in the particles. Particle movement towards regions of high electric field intensities is called positive DEP and occurs when the interior of the particle is more permissive to the field. The opposite effect is the movement towards lower electric field intensities called negative DEP, when the exterior is more permissive (Hughes, 2003; Jones, 1995; Pohl, 1978). The frequency at which the DEP effect changes from positive DEP to negative DEP or negative DEP to positive DEP is called crossover frequency (Jones, 1995; Pohl, 1978). The DEP force depends on both the gradient of the electric field and electrical properties such as permittivity and conductivity of the particle and medium. It is important to note that the force due to DEP is based on the gradient of electric field and not on the absolute value of electric field at any point. Analysis of movement of the particles in a nonuniform electric field needs an accurate knowledge of the electric field distribution in the system. Different electrode geometries and arrangements are used to produce nonuniform electric field. They are polynomial electrodes, castellated electrodes, interdigited electrodes, and array of electrodes. Each arrangement has its own advantages and disadvantages. Bioparticles can be any shape like spherical, oblate, prolate, disc, rod, etc., with dimensions ranging from micron to nano-scale. Assuming arbitrary shape of bioparticles, here we are providing the time averaged dielectrophoretic force $\mathbf{F}_{DEP}$ acts on any arbitrary shaped particle due to stationary wave nonuniform AC electric field. It is derived with slight modification of $\mathbf{F}_{DEP}$ acting on spherical particles provided by Pohl (1978)

$$\mathbf{F}_{DEP} = \frac{3}{2}(vol)\varepsilon_m Re[K(\omega)]\nabla(\mathbf{E}\cdot\mathbf{E}) \tag{1}$$

where (vol) is the volume of particle, ε_m is the permittivity of medium, $Re[K(\omega)]$ is real part of Clausius-Mossotti (CM) factor and $\mathbf{E}$ is the applied electric field vector. CM factor for any arbitrary shaped particle is given as (Yang & Lei, 2007)

$$K(\omega) = \frac{1}{3}\frac{(\varepsilon_p^{'} - \varepsilon_m^{'})}{\varepsilon_m^{'} + A_\alpha(\varepsilon_p^{'} - \varepsilon_m^{'})} \tag{2}$$

where A_α is the depolarization factor, subscript α relates to axis of the particle x or y or z and $\varepsilon_p^{'}$ and $\varepsilon_m^{'}$ are complex permittivities of particle and medium, respectively. They are given as

$$\varepsilon_p^{'} = \varepsilon_p - j\frac{\sigma_p}{\omega} \tag{3}$$

$$\varepsilon_m^{'} = \varepsilon_m - j\frac{\sigma_m}{\omega} \tag{4}$$

where ε_p and ε_m are permittivity of particle and medium respectively, σ_p and σ_m are conductivity of particle and medium respectively, ω is angular frequency of the applied field and $j = \sqrt{-1}$. Depolarization factor for the CM factor varies according to the shape of the particle which leads to change in DEP force. Yang & Lei (2007) reported the calculation of depolarization factor for ellipsoidal, oblate and prolate spheroid shapes. The sum of different axis depolarization factors for a particle should be unity. Considering a, b, and c as dimensions of the particles in the x, y, and z-axis directions respectively, the depolarization factors are given as

For Sphere $(a = b = c)$:

$$A_x = A_y = A_z = \frac{1}{3} \tag{5}$$

For Oblate spheroid $(a = b > c)$:

$$A_x = A_y = \frac{a^2 c}{2(a^2 - c^2)}\left[\frac{\pi/2}{\sqrt{(a^2 - c^2)}} - \frac{c}{a^2}\right] \tag{6}$$

$$A_z = 1 - 2A_x = 1 - 2A_y \tag{7}$$

For Prolate spheroid $(a > b = c)$:

$$A_x = \frac{b^2}{2a^2 e^3}\left[\ln(\frac{1+e}{1-e}) - 2e\right] \tag{8}$$

$$A_y = A_z = \frac{(1 - A_x)}{2} \tag{9}$$

where eccentricity (e) is given as $\sqrt{(1 - \frac{b^2}{a^2})}$. It is observed that CM factor varies with respect to axis of the particle. But in the microchannel, the direction of DEP force acting on the particle is arbitrary. Hence, average CM factor is considered for the particle for calculating DEP force. From Eqn. (1), it is observed that DEP force becomes less effective for small particles, mainly with molecular sizes and submicron particles where thermal effects are dominant. Most of the conventional DEP experiments demonstrated the response of particles with the change in frequency of the applied electric field to decide the crossover frequencies (Castellarnau et al., 2006). This crossover frequencies can be calculated from complex CM factor $K(\omega)$. If $Re[K(\omega)] \geq 0$, positive DEP occurs, otherwise negative DEP occurs. Theoretically, $Re[K(\omega)]$ varies from -0.5 to +1 (Jones, 1995; Pohl, 1978). The crossover frequency for any arbitrary shaped particle is given as

$$f_c = \frac{1}{2\pi}\sqrt{\frac{(\sigma_m - \sigma_p)[\sigma_m + A_\alpha(\sigma_p - \sigma_m)]}{(\varepsilon_p - \varepsilon_m)[\varepsilon_m + A_\alpha(\varepsilon_p - \varepsilon_m)]}} \tag{10}$$

It is observed that f_c can be calculated only when $\frac{(\sigma_m - \sigma_p)}{(\varepsilon_p - \varepsilon_m)} > 0$. If $\varepsilon_p = \varepsilon_m$, f_c will tend to ∞, and practically, it is not possible to apply such frequency for observing the two types of DEP effects. Bioparticles might be made up of two or three different layers with different conductivity and permittivity values. In such cases, the DEP force shown in Eqn. (1) is still valid, if $\varepsilon_p^{'}$ is replaced with effective complex permittivity $\varepsilon_{peff}^{'}$. For a two layered particle where particle p is surrounded with another layer 2, the effective complex permittivity $\varepsilon_{peff}^{'}$ as given by (Jones, 1995; Yang & Lei, 2007)

$$\varepsilon_{peff}^{'} = \varepsilon_{p2}^{'}\left[\frac{\varepsilon_p^{'} + t_\alpha(\varepsilon_p^{'} + \varepsilon_{p2}^{'})/q_\alpha}{\varepsilon_{p2}^{'} + t_\alpha(\varepsilon_p^{'} + \varepsilon_{p2}^{'})/q_\alpha}\right] \tag{11}$$

where t_α is the thickness of particle layer 2 along x, y, and z-axis, $q_\alpha = a$, b, and c for $\alpha = x, y$, and z, respectively and $\varepsilon_{p2}^{'}$ is the complex permittivity of hydration layer which can be written as

$$\varepsilon_{p2}^{'} = \varepsilon_{p2} - j\frac{\sigma_{p2}}{\omega} \tag{12}$$

where ε_{p2} and σ_{p2} are permittivity and conductivity of layer 2, respectively. The interested reader can refer to Jones (1995) or Yang & Lei (2007) for calculating effectives complex permittivity of three layered particles.

Mathematical modeling

The governing equations for dielectrophoretic transport of particles in aqueous solution require the Laplace equation for calculating electric field distributions in a system, Navier-Stokes equation for calculating fluid velocity distribution in a system and convection-diffusion-migration equation for determining the particles distribution. In the present study, the following assumptions are made: (i) the aqueous solution containing particles flowing through the microchannel are at steady state, incompressible and behave like Newtonian fluids; (ii) no chemical reactions take place between the particles or between the particles and walls of the channel; (iii) Electric double-layer, van der Waals and electrothermal effects are neglected.

2.1 Laplace equation

The electric field distribution in the system created by AC signal is described by the Laplace equation (Masliyah & Bhattacharjee, 2006)

$$\nabla^2 \phi = 0 \tag{13}$$

where ϕ is the applied electric potential. Solving Eqn.(13) with appropriate boundary conditions will provide the potential distribution in the computational domain. This potential distribution is used to calculate the DEP force acting on particles.

2.2 Navier-Stokes equation

For an incompressible flow at low Reynolds number, the steady state continuity and Navier-Stokes equations neglecting inertial and body forces are given by,

$$\nabla \cdot \mathbf{u} = 0 \tag{14}$$

$$\nabla p = \mu \nabla^2 \mathbf{u} \tag{15}$$

2.3 Convection-diffusion-migration equation

The steady state concentration distribution of particles in an aqueous solution with no chemical reactions can be given by convection-diffusion-migration equation as (Masliyah & Bhattacharjee, 2006)

$$\nabla \cdot (\mathbf{u}C) = \nabla \cdot (\mathbf{D} \cdot \nabla C) - \nabla \cdot (\frac{\mathbf{D} \cdot \mathbf{F}_{mig}}{k_B T} C) \tag{16}$$

where $\mathbf{u}$ is the medium velocity vector, C is the concentration of particles, $\mathbf{D}$ is diffusion coefficient tensor, $\mathbf{F}_{mig}$ is the migrational force vector on particles due to DEP, k_B is Boltzmann constant $(1.3806503 \times 10^{-23} m^2 kg s^{-2} K^{-1})$ and T is the ambient temperature. The first term of Eqn. (16) represents the transport due to convection, the second term is the transport due to diffusion, and the third term indicates the transport due to migration. Since the interactions between particles are neglected in the assumptions, diffusion tensor $\mathbf{D}$ can be simplified as the Stokes-Einstein diffusion coefficient D_∞,

$$D_\infty = \frac{k_B T}{f} \tag{17}$$

where $f = 12 A_p \mu / l_c$. Here f is the friction factor, A_p is the projected area of the particle, μ is the dynamic viscosity of medium, and l_c is the characteristic length of particle. Both A_p and l_c depend on the shape of the particle and the direction of flow over it. The particle migration velocity for steady state problem can be given as

$$\mathbf{u}_{mig} = \frac{\mathbf{D} \cdot (\mathbf{F}_{mig})}{k_B T} = \frac{\mathbf{F}_{mig}}{f} \tag{18}$$

Combining and rearranging Eqs. (16-18) gives the following modified steady state convection-diffusion-migration equation

$$\mathbf{u}_{tot} \nabla C = D_\infty \nabla^2 C \tag{19}$$

where $\mathbf{u}_{tot} = \mathbf{u} + \mathbf{u}_{mig}$. Solving Eqn. (19) with appropriate boundary conditions will provide the spatial concentration distribution of particles in the computational domain. This concentration distribution is used to check the effectiveness of applying DEP force for manipulating submicron particles.

2.4 Computational domain

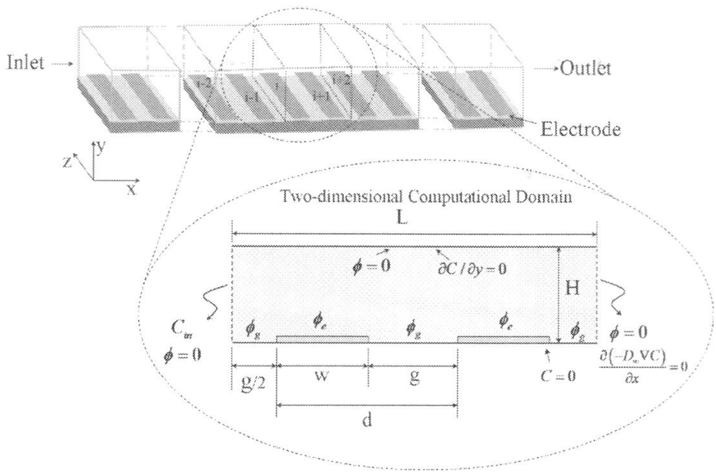

Fig. 1. Schematic view of DEP microfluidic device considered for manipulating the particles. Enlarged view shows the two-dimensional computational domain considered for analysis

Figure 1 depicts the schematic view of the DEP microfluidic system considered for manipulation of microparticles under DEP effects. The device has infinite number of electrodes ($-\infty, \ldots, -3, -2, -1, 0, 1, 2, 3, \ldots, \infty$) on the bottom surface of the microchannel. The enlarged view in Fig.1 shows the two-dimensional computational domain considered for numerical and analytical analysis. Here L is the length of channel considered for computational domain and H is the height. The bottom surface is embedded with array of parallel rectangular microelectrodes of width w and gap g in between the electrodes. The parameter d represents the sum of electrode width w and gap g and ϕ represents the applied electric potential. The notation i and $(i+1)$ represents the ith and $(i+1)^{th}$ electrodes, respectively. Appropriate boundary conditions to solve the above governing equations is also provided in the Fig.1. The remaining boundaries are kept insulated/symmetry for convection-diffusion-migration equation, zero charge/symmetry for Laplace equation and no-slip boundary conditions at walls for Navier-Stokes equation.

2.5 Solution methodology

The procedure for solving the concentration field is divided into three steps: (i) evaluating the electric field distribution in the system using Eqn. (13); (ii) evaluating the flow field velocity distribution in the system using Eqns. (14) and (15); (iii) evaluating the particle spatial concentration distribution using Eqn. (19). Step (i) and (ii) are solved independently, because electrical body forces in the system are neglected. The solution obtained in step (i) is used to find the DEP force. Solutions obtained in step (i) and step (ii) are incorporated into the Eqn. (19) to calculate concentration distribution of particles in the system under negative DEP effects.

The potential distribution is solved analytically as well as numerically. The analytical expression for potential, electric field and DEP force distributions in a microchannel containing parallel array of electrodes at the bottom surface has been already reported in many research papers on the basis of charge density method (Wang et al., 1993), Green's theorem (Clague & Wheeler, 2001; Molla & Bhattacharjee, 2005a;b; Wang et al., 1996), conformal mapping (Manuel & Clague, 2000) and Fourier series (Morgan et al., 2001). The closed form solutions are also developed for electric field and DEP forces by Morgan et al. (2001) and Chang et al. (2003). Wang et al. (1996) compared the analytical solution from Green's Theorem based method with charge density method, whereas Green et al. (2002) compared the analytical solution from Fourier series method with numerical solution solved by finite element method. Clague & Wheeler (2001), and Crews et al. (2001) studied the effect of electrode dimensions, channel height and applied voltage on gradient of squared electric field. Molla & Bhattacharjee (2005a;b) compared the Green's theorem based analytical and finite element based numerical solutions as well as studied the effect of applied voltages and frequencies on DEP force. In the present study, a simple and modified analytical expressions for electric field and gradient of squared electric field squared are derived based on Green's theorem method. In addition, a mesh independent numerical solution using finite element method is also solved. These analytical and numerical solutions are compared with Fourier series method (Morgan et al., 2001) and closed form solutions (CFS) by Morgan et al. (2001) and Chang et al. (2003).

Here, the analytical expressions for potential, electric field and gradient of squared electric field using Green's theorem method is derived. The potential and electric field distributions along the length of the electrodes are uniform for array of parallel rectangular electrodes. Therefore, the in-plane dimension of the system is neglected here. The Laplace equation for two-dimensional system as shown in Fig.1 is solved. Sinusoidal voltage of phase difference $2\pi/n$ and angular frequency ω are applied on the electrodes for producing nonuniform electric field. For particles under stationary wave DEP, value of n will be 2 (Clague & Wheeler, 2001; Molla & Bhattacharjee, 2005b; Wang et al., 1996). The analytical solution for the Laplace equation using Green's theorem for upper half-space, $y \geq 0$ is given as

$$\phi(x,y) = \frac{y}{2\pi} \int \frac{\phi dx_0}{[(x-x_0)^2 + y^2]} \tag{20}$$

where x_0 represents the point in x direction on the electrode plane and ϕ represents the surface potential on the electrode plane. The potential distribution is solved by piecewise integration of Eqn. (20) with surface potential boundary conditions on electrode plane. Assuming the linear variation of surface potential at gap between the electrodes (Chang et al., 2003; Clague & Wheeler, 2001; Crews et al., 2001; Green et al., 2002; Molla & Bhattacharjee, 2005a;b; Morgan et al., 2001; Wang et al., 1996), the surface potential boundary conditions on electrodes and gap between electrodes are given as

$$\phi_e(x_0) = \phi cos\left(\omega t + \frac{2\pi i}{n}\right) \tag{21}$$

$$\phi_g(x_0) = \phi\left\{S\left[x_0 - (id + \frac{w}{2})\right] + cos\left(\omega t + \frac{2\pi i}{n}\right)\right\} \tag{22}$$

where $S = \{cos(\omega t + 2\pi(i+1)/n) - cos(\omega t + 2\pi i/n)\}/g$, the limits of x_0 for electrodes varies from $id - w/2$ to $id + w/2$ and the limits of x_0 for gap between the electrodes varies from $id + w/2$ to $(i+1)d - w/2$. Here i is the ith electrode and varies from $-\infty$ to $+\infty$. Substituting the Eqns.(21) and (22) into Eqn. (20) and integrating yields the potential distribution expression as

$$
\begin{aligned}
\phi(x,y\geq 0) =& \frac{1}{\pi}\sum_{i=-\infty}^{\infty}\left\{-\phi_e(x)\left(tan^{-1}\left[\frac{x-q_i}{y}\right]-tan^{-1}\left[\frac{x-p_i}{y}\right]\right)\right\}\\
&+\frac{1}{\pi}\sum_{i=-\infty}^{\infty}\left\{+\phi_g(x)\left(tan^{-1}\left[\frac{x-q_i}{y}\right]-tan^{-1}\left[\frac{x-p_{i+1}}{y}\right]\right)\right.\\
&\left.-\frac{Sy}{2}\left(ln\left[(x-q_i)^2+y^2\right]-ln\left[(x-p_{i+1})^2+y^2\right]\right)\right\}
\end{aligned}
\tag{23}
$$

where $p_i = id - w/2$, $q_i = id + w/2$, and $p_{i+1} = (i+1)d - w/2$. Electric field distribution in the system can be calculated from the above potential distribution expression using $\mathbf{E} = -\nabla\phi$. The term $\nabla(\mathbf{E}\cdot\mathbf{E})$ in Eqn. (1) can be expressed for a two-dimensional computational domain as follows:

$$
\frac{\partial}{\partial x}(\mathbf{E}\cdot\mathbf{E}) = 2(E_x\frac{\partial E_x}{\partial x}+E_y\frac{\partial E_y}{\partial x})
\tag{24}
$$

$$
\frac{\partial}{\partial y}(\mathbf{E}\cdot\mathbf{E}) = 2(E_x\frac{\partial E_x}{\partial y}+E_y\frac{\partial E_y}{\partial y})
\tag{25}
$$

where E_x is electric field in the x direction, E_y is electric field in the y direction.
The expressions E_x, E_y, $\partial E_x/\partial x$, $\partial E_y/\partial x$, $\partial E_x/\partial y$ and $\partial E_y/\partial y$ are derived by differentiating the potential distribution function given in Eqn. (23). The expressions derived for potential, electric field in x and y directions are similar to the Wang et al. (1996), Clague & Wheeler (2001) and Molla & Bhattacharjee (2005a;b) with different notation. Here the simplified and modified expressions are provided. The following expressions can be used to calculate the DEP forces by substituting into Eqn. (1)

$$
\begin{aligned}
E_x =& \frac{1}{\pi}\sum_{i=-\infty}^{\infty}\left\{\phi_e(x)y\left(\frac{1}{y^2+(x-q_i)^2}-\frac{1}{y^2+(x-p_i)^2}\right)\right\}\\
&+\frac{1}{\pi}\sum_{i=-\infty}^{\infty}\left\{-\phi_g(x)y\left(\frac{1}{y^2+(x-q_i)^2}-\frac{1}{y^2+(x-p_{i+1})^2}\right)\right.\\
&+Sy\left(\frac{x-q_i}{y^2+(x-q_i)^2}-\frac{x-p_{i+1}}{y^2+(x-p_{i+1})^2}\right)\\
&\left.-S\left(tan^{-1}\left[\frac{x-q_i}{y}\right]-tan^{-1}\left[\frac{x-p_{i+1}}{y}\right]\right)\right\}
\end{aligned}
\tag{26}
$$

$$
\begin{aligned}
E_y =& \frac{1}{\pi}\sum_{i=-\infty}^{\infty}\left\{-\phi_e(x)\left(\frac{x-q_i}{y^2+(x-q_i)^2}-\frac{x-p_i}{y^2+(x-p_i)^2}\right)\right\}\\
&+\frac{1}{\pi}\sum_{i=-\infty}^{\infty}\left\{+\phi_g(x)\left(\frac{x-q_i}{y^2+(x-q_i)^2}-\frac{x-p_{i+1}}{y^2+(x-p_{i+1})^2}\right)\right.\\
&+Sy^2\left(\frac{1}{y^2+(x-q_i)^2}-\frac{1}{y^2+(x-p_{i+1})^2}\right)\\
&\left.+\frac{S}{2}\left(ln\left[(x-q_i)^2+y^2\right]-ln\left[(x-p_{i+1})^2+y^2\right]\right)\right\}
\end{aligned}
\tag{27}
$$

$$
\begin{aligned}
\frac{\partial E_x}{\partial x} &= -\frac{\partial E_y}{\partial y} \\
&= \frac{1}{\pi} \sum_{i=-\infty}^{\infty} \left\{ -2\phi_e(x) y \left(\frac{x-q_i}{[y^2+(x-q_i)^2]^2} - \frac{x-p_i}{[y^2+(x-p_i)^2]^2} \right) \right\} \\
&+ \frac{1}{\pi} \sum_{i=-\infty}^{\infty} \left\{ +2\phi_g(x) y \left(\frac{x-q_i}{[y^2+(x-q_i)^2]^2} - \frac{x-p_{i+1}}{[y^2+(x-p_{i+1})^2]^2} \right) \right. \\
&+ Sy \left(\frac{y^2-(x-q_i)^2}{[y^2+(x-q_i)^2]^2} - \frac{y^2-(x-p_{i+1})^2}{[y^2+(x-p_{i+1})^2]^2} \right) \\
&\left. -2Sy \left(\frac{1}{y^2+(x-q_i)^2} - \frac{1}{y^2+(x-p_{i+1})^2} \right) \right\}
\end{aligned}
\tag{28}
$$

$$
\begin{aligned}
\frac{\partial E_x}{\partial y} &= \frac{\partial E_y}{\partial x} \\
&= \frac{1}{\pi} \sum_{i=-\infty}^{\infty} \left\{ -\phi_e(x) \left(\frac{y^2-(x-q_i)^2}{[y^2+(x-q_i)^2]^2} - \frac{y^2-(x-p_i)^2}{[y^2+(x-p_i)^2]^2} \right) \right\} \\
&+ \frac{1}{\pi} \sum_{i=-\infty}^{\infty} \left\{ +\phi_g(x) \left(\frac{y^2-(x-q_i)^2}{[y^2+(x-q_i)^2]^2} - \frac{y^2-(x-p_{i+1})^2}{[y^2+(x-p_{i+1})^2]^2} \right) \right. \\
&-2Sy^2 \left(\frac{x-q_i}{[y^2+(x-q_i)^2]^2} - \frac{x-p_{i+1}}{[y^2+(x-p_{i+1})^2]^2} \right) \\
&\left. +2S \left(\frac{x-q_i}{y^2+(x-q_i)^2} - \frac{x-p_{i+1}}{y^2+(x-p_{i+1})^2} \right) \right\}
\end{aligned}
\tag{29}
$$

Analytical methods give exact solution to the potential and electric field distributions in the system as well as DEP force on the particles. This analytical method is only applicable to simplified geometries (mainly two-dimensional) like infinite array of parallel electrodes. However, most of the applications, electrode geometries and layouts are different and not possible to simplify as two-dimensional models. Solving the two-dimensional convection-diffusion-migration equation by analytical methods is a tedious process due to elliptical nature of equation. Therefore, numerical method is implemented to obtain approximate solutions for electric field and particle concentration distributions in the system. The governing equations and the boundary conditions described earlier are implemented in a finite element based software COMSOL Multiphysics version 3.5a (COMSOL, Inc., Burlington, MA, USA), to study the dielectrophoretic behavior of microparticles. To obtain the numerical solution, only two electrodes are used for simulations instead of array of electrodes as it is periodic in nature (as shown in Fig.1). The two-dimensional computational domain is discretized with quadrilateral elements. The electrode edges are discretized with finer elements to capture the effect of high intensity electric field. The model uses Lagrange-quadratic elements for calculating parameters inside the domain like electric potential, electric field, etc. The structured (mapped) mesh scheme is used to discretize the computational domain. The simultaneous linear equations produced by the finite element method are solved using direct elimination solver (PARDISO). A mesh independent finite element solution is achieved with around 12,000 elements. The convection-diffusion-migration model is solved with small artificial isotropic diffusion (= 0.05) to improve the convergence and to reduce the oscillations in concentration profile (Molla & Bhattacharjee, 2007).

2.6 Modeling results

Results for the dielectrophoretic behavior of the bioparticles in aqueous solution are presented in this section. All the results shown for the case when the width of the electrode is equal to gap between the electrodes ($W = G$). Similar results are observed for other electrode configurations ($W < G$ and $W > G$), which are not described here for the sake of brevity. Thickness of the electrodes is assumed to be very small as compared to the height of channel and hence neglected in the simulations. The height of the channel is three times the width of electrodes ($H = 3W$).

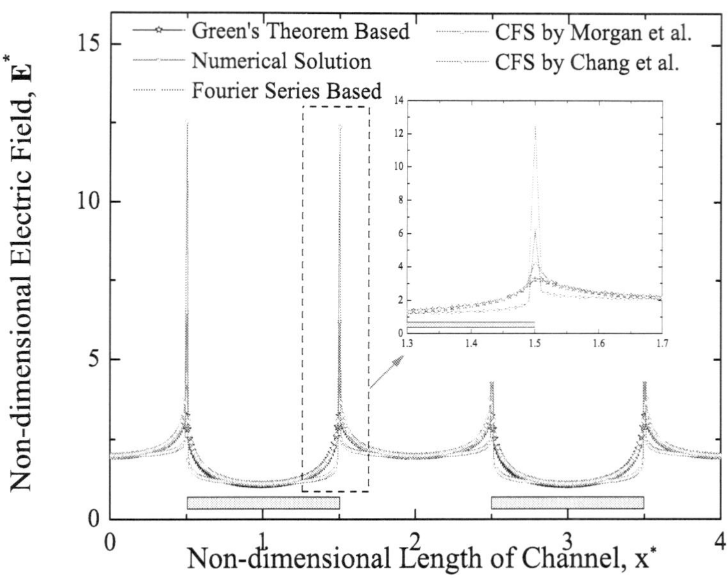

Fig. 2. Comparison of non-dimensional electric field along the length of channel near the electrodes for different solution methods

Figure 2 shows the comparison of non-dimensional electric field along the length of channel near the electrodes for Green's theorem based analytical solution, Fourier series based analytical solution (Morgan et al., 2001), finite element based numerical solution, CFS by Morgan et al. (2001) and CFS by Chang et al. (2003). The horizontal axis in this figure shows the non-dimensional length of the channel (x^*), whereas vertical axis shows the non-dimensional electric field ($\mathbf{E}^*$). The different symbols in the figure indicates the different solution methods. The electric field is maximum at the edges of the electrodes and minimum else where. But the magnitude of the electric field at the center of the electrode is very less than the electric field at the mid point of the gap between the electrodes. The excellent agreement is observed between Green's theorem based analytical solution and finite element based numerical solution. However, slight discrepancies are identified at the edge of the electrode for Green's theorem based/numerical solution with Fourier series based analytical solution and CFS by Chang et al. The peak magnitude for non-dimensional electric field is observed for CFS by Chang et al. compared with other solution methods. CFS by Morgan et al. (2001) has slight flat profile along the electrodes/gap between electrodes compared to semi circular curved profile of non-dimensional electric field for other solution methods.

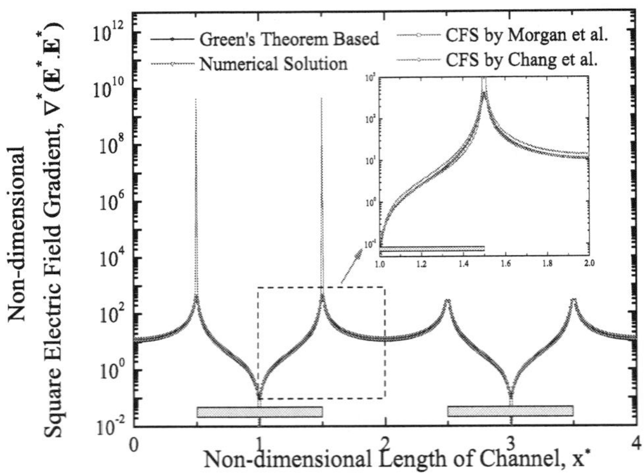

Fig. 3. Comparison of non-dimensional squared electric field gradient along the length of channel near the electrodes for different solution methods

As discussed earlier, DEP force depends on the volume of particle, real part of the CM factor and the gradient of squared electric field. Since the effect of presence of microparticles on electric field is neglected, gradient of squared electric field is independent of shape, size, and properties of particles. Hence, the variation of squared electric field gradient along the length of channel and height of the channel is studied. Figure 3 illustrates the comparison of non-dimensional squared electric field gradient with respect to length of channel near the electrode plane for Green's theorem-based analytical solution, numerical solution based on COMSOL, CFS by Morgan et al. (2001) and CFS by Chang et al. (2003). The horizontal axis in this figure shows the non-dimensional length of the channel (x^*) and vertical axis shows the non-dimensional squared electric field gradient ($\nabla^*(\mathbf{E}^*\cdot\mathbf{E})^*$). The different solution methods are indicated with different symbols in Fig. 3. The results show that the squared electric field gradient is maximum at the edges of the electrodes and minimum elsewhere. The magnitude of non-dimensional squared electric field gradient is in the range of 10^{-1} to 10^{10} for an applied electric potential of $\phi^* = 1$. The attraction or repulsion of particles can be achieved significantly due to large amount of electric field at the edges of the electrodes. The variation profile of non-dimensional squared electric field is almost matches with that of Green's theorem-based solution, numerical solution, and CFS by Morgan et al. (2001) and

Chang et al. (2003). The Fourier series-based solution is not compared here due to some large discrepancies with other solution methods. The excellent agreement is identified with Green's theorem-based solution and numerical solution, whereas some slight difference in non-dimensional squared electric field gradient is observed along the length of the channel (except the edges of electrode) with other solution methods. CFS by Chang et al. (2003) and Morgan et al. (2001) provide the maximum non-dimensional squared electric field gradient at the edges of the electrode compared to that of Green's theorem method and finite element method.

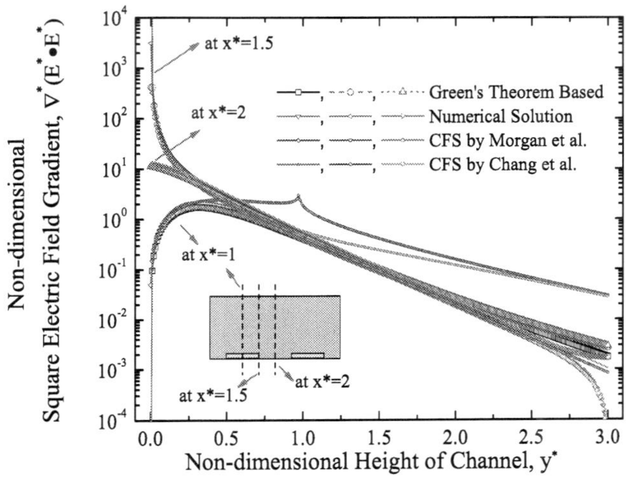

Fig. 4. Comparison of non-dimensional squared electric field gradient along the height of channel at edge of the electrode, mid point of the electrode and mid point of gap between the electrodes for different solution methods

Figure 4 depicts the comparison of non-dimensional squared electric field gradient with respect to the height of channel at electrode edge, mid point of electrode and mid point of gap between the electrodes with different solution methods. The horizontal axis in this figure shows the non-dimensional height of the channel (y^*) whereas vertical axis shows the non-dimensional squared electric field gradient ($\nabla^*(\mathbf{E}^*\cdot\mathbf{E})^*$). The non-dimensional squared electric field gradient decays exponentially along the height of channel at the edges of the electrodes. At mid point of electrodes, the squared electric field gradient increases exponentially $y^* = 0.32$ and then linearly decreased along the height of channel. The linear decaying of squared electric field is observed at the mid point of gap between the electrodes. At the height $y^* = 1.25$, the gradient of squared electric field is constant throughout the channel length and magnitude is decreased along the height of channel. This decides the effectiveness of DEP force in the channel. The profiles for variation of non-dimensional squared electric field gradient with different solution methods are matched for all the cases. There is some discrepancy with profiles along the height of channel at mid point of electrodes for Green's theorem-based solution or numerical solution with CFS by Morgan et al. (2001) and Chang et al. (2003).

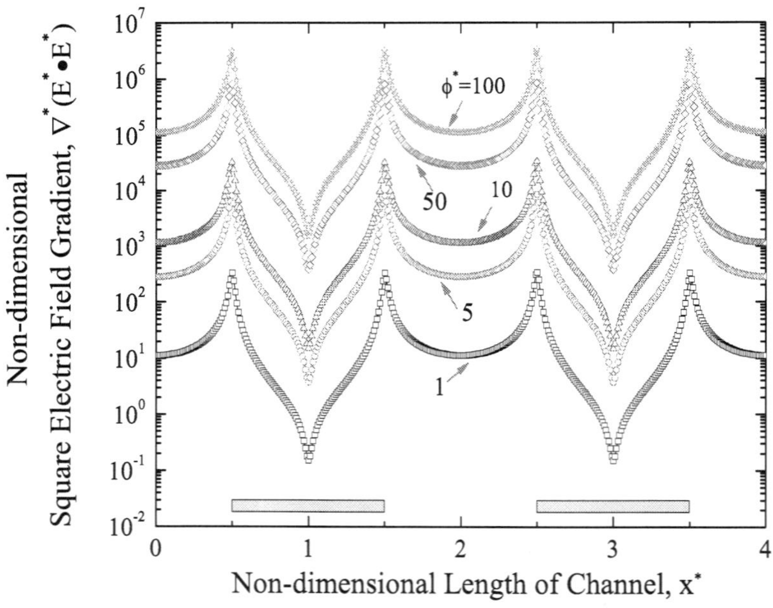

Fig. 5. Comparison of non-dimensional squared electric field gradient along the length of channel near the electrodes for different non-dimensional applied voltages

Figure 5 shows the dependence of non-dimensional squared electric field gradient on applied voltage along the length of channel near the electrodes. The horizontal axis in this figure shows the non-dimensional length of the channel (x^*), whereas vertical axis represents the non-dimensional gradient of the squared electric field. Different symbols indicate the different voltages in the figure. It is observed that squared electric field gradient is directly proportional to the applied voltage. The magnitude of peak non-dimensional squared electric field gradient is increased from 3×10^2 to 3×10^6 for an increase in non-dimensional applied voltage (ϕ^*) from 1 to 100, respectively.

Figure 6(a) and 6(b) shows the comparison of DEP velocity under positive and negative DEP effects, respectively. Arrows in figures indicate the direction of particles movement due to DEP force. The length of the arrow does not indicate the magnitude of the DEP velocity. Contours in the figure indicate the constant DEP velocities along the curves. In Fig. 6(a), converging of arrows at electrode edges indicate the collection of particles in that area, which can be used as concentration regions (or collectors). In Fig. 6(b), the direction of the particle movement has changed and the particles are being repelled from the electrode. As this is a closed channel, the particles are collecting at the top wall of the channel and at a position

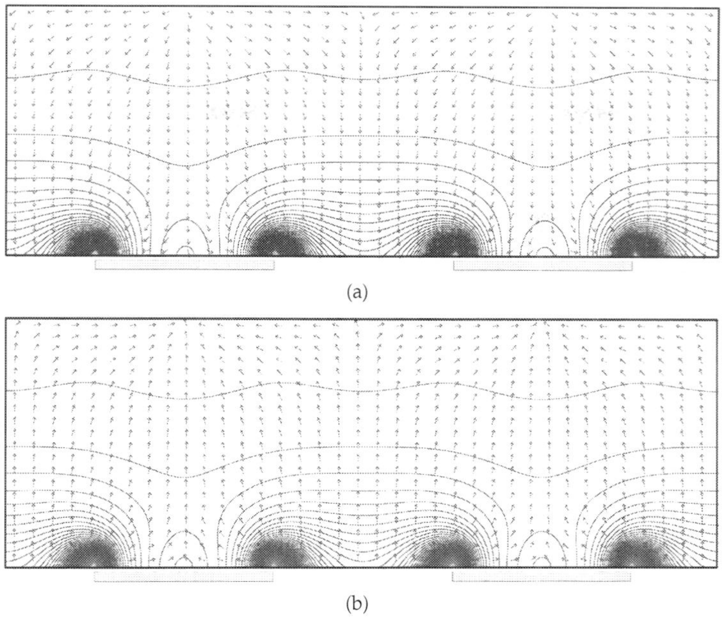

Fig. 6. Comparison of DEP velocity contour and arrow plots; (a) under positive DEP effect (b)under negative DEP effect

parallel to the mid-point of the electrode. The region where the particles are collecting is called concentrating regions.

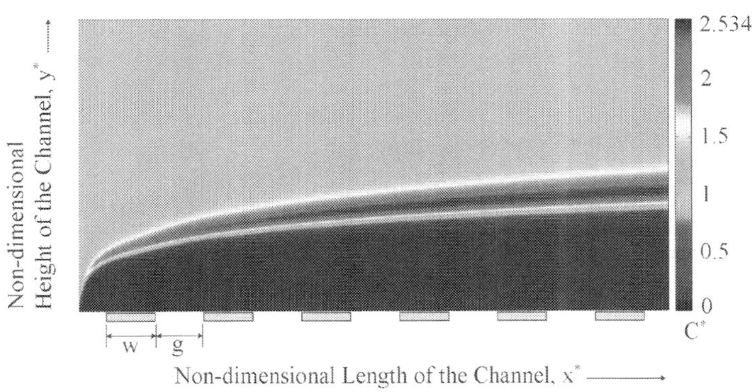

Fig. 7. Variation of mass concentration of the particles inside the microchannel under the influence of DEP and flow field along the channel

Figure 7 shows the variation of non-dimensional concentration of particles inside the microchannel. The particles are levitated to certain height due to repulsive DEP forces. This analysis is applied to myoglobin (Gunda & Mitra, 2009; 2010b) to study the behavior of myoglobin in microchannel. In their study, a channel of 400 nm length and 300 nm height with 100 nm width electrodes and 100 nm gap is utilized to create nonuniformities in the electric field gradients. Maximum concentration distribution of the myoglobin was found at 240 nm, the channel height from the bottom wall under 10 Vpp, and 1 kHz AC voltage and frequency respectively. Both, positive and negative DEP effects were observed at 50 MHz and 1 kHz AC frequency respectively (Gunda & Mitra, 2009; 2010b).

3. Materials and methods

DEP microfluidic device can be fabricated using glass, PDMS and silicon materials. Experimental details of fabrication of channels and microelectrodes on PDMS and glass materials, respectively can be found at Gunda et al. (n.d.). In this chapter, we are providing the fabrication of DEP chip with two glass substrates.
Fabrication of DEP microfluidic device with two glass substrates with a network of microchannels, fluidic and electrical ports in top substrate and different set of microelctrodes in bottom substrates is described in this section. Initially, the layout of microelectrode configuration (rectangular array of electrodes) and microchannel are designed with the L-Edit MEMS Design software (MemsPRO v6, Tanner Research, Inc., CA) and then exported to Laser Pattern Generator (Heidelberg DWL-200, Heidelberg Instruments, Germany) for fabricating the chrome masks. These chrome masks are used in the photolithography process to transfer the structures on the glass substrates.

3.1 Fabrication of microelectrodes

Fabrication of microelectrodes on glass substrate is described in this section. Piranha (H_2SO_4:H_2O_2 of 4:1 by volume)cleaned borofloat glass wafer (Paragon Optical Company, Inc., PA) of 4 $in \times 4$ in and 1.1 mm thick is taken and a layer of 40 nm chromium and 200 nm gold sequentially deposited using planar magnetron sputtering system. The gold coated glass wafer is then spin-coated with a layer of $1 - 2$ μm positive photoresist(PPR)(HPR 504, Fujifilm Electronic Materials, Inc., Arizona) using Solitec resist spinner (Model 5110-CD, Solitec Wafer Processing, Inc., CA). Then, the PPR coated wafer is soft-baked at 110 ^oC for 90 s on a Solitec vacuum hot plate (Solitec Wafer Processing, Inc., CA). Using mask aligner, the spin-coated wafer is exposed to UV illumination (350-400 nm) through chrome mask for $2 - 3$ s to transfer the electrode structures on PPR. The wafer is then developed using PPR developer (HPRD 429, Fujifilm Electronic Materials, Inc., Arizona) for $20 - 30$ s. Later, gold and chromium are etched using gold etchant ($KI + I_2 + H_2O$) and chromium etchant ($K_3[Fe(CN)_6] + NaOH + H_2O$), respectively. Acetone is used to strip off the PPR. Finally, the wafer is cleaned in isopropyl alcohol and dried with nitrogen spray. The schematic of process flow for fabrication of microelectrodes is depicted in Fig. 8.

3.2 Fabrication of microchannels

In this section, fabrication of microchannels is described. The process of piranha cleaning and deposition of chromium and gold is similar to above mentioned procedure. Photolithography is carried out using mask containing microchannel structures. The metal etching procedure is the one explained above. Channels are then etched in the borofloat substrate using wet or dry etching methods. Fluidic and electrical ports are drilled using water jet cutting machine (OMAX Corporation, Kent, WA, USA). The schematic of process flow for fabrication of microchannels is depicted in Fig. 10.

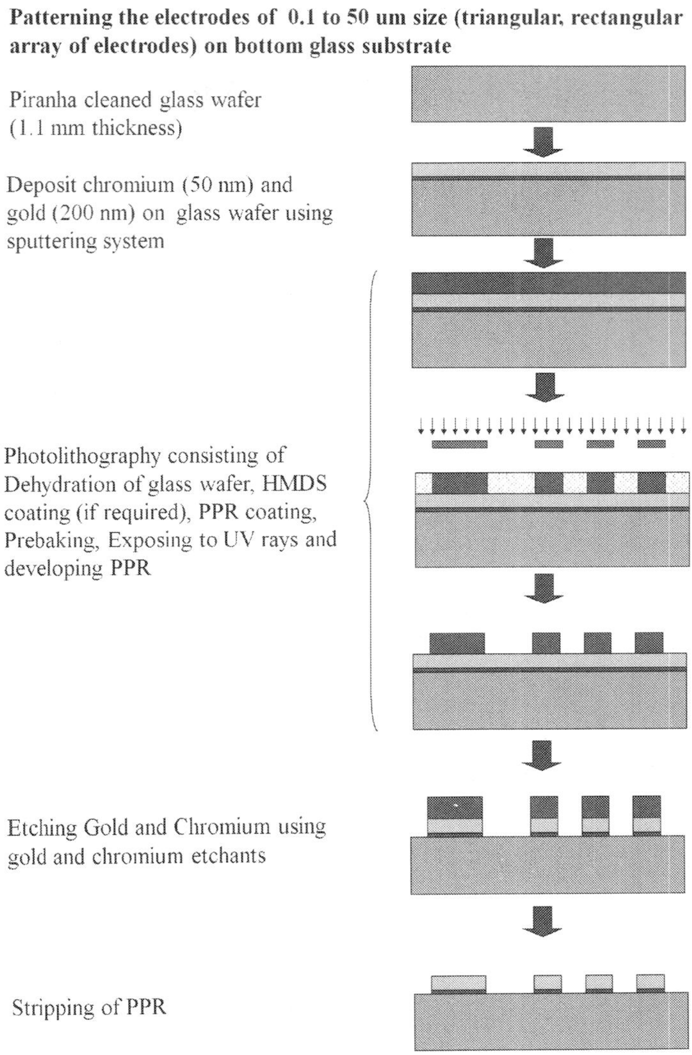

Fig. 8. Process flow for fabrication of microelectrodes

3.3 Bonding of two substrates

The above fabricated substrates are bonded using fusion process to form a closed channel. The schematic of bonded dielectrophoretic microfluidic chip is shown in Fig. 10. Several layouts of chips on glass wafer are diced using a diamond touch dicing saw.

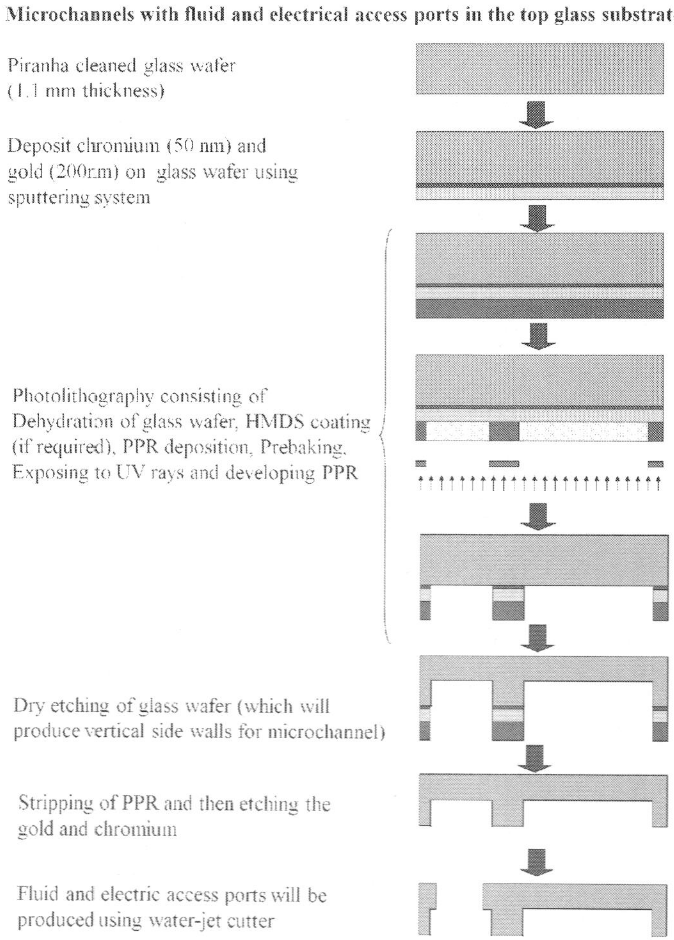

Fig. 9. Process flow for fabrication of microchannels

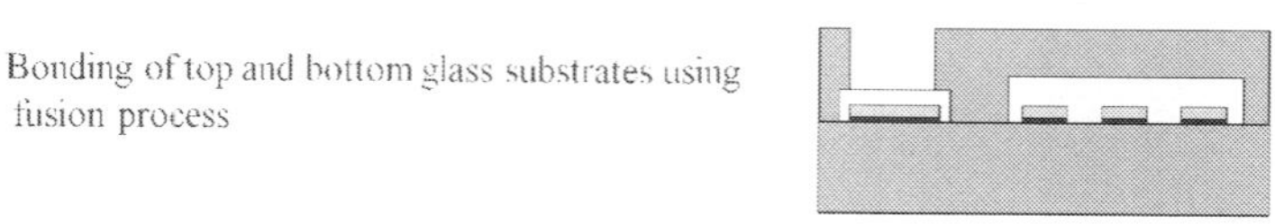

Fig. 10. Schematic of bonded dielectrophoretic microfluidic chip

3.4 Test equipment

Testing of the fabricated device under the influence of DEP phenomena requires AC voltage source generating four phases, high frequency and high voltage sinusoidal signal. Instruments like arbitrary waveform generator and voltage amplifier are used to generate

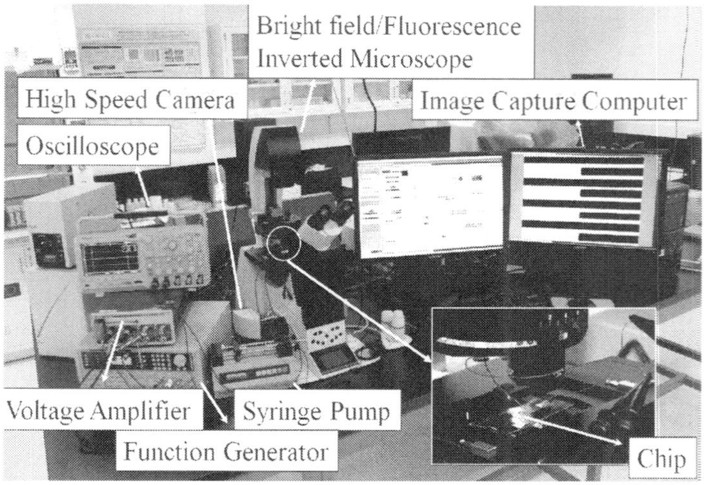

Fig. 11. Testing set-up for DEP experiments

the required AC signals and oscilloscope to check the generated signal for verification. A syringe pump is used to inject the sample into the device. A fully automated bright field and /or fluorescence inverted microscope with high speed monochrome camera is used to observe and capture the process of mixing and separation. The images captured at the detection site of the device are used to quantify the concentration of particles from image processing analysis. The experimental testing set-up discussed above is presented in Fig. 11. The specification and other details of fluidic and electrical connections used in this work can be found in Gunda & Mitra (2010a).

3.5 Experimental results

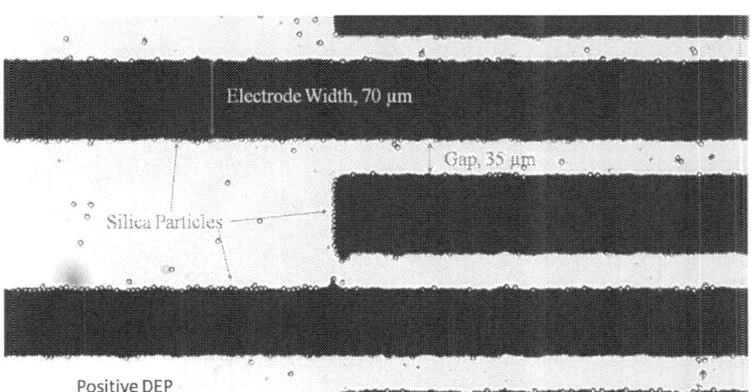

Fig. 12. Positive DEP effect on silica particles

In this section, the results of DEP effects on silica particles are presented. Silica particles of 5 μ diameter are used for these experiments. Both types of DEP effects (positive and negative) are

Fig. 13. Negative DEP effect on silica particles

observed for silica particles. Figure 12 shows the positive DEP effect of silica particles under $5-10\ V$ applied voltage and for the frequency range of 0 to 1 KHz. It is clearly observed that the particles are trapped at the electrode edges. The image is acquired from the inverted microscope where the light source is placed at the top and a capturing camera is placed at the bottom of the chip. Figure 13 shows the negative DEP effect of silica particles under 10 V applied voltage for the frequency range of 10 KHz to 40 KHz. Under negative effects, the particles move from edges of the electrodes to the middle of the electrodes, to the mid-point of the gap between the electrodes. The spreading of the particles on the electrode surface is also observed when the frequency is shifted from 40 KHz to 60 KHz.

4. Conclusion

Mathematical models for dielectrophoretic transport of bioparticles in a microchannel have been developed. Experiments have been carried out to demonstrate the manipulation of silica particles using DEP. Positive and negative DEP effects on silica particles have been identified.

5. Acknowledgment

The authors gratefully acknowledge the financial support of Alberta Ingenuity Fund in the form of the scholarship provided to NSKG. The authors also would like to acknowledge CMC Microsystems for their help and support in setting up test set-up for DEP experiments. CMC is a non-profit corporation funded by the Natural Sciences and Engineering Research Council of Canada (NSERC), with matching contributions from industry.

6. References

Basuray, S. & Chang, H.-C. (2010). Designing a sensitive and quantifiable nanocolloid assay with dielectrophoretic crossover frequencies, *Biomicrofluidics* 4(1): 013205.

Bunthawin, S., Wanichapichart, P., Tuantranont, A. & Coster, H. G. L. (2010). Dielectrophoretic spectra of translational velocity and critical frequency for a spheroid in traveling electric field, *Biomicrofluidics* 4(1): 014102.

Castellarnau, M., Errachid, A., Madrid, C., Juarez, A. & Samitier, J. (2006). Dielectrophoresis as a tool to characterize and differentiate isogenic mutants of escherichia coli, *Biophys J* 91: 3937–3945.

Chang, D. E., Loire, S. & Mezic, I. (2003). Closed-form solutions in the electrical field analysis for dielectrophoretic and travelling wave inter-digitated electrode arrays, *J Phys D: Appl Phys* 36: 3073–3078.

Church, C., Zhu, J., Wang, G., Tzeng, T.-R. J. & Xuan, X. (2009). Electrokinetic focusing and filtration of cells in a serpentine microchannel, *Biomicrofluidics* 3(4): 044109.

Clague, D. S. & Wheeler, E. K. (2001). Dielectrophoretic manipulation of macromolecules: The electric field, *Phys Rev E: Stat Nonlinear Soft Matter Phys* 64: 026605.

Crews, N., Darabi, J., Voglewede, P., Guo, F. & Bayoumi, A. (2001). An analysis of interdigitated electrode geometry for dielectrophoretic particle transport in micro-fluidics, *Scand J Clin Lab Invest* 61: 95–102.

Du, J.-R., Juang, Y.-J., Wu, J.-T. & Wei, H.-H. (2008). Long-range and superfast trapping of dna molecules in an ac electrokinetic funnel, *Biomicrofluidics* 2(4): 044103.

Ferrier, G. A., Hladio, A. N., Thomson, D. J., Bridges, G. E., Hedayatipoor, M., Olson, S. & Freeman, M. R. (2008). Microfluidic electromanipulation with capacitive detection for the mechanical analysis of cells, *Biomicrofluidics* 2(4): 044102.

Gagnon, Z., Mazur, J. & Chang, H.-C. (2009). Glutaraldehyde enhanced dielectrophoretic yeast cell separation, *Biomicrofluidics* 3(4): 044108.

Green, N. G., Ramos, A. & Morgan, H. (2002). Numerical solution of the dielectrophoretic and traveling wave forces for interdigitated electrode arrays using the finite element method, *Journal of Electrostatics* 56: 235–254.

Gunda, N. S. K. & Mitra, S. K. (2009). Modeling of dielectrophoresis for myoglobin molecules in a microchannel with parallel electrodes, Proceedings of the ASME 2009 International Mechanical Engineering Congress and Exposition, Lake Buena Vista, Florida, USA, November 13-19, IMECE2009-10765.

Gunda, N. S. K. & Mitra, S. K. (2010a). Experimental investigation of dielectrophoretic behaviour of myoglobin and silica particles on a microelectrode chip, Proceedings of ASME 2010 3rd Joint USEuropean Fluids Engineering Summer Meeting and 8th International Conference on Nanochannels, Microchannels, and Minichannels, Montreal, Canada, August 2-4, FEDSM-ICNMM2010- 30306.

Gunda, N. S. K. & Mitra, S. K. (2010b). Modeling of dielectrophoretic transport of myoglobin molecules in microchannels, Biomicrofluidics 4(1): 014105.

Gunda, N. S. K., Mitra, S. K. & Bhattacharjee, S. (2009). Dielectrophoretic mixing with novel electrode geometry, Proceedings of the ASME 2009 Fluids Engineering Division SummerMeeting, FEDSM09, Vail, Colorado, August 2-6, FEDSM2009-78260.

Gunda, N. S. K., Mitra, S. K. & Rao, V. R. (2009). Fabrication of dielectrophoretic microfluidic Device, Proceedings of the Seventh International ASME Conference on Nanochannels, Microchannels and Minichannels, Pohang, South Korea, June 22-24, ICNMM2009-82170.

Hughes, M. P. (2003). *Nanoelectromechanics in Engineering and Biology*, CRC Press, Boca Raton.

Hwang, H., Lee, D.-H., Choi, W. & Park, J.-K. (2009). Enhanced discrimination of normal oocytes using optically induced pulling-up dielectrophoretic force, *Biomicrofluidics* 3(1): 014103.

Jones, T. B. (1995). *Electromechanics of particles*, Cambridge University Press.

Lewpiriyawong, N., Yang, C. & Lam, Y. C. (2008). Dielectrophoretic manipulation of particles in a modified microfluidic h filter with multi-insulating blocks, *Biomicrofluidics* 2(3): 034105.

Lin, J. T. Y. & Yeow, J. T. W. (2007). Enhancing dielectrophoresis effect through novel electrode geometry, *Biomed Microdevices* 9(6): 823–831.

Manuel, G. & Clague, D. (2000). The 2d electric field above a planar sequence of independent strip electrodes, *J Phys D: Appl Phys* 33: 1747–1755.

Masliyah, J. & Bhattacharjee, S. (2006). *Electrokinetic and Colloid Transport Phenomena*, Willey Interscience, Hoboken, New Jersey.

Molla, S. H. & Bhattacharjee, S. (2005a). Prevention of colloidal membrane fouling employing dielectrophoretic forces on a parallel electrode array, *J Membr Sci* 255: 187–199.

Molla, S. H. & Bhattacharjee, S. (2005b). Simulations of a dielectrophoretic membrane filtration process for removal of water droplets from water-in-oil emulsions, *J Colloid Interface Sci* 287: 338–350.

Molla, S. H. & Bhattacharjee, S. (2007). Dielectrophoretic leviation in the presence of shear flow: Implications for colloidal fouling of filtration membranes, *Langmuir* 23(21): 10618–10627.

Morgan, H., Alberto, G. I., David, B., Green, N. G. & Ramos, A. (2001). The dielectrophoretic and traveling wave forces generated by interdigited electrode arrays: Analytical solution using fourier series, *J Phys D: Appl Phys* 34: 1553–1561.

Nguyen, N. T. & Werely, S. T. (2006). *Fundamentals and Applications of Microfluidics*, Artech House, Boston.

Parikesit, G. O. F., Markesteijn, A. P., Piciu, O. M., Bossche, A., Westerweel, J., Young, I. T. & Garini, Y. (2008). Size-dependent trajectories of dna macromolecules due to insulative dielectrophoresis in submicrometer-deep fluidic channels, *Biomicrofluidics* 2(2): 024103.

Pohl, H. A. (1978). *Dielectrophoresis*, Cambridge University Press.

Wang, X. B., Huang, Y., Burt, J. P. H., Markx, G. H. & Pethig, R. (1993). Selective dielectrophoretic confinement of bioparticles in potential energy wells, *J Phys D: Appl Phys* 26: 1278–1285.

Wang, X., Wang, X. B., Becker, F. F. & Gascoyne, R. C. P. (1996). A theoretical method of electric field analysis for dielectrophoretic electrode arrays using green's theorem, *J Phys D: Appl Phys* 29: 1649–1660.

Wei, M.-T., Junio, J. & Ou-Yang, H. D. (2009). Direct measurements of the frequency-dependent dielectrophoresis force, *Biomicrofluidics* 3(1): 012003.

Yang, C. Y. & Lei, U. (2007). Quasistatic force and torque on ellipsoidal particles under generalized dielectrophoresis, *J Appl Phys* 102: 094702.

Yang, F., Yang, X., Jiang, H., Bulkhaults, P., Wood, P., Hrushesky, W. & Wang, G. (2010). Dielectrophoretic separation of colorectal cancer cells, *Biomicrofluidics* 4(1): 013204.

Zhu, X., Yi, H. & Ni, Z. (2010). Frequency-dependent behaviors of individual microscopic particles in an optically induced dielectrophoresis device, *Biomicrofluidics* 4(1): 013202.

18

Role of Proteins on the Electrochemical Behavior of Implanted Metallic Alloys, Reproducibility and Time-Frequency Approach from EIS (Electrochemical Impedance Spectroscopy)

Geringer Jean and Navarro Laurent
Center for Health Engineering, Biomechanics and Biomaterials Department,
Bio-Tribocorrosion lab, UMR CNRS 5146, IFR 143,
Ecole Nationale Supérieure des Mines de Saint-Etienne, ENSM-SE
France

1. Introduction

Metallic alloys are commonly used in orthopedic implants. Some attempts were investigated for replacing the human organs or joints. Without being exhaustive, some key points of the history of the orthopedic implants could be presented (Callaghan, 2007):

- In 1826, the first pseudoarthrosis was practiced by J. Barton with a wood piece of the hip joint;
- In 1891, the first femoral head in ivory was implanted by T. Gluck (Gluck, 1890);
- In 1923, the "Molded arthroplasty" using hollow hemisphere made of glass was practiced by M.N. Smith-Petersen;
- In 1936, the first acrylic femoral stem was implanted by Judet's brothers.

One might suggest the implanted materials are close to the organic materials in terms of natural origin. The last one, acrylic polymer, would be a dedicated material because their mechanical properties are close to the ones of bone. However the mechanical and tribological properties are not sufficient for being enough resistant. Thus the metallic implants were investigated because of their better mechanical properties, elastic modulus and tensile strength. Following, few important dates are suggested:

- In 1938, M.N. Smith-Petersen used the Vitallium® made of Co-Cr-Mo, Cobalt-Chromium-Molybdenum, alloy for the femoral stem;
- In 1949, Judet's brothers implanted the first total hip arthroplasty (Judet, 1949);
- Finally, in 1962, Sir J. Charnley imposed the low friction arthroplasty with a femoral stem made of 316L stainless steel (Charnley, Livingstone, 1970; Charnley, Springer, 1970).

Finally 3 main materials are implanted as femoral stem or metallic components: the titanium alloy, Ti-6Al-4V, the stainless steel, 316L SS, and the cobalt-chromium alloy (Park, 1992). The first one is dedicated to the femoral stem, the second one is used as material for manufacturing femoral stem, metal back and possibly the head for Metal on Polymer, MoP,

contact, the third metal could be investigated as the Head and cup assembly for Metal on Metal, MoM, assembly, the head component for MoP assembly and no frequently the femoral stem. Figure 1 highlights the different assemblies involved in the femoral stem. The ceramic material will not be presented in this work.
From this point, we will focus on the metallic alloys that are involved in implants and specifically hip implants. Obviously metallic materials are not originally exhibited in human body. The interactions with human organic substances, proteins, phosphate ions and so on, should play a key role in the materials lifetime. The physical and chemical reactions are numerous and the passivity of the metallic alloys is submitted to the influence of the liquid medium. Some electrochemical investigations were carried out for understanding and predicting the passivity of alloys.

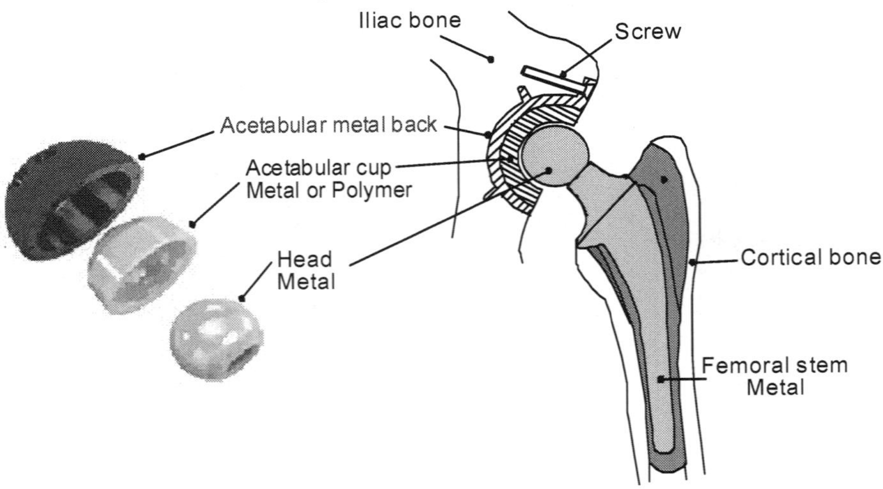

Fig. 1. Scheme of a femoral stem and the components

Normally the materials are fixed in the bone by adhesion of cells as osteoblasts. Due to the difference of mechanical properties between materials in contact (femoral stem of 316L and femoral bone for instance), the debonding is promoted during human gait (Pellier, 2011). The difference of the elastic modulii is of the order of magnitude of 100. Thus the friction under small displacements, i.e. the fretting corrosion (Barril, 2002; Bethune, 1968; Eden, 1911; Geringer, 2005; Geringer, 2006; McDowell, 1953; Tomlinson, 1927; Tomlinson, 1939; Uhlig, 1954; Waterhouse, 1955; Waterhouse, 1980), could occur. One will not pay attention on this point in this work. However it is worth noting that fretting corrosion is the topic of research works. Thus some investigations are in progress for understanding the role of proteins on the lifetime of metals that are submitted to fretting. Finally we will focus our attention only on the passivity of the alloy submitted to pure corrosion.
Understanding corrosion reactions and factors that promote the corrosion degradations is a challenging goal. The titanium alloy is particularly interesting because of this

biocompatibility. Cells and tissues adhere friendly to this metallic alloy (Dowson, 1981; Bronzino, 1995). The surface state, it means the roughness, of the titanium alloy material plays a significant role on the passivity. Indeed, polished surfaces of Ti-6Al-4V involve a decreasing of the current density, 2 orders of magnitude, in distilled water at 22°C (Kirbs, 2003). However, in Phosphate Buffered Solution (PBS), at 22°C, the potential of corrosion is close to -300 mV/SCE (Standard Calomel electrode) and no effect of the roughness was highlighted (Kirbs, 2003). The investigations about the proteins effect were pointed out with synovial liquid, coming from joint puncture of human patients, bovine serum and urine. Finally the passivity was the worst one for the synovial liquid compared to the other media (Hsu, 2004). These experiments were carried out at different temperatures and the current density increases, i.e. the passivity decreases, when the temperature of electrochemical investigations increases (Hsu, 2004). About the local mechanisms of adsorption and corrosion, the double layer, i.e. the first layer of adsorbed species and ions on the surface of the pristine metal, is constituted by hydroxyl ions. The charge transfer occurs through this layer. The proteins promote the diffusion of metallic cations for pH lower than 7. Beyond 7, i.e. between 7 and 9, the proteins play the role of protective layer against the dissolution of metal. The layer on the metal surface is mechanically less resistant than the one after dousing in solution of proteins, results coming from the measurement of hardness (Khan, 1999).

The Electrochemical Impedance Spectroscopy, EIS, is a useful tool to describe the close interface between metal and solution (Dygas, 1999; Harrington, 2001; Macdonald, 1998; Orazem, 2004). This experimental technique allows modeling the electrical circuit constituting by metal-interface-solution thanks to the impedance measurements, i.e. the transfer function between the imposed voltage, imposed physical parameter, and the measured current density, measured parameter. The most basic electrical circuit is constituted by the R_{sol} (resistance of the solution) in serie with an association in parallel with a polarization resistance, R_{pol}, and a capacitor, C, or a constant phase element, Q, to take into account the non uniform behavior of the capacitor, $R_{sol}(R_{pol}//C)$. This circuit highlights one time constant and one interface is modeled. Two time constants indicate a layer that is constituted by two interfaces. From this useful kind of investigations, two time constants were highlighted on the Ti-6Al-4V alloy: the first layer is the thickness of oxides and the second one is the adsorbed proteins (Pan, 1996; Tamilselvi, 2006). When a solution constituted by phosphate ions, from PBS solution, and proteins, the equivalent electrical circuit with two constant times fits well (Zaveri, 2008). A competitive adsorption does exist between the one of phosphate ions and the one of proteins. Consequently the EIS measurements could be interpreted differently due to close experimental conditions but the reproducibility is not studied (Ouerd, 2007; Zaveri, 2008)). To conclude on this part, it is worth noting that the quantity of the adsorbed proteins was investigated. On pristine pure titanium, the quantity of proteins is within the range of 1.8 and 2.89 μg.cm^{-2}, in a solution of proteins and phosphate ions at 37°C (Cai, 2006; Yan, 2008). These results were obtained thanks to measuring by UV spectrometry the quantity of free proteins in solution, taking into account the known quantity of initial concentration of proteins. The adsorbed concentration of proteins was determined by the difference between the initial and the free concentration of proteins. The same type of investigations was carried out except about the measurement of the concentration of the adsorbed proteins (Payet, 2008). This measurement was carried out thanks to a quartz microbalance. The authors found a value of 0.71 ± 0.07 μg.cm^{-2}. The gap between both values is about 3 or 4. The non direct measurement technique should involve a huge discrepancy compared to the second one. Moreover the surface state is not controlled in these experiments. This key point should be relevant for this kind of investigations. Finally in order to improve the corrosive resistance of the Ti-6Al-4V a coating should be added on the surface, i.e. TiN (Liu, 2003). The problem of this approach is that sometimes the coating is not biocompatible.

In this section, we will present the passive behavior of Co-Cr and 316L alloys from bibliographical results. Numerous experiments were carried out on the Co-Cr alloys. The passivity of Co-Cr-Mo alloy with proteins, bovine serum or albumin, and phosphate ions was hugely investigated thanks to EIS experiments. In a Phosphate Buffered Solution, the Co-Cr-Mo alloy exhibits an enrichment of the chromium content of the oxides film. The Cobalt is dissolved preferentially compared to the other elements (Ouerd, 2008). For solution constituted by bovine serum and phosphate ions, the polarization resistance increases when the concentration of phosphate ions increases. It is worth noting that the bovine serum does not play any significant role on the corrosion of the Co-Cr alloy. No obvious impact of the bovine serum was highlighted. The competitive adsorption, ions and proteins, was investigated by Munoz et al (Munoz, 2007). The phosphate ions influence the corrosion resistance of the Co-Cr alloy. The highest is the concentration of phosphates; the highest is the corrosion resistance. To confirm the previous study (Ouerd, 2008), the present study does not show an influence of proteins. The state of the passive film does hugely influence the action of proteins. Finally, the inhibitor role of phosphate, resp albumin, was found to be anodic, resp. cathodic for Co-Cr and 316L SS (Valero, 2008). About the polarization resistance, the effect of albumin is opposite on both metallic alloys. This protein decreases the polarization resistance for 316L and it decreases the resistance of Co-Cr. Both metallic alloys are not sensitive to the albumin effect. The passivation state of the metallic alloys, before the tests, should play a significant role on the effect of proteins on the alloy.

To conclude, numerous factors are involved in the electrochemical behavior of the metallic alloys. Moreover the time dependence of the proteins effect was not really investigated. We suggest studying the influence of proteins and ions with different solutions. Thus the time dependence, i.e. the time-frequency response, for a couple of metallic alloy/solution should provide significant results for understanding the influence of proteins. The physiological liquid contains phosphate ions in the PBS solution; this kind of solution will be studied. The hip implant could be tested with the ISO 14242 close to the actual conditions. Thus the bovine serum, in this typical test, contains sodium azide. This salt and specifically the ions N_3^- could involve a different reaction related to corrosion of the metallic alloy. We will pay attention on this specific point.

2. Materials and methods

2.1 The materials

The investigated metallic alloys are Ti-6Al-4V, titanium alloy, Co-Cr-Mo alloy and the 316L, stainless steel alloy. The Table 1 exhibits the composition of these alloys. They were obtained by spark optical emission spectrometry. The compositions are related to the specifications of ASTM F136 for Ti-6Al-4V (TA6V), ASTM standards: ASTM A240 for 316L stainless steel alloy; and finally ASTM F1537 for Co-Cr alloy. The measured compositions are in agreement with the ones from the ASTM standards, except for 316L alloy for which the Ni content is 4% higher than the maximum value.

Ti-6Al-4V alloy

Elements	Al	V	Fe	O	Cr	Ni	C	N	Ti
Composition (% w/w or ppm)	5.91%	3.87%	1096 ppm	1038 ppm	137 ppm	125 ppm	124 ppm	53 ppm	Bal

316L SS

Elements	Cr	Ni	Mo	Mn	Si	Cu	C	P	S	Fe
Composition (% w/w)	17.05	14.55	2.80	1.73	0.40	0.10	0.02	0.02	<0.01	Bal.

Co-Cr-Mo alloy

Elements	Cr	Mo	Mn	Si	Ni	C	Al	Co
Composition (% w/w)	28.50%	5.87%	0.78	0.46	0.25	0.037	0.02	Bal

Table 1. Composition of the metallic alloys.

The final polishing step after manufacturing samples is a key step for controlling the surface state and especially the roughness that could play a significant role on the corrosion reactions. Following steps were carried out on metal samples: the abrasive grid paper 4000, the 6 µm, 3 µm and 1 µm diamond paste with around duration of 5 minutes.

2.2 Solutions

Table 2 exhibits the compositions of the chosen solutions. Six solutions, desionized water, Ringer solution, Phosphate Buffered solution (PBS), PBS + bovine serum, PBS + bovine

Weight concentration g.L-1	NaCl	KCl	$CaCl_2 2H_2O$	$NaHCO_3$	KH_2PO_4	Na_2HPO_4	Albumin	Bovine serum	NaN_3
Solution 1 desionized water									
Solution 2 Ringer solution	8,500	0,250	0,220	0,150					
Solution 3 PBS solution	8,192	0,223			0,136	1,420			
Solution 4 PBS+Alb solution	8,192	0,223			0,136	1,420	1,000		
Solution 5 PBS + serum	8,192	0,223			0,136	1,420		18,5	
Solution 6 PBS + serum + NaN_3	8,192	0,223			0,136	1,420		18,5	1,000

Table 2. Constituents of the 6 investigated solutions; PBS: Phosphate Buffered solution, Alb: Albumin, serum: bovine serum or calf serum, NaN_3: Sodium azide

serum + NaN_3 (sodium azide) allow testing the influence of ions, the pure albumin (Albumin fraction V extracted from bovine serum, model protein) and the proteins from bovine serum (calf serum heat inactivated, PAA, triplicated filtering with a porosity of 0.1 µm). This last solution is the reference solution for testing the prosthetic hip implant according to the ISO standard 14242. Sodium azide is mentioned in this procedure as an antioxidant for preventing the degradations of the bovine serum. It is constituted by 74 $g.L^{-1}$ of total proteins. More precisely the serum contains 35 $g.L^{-1}$ of albumin, 9 $g.L^{-1}$ of α-globulin, 11 $g.L^{-1}$ of β-globulin and 19 $g.L^{-1}$ of γ-globulin. The bovine serum was diluted by 4 in the studied solution. The temperature of experiments was of 37 ± 1 °C during all electrochemical measurements. To conclude these solutions were selected because they highlight the potential interest for studying the corrosion resistance (Geringer, 2007).

2.3 Electrochemical conditions

The table 3 summarizes the relevant elements about the electrochemical device. The key points are the sizes and the positioning of the electrodes, working and counter electrodes

Potentiostat	Parstat 2263
Size of the working electrode, WE	7.07 cm^2; diameter of 30mm
Reference electrode, RE	SCE; 0.250 V/SHE
Counter electrode, CE	Platinium wire, circle with a diameter of 25 mm
Distance RE-WE	10 ± 2 mm
Volume of solution	60 ± 2 mL
pH of solution	7,6 ± 0,1
Temperature	37 ± 1 °C
Device with thermostat	Double wall

Table 3. Experimental conditions; SCE: Standard Calomel Electrode; SHE: Standard Hydrogen Electrode

From the bibliographical study, the adsorption effect of phosphates ions and proteins is confused. It depends from the conditioning of the materials, polishing, storage, and first step of the electrochemical conditions. Consequently a particular attention was paid on this first step because it will determine the further chemical and electrochemical reactions. Before performing the following experiments of EIS, a cathodic polarization was carried out for each test.

Finally four types of experiments were performed:

1. Applied potential -1 V/SCE during 5 minutes
2. Free corrosion potential or Open Circuit Potential, OCP, during 2 hours, conditioning of the materials
3. Loop that will be repeated 120 times:
4. EIS, from 100 kHz to 0 Hz, 20 pts/decade, voltage amplitude of ± 10 mV, Data quality of 15 (Influence on the duration of measurements), Open circuit potential is the potential of measurement
5. OCP during 2 min
6. OCP during 26 hours

The Data quality parameter plays a significant role on the reproducibility of measurements. The increasing of this parameter involves the increasing of the number of the measurements.

For a same frequency and a couple of (U, I), the duration of measurements increases but the ratio signal/noise decreases. Considering this point, the measurements are more accurate than the usual ones without working with high Data quality value. Moreover the experiments were repeated 3 times, exactly in the same conditions, experiences and quality of measurements. The double wall, electrical connections, samples and the electrodes (working and counter) are isolated from outside waves by a Faraday cage. Moreover the potentiostat performed measurements with a floating mass for avoiding the leakage current. Finally, a particular attention was paid on the statistical analysis. As we mentioned, the triplicated measurements (new samples and new measurements) allow involving an average value and a standard deviation. The reproducibility was thus investigated.

3. Raw results

3.1 Comparison of the results in the X-Y plane

The Figure 2 a) shows the Nyquist Diagram from a sample of Ti-6Al-4V immersed in desionized water. The time 0h is related to the 3rd sequence and the 1st experiment of EIS, i.e. after 2 hours of Open Circuit Potential. The time 12.5 his related to the 120th experiment of EIS. The electrochemical behavior is different according to the time. The capacitive loop decreases. The oxides layer and the double layer protect less the metal against corrosion. The Figure 2 b) highlights the evolution of the module and the phases for the same experiment. In the frequency range, the evolution of the module does not exhibit any significant change. On the contrary, the phase decreases slightly from the first to the 120th experiment at low frequencies. The evolution of the phase is more accurate than the one of the module.

The huge interest for presenting 120 experiments is getting information about the kinetic evolution of the competitive effect of adsorption of ionic species, phosphates and chlorides, and the organic species, albumin and proteins more generally in the bovine serum. However graphics are not common. It is the reason why 3D graphics are suggested in this study. The plane is time-frequency (X-Y plane) and the Z coordinates are the modules or the phases thanks to a Matlab® program from raw data. From Figure 2b), it is possible to get the Figure 3a) and the Figure 3b) is the projection in the X-Y plane time-frequency. The module, for instance, will be presented in ohm, Ω, and the surface was equal for each experiment to 7.07 cm².

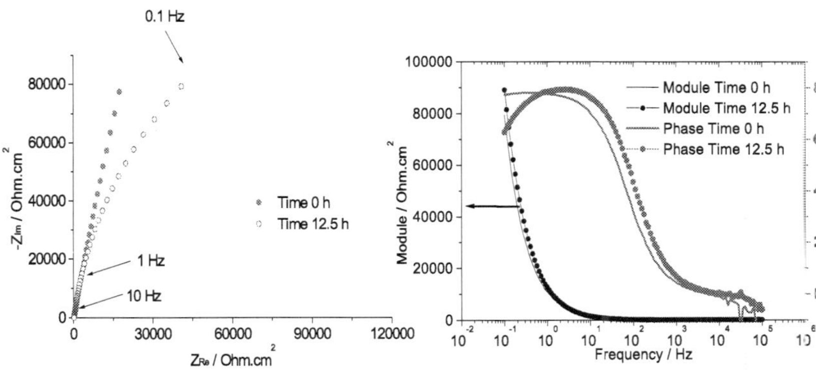

Fig. 2. Nyquist diagram related to a sample of Ti-6Al-4V in desionized water; time 0h: 1st experiment of EIS; time 12.5h: 120th experiment of EIS; b) Modules and phases of the same experiment

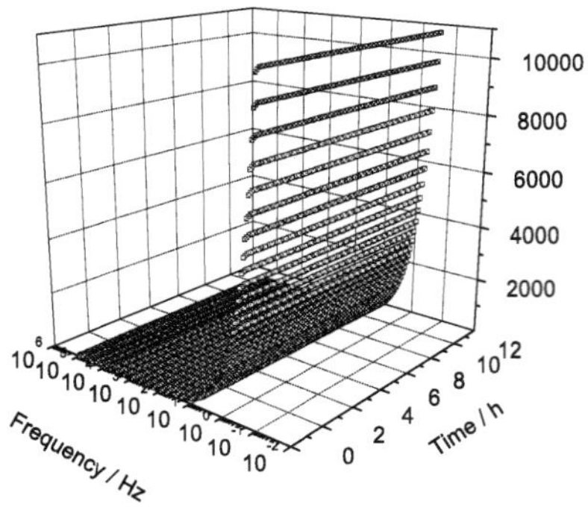

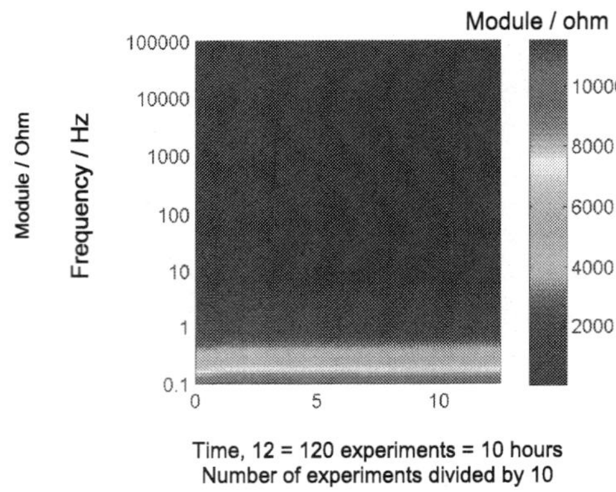

Fig. 3. a) Evolution of the average module (3 experiments) from EIS experiments in desionized water vs. time and vs. frequency; b) Evolution of the average module in desionized water, projection in the plane time-frequency, color corresponds to the module

Thus one might suggest to represent the evolution of modules, phases and the variation coefficient or the coefficient of variation (standard deviation divided by the average value) of the three experiments obtained in the same conditions. The comparison was carried out between the 6 solutions that were presented in the Table 2. The experiments in the desionized water will be considered as the reference ones. The differences between the modules of solutions 2 to 6 and the reference solution, solution 1, will be presented in order to compare the evolutions according to the time. Only the significant results will be presented in this study.

3.2 Results from Ti-6Al-4V; 316L; Co-Cr-Mo

First of all, the results from the Ringer solution and the desionized water are the same. Thus the media with PBS + serum and PBS + serum + NaN_3 do not exhibit significant differences. Consequently these media will not be compared in this study

3.2.1 Ti-6Al-4V

First of all, the results from the Ringer solution and the desionized water are the same. Consequently they will not be compared in this study. The Figure 4a) shows the evolution of the modules in the plane time-frequency for the 120 experiments. The results for the frequencies higher than 10 kHz exhibit the highest values of the variation coefficient. The value is not so significant, i.e. always lower than the one at 1 %. However this trend is always the same for all metals, see Figure 6a) and Figure 8a).
However the Figure 5a) exhibits the difference between the average value of the module in the considered medium and the one in desionized water. This particular evolution presents that the difference is always negative. It means that the module in all media is lower than the one in the desionized water. The more the module is high, the more the medium is protective for the considered metal. Consequently the most protective medium is the water for the Ti-6Al-4V. Ions, like in PBS, or ions and proteins, i.e. PBS + Albumin and PBS + serum (calf serum), promote the dissolution of the metal Ti-6Al-4V.

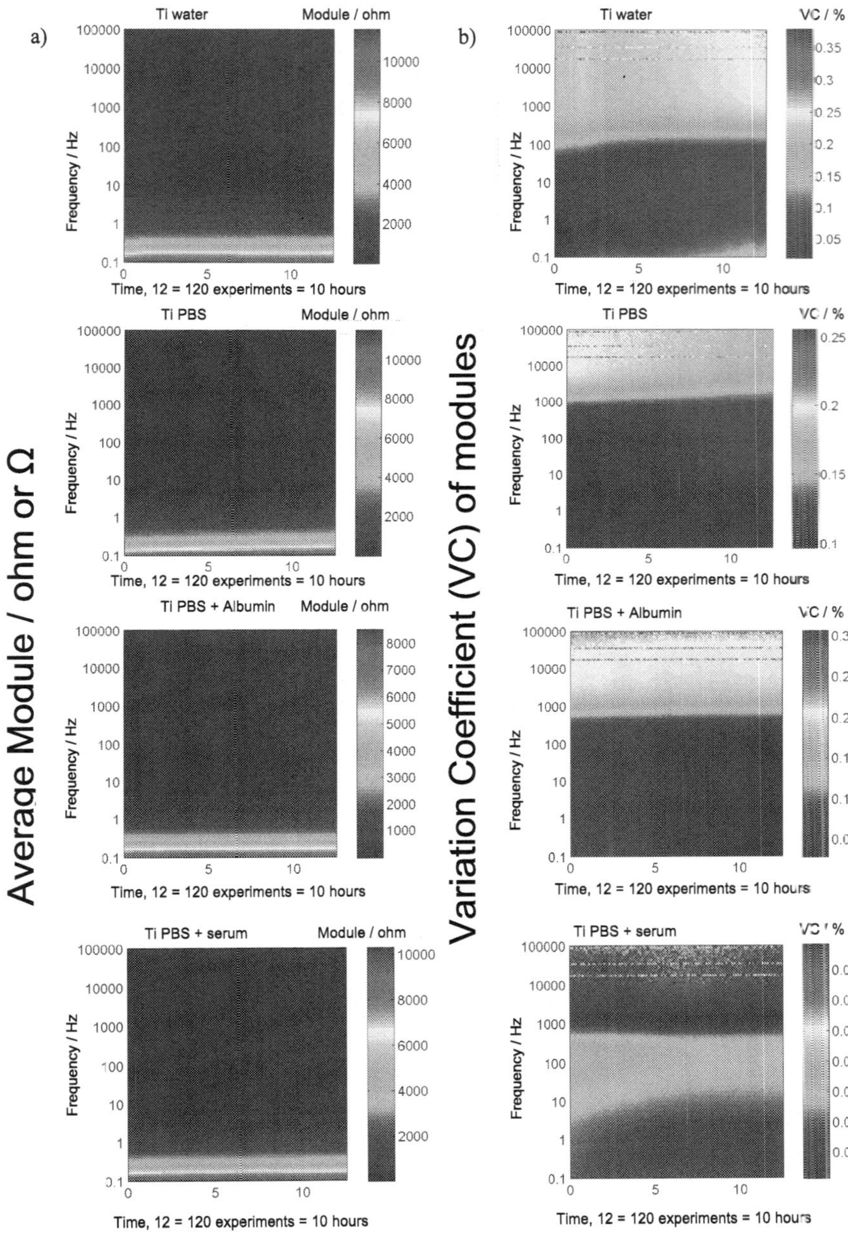

Fig. 4. a) average modules from experiments: water (desionized water), PBS (Phosphate Buffered solution), PBS + Albumin, PBS + serum (bovine serum); b) variation coefficient (VC) from the same solutions than a); time-frequency plane; Ti-6Al-4V alloy.

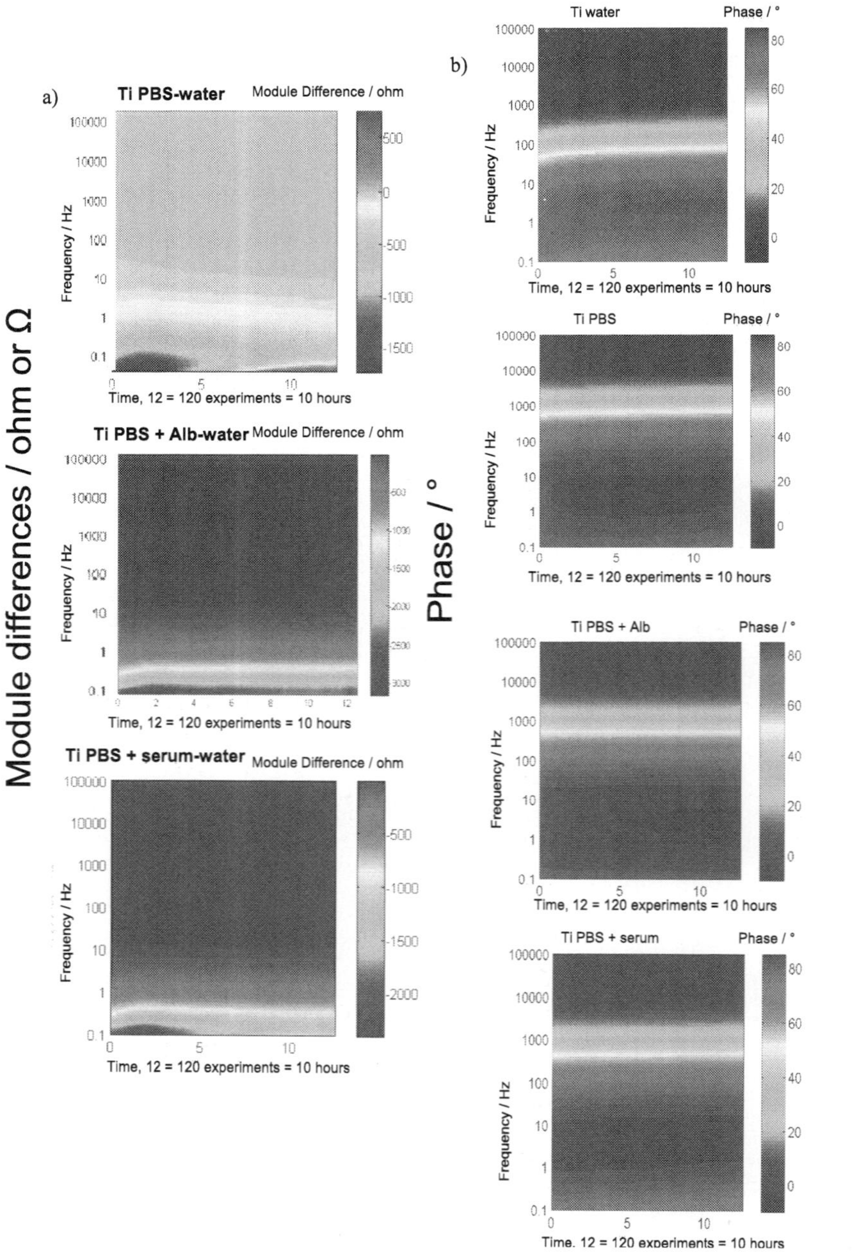

Fig. 5. a) differences of modules for 3 combinations; b) Phase / ° for; the solutions are the same than the ones from Figure 4; time-frequency plane; Ti-6Al-4V alloy.

From Figure 5b), the evolution of the phase shows interesting results. The phase reaches a maximum of 90 °, related to the behavior of a capacitance, for the desionized solution. However, considering the other media, the phase is maximum, i.e. equal to 80-90 ° and it never decreases at low frequencies. One may suggest that the electrochemical behavior is close to a capacitance when the media are PBS, PBS + Albumin or PBS + calf serum.
Thus the module is lower for the Ti-6Al-4V in media with ions and proteins but otherwise the phase is higher in the media with ions and ions + proteins (Albumin or calf serum). The capacitive behavior is promoted by the ions and proteins and the resistance of the electrochemical layer at the surface of the implant made of Ti-6Al-4V. The variations are weak because if one extrapolates the data with an equivalent electrical circuit, taking into account the discrepancies of measurements and calculations, no significant evolution of the polarization resistance and the capacitances were highlighted.
This approach shows, for Ti-6Al-4V, the electrochemical evolution of the surface, during the 10 hours of the experiments, is different: the ions and the combination of ions and proteins decrease significantly the module at low frequencies. Moreover the phase did not decrease even at low frequencies, in media with ions and ions+proteins. The capacitance of the metallic surface is higher in these media than the one in water.

3.2.2 316L SS

The Figure 6a) shows that the module calculated in the PBS + serum solution is higher than the ones calculated in other solutions. The variation coefficient, Figure 6b), highlights that the desionized water involves the highest discrepancies. The electrochemical system is submitted to fluctuations. One might suggest that the corrosion did not occur continuously. However the ions and the proteins could decrease the random specification of the corrosion process compared to the corrosion in other media.
The difference of modules shows that the PBS + serum - water is positive. Thus the module of this typical experiment is higher than the ones from the water test. Finally the phase highlights the main difference of the electrochemical behavior. The maximum of the phase is reached for the media of PBS + serum and PBS + Albumin at the highest frequency of 100 Hz. For the media PBS, the maximum of the phase is reached around 1 Hz and it decreases from 1 Hz to 0.1 Hz. Consequently the capacitive behavior is promoted preferentially in the medium containing the proteins solutions even according to the time. This evolution corroborates the highest modules showed in the Figure 6a). Thus the proteins promote a protective effect on the 316L surface.

3.2.3 Co-Cr-Mo alloy

The Figure 8a) presents the evolution of the module for the same media than the previous studies for the Co-Cr-Mo medium. The water, PBS and PBS + Albumin media do not exhibit significant differences for the module evolution. However the PBS + serum medium promotes the highest module. The evolution of the variation coefficient is the lowest for the PBS solution. This medium induces a very good reproducibility. The process of adsorption of proteins should be not delayed. For the other media, the variation coefficient is approximately equal to 0.3-0.4 for the highest values at the highest frequencies.
The Figure 9a) confirms that the results from the Figure 8a). The difference of the modules between PBS + serum and water is positive and it is related to the protective effect of the serum. The Figure 9b) presents the evolution of the phase for the Co-Cr alloy. The phase reaches the maximum of 90° according to the time, i.e. after 2 hours for PBS + Albumin and PBS + serum.

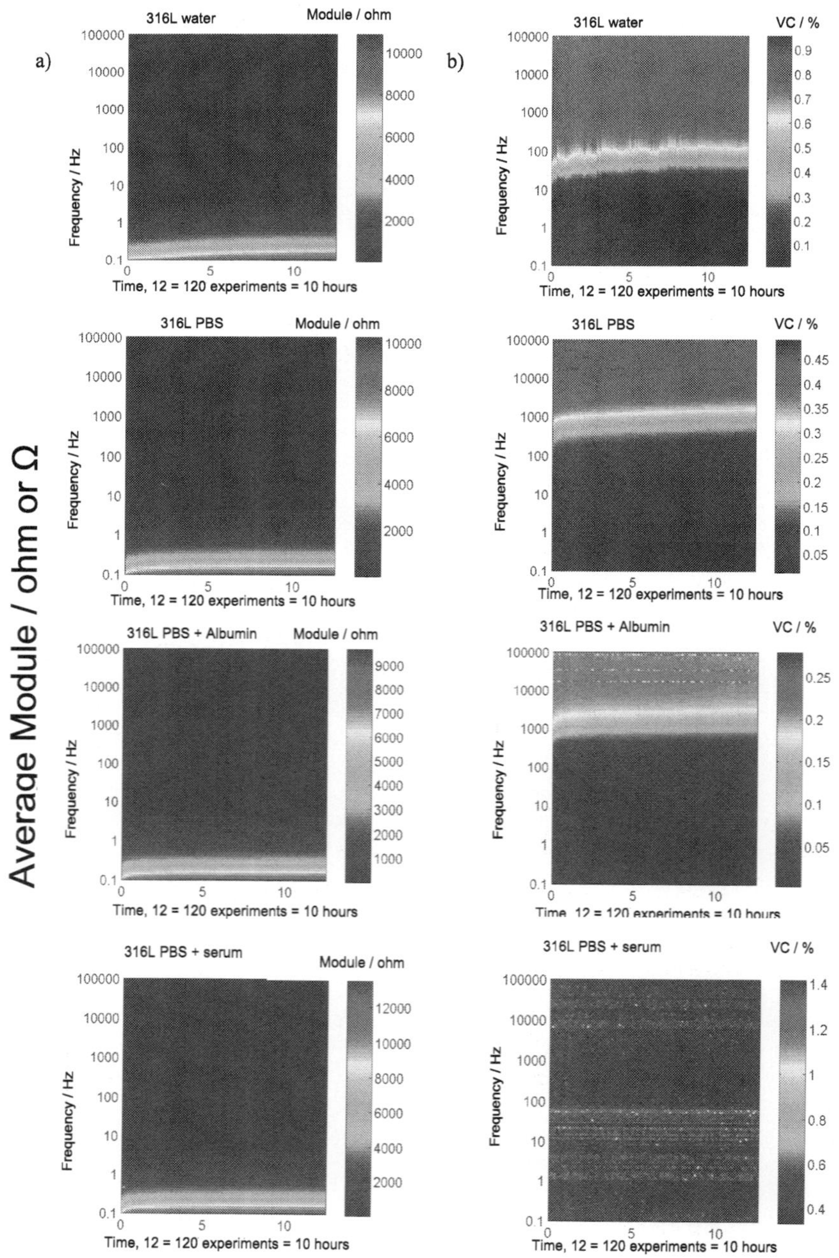

Fig. 6. a) Average modules, same solutions than the Figure 4; b) variation coefficient (VC) from the same solutions than a); time-frequency plane; 316L SS alloy.

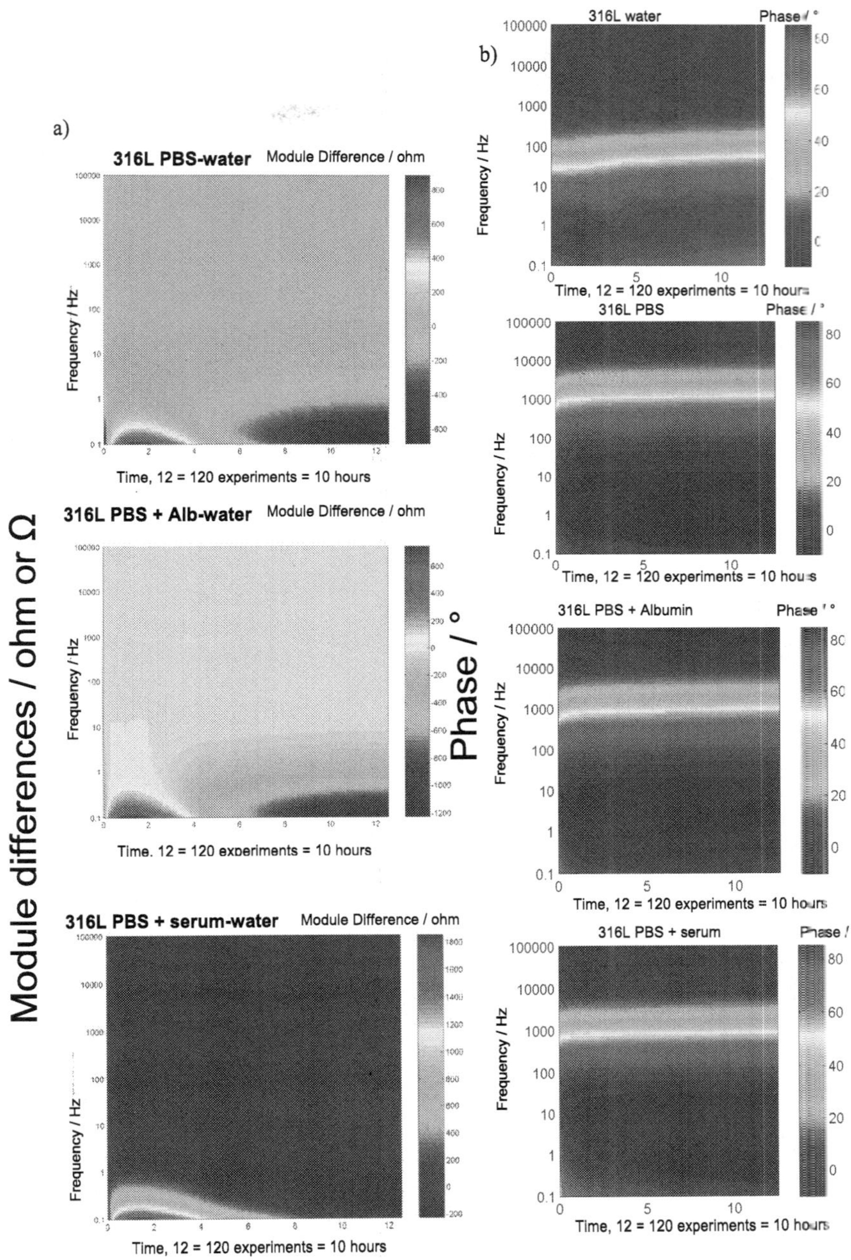

Fig. 7. a) differences of modules for 3 combinations; b) Phase / ° for; the solutions are the same than the ones from Figure 4; time-frequency plane; 316L SS alloy.

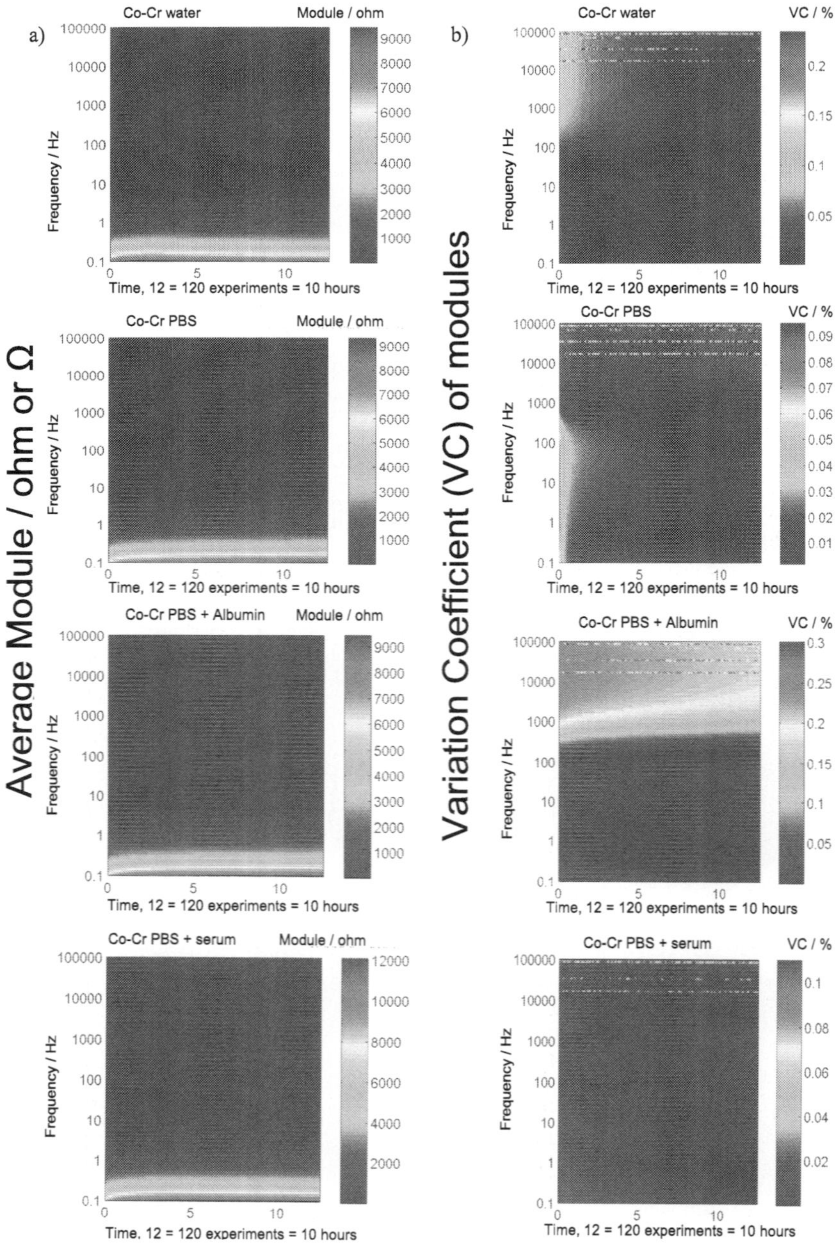

Fig. 8. a) Average modules, same solutions than the Figure 4; b) variation coefficient (VC) from the same solutions than a); time-frequency plane; Co-Cr alloy.

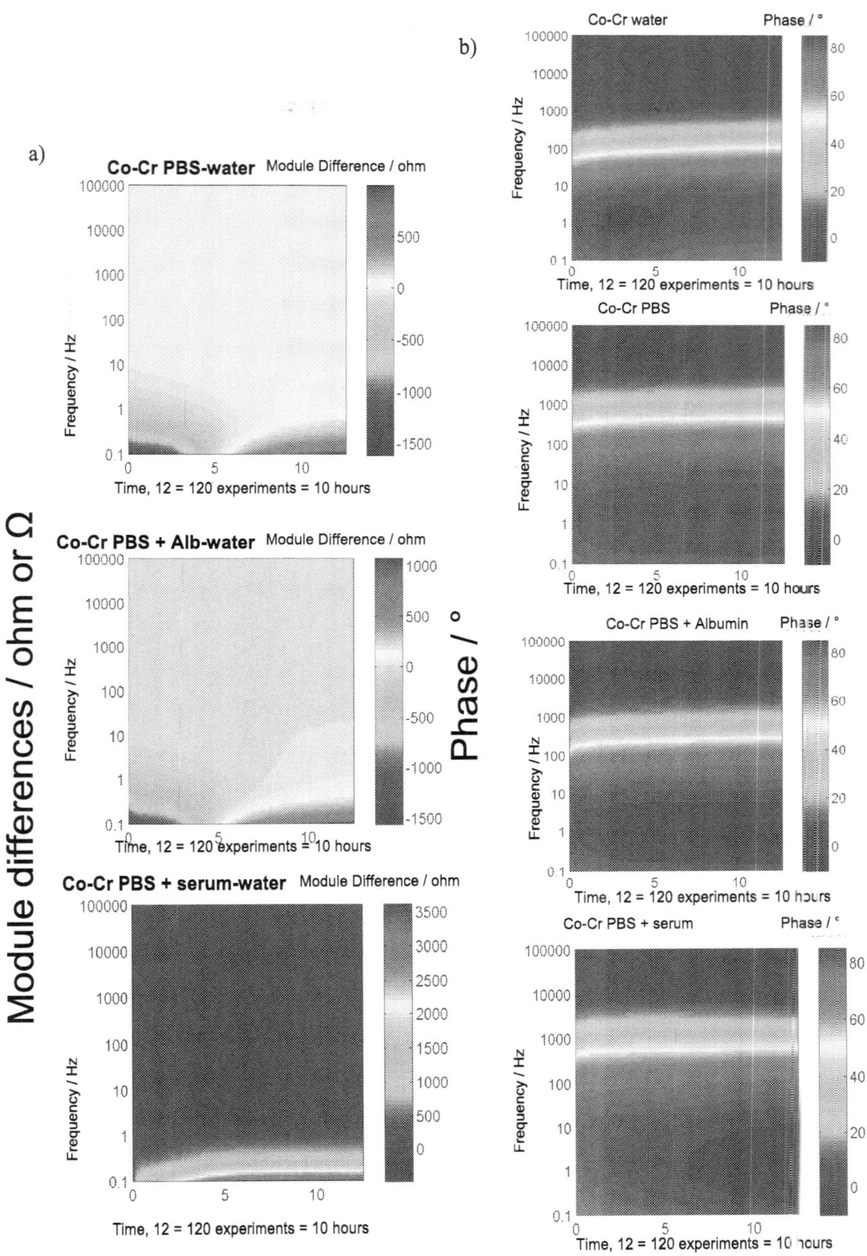

Fig. 9. a) differences of modules for 3 combinations; b) Phase / ° for; the solutions are the same than the ones from Figure 4; time-frequency plane; Co-Cr alloy.

Finally the most protective medium is PBS + serum for the Co-Cr-Mo alloy and the 316L SS due to the highest modules, the difference is the highest between modules of PBS+ serum and modules of water for these two alloys. The highest modules differences are the ones of Co-Cr-Mo. This result confirms the approach of Valero et al [40]. Additionally the phase is the highest too for the combination PBS + serum and Co-Cr-Mo and PBS + serum and 316L. This typical evolution corroborates the conclusion from the evolution of the modules. On the contrary, the Ti-6Al-4V seems to be the less protected in the media with proteins, negative difference of modules. These results confirm the choice of 316L SS and Co-Cr-Mo alloys that have the better corrosion resistance in a medium with proteins. These evolutions are assessed by the time evolution and the particular time-frequency 3D graphs. For both alloys, taking into account the time-frequency evolution of the modules differences and the one of the phases, the most significant information of the EIS investigations is highlighted. Distinguishing the corrosion behavior of alloys is quite possible. From this study, the alloys are ranked from the less protected to the more protected: Ti-6Al-4V < 316L < Co-Cr-Mo.

4. Biocorrosion of implants - Discussion and future directions

The new approach, suggested in this work, shows relevant results from the investigations according to the time-frequency plane. A study of reproducibility, *a minima,* 3 tests, is necessary for highlighting the right evolution. We described a tool from EIS investigations for better understanding the behavior of metal in solution. This method could be used at applied potentials and with different solutions or coatings on surfaces that could be issued from usual materials or biological materials as cells.

The role of proteins is relevant for the corrosive behavior of metals, the results presented in this work highlights these key points. The following investigations should be focused on the influence of cells on the corrosive behavior of metals. Due to the reactions of cells submitted to stress, electrical or mechanical, some oxidative species could be produced, especially the Reactive Oxidative Species, ROS. It has been showed the corrosion resistance of the Co-Cr alloy is lower with macrophages cells from Lin et al (Lin-Journal of Orthopedic Research, 2004). The ROS species, as H_2O_2, promote the corrosion of the Co-Cr alloy. The suggested method in this work should be applied for investigating the time dependence of the cells behavior. Moreover the Ti-6Al-4V alloy is submitted to the same decrease of the corrosion resistance when macrophages are deposited on the alloy surface. The macrophages are liberated when debris or metal ions or metal complexes are released in a corrosive medium in the *in vivo* behavior. Thus the surface composition of the titanium alloy changes according to the presence of macrophages. Performing the protection of this alloy is more and more difficult with macrophages cells (Lin-Applied Surface Science, 2004). It is worth noting that the presence of chlorides does not promote the resistance against corrosion because the passive film is less protective than the one without chlorides (Marino, 2006). Our study highlights that the Ti-6Al-4V alloy is less protected in a medium containing proteins. It suffers from the comparison with 316L SS and Co-Cr-Mo alloys. Finally the typical study that is focused on the role of cells on the corrosive behavior of metallic alloys should be emphasized with a study with different cells (Oshida, 2007). The corrosive behavior of metallic alloys should be studied in *in vivo* conditions. The first step should be the corrosion investigations in fresh tissues coming from hip joint for instance. The second step could be related to the animal experiments and measuring the electrochemical behavior should be measured according to the validation of protocols. Finally one might suggest the experiments in human cases. One should think about the electrochemical investigations of implants in human body will add actual information about the lifetime of the metallic implants. The tissue is typical to the human body and all reactions are specific to the surrounding environment of an articulation for instance. With these typical experiments ethic problems are significantly highlighted. One should preserve the health state, the safety and the integrity of patients from which the agreement should be obtained. It was mentioned that this kind of experiments was substantially investigated 30 years ago (Steinemann, 1980). For a short duration of experiments, these investigations, in human body, were performed with Nitinol alloy involved in manufacturing stents dedicated for blocked arteries (Pertile, 2008). The short experiments do not allow predicting the corrosive behavior for a long time. The experiments of a long duration should be considered for understanding the corrosive behavior, OCP and EIS investigations.

New alloys are suggested for replacing the bone for instance. Magnesium alloys have the same mechanical properties than the ones of bone. However they are submitted to severe corrosion reactions, one might suggest that this alloy could be completely dissolved for allowing the rebuilding of the bone matrix. Some questions are related to the toxicity of the corrosion reactions and the degradations of products. The scientist and surgical communities pay attention on this risk assessment of this new alloy (Yuen, 2010). Thus some alloys are implanted, Titanium, Co-Cr and 316L SS alloys and implanting new alloys as Magnesium alloys is a huge challenge. One should expect that some investigations are needed about the already implanted alloys. The electrochemical behavior and specifically the corrosion in tissues are not well described according to the time. Consequently the time-frequency analysis should get additional information about the corrosive of these implanted alloys.

In the introduction part, the fretting behavior was highlighted. Indeed about implants, one may suggest that, after debonding between bone and implants, the fretting, friction under small displacements or friction, should be triggered. Some questions are related to the behavior of implants in a physiological liquid with proteins for example. In fretting conditions the degradation of the Ti-6Al-4V alloy does not suffer any effect of proteins. On the contrary, the corrosion rate of the 316L, submitted to fretting degradations, decreases according to the proteins concentration (Williams, 1988). The same trend was highlighted in the results presented in this paper, without fretting. Moreover the corrosion rate of a 316L submitted to fretting corrosion decreases with the concentration of albumin[7]. The future directions about this kind of investigations are related to the role of proteins for a better understanding and the role of cells, specifically the ROS on the corrosion and the friction-corrosion (and fretting-corrosion) investigations.

Finally one should pay attention on the electrical equivalent circuit. Normally the Nyquist diagrams, from EIS analyses, could be interpreted thanks to an electrical equivalent circuit, $R_{sol}(C//R_{pol})$, for example. More complex electrical circuits could be investigated for interpreting the diagrams, especially Warburg impedance that is dedicated to simulate the diffusion of species. Each time, the point is: is the electrical circuit relevant with the electrochemical interface at the metal surface? As we did not practice additional investigations about the oxides film or the layer on the metal surface, we prefer to draw conclusions from the modules and the phases and not on the evolutions of the electrical components of the non realistic circuit.

5. Conclusions and outlooks

This work was dedicated to study the corrosion resistance of the metallic alloys with synthetic solutions for mimicking the physiological liquid. A new approach allows

describing the evolution of modules and phases in the plane time-frequency. These graphs become from the Electrochemical Impedance Spectroscopy investigations.
The results show significantly that the Ti-6Al-4V alloy is the less protected alloy. The Co-Cr alloy seems to be the most resistant. Moreover the proteins allow increasing the passivity of Co-Cr and 316L alloys. The new approach highlights the particular evolution according to the time. Thus the electrochemical behavior is stabilized after 5 hours. The best material, from this study, is the Co-Cr alloy, about the electrochemical behavior.
The corrosion resistance in a physiological liquid is the first element about the quality of an implanted metallic material. Afterwards the behavior during fretting corrosion or friction corrosion is a key point about the lifetime of a metallic implant. The first results, in fretting corrosion[7], show that proteins decrease the corrosive behavior but it increases the mechanical wear. Understanding the influence of proteins during fretting-corrosion is a goal in next years for all implanted alloys. From the point of view of the understanding of physic phenomena, the synergisms between the mechanical and the corrosive degradations have to be investigated. The corrosive characterization is carried out from this work and the previous ones.
On this related field proteins-metal-friction some investigations are in progress.

6. Acknowledgement

The authors are grateful to A. Gault and B. Allirand for manufacturing the electrochemical cell. Moreover they want to acknowledge Pr. D.D. Macdonald for fruitful discussions.

7. References

Barril, S.; Debaud, N.; Mischler, S. & Landolt, D. (2002) A tribo-electrochemical apparatus for in vitro investigation of fretting-corrosion of metallic implant materials. *Wear*, 252, pp. 744-754.

Bethune, B. & Waterhouse, R.B. (1968) Electrochemical studies of fretting corrosion. Wear, 12, pp. 27-34

Bronzino, J.D. (1995) The Biomedical Engineering Handbook, CRC Press, pp. 540-542, Boca Raton Florida

Cai, K.; Frant, M.; Bossert, J.; Hildebrand, G.; Liefeith, K. & Jandt K.D. (2006), Surface functionalized titanium thin films: Zeta-potential, protein adsorption and cell proliferation. *Colloids and Surfaces B: Biointerfaces*, 50, pp. 1-8

Callaghan, J.J.; Rosenberg, A.G. & Rubash, H.E. (2007) *The adult hip*, Eds Wolters Kluwer Health Lippincott Williams & Wilkins, pp. 7-14, Philadelphia PA,

Charnley J. (1970) *Acrylic cement in orthopaedic surgery*, Eds: Livingstone Ltd, Edinburgh, London

Charnley J. (1970) *low friction arhtroplasty of the hip*, Eds Springer-Verlag, New York

Dowson, D. & Wright, V. (1981) *An introduction to the biomechanics of joints and joint replacement*, Eds Mechanical Engineering Publications, pp. 174, London

Dygas, J.R. & Breiter, M.W. (1999) Variance of errors and elimination of outliers in the least squares analysis of impedance spectra. *Electrochimica Acta*, 44, pp. 4163-4174

Eden, E.M.; Rose, W.N. & Cunningham, F.L. (1911) The endurance of metals. *Proc. Instn Mech. Engers*, 4, pp. 839-974

Geringer, J.; Forest, B. & Combrade, P. (2005) Fretting corrosion of materials used as orthopaedic implants. *Wear*, 259, pp. 943-951.

Geringer, J.; Forest, B. & Combrade, P. (2006) Wear analysis of materials used as orthopaedic implants. *Wear*, 261, pp. 971-979

Geringer, J.; Normand, B.; Diemiaszonek, R.; Alemany-Dumont, C. & Mary, N. (2007) Electrochemical impedance spectroscopy on Co-Cr-Mo alloy in two media simulating physiological liquid. Matériaux et Techniques, 95, pp. 417-426

Gluck T. (1890). Die invaginations methode der Osteo- und Arthroplastik. *Berl Klin Wochenschr,* 28, pp. 732-736

Harrington, D.A. & van den Driessche, P. (2001) Stability and electrochemical impedance of mechanisms with a single adsorbed species. *Journal of Electroanalytical Chemistry,* 501, pp. 222-234.

Hsu, R.W-W.; Yang, C-C.; Huang, C-A. & Chen, Y-S. (2004) Electrochemical corrosion properties of Ti-6Al-4V implanet alloy in the biological environment. *Materials Science and Engineering A,* 380, pp. 100-109

Judet, R. & Judet, J. (1949), Essais de reconstruction prothétique de la hanche après résection de la tête fémorale. *Journal de chirurgie,* 65, pp. 17-24

Khan, M.A.; Williams, R.L. & Williams, D.F. (1999) The corrosion behaviour of Ti-6Al-4V, Ti-6Al-7Nb and Ti-13Nb-13Zr in protein solutions. *Biomaterials*, 20, pp. 631-637

Kirbs, A.; Lange, R.; Nebe, B.; Rychly, R.; Baumann, A.; Neumann, H.G. & Beck, U. (2003) Methods for the physical and chemical characterisation of surfaces of titanium implants. *Materials Science and Engineering C,* 23, 425-429

Lin, H-Y. & Bumgardner, J.D. (2004) Changes in surface composition of the Ti-6Al-4V implanet alloy by cultured macrophage cells. *Applied Surface Science*, 225, pp. 21-28

Lin, H-Y. & Bumgardner, J.D. (2004) In vitro biocorrosion of Co-Cr-Mo implanet alloy by macrophage cells. *Journal of Orthopaedic Research*, 22, pp. 1231-1236

Liu, C.; Bi, Q. & Matthews, A. (2003) Tribological and electrochemical performance of PVD TiN coatings on the femoral head of Ti-6Al-4V artificial hip joints. *Surface and Coatings Technology*, 163-164,pp. 597-604

Macdonald, D.D.; Sikora, E. & Engelhardt, G. (1998) Characterizing electrochemical systems in the frequency domain. *Electrochimica Acta*, 43, pp. 87-107

Marino, C-E.B.; Biaggio, S.R.; Rocha-Filho, R.C. & Bocchi, N. (2006) Voltammetric stability of anodic films on the Ti6Al4V alloy in chloride medium. *Electrochimica Acta,* 51, pp. 6580-6583

McDowell, O.J. (1953) *Fretting corrosion tendencies of several combinations of materials, Symposium on fretting corrosion*, ASTM Philadelphia, pp. 40-53.

Munoz, A.I. & Mischler, S. (2007) Interactive Effects of Albumin and Phosphate Ions on the Corrosion of CoCrMo Implanet Alloy. *Journal of The Electrochemical Society,* 154, pp. C562-C570

Orazem, M. (2004) Systematic approach toward error structure identification for impedance spectroscopy. *Journal of Electroanalytical Chemistry*, 572, pp. 317-327.

Oshida, Y. (2007) *Implanet-Related Biological Reactions,* In: Bioscience and Bioengineering of Titanium Materials, Elsevier, pp. 157-214, Oxford UK

Ouerd, A.; Alemany-Dumont, C.; Berthomé, G.; Normand, B. & Szunerits, S. (2007) *Journal of The Electrochemical Society*. 154, pp. C593-C601

Ouerd, A.; Alemany-Dumont, C.; Normand, B. & Szunerits S. (2008) Reactivity of CoCrMo alloy in physiological medium: Electrochemical characterization of the metal/protein interface. *Electrochimica Acta* 53, pp. 4461-4469

Pan, J.; Thierry, D. & Leygraf, C. (1996) Integrated AFM and SCEM for in situ studies of localized corrosion of Al alloys. *Electrochimica Acta*, 41, pp. 1143-1153

Park, J.B. & Lakes, R.S. (1992) *Biomaterials an Introduction*, 2nd ed. Plenum Press, pp. 83-88, New York

Payet, V.; Brunner, S.; Galtayries, A.; Frateur, I. & Marcus P. (2008) Cleaning of albumin-contaminated Ti and Cr surfaces: an XPS and QCM study. *Surf. Interface Anal*, 40, pp. 215-219

Pellier, J.; Geringer, J. & Forest, B. (2011) Fretting-corrosion between 316L SS and PMMA. Influence of ionic strength, protein and electrochemical conditions on material wear. Application to orthopedic implants. *Wear in press*

Pertile, L.B.; Silva, P.M.S; Peccin, V.B.; Peres, R.; Silveira, P.G.; Giacomelli, C.; Giacomelli, F.C.; Fredel, M.C. & Spinelli, A. (2008) In vivo human electrochemical properties of a NiTi-based alloy (Nitinol) used for minimally invasive implants. *Journal of Biomedical Materials Research Part A*, 89, pp. 1072-1078

Steinemann, S.G. (1980) *Evaluation of Biomaterials-Corrosion of Surgical Implants-in vivo and in vitro tests*, In: G.D. Winter, J.L. Leray, K. de Groot, John Wiley & Sons Ltd, pp. 2-33, New York USA

Tamilselvi, S.; Raman, V. & Rajendran N. (2006) Corrosion behaviour of Ti–6Al–7Nb and Ti–6Al–4V ELI alloys in the simulated body fluid solution by electrochemical impedance spectroscopy. *Electrochimica Acta*, 52, pp. 839-846

Tomlinson, G.A. (1927) The rusting of steel surfaces in contact. *Proc. Roy. London Ser. A.*, 115, pp. 472-483

Tomlinson, G.A.; Thorpe, P.L. & Gough, H.J. (1939) An investigation of fretting corrosion of closely fitting surfaces. *Proceedings of the Institution for Mechanical Engineers*, 141, pp. 223-249

Uhlig, H.H. (1954) Mechanism of fretting corrosion. *Journal of Applied Mechanics*, 21, pp. 401-407

Uhlig, H.H. (1979) Passivity in metals and alloys. *Corrosion Science*, 19, pp. 777-791

Valero, C. & Munoz, A.I. (2008) Electrochemical characterisation of biomedical alloys for surgical implants in simulated body fluids. Corrosion Science, 50, pp. 1954-1961

Waterhouse, R.B. (1955) Fretting corrosion. *Proceedings of the Institution for Mechanical Engineers*, 169, pp. 1159-1172

Waterhouse, R.B. (1977) The role of adhesion and delamination in the fretting wear of metallic materials. *Wear*, 45, pp. 355-364

Waterhouse, R.B. & Lamb, M. (1980) Fretting corrosion of orthopaedic implanet materials by bone cement. *Wear*, 60, pp. 357-368

Williams, R.L.; Brown, S.A. & Merritt, K. (1988) Electrochemical studies on the influence of proteins on the corrosion of implanet alloys. *Biomaterials*, 9, pp. 181-186

Yan, H.; Xiaoying, L.; Jingwu, M. & Nan H. (2008) In vitro investigation of protein adsorption and platelet adhesion on inorganic biomaterial surfaces. *Applied surface Science*, 255, pp. 257-259

Yuen, C.K. & Ip, W.Y. (2010) Theoretical risk assessment of magnesium alloys as degradable biomedical implants. *Acta Biomaterialia*, 6, pp. 1808-1812

Zaveri, N.; Mahapatra, M.;. Deceuster, A.; Peng, Y; Li, L. & Zhou A. (2008) Corrosion resistance of pulsed laser-treated Ti-6Al-4V implanet in simulated biofluids, *Electrochimica Acta*, 53, pp. 5022-5032